Simultaneous EEG and fMRI

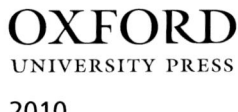

Simultaneous EEG and fMRI

Recording, Analysis, and Application

EDITED BY:

Markus Ullsperger, MD, PhD
Biological Psychology / Donders Centre for Cognition
Radboud University Nijmegen
Nijmegen, The Netherlands; and
Max Planck Institute for Neurological Research
Cologne, Germany

Stefan Debener, PhD
Institute of Psychology
Carl von Ossietzky University Oldenburg
Oldenburg, Germany; and
Biomagnetic centre
Hans Berger Clinic for Neurology
University Hospital Jena
Jena, Germany

OXFORD
UNIVERSITY PRESS

2010

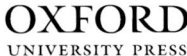
OXFORD
UNIVERSITY PRESS

Oxford University Press, Inc., publishes works that further
Oxford University's objective of excellence
in research, scholarship, and education.

Oxford   New York
Auckland   Cape Town   Dar es Salaam   Hong Kong   Karachi
Kuala Lumpur   Madrid   Melbourne   Mexico City   Nairobi
New Delhi   Shanghai   Taipei   Toronto

With offices in
Argentina   Austria   Brazil   Chile   Czech Republic   France   Greece
Guatemala   Hungary   Italy   Japan   Poland   Portugal   Singapore
South Korea   Switzerland   Thailand   Turkey   Ukraine   Vietnam

Published by Oxford University Press, Inc.
198 Madison Avenue, New York, New York 10016
www.oup.com

Oxford is a registered trademark of Oxford University Press

Library of Congress Cataloging-in-Publication Data
Simultaneous EEG and fMRI : recording, analysis, and application / edited by
Markus Ullsperger, Stefan Debener.
p.   ;   cm.
Includes bibliographical references and index.
ISBN 978-0-19-537273-1 (alk. paper)
1. Electroencephalography.   2. Brain—Magnetic resonance imaging.
I. Ullsperger, M. (Markus)   II. Debener, Stefan.
[DNLM: 1. Electroencephalography.   2. Magnetic Resonance Imaging.
3. Brain—physiology. WN 185 S614 2010]
QP376.5.S56 2010
616.8'047547—dc22
2009029992

9   8   7   6   5   4   3   2

Printed in the United States of America
on acid-free paper

Preface

One of the major challenges in science is to study and understand the human brain. Numerous methods have been developed and employed to examine different aspects of brain functions. To study systemic interactions in brain networks in vivo, non-invasive methods such as electroencephalography (EEG) and functional magnetic resonance imaging (fMRI) have been used with great success. However, each of these methods can map only certain, quite selective aspects of brain function while missing others; and the inferences on neuronal processes and information flow are often indirect. To overcome these shortcomings of single methods, researchers have attempted to combine methods in order to make optimal use of their advantages while compensating for their disadvantages. Hence, it is not surprising that since the introduction of fMRI as a neuroimaging method the possibilities of combinations with EEG have been explored. In the meantime, numerous technical issues have been solved, such that relatively easy-to-use equipment for simultaneous recordings has become commercially available. As a result, the number of publications on simultaneous EEG/fMRI has increased dramatically in recent years. Moreover, the focus of the published reports has shifted and expanded from demonstrating technical feasibility to methodological issues of artifact control, new ways of analyzing and integrating the data, and—probably most exciting—to applications for scientific and clinical questions. Scientific research topics addressed with EEG/fMRI cover a broad range from physiological questions on the bases of the two recorded signals and their relationship via questions about the relationship of ongoing and task-related brain activity to specific questions on the mechanisms of certain cognitive functions. Clinically oriented EEG/fMRI research has focused on diagnostics in epilepsy; but recently other topics such as anesthesiology and pain research have been added. We predict a steep increase in the use of combined EEG/fMRI and observe that more and more imaging centers are acquiring the necessary equipment and know-how.

This book is intended to aid researchers who plan to set up a simultaneous EEG-fMRI laboratory and those who are interested in integrating electrophysiological and hemodynamic data. As will be obvious from the different chapters, this is a dynamically developing field in which several approaches are being tested, validated, and compared. Currently, there is no one best solution for all problems available, but many promising techniques are emerging. This book gives a comprehensive overview of these techniques. In addition, it points to open questions and directions for future research.

Part 1 is dedicated to the physiological basics of both EEG and fMRI techniques. Only a comprehensive understanding of the signals we record and their relationship to the underlying neuronal activity enables us to make inferences and eventually optimally combine the two methods. C. Michel and D. Brandeis introduce the basics of scalp-recorded EEG, and J. Goense and N. Logothetis present current knowledge on the relation of the blood oxygen level dependent (BOLD) signal measured with fMRI and neuronal activity. A. Snyder and M. Raichle put these physiological considerations into a broader context and discuss why, when, and how the two modalities can and should be combined optimally.

Part 2 is intended to help set up a laboratory allowing for simultaneous recordings. I. Gutberlet provides an overview of currently available systems allowing EEG recordings in the MR environment and gives an outlook on ongoing technical developments and innovations. Moreover, important safety aspects are discussed that every researcher intending to record EEG in the MR scanner should be aware of. A. P. Bagshaw and C-G. Benár elaborate on different scanning strategies with respect to the potential applications. One of the major problems in simultaneous EEG/fMRI data has been different artifacts that need to be avoided or removed. Remarkable progress has been made in off-line artifact control and denoising of the EEG data. S. Debener and colleagues give a comprehensive introduction to the state of the art in cleaning up EEG data recorded during fMRI. Less often discussed, but of substantial importance, is the influence of the EEG equipment on MRI image quality. K. Mullinger and R. Bowtell address this issue.

Once the data have been denoised, the two modalities need to be integrated to make use of the advantages of both methods. The chapters in Part 3 present and discuss different analysis and integration approaches and techniques. Several chapters are dedicated to independent component analysis (ICA), a blind source separation technique that has yielded neurobiologically plausible solutions. S. Debener and colleagues report on the use of ICA for EEG analyses; and G. Valente, E. Formisano, and colleagues demonstrate the application of ICA to fMRI data. M. Ullsperger presents a straightforward way of integrating EEG and fMRI and a selective review of recent applications of a particular technique, EEG-informed fMRI analysis. Further recent methodological advances, such as parallel and joint ICA of EEG and fMRI data, appear to open novel and promising methods of data fusion. Two chapters, by V. D. Calhoun and T. Eichele, are dedicated to these analysis methods, which can be applied to many kinds of multimodal data sets beyond EEG/fMRI. While most EEG-informed fMRI analyses make use of a predefined hemodynamic response function, the chapter by de Munck and colleagues demonstrates how EEG data can be used to better estimate the hemodynamic response. However, a number of variables can make it advantageous to record EEG and fMRI in separate sessions, and other measures of brain electrical activity such as magnetoencephalography (MEG) have to be acquired separately. M. Wibral and colleagues review and discuss the recent advances in integrating these data with fMRI. Finally, two chapters by S. J. Kiebel and colleagues and K.E. Stephan and K. Friston provide an overview on the analysis of functional and effective connectivity using EEG, MEG, and fMRI data. These techniques are important to test hypotheses on the information processing steps in large networks.

Part 4 contains two chapters dedicated to applications of simultaneous EEG and fMRI. M. Siegel and T. Donner discuss the analysis of oscillatory patterns in electrophysiological measures and their relationship to the fMRI and review a range of applications of the EEG/fMRI approach in this field. Finally, H. Laufs and R. Thornton discuss the clinical application of EEG/fMRI with a focus on epilepsy.

We believe that the development of multimodal noninvasive imaging using EEG and fMRI is still in its early days. A number of questions remain to be explored, and we look forward to the many new insights that will be gathered in the coming years. We wish all readers success and fun with applying this exciting combination of methods.

Acknowledgments

We would like to thank the authors for their valuable contributions to this volume.

We would also like to thank the referees for their help in achieving high clarity despite the complexity of the presented topics: Andrew Bagshaw, Christoph Bledowski, Vince D. Calhoun, Tom Eichele, Jean Gotman, Ingmar Gutberlet Barry Horwitz, René J. Huster, Cornelia Kranczioch, Julie Onton, Rey Ramirez, Claudia Tesche, Michael Wibral, Herbert Witte.

Finally, we thank Oxford University Press for their support during the different phases of this book.

Contents

Contributors

Andrew P. Bagshaw, PhD
School of Psychology
University of Birmingham
Birmingham, UK

Christian-G. Bénar, PhD
INSERM, Epilepsy and Cognition Laboratory
Timone Faculty of Medicine
Marseille, France

Christoph Bledowski, PhD
Institute of Medical Psychology (IMP)
Goethe University
Frankfurt am Main, Germany

Richard Bowtell, PhD
Sir Peter Mansfield Magnetic Resonance Centre
School of Physics and Astronomy
University of Nottingham
Nottingham, UK

Daniel Brandeis, PhD
Department of Child and Adolescent
Psychiatry
University of Zurich
Zürich, Switzerland; and
Department of Child and Adolescent Psychiatry
and Psychotherapy
Central Institute of Mental Health Mannheim
Mannheim, Germany

Vince D. Calhoun, PhD
The Mind Research Network
Department of ECE
University of New Mexico
Albuquerque, NM

Fernando Henrique Lopes da Silva, MD, PhD
Swammerdam Institute for Life Sciences
University of Amsterdam
Amsterdam, The Netherlands

Stefan Debener, PhD
Institute of Psychology
Carl von Ossietzky University Oldenburg
Oldenburg, Germany; and
Biomagnetic Center
Department of Neurology
Friedrich-Schiller-University
University Hospital Jena
Jena, Germany

Federico de Martino, PhD
Maastricht Brain Imaging Center (M-BIC)
Department of Cognitive Neurosciences
University of Maastricht
Maastricht, The Netherlands

JC de Munck, PhD
Department of PMT
VU University Medical Center
Amsterdam, The Netherlands

Tobias H. Donner, MD, PhD
Department of Psychology and Center for Neural
Science
New York University
New York, NY; and
Department of Psychology
University of Amsterdam
Amsterdam, The Netherlands

Tom Eichele, MD, PhD
Department of Biological and Medical Psychology
University of Bergen
Bergen, Norway; and
Mind Research Network
Albuquerque, NM

Fabrizio Esposito, PhD
Maastricht Brain Imaging Center (M-BIC)
Department of Cognitive Neurosciences
University of Maastricht
Maastricht, The Netherlands

Elia Formisano, PhD
Maastricht Brain Imaging Center (M-BIC)
Department of Cognitive Neurosciences
University of Maastricht
Maastricht, The Netherlands

Karl J. Friston, MD
The Wellcome Trust Centre for Neuroimaging
University College London
London, UK

Marta I. Garrido, PhD
The Wellcome Trust Centre for Neuroimaging
University College London
London, UK

Rainer Goebel, PhD
Maastricht Brain Imaging Center (M-BIC)
Department of Cognitive Neurosciences
University of Maastricht
Maastricht, The Netherlands

Jozien Goense, PhD
Department of Physiology of Cognitive Processes
Max Planck Institute for Biological Cybernetics
Tuebingen, Germany

SI Gonçalves
Department of PMT
VU University Medical Center
Amsterdam, The Netherlands

Ingmar Gutberlet, PhD
Brain Products GmbH
Gilching, Germany; and
BlindSight GmbH
Schlitz, Germany

Stefan J. Kiebel, PhD
Max Planck Institute for Human Cognitive and Brain Sciences
Leipzig, Germany

Helmut Laufs, MD
Klinik für Neurologie und Brain Imaging Center
Goethe-Universität
Frankfurt am Main, Germany

Nikos K. Logothetis, PhD
Department of Physiology of Cognitive Processes
Max Planck Institute for Biological Cybernetics
Tuebingen, Germany; and
Imaging Science and Biomedical Engineering
University of Manchester
Manchester, UK

R. Mammoliti
Department of PMT, VU University Medical Center
Amsterdam, The Netherlands; and
Dipartimento di Scienze Neurologiche e Cardiovascolari
Universitàdi Cagliari
Monserrato, Italy

Christoph M. Michel, PhD
Department of Neuroscience
Head of the Functional Brain Mapping Laboratory
Director, EEG-core of the Lemanic Biomedical Imaging Center
Geneva University
Geneva, Switzerland

Matthias Moosmann, PhD
Department of Biological and Medical Psychology
University of Bergen
Bergen, Norway

Karen Mullinger, PhD
Sir Peter Mansfield Magnetic Resonance Centre
School of Physics and Astronomy
University of Nottingham
Nottingham, UK

P. Ossenblok, MD
Epilepsy Centre
Kempenhaeghe, Heeze, The Netherlands

Marcus E. Raichle, MD
Mallinckrodt Institute of Radiology and Department of Neurology
Washington University School of Medicine
St Louis, MO

Till R. Schneider
Department of Neurophysiology and Pathophysiology
University Medical Center Hamburg-Eppendorf
Hamburg, Germany

Markus Siegel, MD, PhD
The Picower Institute for Learning and Memory
Department of Brain and Cognitive Sciences
Massachusetts Institute of Technology
Cambridge, MA

Abraham Z. Snyder, MD, PhD
Mallinckrodt Institute of Radiology and Department of Neurology
Washington University School of Medicine
St Louis, MO

Klaas Enno Stephan, MD, Dr. Med, PhD
Laboratory for Social and Neural Systems Research
Institute for Empirical Research in Economics
University of Zurich, Switzerland

Jeremy Thorne
Biomagnetic Center
Department of Neurology
Friedrich-Schiller-University
University Hospital Jena
Jena, Germany; and
Institute of Psychology
Carl von Ossietzky University Oldenburg
Oldenburg, Germany

Rachel Thornton
Department of Clinical and Experimental Epilepsy
Institute of Neurology
University College London
London, UK

Georg Turi, MSc
Department of Neurophysiology
Max-Planck-Institute for Brain Research
MEG Unit, Brain Imaging Center (BIC)
Goethe University
Frankfurt am Main, Germany

Markus Ullsperger, MD, PhD
Biological Psychology / Donders Centre for Cognition
Radboud University Nijmegen
Nijmegen, The Netherlands; and
Max Planck Institute for Neurological Research
Cologne, Germany

Giancarlo Valente, PhD
Maastricht Brain Imaging Center (M-BIC)
Department of Cognitive Neurosciences
University of Maastricht
Maastricht, The Netherlands

PJ van Houdt
Department of PMT
VU University Medical Center
Epilepsy Centre
Kempenhaeghe, Heeze, The Netherlands.

Filipa Campos Viola
Biomagnetic Center
Department of Neurology
Friedrich-Schiller-University
University Hospital Jena
Jena, Germany; and
Institute of Psychology
Carl von Ossietzky University Oldenburg
Oldenburg, Germany

Michael Wibral, PhD
MEG Unit, Brain Imaging Center (BIC)
Goethe University
Frankfurt am Main, Germany

Lei Wu
Mind Research Network
Albuquerque, NM

Simultaneous EEG and fMRI

Part 1 ⸬

Physiological Basics of EEG and fMRI

1.1

Christoph M. Michel and Daniel Brandeis

The Sources and Temporal Dynamics of Scalp Electric Fields

Introduction

Neuronal activity in the brain induces electric fields that extend to the surface of the head, where they give rise to a specific topographical distribution. These scalp potential maps can be sampled accurately, provided that sufficient electrodes cover the whole head surface. Such scalp EEG mapping is the precursor of electric source imaging, which estimates the source distribution in the brain. EEG mapping and source estimation has matured to become a true neuroimaging procedure. The specific advantage is that neuronal activity is recorded directly and with a very high temporal resolution. However, the limited spatial resolution has prompted recent efforts to combine electrical neuroimaging with fMRI. High-resolution EEG recordings in the scanner are now possible, and powerful artifact correction algorithms exist. Spatial analysis of such EEG during scanning allows direct comparison with the hemodynamic response, provided that differences regarding the generation and the spatiotemporal properties of the EEG and fMRI signals are understood. Concerning the EEG, it is critical to understand which neural events are detectable at which spatial scales. Because of the unique high temporal resolution of the EEG, electrical neuroimaging not only concerns the localization, but also the temporal dynamics of the neuronal activation. One of the best-known temporal characteristics of electrical activity is the prominent rhythmic oscillation in different frequency ranges. Understanding the intrinsic rhythmic properties of cortical or subcortical-cortical networks can help to constrain electric neuroimaging to certain frequency ranges of interest, analogous to the spatial "regions of interest." Such insights can also help to optimize spatial analysis for operation in the frequency domain. For both oscillatory and transient EEG, the spatial analysis of the EEG also reveals a common, characteristic temporal evolution of the electric fields: instead of continuous smooth transitions between field configurations, sharp transitions separate discrete segments of electrical stability. These periods of stable electric field configurations are called functional microstates. Microstates have been proposed to reflect particular information processing steps, and to form the basic building blocks of the content of consciousness. This chapter focuses on these spatiotemporal aspects of the EEG, and discusses the most important findings concerning the oscillations and the temporal dynamics of electrical activity.

Neuronal Generators

Different spatial and temporal scales reflecting increasing integration characterize the dominant neuroelectric events in intracellular, extracellular, and scalp recordings. The action potentials, which mainly reflect neuronal output, are responsible for fast neural communication along the axons. They dominate the intracellular recordings, and make up the multi-unit activity (MUA) defined as frequencies above 300 Hz in extracellular recordings. These large spikes reflect changes of more than 80 mV in under 2 ms at the cell membrane. However, they play a minor role in EEG and event-related potential (ERP) recordings, mainly because they fall off rapidly to a tenth ($< 60\ \mu V$) outside a 50 μm radius (Henze et al., 2000). Scalp electrodes for EEG recording are at a distance of several cm from the neurons. For this reason, individual spikes cannot be measured from EEG electrodes. Also, the short spike duration makes temporal summation less likely. As a consequence, action potentials, and more generally electrical activity in white matter structures, contribute little to the EEG. However, even the small contributions of summated spikes may be isolated through averaging techniques. This is well illustrated by the averaged scalp ERP following median nerve stimulation. Averaging reveals that its initial phase contains small, high-frequency oscillations (0.2 μV at 600Hz), which presumably reflect summated population spike activity in the thalamus (Gobbele et al., 1998). The main sources of the EEG are the slower (<250 Hz) local field potentials (LFP). Such field potentials mainly reflect neuronal input from postsynaptic potentials, and show more spatial and temporal summation than the spikes. Because these postsynaptic potentials only originate in gray matter, electrophysiological source models can be constrained to gray matter structures as the solution space. This anatomical separation is particularly important because functional separation between spikes and field potentials is not always possible. Spike and LFP acivities often correlate among each other, as well as with metabolic demand (Logothetis et al., 2001).

Because of the distance of the scalp electrode to the neurons, and because of the important attenuation of the field due to the electrical resistivity of the skull, scalp EEG generation must involve LFP summation. The major generators of the scalp EEG are therefore extended patches of gray matter, polarized through synchronous synaptic input either in an oscillatory fashion or as transient evoked activity (Shah et al., 2004). In the cortex, such patches contain thousands of cortical columns. In these columns, large pyramidal cells are aligned perpendicularly to the cortical surface. Models that consider the realistic cell geometries suggest that not only apical but also basal dendrites of the neurons may contribute to the EEG (Murakami and Okada, 2006). When these cells are activated, extracellular currents flow between the different layers of the columns. Reverse intracellular currents match these. Thus the variable generator regions lead to a variety of

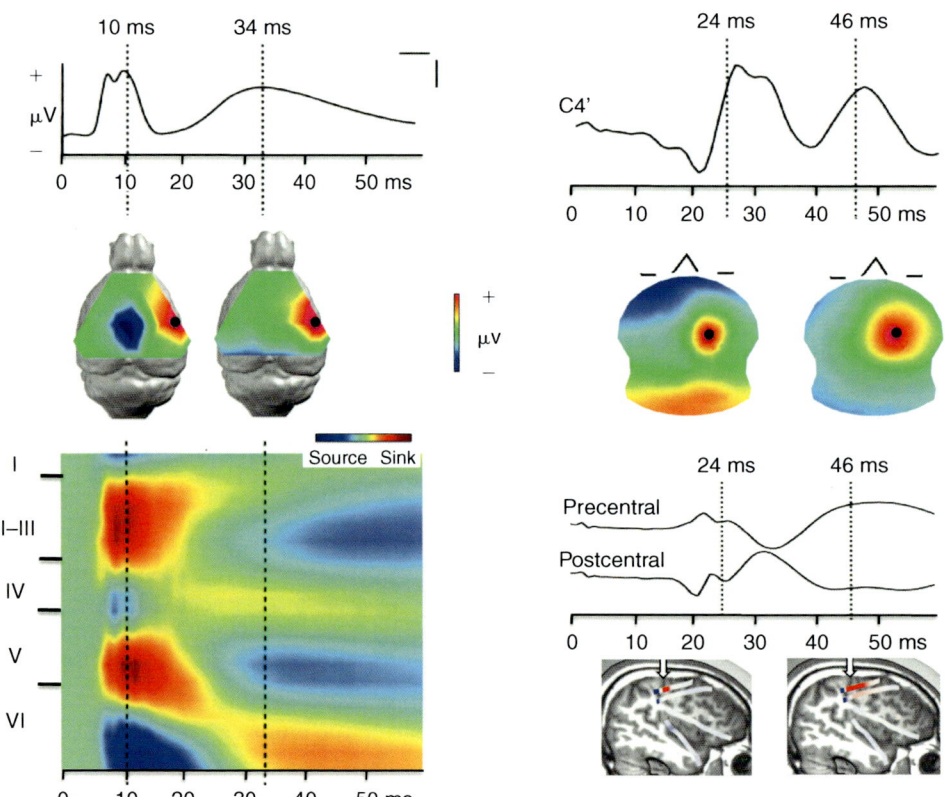

Figure 1.1.1. Extra- and intracranial recordings of somatosensory evoked potentials (SEP) in mice and in humans. **Left top:** Grand average epicranial waveform at one electrode and instant 32-channel maps of left whisker–evoked SEP in mice (the position of the electrode is marked in the maps. Note the same polarity and amplitude of the voltage at this location for the two selected time points. **Left bottom:** Grand average whisker-evoked current source density profile in mouse primary somatosensory cortex (SI) recorded from 16 electrodes in different laminar positions. Note the different source-sink profiles for the two time points that produced the same (positive) surface potential. **Right top:** Grand average waveform of one electrode (C4') and instant maps of 256-channel SEP to electrical left median nerve stimulation in 44 healthy human subjects. **Right bottom:** Average waveforms of SEP to electrical stimulation of the left median nerve in an epileptic patient implanted with subdural electrode strips spanning the central sulcus (indicated by an arrow). The blue and red coding on the strips indicate negative and positive potentials. Note that both the scalp and the subdural recordings indicate the same potentials for the two time points, similar to the mouse recording, suggesting that these time points are also generated by different laminar source-sink profiles in the cortex. Reprinted from *Neuroimage* 42. Megevand P, Quairiaux C, Lascano AM, Kiss JZ, Michel CM. A mouse model for studying large-scale neuronal networks using EEG mapping techniques, 591–602, 2008 with permission from Elsevier.

laminar potentials and variable current density distributions. While evoked activity often starts with prominent current sinks in cortical layer IV (Mitzdorf, 1985; Schroeder et al., 1998), more variable laminar distributions of sinks and sources characterize later components of the evoked potentials (Megevand et al., 2008b) as well as spontaneous (Bollimunta et al., 2008) and epileptic activity (Ulbert et al., 2004).

The surface EEG does not allow to distinguish between the various possible arrangements of sinks and sources in the different cortical layers (Mitzdorf, 1985). Even for a given EEG frequency and brain system, different laminar distribution may characterize different subregions of the active network. This is well illustrated by a recent analysis of the most prominent oscillatory EEG activity in the visual system, the posterior alpha rhythm (8-10Hz). Laminar recordings of alpha from spontaneously behaving monkeys revealed that current density profiles differ across visual regions. Alpha was dominated by activity of deeper (granular and infragranular) layers in lower-order visual areas, but by activity of more superficial (supragranular) layers in the higher inferotemporal visual regions (Bollimunta et al., 2008). The scalp EEG topography does not readily identify such different activity profiles in the cortex. This fact is illustrated in Figure 1.1.1 (Megevand et al., 2008): Somatosensory evoked potentials (SEP) after whisker stimulation were recorded from the scalp and in the cortex of anesthetized mice. The 32 epicranial electrodes covered the scalp, while 16 intracranial electrodes spanned the different cortical layers. It can be easily seen that the scalp potential map can have similar scalp topographies with similar polarities at different moments in time, but the source-sink distribution across the different layers are completely different for these maps. Human scalp and subdural SEP recordings also show similar map topographies at different time points and are probably also generated by different source-sink distributions. The reason for this insensitivity of the scalp EEG to the intracolumnar source-sink distribution is that the scalp potentials represent only the summated field at a distance. This corresponds to the open field dipolar component of the complex multipolar current generators within the different cortical layers (Tenke et al., 1993). There is therefore no simple way to relate a given polarity of the scalp potential to the activity at a specific level of the dendrites. In addition, there have been studies showing that early scalp evoked potential components can be related to presynaptic activation of the thalamocortical afferents and excitatory postsynaptic potentials on the stellate cells in area 4C (Steinschneider et al., 1992; Tenke et al., 1993). These results suggest that not only cortical pyramidal cells are generating potential fields that can be detected by the EEG. Thus, the scalp potential represents a weighted sum of all active currents within the brain that generate open fields. The sum of all these open field generators form what is often called an equivalent dipole generator (Scherg et al., 1989). The current dipoles are thus used as simple, idealized models describing strength, orientation, and localization of the sum of the volume-conducted open field activity of all layers of the cortical or subcortical brain structures.

Sources and Spatial Scales of EEG and ERP Activity

Modeling the sources of normal EEG and ERP activity at the scalp usually results in equivalent current dipoles of up to 10 nA for evoked activity, and up to 100 nA for spontaneous activity. This holds for both the EEG and the MEG (magnetoencephalogram) due to the magnetic field generated by the same current dipoles (Hämäläinen et al., 1993; Murakami and Okada, 2006). Based on the properties of single post-synaptic potentials, this strength corresponds to about 1 million synapses in a cortical area of 40–200 mm^2 (Hämäläinen et al., 1993), and would mean that less than 1% of the synapses contribute to the EEG at any given moment. This estimate is also consistent with laminar recording of current source density. However, these recording are usually one-dimensional and fail to reveal the spatial extent of laminar sources and sinks. As a consequence, independent estimates regarding degree and spatial extent of postsynaptic neural synchronization represented by a scalp event are difficult. Even stronger activity than during spontaneous oscillations is observed during epileptic seizures and during slow wave sleep, particularly in children. These large activities can exceed 500 μV at the scalp for spontaneous or pathological EEG activity. They are thought to result from mass action due to a large extent and/or a high degree of synchronization.

The few clinical studies that have combined intracranial with scalp recordings in epilepsy patients for diagnostic purposes provide the most crucial information about the spatial scale of intracranial synchronization in relation to the scalp EEG. This holds even though such EEG is often abnormally synchronized, and despite the limited intracranial coverage confined to the small portion of the brain determined by clinical principles. The findings illustrate the strikingly different spatial scale of synchronization in intracranial and scalp EEG.

In intracranial recordings, focal interictal spike activity is often limited to less than 3 cm (as measured with multicontact electrodes spaced 0.5–1 cm apart) (Lantz et al., 1996), or to less than 6 cm^2 on an electrode grid. Such focal activity is usually not detected in the scalp EEG, even though the intracranial amplitudes can reach 50–500 μV (Lantz et al., 1996; Nayak et al., 2004; Tao et al., 2005; Zumsteg et al., 2006). This intracranial focality is also evident in correlations within intracortical grids, which typically fall off sharply outside regions of 2–5 cm diameter (Schevon et al., 2007).

To give rise to the typical scalp EEG, more widespread activation is necessary. At least 4–6 cm^2 of synchronously activated brain tissue seem to be needed to generate 10–20 μV at the scalp (Hämäläinen et al., 1993; Kobayashi et al., 2005; Murakami and Okada, 2006). This corresponds well to the original 6 cm^2 estimate for a model generator inside a skull to generate 25 µV at the outside (Cooper et al., 1965). More recent studies using intracranial grids with epilepsy patients even suggest that at least 10 cm^2 of cortex must exhibit synchronized epileptiform activity to generate reliably detectable scalp potentials, while synchronization of under 6 cm^2 is rarely detectable (Tao et al., 2005). Such estimates may be somewhat inflated due to the use of isolating grids, which dramatically attenuate the scalp potentials (Zhang et al., 2006). Intracranial occipital recordings of the spontaneous human EEG rhythm suggests a similar synchronization over a few cm, and some sharp polarity reversals within about 1–2 cm (Perez-Borja et al., 1962). Averaging can retrieve much smaller activities at the scalp (< 0.5 µV as for the brain stem potentials), provided they are systematically time locked to external (or to larger intracranial) events.

Spatial Field Distributions

Even extended synchronization would go undetected in the scalp EEG or ERP if its geometry were dominated by opposing directions. This would lead to full cancellation due to linear summation of the "closed" local fields. As a consequence, patches of synchronously polarized brain tissue must not only cover a considerable area but also need one dominant orientation to result in a "far field" at the scalp. Flat, extended, polarized patches of cortical tissue best meet this constraint and thus represent the optimal source geometry for scalp EEG and ERPs.

Fortunately, the cortex contains substantial portions that are nearly flat or have at least a clear main orientation, and are often activated synchronously. Cortical polarizations of gyral crowns and fundi are predominantly radial with regard to the skull, but mainly tangential on the sulcal walls. Both types of polarization give rise to characteristic EEG maps with distinct scalp distributions (Figure 1.1.2). In contrast, only tangential polarization generates MEG maps. Small spherical brain structures generate only "closed fields" because of dominant sources with opposite orientations. Whether heavily folded structures like the cerebellum generate detectable scalp EEG has long been debated. However, recent reports of consistent cerebellar activation (Timmermann et al., 2002; Ioannides and Fenwick, 2004; Martin et al., 2006), and task-specific activations of mesial temporal structures (James et al., 2008) strongly suggest that these structures also generate scalp EEG. Even better evidence comes from simulations (Attal et al., 2007) and recordings in patients with epilepsy (Lantz et al., 2001a; Michel et al., 2004a) suggesting that activity from hippocampus and amygdala can be detected by EEG and MEG,

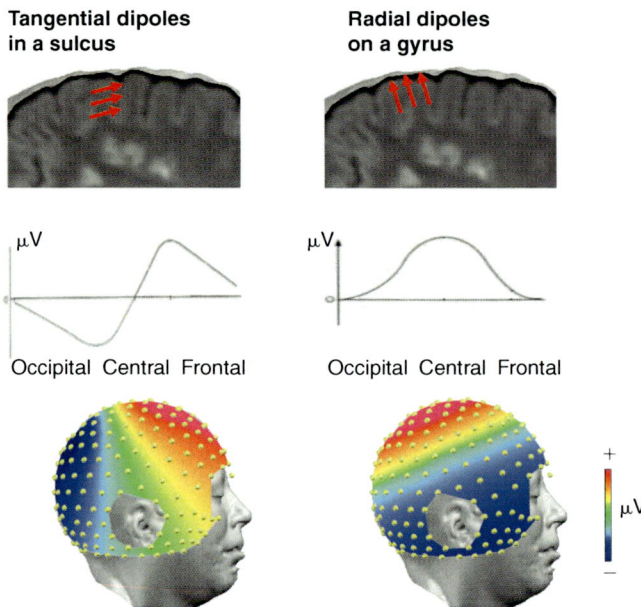

Figure 1.1.2. Sources and corresponding EEG scalp potential maps. The mass activity of aligned pyramidal neurons lead to volume currents that can be modeled as pointlike polarization dipoles. Pyramidal neurons located in a sulcus will lead to tangential dipoles, those located on a gyrus to radial dipoles. These dipoles induce electric potentials that spread to the surface and generate the potential fields with negative and positive polarities. In the case of tangential dipoles illustrated here, electrodes over occipital cortex will measure the negative part of the field, electrodes over frontal cortex the positive part. Electrodes located above the active neurons will measure zero potential. In the case of radial dipoles, the electrodes over the active area will record maximal positive potential, while the lowest temporal electrodes will pick up some part of the negative potential of the field (note that the maximal negativity cannot be measured in this case). The maps on the bottom show these two completely different configurations made by generators in the same brain area but with different orientation.

even though these mesial temporal structures are deep and strongly folded.

Knowing the intracranial potential distribution along with the shape and the conductivity distribution of the head (including scalp, skull, and brain) is sufficient to compute the electric scalp field without ambiguity, using so-called forward solutions. However, it is obviously unrealistic to obtain and validate a fully accurate description of the three-dimensional electrical distribution down to the spatial submillimeter scale.

It is thus of key importance to identify sensible spatial constraints on potential scalp EEG generators that suppress irrelevant detail at the microscopic level but retain all relevant details at a more macroscopic spatial scale that determines the forward solutions of the scalp EEG, such as the constraints on spatial extent and geometry discussed above. However, it is equally important to avoid invalid spatial constraints. An example is that EEG generators can not be constrained to those parts of the brain that are closest to the electrodes, as has often been assumed. Instead the EEG displays considerable sensitivity to deep sources, even more than the MEG. While local field potentials indeed fall off rapidly within the brain, far less attenuation is observed when recording across skull and scalp. The reason is that the lower conductivity of the skull (compared to brain and scalp) attenuates superficial sources more strongly than deep ones, thus acting like a spatial low-pass filter. This property causes strong blurring and attenuation of the focal superficial fields but has less of an effect on the more diffuse ("low spatial frequency") fields from deeper sources. Intracranial and scalp recordings of the potential distribution induced by intracranial stimulation in patients (Smith et al., 1983) confirm this behavior, and closely match predictions based on forward solutions using a dipole model. A core finding is that the attenuation of scalp voltages generated by the deepest compared to those generated by the most superficial sources in the brain can be as low as a factor of 2, while it would reach at least a factor of 7 if the skull had the same conductivity as the brain. Neglecting deep EEG sources in a model would thus be an invalid constraint. Instead, the role of skull conductivity, which determines the relative sensitivity to superficial versus deep sources, should be examined more systematically. This is particularly relevant for developmental studies with infants (Lai et al., 2005), as their higher skull conductivity emphasizes superficial over deep sources and lowers correlation or coherence estimates between electrodes (Grieve et al., 2003).

Taken together, spatial considerations derived from basic neurophysiology and from intracranial recordings provide some strong constraints on the major EEG and ERP generators, which reflect dynamic, synchronous polarization of spatially aligned neurons in extended gray matter networks. However, further putative constraints claiming a dominant orientation, insensitivity to deep structures, or a general laminar structure of EEG and ERP generators are not sufficiently supported. Recent evidence suggests that a considerably larger range of brain structures, layers, and cell types than previously thought can contribute to both event-related and spontaneous EEG phenomena.

Oscillations in Brain Networks

The most prominent features of EEG scalp potential waveforms are the oscillations at multiple frequencies. Distinct dominant electrical brain oscillations characterize different brain states ranging from alert wakefulness to deep sleep. Consequently, quantitative EEG analysis is often made according to the spectral content of the signals. Even though such analyses have revealed important results, they can also lead to erroneous conclusions when neglecting the fact that a given frequency band can reflect distinct phenomena originating from different sources. Therefore, frequency analysis of the EEG is highly ambiguous unless all oscillations originate from a single source, which is an unlikely assumption for typical brain states. This ambiguity is particularly pronounced when analyses are restricted to certain electrode locations or to averages over several electrode positions. It also limits the interpretation of correlations between the power variations of certain EEG rhythms and the BOLD signal measured in the fMRI. Before discussing the limitation of such studies, a brief summary of the possible generators and the functional significance of the different rhythms is provided. For more details the reader is referred to the excellent work of György Buzsáki, particularly *Rhythms of the Brain* (Buzsáki, 2006).

Here we use the conventional separation of frequency bands or dominant frequencies, since they are typically associated with different brain states (Klimesch, 1999; Engel et al., 2001). However rhythms of different frequencies can coexist and interact with each other (Steriade, 2001; Csicsvari et al., 2003) to produce a much wider range of brain states. Also, frequencies outside the conventional EEG frequency range can be recorded and might turn out to have functional significance (Gonzalez et al., 2006; Martuzzi et al., 2008).

Delta Rhythms

Delta waves are defined as rhythms with frequencies below 4 Hz (IFSECN, 1974). They are typically attributed to stage 3 and 4 of sleep (slow wave sleep) in human adults. Delta waves during slow wave sleep typically localize to midline cingulate structures, with stable microstate-like distributions but also distinct trajectories (Murphy et al., 2009). Their amplitude increases after sleep deprivation and reaches particularly high values in children. During wakefulness, delta activity mainly characterizes pathological states in adults, but is still normal in young children. In animal models, generators of delta activity have been demonstrated in the thalamus. Intrinsic clock-like oscillations within the delta frequency range can be recorded in thalamic neurons (Leresche et al., 1990; McCormick and Pape, 1990) that project to various regions of the cortex (thalamo-cortical neurons). However, in intact thalamo-cortical loops these oscillations are suppressed by the ongoing cortical activity (Nita et al., 2003). It is therefore questionable whether these intrinsically generated thalamic rhythms play a role in the generation of the slow waves observed on the level of the human EEG. On the other hand, a second type of slow wave exists during sleep that is generated by the cortex (Timofeev et al., 1996; Sanchez-Vives and McCormick, 2000). The frequency of this cortical delta is typically below 1 Hz and can be measured in both animals (Amzica and Steriade, 1997; Massimini et al., 2003) and humans using EEG (Achermann and Borbely, 1997; Molle et al., 2002) and MEG (Simon et al., 2000). It has been proposed that glial cells might also be involved in the control of the pace of these cortical slow wave oscillations (Amzica and Massimini, 2002; Amzica et al., 2002). In order to determine brain areas that might be involved in the generation of the delta waves recorded with the EEG, simultaneous

EEG-fMRI studies during sleep have been performed. Significant increases in BOLD response associated with delta and slow waves have been found in an extended network including several cortical areas such as the inferior frontal, medial prefrontal, precuneus, and posterior cingulate (Dang-Vu et al., 2008). Since these areas partially overlap with the waking default network (Fox and Raichle, 2007; Raichle and Snyder, 2007), it has been suggested that slow wave sleep is an active state during which brain activity is consistently synchronized in specific cerebral regions. Other studies however found reduced activity in several cortical regions as well as in limbic, thalamic, and midbrain structures that correlated with delta power during sleep (across all non-REM sleep stages) (Kaufmann et al., 2006). A recent EEG-fMRI study (Tyvaert et al., 2008) again showed positive rather than negative correlation of BOLD with delta rhythms. The positive correlations were mostly cortical, but rather heterogenous across subjects. The authors interpreted these variable results with the heterogeneity of different delta rhythms that might be present during a prolonged recording. This is indeed an important point, which underlines that different networks can generate the same rhythm, and should be separated by electrical neuroimaging. In addition to the different possible location of the generators, the potential distinction of two types of faster and slower delta waves, one generated by the thalamus and the other by the cortex should be tested systematically, although the current evidence for distinct generators in human sleep EEG remains limited.

Theta Rhythms

Theta rhythms denote oscillations in the frequency range of 4 to 7 Hz. They are more prominent in infancy and childhood, as well as during drowsiness and in sleep. In the EEG of awake adults, theta activity dominating at mid-frontal electrodes (frontal midline theta waves) are well described and are related to cognitive activities, especially in tasks that involve working memory (Klimesch, 1999; Mitchell et al., 2008). Consequently, the relation between the well-known theta activity in the hippocampus and the frontal midline theta is still debated (Mitchell et al., 2008). Theta increases at mid-frontal electrodes with increased memory load (Gevins et al., 1997). Dipole and distributed source models of theta scalp maps revealed generators in dorsal anterior cingulate cortex (Onton et al., 2005). In line with these findings, memory load also correlates with intracranial frontal midline theta in patients (Meltzer et al., 2008), and with frontal midline fMRI memory load effects (Meltzer et al., 2007). Involvement of posterior sites during memory retrieval attempts have also been described (Sauseng et al., 2002; Klimesch et al., 2005). Frontal theta EEG changes are correlated with power changes in the alpha band (Klimesch et al., 2005), and it is often phase locked to high frequency gamma activity (Lakatos et al., 2005), giving rise to an "oscillatory hierarchy." Simultaneous EEG-fMRI during wakefulness found positive correlations between theta activity and BOLD response in the insular cortex, the hippocampus, superior temporal areas, the cingulate cortex, as well as superior parietal, and frontal areas (Sammer et al., 2007). These authors concluded that theta band oscillations represent "dynamic functional binding of widely distributed cortical assemblies, essential for cognitive processing." However, other studies found no correlation between theta activity and BOLD response (Laufs et al., 2003b), or found only negative correlations in areas that again partly overlap with the default mode network (Scheeringa et al., 2008a), which was interpreted as a general reduction of alertness (Tyvaert et al., 2008).

Theta during wakefulness is different from the theta during sleep. The theta activity recorded in the human hippocampus during REM sleep and during transitions from sleep to wake were not coupled with the theta activity observed in frontal and temporal cortex in the sleep-wake transition (Cantero et al., 2003). This indicates that, as for the delta activity, different theta generators exist in the human brain and are active in different brain states.

Alpha Rhythms

The alpha rhythm (oscillations between 8 and 12 Hz) was the first described EEG oscillation (Berger, 1929). Despite this long history, the functional significance and the neuronal generators of these rhythms are still largely unknown (Buzsáki, 2006; Klimesch et al., 2007). In addition to thalamic generators (Lopes da Silva et al., 1980), alpha is also generated in different cortical populations and shows slightly different frequency characteristics in different cortical areas (Lopes da Silva, 1991; de Munck et al., 2007a). Cortical alpha rhythms may also result from an interaction between thalamo-cortical and cortico-cortical mechanisms (Lopes da Silva et al., 1980; Suffczynski et al., 2001). Alpha-band power at rest or baseline was found in different EEG studies to be stable within individuals over time (Hanslmayr et al., 2007; Klimesch et al., 2007; Napflin et al., 2007), indicating that alpha-power might reflect a traitlike variable in each individual. Combined EEG-fMRI studies consistently revealed positive correlation of alpha power with BOLD in the thalamus and negative correlation (i.e., BOLD decrease with increasing alpha power) in occipital, parietal, and frontal cortical regions (Laufs et al., 2003a; Goncalves et al., 2006; Laufs et al., 2006; de Munck et al., 2007b; Tyvaert et al., 2008). These are again areas that overlap with the default network, as already described for the slower frequencies above.

The early observation that alpha is the most prominent oscillatory frequency over occipital cortex during rest and with eyes closed led to the conclusion that alpha was an idling rhythm involved in active suppression of sensory input (Worden et al., 2000). Demonstrating alpha suppression after eye opening, visual stimulus presentation, and during mental activity reinforced this hypothesis. In addition, the results of combined transcranial magnetic stimulation (TMS) and EEG studies showed that visual cortical excitability as measured by TMS-induced phosphene perception is dependent on the momentary alpha desynchronization before the TMS pulse is delivered (Romei et al., 2007).

But alpha is not only an occipital rhythm indicating low level of arousal. Alpha oscillations also occur over frontal cortex, i.e., the frontal eye fields, as well as over sensory motor cortex and the supplementary motor area (named the mu rhythm) (Pfurtscheller and Andrew, 1999), and over primary auditory cortex (Hari and Salmelin, 1997). In these studies, the most prominent feature was the blocking of the spontaneous alpha rhythm by activity. However, the studies also showed suppression of the mu rhythm that began before a movement was planned over related cortical areas (Pfurtscheller et al., 1997). The reduction of alpha-power was subsequently related to be a functional correlate of brain activation or a state of high cortical excitability (Pfurtscheller and Lopes da Silva, 1999; Klimesch et al., 2007). The so-called alpha suppression was long considered as the prevailing functional correlate of cortical activation. Also, increased alpha synchronization was described for a long time exclusively as a cortical idling phenomenon (Pfurtscheller, 1992) despite early findings of task-induced increases of alpha-band power, which argued against a pure idling hypothesis (Klimesch, 1999). Such relative increases in alpha power were also described during retention and with increasing working memory load (Jensen et al., 2002; Jokisch and Jensen, 2007; Michels et al., 2008). Again, different alpha distributions are found during wakefulness and slow wave sleep (Ehrhart et al., 2000).

The role of alpha increase and decrease has also been extensively studied in relation to modulation of visual spatial attention. In typical cued attention tasks, alpha power decreases just before a target appears, occurring over visual cortex contralateral to the attended hemifield (Sauseng et al., 2005; Yamagishi et al., 2005; Thut et al., 2006), thus indicating anticipatory activity over areas preparing to process the target. On the other hand, alpha-band power increases over posterior sites contralateral to the unattended location (i.e., ipsilateral to the attended position), which might serve to actively suppress visual input from task-irrelevant or unattended positions (Worden et al., 2000; Kelly et al., 2006; Rihs et al., 2007, 2009) (Figure 1.1.3). Increases in alpha amplitude over occipital cortex were also found using cross-modal attention paradigms when attention was directed to auditory inputs (Foxe et al., 1998; Fu et al., 2001).

The conclusion is that again (as for the slower frequencies described before) there is no single alpha rhythm in the brain. Alpha rhythms appear in different brain areas, and have different behavioral significance as well as different laminar generators. This was most impressively demonstrated in the work of Bollimunta et al. (2008), where intracranial activity was recorded from different visual areas of spontaneously behaving monkeys. The combination of laminar current source density analysis and multiunit activity clearly revealed different local pacemaking generators for the alpha rhythm in area V2 and V4 of the visual cortex as compared to the generators in the inferotemporal cortex. The current density

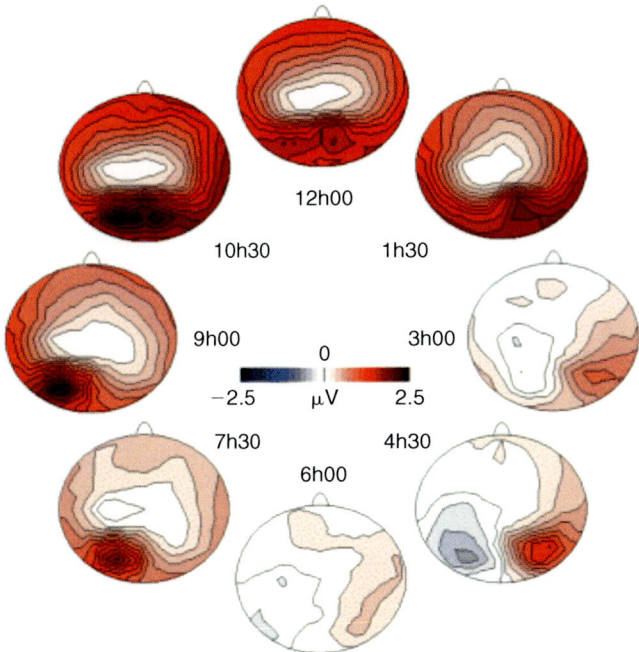

Figure 1.1.3. Alpha-band synchronization as index of selective inhibition. Subjects viewed a central fixation cross surrounded by eight light grey squares placed in a clock-face arrangement indicating possible target locations. A shortly flashed central arrow then pointed to the to-be-attended position, which varied randomly across trials. After 1300 ms a visual stimulus appeared, more often at cued than noncued locations, and represented either a go or nogo target. The response for go targets was to press a button. The figure shows the analysis of the EEG alpha activity in the last 250 ms of the cue-target interval, i.e., when anticipating a cued target. The maps show the relative changes in alpha-band activity over the entire electrode array (128 electrodes) for each of the eight cued and attended positions. Red indicates alpha increase (synchronization), blue alpha decrease (desynchronization). Alpha synchronization showed a retinotopically organized pattern over posterior recording sites that depended in location on the laterality, horizontal offset, and elevation (upper vs. lower visual field) of the attention focus. The synchronization was found contralaterally to the unattended space, providing evidence that alpha synchronization serves to actively suppress visual input from unattended positions. Reprinted from Rihs TA, Michel CM, Thut G (2007) Mechanisms of selective inhibition in visual spatial attention are indexed by alpha-band EEG synchronization. Eur J Neurosci 25:603–610 with permission from John Wiley & Sons, Inc.

profiles are dominated by deeper (granular and infragranular) layers in lower-order visual areas, but by activity in more superficial (supragranular) in the higher inferotemporal visual regions. This finding has profound implication for interpretation of scalp EEG recordings, since the net dipole fields of the alpha activity might be different for different brain areas and might thus contribute differently to the scalp EEG alpha rhythm. It is obvious that these implications also affect the combined EEG-fMRI studies since it means that correlations between alpha activity and the BOLD response will depend on the brain region from which the alpha activity was recorded.

Fast and Ultra-Fast EEG Rhythms

Already in the first reports on the EEG, Hans Berger (Berger, 1929) distinguished the large alpha waves from small fast waves that he termed "beta waves." He described the beta waves as the "concomitant phenomenon of mental activity" (Berger, 1938). Beta activity (15–30 Hz) is generally considered as an activation or arousal response of the cortex initiated by brainstem structures that suppress slower EEG rhythms (Buzsáki et al., 1988). Combined EEG-fMRI studies found correlation between beta power and BOLD response in the posterior cingulate and precuneus as well as the temporo-parietal and dorsomedial prefrontal cortex (Laufs et al., 2003b), areas that are concomitantly considered as the default mode of brain function, i.e., the brain areas that are active when the subject is left undisturbed and performs complex reflections and abstractions of the outer world without external input (Raichle et al., 2001; Buckner et al., 2008). This is distinct from the beta band oscillations observed in the sensorimotor system during motor activity, where beta rhythms in somatosensory and motor cortex are synchronized, allowing to relate the sensory input with the motor command (Baker, 2007). Thus again, as for the other frequency bands, Beta activity has a variety of distinct functional significance and distinct generators depending on the functional state of the brain.

The most widely studied rhythms in relation to sensory and cognitive brain functions are the so called gamma-activities in the range from around 30 to 100 Hz. It was proposed that synchronization of distant brain areas in the gamma frequency range allows functional aggregation of these areas into a large-scale network, with the purpose of creating a global percept of different features, i.e., serving as a basic mechanism for figure-ground distinction and feature binding (von der Malsburg and Schneider, 1986; Singer, 1999). The involvement of gamma band oscillations in such elaborate aspects of information processing is, however, arguable. On the one hand, gamma oscillations are intrinsic properties of thalamocortical and cortical networks and present during states such as sleep and deep anesthesia, where conscious cognitive processing is absent (Steriade and Amzica, 1996; Steriade et al., 1996). On the other hand, recent EEG studies showed that some of the induced gamma activity that was attributed to feature binding generated in visual cortical areas were in fact artifacts of miniature saccades evoked by the stimuli (Yuval-Greenberg et al., 2008). In addition, a strong link between gamma band oscillations and facial muscle activity during cognitive tasks was confirmed by showing that such oscillations disappear despite normal cognitive performance when the muscles are paralyzed (Whitham et al., 2008). While these findings may invalidate some conclusions of previous studies on evoked gamma activity, they do not put into question the fact that gamma oscillations can reflect a state of high neuronal excitability involved in complex brain processes, and that a cortical origin of some EEG gamma band oscillations can (and must) be demonstrated through topographic analyses and source estimates (Fries et al., 2007). The fact that muscular artifacts may be misinterpreted as neuronal activity demonstrates the caution required when recording and interpreting EEG recordings from selected channels. The influence of the reference electrode on spectral parameters and the contribution of non-neuronal electrical activity to the EEG signal requires careful consideration. Proper spatial sampling and source estimation of oscillations is particularly important to disambiguate the relation between the scalp signals and generators in the brain.

Functional Microstates of the Brain

As described in the previous chapter, the rhythmic oscillations of the electrical neuronal activity in the different frequency ranges are obviously linked to different functional states of the brain. These frequency-specific oscillations have repeatedly been correlated with the hemodynamic response measured with the fMRI in order to discover the brain regions that may be generating or modulating these brain rhythms. Thereby, the EEG recorded in the scanner is frequency-transformed, and power of the selected frequencies and channels is convolved with the (much slower) hemodynamic response function at each voxel (Goldman et al., 2002; Laufs et al., 2003a; Laufs et al., 2006; Difrancesco et al., 2008; Scheeringa et al., 2008b). However, this type of analysis of the EEG not only assumes stationary of the signal in time but also in space. In other words, only one process is assumed to oscillate per frequency, expressed in all electrodes in the same way over the whole analysis period. This assumption is problematic, as the spatial analysis of the EEG clearly shows changes in EEG map topography while the spectral power in the different frequencies remains stable (Lehmann et al., 1987; Koenig et al., 2001; Koenig et al., 2005a). These changes in map topography reflect different distributions of neuronal generators that contribute to a given oscillatory behavior. Different networks can thus contribute to one given rhythm observed at a given electrode. From a functional point of view, important changes in brain functioning thus need not be related to changes of oscillations frequency, and may go undetected when looking at single channel oscillations only. In addition, rapid functional changes of the brain state may not be well represented in classical frequency domain analysis of the EEG.

Determination of changes in EEG map topography over time requires spatial rather than frequency-domain analysis. It is thus a problem related to pattern recognition rather than to time series analysis. The pattern analysis compares the spatial configuration of the momentary potential maps time point for time point and looks for moments of significant topographic changes. Using such spatiotemporal analysis methods, it has been shown that the spontaneous ongoing EEG usually consists of sequential segments of stable map configurations that last about 80–120 ms and that are separated by short periods of rapid transition between the configurations (Lehmann, 1971; Lehmann et al., 1987; Strik and Lehmann, 1993). Periods of transition typically happen during low global strength of the field, while peaks of field strength characterize periods of topographic stability (Figure 1.1.4). Stability of field configuration is defined independent of field strength, and usually also independent of polarity when focusing on oscillations. Polarity reversals of the same field configuration are due to the intrinsic oscillatory activity of the generator processes as described above. The observation of discontinuous changes of field configuration has led to the concept of *functional microstates* of the brain (Lehmann, 1971; Lehmann et al., 1987). It has been proposed that these microstates represent the basic building blocks of human mentation, i.e. the basic elements of conscious thinking and information processing (Lehmann, 1992; Lehmann et al., 1998; Changeux and Michel, 2004; Lehmann et al., 2009). Pattern recognition algorithms have been used to classify the map configurations of the different microstates. The results indicate that a limited number of configurations exist, and that these configurations follow each other according to systematic transition preferences

(Wackerman et al., 1993; Pascual-Marqui et al., 1995). The temporal syntax of these microstates (i.e., their succession and duration) is altered in several pathological conditions such as depression (Strik et al., 1995), dementia (Strik et al., 1997; Koenig et al., 2005b), schizophrenia (Koenig et al., 1999; Lehmann et al., 2005) and epilepsy (Lantz et al., 2001b), as well as after drug intake (Lehmann et al., 1993; Kinoshita et al., 1995). In normal subjects, the duration and frequency of appearance of the four most dominant microstate configurations varies with age, as shown in a analysis of EEG from 496 subjects (Koenig et al., 2002).

The topographic analysis of the EEG shows that the EEG can be parsed into a series of microstates with distinct topographies. These microstates are largely independent of the frequencies of the EEG oscillations. Topographic time-frequency decomposition shows that several processes can operate in the same frequency range, but differ in topography (Koenig et al., 2001; Koenig et al., 2005a). EEG-fMRI comparisons using FFT analysis methods for the EEG will therefore collapse different functional states of the brain that take

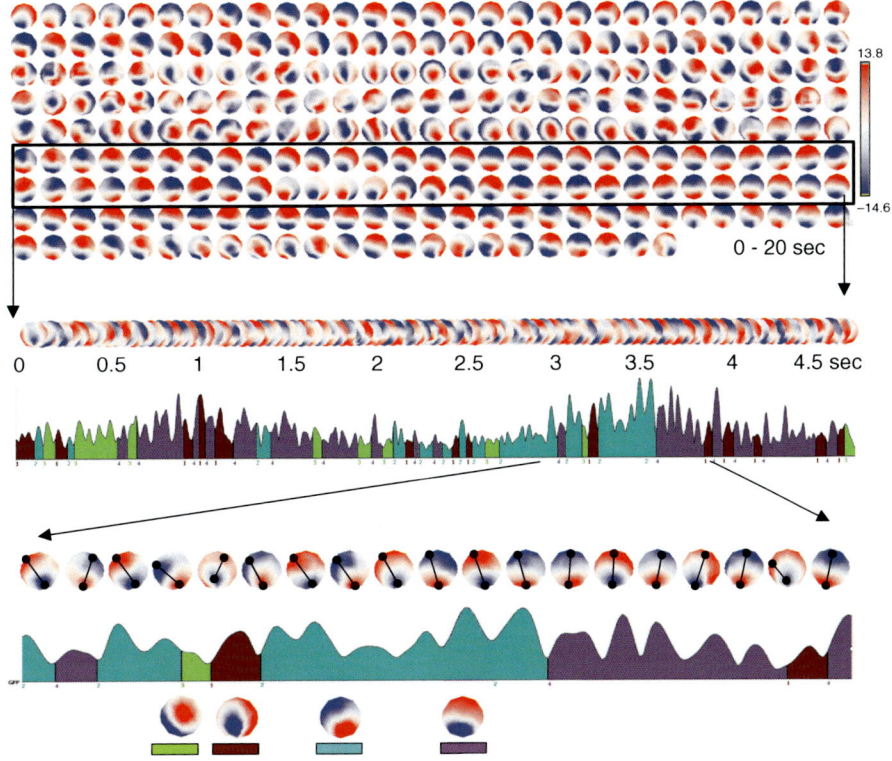

Figure 1.1.4. Microstate segmentation of spontaneous EEG. A 42-channel eyes-closed EEG of 20 seconds is shown on top in terms of a series of scalp potential maps (only around every twentieth map is shown, for space reasons). A part of this map series (5 seconds) is shown in more detail below (still less than what has been sampled in reality). All the 1280 maps of this 5-second period were subjected to a k-means cluster analysis that identified the four maps shown on the bottom. Each of these four maps was repeatedly present during a short period of time (in average around 100 ms). These periods are marked under the global field power curve as colored segments representing the four maps. A short period is enlarged to illustrate the topographic stability during such periods: The landscape of the maps, e.g., the position of the maximum and minimum, remains stable during such a period, only the polarity changes due to the intrinsic oscillatory activity of the generator processes. These segments of stable potential maps have been labeled the *functional microstates*. Adapted from Michel et al. (2009).

place in the subsecond range. These slower global variations of the strength of oscillations might correlate with certain fMRI-defined stable resting state networks of the brain as described above. However, the large-scale neurocognitive networks of the brain that underly human brain function have to grant both, stability and plasticity, and thus have to adapt rapidly depending on the momentary cognitive thought (Bressler, 1995; Bressler and Tognoli, 2006). The corresponding subsecond changes of network functions cannot be studied with hemodynamic or metabolic functional imaging methods that work in the range of seconds or more. Such rapid changes are also missed by conventional EEG frequency power analysis integrating activity over seconds. The spatial analysis of the EEG using pattern recognition algorithms captures them much better, because it measures the activity of large-scale neuronal networks at any moment in time with millisecond resolution. The observation of noncontinuous variation of EEG microstates in the subsecond time range corresponds well to the proposal that neurocognitive networks evolve through a sequence of quasi-stable coordination states, rather than through a continuous flow of neuronal activity (Grossberg, 2000; Bressler and Tognoli, 2006; Fingelkurts, 2006). In the neuronal workspace model of consciousness (Baars, 2002; Dehaene et al., 2003), it is proposed that episodes of coherent activity last a certain amount of time (around 100 ms) and are separated by sharp transitions and that only one such workspace representation is active at any given time (Baars, 2002; Dehaene et al., 2003). This model adequately fits the observation of functional microstates of the brain described above (Changeux and Michel, 2004).

EEG Source Imaging

The topographical analysis of the scalp potential map is the first step toward the use of EEG as a functional imaging procedure. Differences in map topographies directly indicate differences in configuration (or weighting) of the neuronal generators in the brain. The second step of electrical neuroimaging concerns the determination of the generators in the brain that gave rise to a given scalp potential map. It is well known that this problem has no unique solution. An infinite number of source distributions can generate the same scalp potential map. This so-called inverse problem can only be solved by incorporating certain a priori assumptions about the sources. Such assumptions are either purely mathematical, or incorporate some of the physiological knowledge about the generators of the EEG described above. The interested reader can find several comprehensive reviews on EEG source imaging (Grave de Peralta Menendez and Gonzalez Andino, 1998; Pascual-Marqui, 1999; Baillet et al., 2001; He and Lian, 2002; Michel et al., 2004b; He and Lian, 2005).

Early source localization attempts have focused on overdetermined source models. This was achieved by limiting the

number of sources so that the number of unknown parameters is less than or equal to the number of recording electrodes. Non-linear search algorithms then find the optimal location and orientation of the dipoles generating the scalp potential distribution which best resembles the actually measured map. The major limiting factor of this type of algorithm is the fact that the number of dipoles has to be small and known a priori. Multiple signal classification techniques (Mosher and Leahy, 1998), spatiotemporal decomposition approaches (Koles and Soong, 1998) or independent component analysis (Kobayashi et al., 2002) have been proposed to automatically determine the optimal (though limited) number of sources. Some authors proposed to use other functional imaging methods like fMRI to define the number and location of the active sources and then use the EEG merely to look at the temporal dynamic of these fixed sources (Menon et al., 1997; Korvenoja et al., 1999; Murray et al., 2002). This is not without risk, given the still unclear relationship between hemodynamic and electrophysiological activities (Logothetis et al., 2001), and given the fact that short-lasting EEG events might not reach significance level in fMRI thresholding (Vitacco et al., 2002). Such systematic differences in sensitivity may result in genuine discrepancies between the EEG and fMRI-based results that are highly informative (Brem et al., 2009). The fundamental problem of determining the number of dipoles a priori has made the overdetermined source models rather unreliable. Therefore attempts have been made to develop underdetermined source models where other constraints than the number of sources are incorporated. These so-called distributed source models reconstruct brain electric activity in each point of a large three-dimensional grid of solution points, using a dipolar source of a given strength and orientation on each grid point. Since such models lead to a highly underdetermined inverse problem, additional a priori constraints are needed. Different such a priori assumptions have been proposed in the literature, most prominent the so-called minimum norm assumption, which searches for the 3D current distribution that has minimal overall intensity or power (Hämäläinen and Ilmoniemi, 1984). Since this assumption leads to an excessive estimation of superficial sources, additional weighting strategies have been proposed, most well-known the so-called Laplacian weighted minimum norm algorithm that is implemented in the LORETA software (Pascual-Marqui et al., 1994). The Laplacian weighting, which leads to a smoothing of the solution in space is justified by the parallel oriented and synchronized local neuronal activity. Because LORETA blurs the solution rather strongly (Fuchs et al., 1999), other constraints have been proposed, such as the autoregressive average implemented in the LAURA algorithm (Grave de Peralta Menendez et al., 2001). The differently weighted minimum norm algorithms give rather comparable results with slight differences in the relative strength of the different sources (Schulz et al., 2008) (Figure 1.1.5).

The distributed inverse solutions applied to high resolution EEG has proven to very reliably localize electrical neuronal activity. This has mainly been demonstrated in studies on epileptic patients, where localization precision was as high

Semantic Incongruency Effect

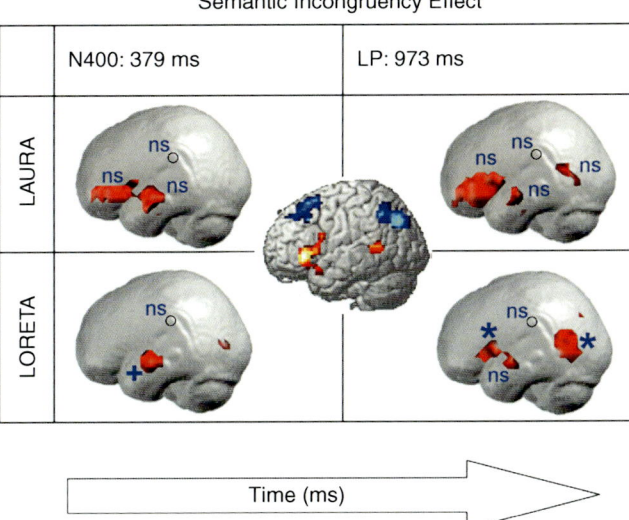

Time (ms)

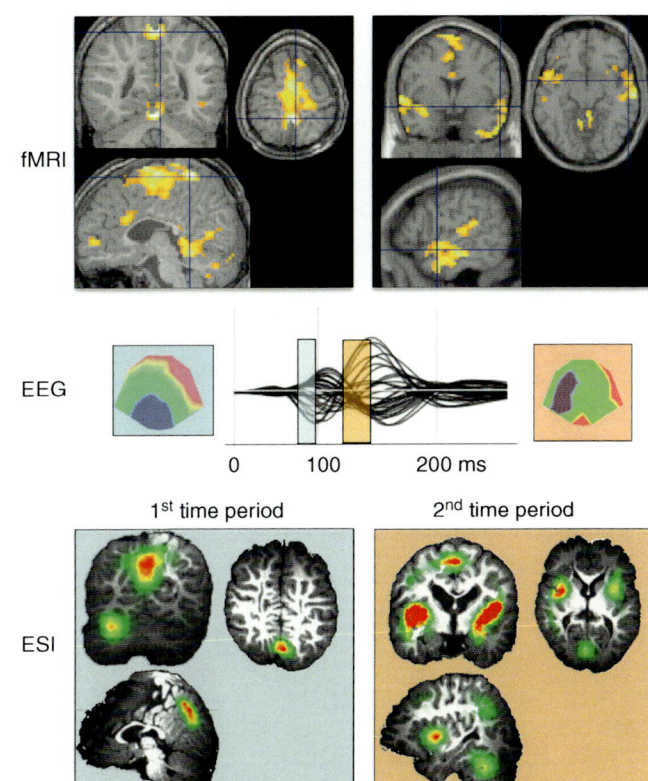

Figure 1.1.5. Comparison of ERP source imaging and fMRI in a sentence reading task performed by N = 52 children for the ERP and N = 37 children for the fMRI (Schulz et al., 2008). The effects of semantic incongruity (contrasting activity for incongruent vs. congruent sentence endings) are shown for two different distributed linear inverse solutions, LORETA (top) and LAURA (bottom) at two different time periods. Current source density at these time periods was tested vs. time zero in the voxels showing local maxima for the grand mean incongruency effect. Significance of the effects is indicated in the figure (*: p < 0.05, +: p < 0.11; ns: not significant). The center inset shows the fMRI analysis (p <.001 uncorrected, red for positive, blue for negative BOLD effect). Note the comparable results of the two inverse solutions (though different in relative strength) and the comparable results of the ERP inverse solutions and the positive BOLD in the fMRI (though resolved in time with the ERPs). From Brandeis D, Michel CM, Gianotti LRR (2009) Integration with Other Functional Imaging Methods. In: Electrical Neuroimaging (Michel CM, Koenig T, Brandeis D, Gianotti LRR, Wackermann J, eds), with permission from Cambridge University Press.

Figure 1.1.6. fMRI and electric source imaging (ESI) of interictal spikes in a patient with partial epilepsy. The 30-channel EEG recorded in the 3T scanner was analyzed for the same spikes that were used for the fMRI analysis, after proper elimination of scanner and heartbeat artifacts. The top shows the result of the fMRI analysis. Several areas showed significant BOLD effects related to the spikes, including medial centro-parietal as well as bilateral temporal areas, making interpretation in terms of primary epileptic focus difficult. The ESI of the averaged spike shows the same active areas but resolving them in time: the medial centro-parietal area is active at the rising phase of the spike, while the bilateral temporal areas are propagation areas becoming active during later phases of the discharge, leading to the conclusion that the medial centro-parietal area represents the primary focus. Data recorded by Dr. Michael Siniatchkin from the Neuropediatric Department, Christian-Albrechts-University, Kiel, Germany. For details and additional examples see Groening et al. (2009).

as with other functional imaging procedures and where verification of the correctness of the localization was based on postoperative outcome or direct intracranial recordings in the same patients (Michel et al., 1999; Lantz et al., 2003a; Lantz et al., 2003b; Holmes et al., 2004; Michel et al., 2004a; Zumsteg et al., 2005; Sperli et al., 2006; Zumsteg et al., 2006) (Figure 1.1.6). Applications to sensory as well as cognitive evoked potentials have also repeatedly shown the validity of these localization procedures (Michel et al., 2001; Blanke et al., 2005; Murray et al., 2006; Stein et al., 2006; De Santis et al., 2007; Britz et al., 2008; James et al., 2008; Murray et al., 2008; Schulz et al., 2008). Thereby, so-called source waveforms are directly analyzed, i.e., the current density of a certain brain region is estimated at each time point and the temporal variation of the activity in this region is analyzed and compared between experimental conditions or between task demands. Direct comparison of electric source imaging with fMRI has generally shown very good correspondence,

although important differences in sensitivities have also been reported (Groening et al., 2009; Vulliemoz et al., 2009). In the typical case of converging network localizations, the combination of the two techniques will be particularly valuable to achieve high spatial and temporal resolution for functional neuroimaging (see the examples in Figures 1.1.5 and 1.1.6). This joint resolution advantage should be particularly prominent for the high-resolution EEG recorded during fMRI scanning, because these simultaneous recordings ensure identical conditions and brain states. Such "contaminated" EEG can now be cleaned with powerful denoising algorithm and can then be analyzed like EEG recorded outside the scanner (Figure 1.1.6).

The power of EEG as a functional neuroimaging method is unfortunately still largely underestimated. Many impressive experimental and clinical EEG studies using these tools have not received the attention they merit. The reason is manifold. First, functional magnetic resonance imaging has received a unique status of being able to reduce brain activity to the underlying neural sources nonambiguously. Second, misinterpretations of EEG and evoked potential waveforms due to a lack of understanding the spatial properties of electromagnetic fields, and the influence of non-neuronal signals, resulted in some incorrect claims regarding localization abilities and limitations. Third the EEG is somehow harmed by history. The term EEG is still often related to the art of interpreting grapho-elements by skilled clinicians and neurophysiologists. The magnetoencephalogram (MEG) that basically measures the same signals with the same limitations does not suffer from this history and is more easily considered as a neuroimaging method (e.g., by public encyclopedias such as Wikipedia). Both approaches require that the data be correctly interpreted on the basis of proper knowledge about the generation and propagation of electric and magnetic neuronal activity in the human brain. In this chapter, we have attempted to correct this historical view of the EEG, and demonstrate that spatial EEG analysis has matured to become a powerful, flexible, and affordable neuroimaging method with unique strengths.

REFERENCES

Achermann P, Borbely AA (1997) Low-frequency (< 1 Hz) oscillations in the human sleep electroencephalogram. Neuroscience 81:213–222.

Amzica F, Steriade M (1997) The K-complex: its slow (<1-Hz) rhythmicity and relation to delta waves. Neurology 49:952–959.

Amzica F, Massimini M (2002) Glial and neuronal interactions during slow wave and paroxysmal activities in the neocortex. Cereb Cortex 12:1101–1113.

Amzica F, Massimini M, Manfridi A (2002) Spatial buffering during slow and paroxysmal sleep oscillations in cortical networks of glial cells in vivo. J Neurosci 22:1042–1053.

Attal Y, Bhattacharjee M, Yelnik J, Cottereau B, Lefevre J, Okada Y, Bardinet E, Chupin M, Baillet S (2007) Modeling and detecting deep brain activity with MEG & EEG. Conf Proc IEEE Eng Med Biol Soc 2007:4937–4940.

Baars BJ (2002) The conscious access hypothesis: origins and recent evidence. Trends Cogn Sci 6:47–52.

Baillet S, Mosher JC, Leahy RM (2001) Electromagnetic brain mapping. IEEE Signal Processing Magazine:14–30.

Baker SN (2007) Oscillatory interactions between sensorimotor cortex and the periphery. Curr Opin Neurobiol 17:649–655.

Berger H (1929) u?ber das Elektroenkephalogramm des Menschen. Archiv fu?r Psychiatrie und Nervenkrankheiten 87:527–570.

Berger H (1938) Ueber das Elektrenkephalogramm des Menschen. Vierzehnte Mitteilung. Arch Psychiat Nervenkr 108:407–431.

Blanke O, Mohr C, Michel CM, Pascual-Leone A, Brugger P, Seeck M, Landis T, Thut G (2005) Linking out-of-body experience and self processing to mental own-body imagery at the temporoparietal junction. J Neurosci 25:550–557.

Bollimunta A, Chen Y, Schroeder CE, Ding M (2008) Neuronal mechanisms of cortical alpha oscillations in awake-behaving macaques. J Neurosci 28:9976–9988.

Brandeis D, Michel CM, Gianotti LRR (2009) Integration of electrical neuroimaging with other functional imaging methods. In: Electrical neuroimaging (Michel CM, Koenig T, Brandeis D, Gianotti LRR, Wackermann J, eds), pp. 215-232. Cambridge: Cambridge University Press.

Brem S, Halder P, Bucher K, Summers P, Martin E, Brandeis D (2009) Tuning of the visual word processing system: distinct developmental ERP and fMRI effects. Hum Brain Mapp 30:1833–1844.

Bressler SL (1995) Large-scale cortical networks and cognition. Brain Res Brain Res Rev 20:288–304.

Bressler SL, Tognoli E (2006) Operational principles of neurocognitive networks. Int J Psychophysiol 60:139–148.

Britz J, Landis T, Michel CM (2008) Right parietal brain activity precedes perceptual alternation of bi-stable stimuli. Cereb Cortex 19:55–65.

Buckner RL, Andrews-Hanna JR, Schacter DL (2008) The brain's default network: anatomy, function, and relevance to disease. Ann N Y Acad Sci 1124:1–38.

Buzsáki G. (2006) Rhythms of the brain. Oxford: Oxford University Press.

Buzsáki G, Bickford RG, Ponomareff G, Thal LJ, Mandel R, Gage FH (1988) Nucleus basalis and thalamic control of neocortical activity in the freely moving rat. J Neurosci 8:4007–4026.

Cantero JL, Atienza M, Stickgold R, Kahana MJ, Madsen JR, Kocsis B (2003) Sleep-dependent theta oscillations in the human hippocampus and neocortex. J Neurosci 23:10897–10903.

Changeux J-P, Michel CM (2004) Mechanism of neural integration at the brain-scale level. In: Microcircuits (Grillner S, Graybiel AM, eds), pp. 347–370. Cambridge: MIT Press.

Cooper R, Winter AL, Crow HJ, Walter WG (1965) Comparison of subcortical, cortical and scalp activity using chronically indwelling electrodes in man. Electroencephalogr Clin Neurophysiol 18:217–228. Csicsvari J, Jamieson B, Wise KD, Buzsaki G (2003) Mechanisms of gamma oscillations in the hippocampus of the behaving rat. Neuron 37:311–322.

Dang-Vu TT, Schabus M, Desseilles M, Albouy G, Boly M, Darsaud A, Gais S, Rauchs G, Sterpenich V, Vandewalle G, Carrier J, Moonen G, Balteau E, Degueldre C, Luxen A, Phillips C, Maquet P (2008) Spontaneous neural activity during human slow wave sleep. Proc Natl Acad Sci U S A 105:15160–15165.

de Munck JC, Goncalves SI, Huijboom L, Kuijer JPA, Pouwels PJW, Heethaar RM, Lopes da Silva FH (2007a) The hemodynamic response of the alpha rhythm: an EEG/fMRI study. NeuroImage 35:1142.

de Munck JC, Goncalves SI, Huijboom L, Kuijer JP, Pouwels PJ, Heethaar RM, Lopes da Silva FH (2007b) The hemodynamic response of the alpha rhythm: an EEG/fMRI study. Neuroimage 35:1142–1151.

De Santis L, Spierer L, Clarke S, Murray MM (2007) Getting in touch: segregated somatosensory what and where pathways in humans revealed by electrical neuroimaging. Neuroimage 37:890–903.

Dehaene S, Sergent C, Changeux JP (2003) A neuronal network model linking subjective reports and objective physiological data during conscious perception. Proc Natl Acad Sci U S A 100:8520–8525.

Difrancesco MW, Holland SK, Szaflarski JP (2008) Simultaneous EEG/functional magnetic resonance imaging at 4 Tesla: correlates of brain activity to spontaneous alpha rhythm during relaxation. J Clin Neurophysiol 25:255–264.

Ehrhart J, Toussaint M, Simon C, Gronfier C, Luthringer R, Brandenberger G (2000) Alpha activity and cardiac correlates: three types of relationships during nocturnal sleep. Clin Neurophysiol 111:940–946.

Engel AK, Fries P, Singer W (2001) Dynamic predictions: oscillations and synchrony in top-down processing. Nat Rev Neurosci 2:704–716.

Fingelkurts AA (2006) Timing in cognition and EEG brain dynamics: discreteness versus continuity. Cogn Process 7:135–162.

Fox MD, Raichle ME (2007) Spontaneous fluctuations in brain activity observed with functional magnetic resonance imaging. Nat Rev Neurosci 8:700–711.

Foxe JJ, Simpson GV, Ahlfors SP (1998) Parieto-occipital approximately 10 Hz activity reflects anticipatory state of visual attention mechanisms. Neuroreport 9:3929–3933.

Fries P, Nikolic D, Singer W (2007) The gamma cycle. Trends Neurosci 30:309–316.

Fu KM, Foxe JJ, Murray MM, Higgins BA, Javitt DC, Schroeder CE (2001) Attention-dependent suppression of distracter visual input can be cross-modally cued as indexed by anticipatory parieto-occipital alpha-band oscillations. Brain Res Cogn Brain Res 12:145–152.

Fuchs M, Wagner M, Köhler T, Wischmann H-A (1999) Linear and nonlinear current density reconstructions. J Clin Neurophysiol 16:267–295.

Gevins A, Smith ME, McEvoy L, Yu D (1997) High-resolution EEG mapping of cortical activation related to working memory: effects of task difficulty, type of processing, and practice. Cereb Cortex 7:374–385.

Gobbele R, Buchner H, Curio G (1998) High-frequency (600 Hz) SEP activities originating in the subcortical and cortical human somatosensory system. Electroencephalogr Clin Neurophysiol 108:182–189.

Goldman RI, Stern JM, Engel J, Jr., Cohen MS (2002) Simultaneous EEG and fMRI of the alpha rhythm. Neuroreport 13:2487–2492.

Goncalves SI, de Munck JC, Pouwels PJ, Schoonhoven R, Kuijer JP, Maurits NM, Hoogduin JM, Van Someren EJ, Heethaar RM, Lopes da Silva FH (2006) Correlating the alpha rhythm to BOLD using simultaneous EEG/fMRI: inter-subject variability. Neuroimage 30:203–213.

Gonzalez SL, Grave de Peralta R, Thut G, Millan Jdel R, Morier P, Landis T (2006) Very high frequency oscillations (VHFO) as a predictor of movement intentions. Neuroimage 32:170–179.

Grave de Peralta Menendez R, Gonzalez Andino SL (1998) A critical analysis of linear inverse solutions. IEEE Trans Biomed Eng 45:440–448.

Grave de Peralta Menendez R, Gonzalez Andino S, Lantz G, Michel CM, Landis T (2001) Noninvasive localization of electromagnetic epileptic activity: I. Method descriptions and simulations. Brain Topogr 14:131–137.

Grieve PG, Emerson RG, Fifer WP, Isler JR, Stark RI (2003) Spatial correlation of the infant and adult electroencephalogram. Clin Neurophysiol 114:1594–1608.

Groening K, Brodbeck V, Moeller F, Wolff S, van Baalen A, Michel CM, Jansen O, Boor R, Wiegand G, Stephani U (2009) Combination of EEG-fMRI and EEG source analysis improves interpretation of spike-associated activation networks in paediatric pharmacoresistent focal epilepsies. Neuroimage 46:827–833.

Grossberg S (2000) The complementary brain: unifying brain dynamics and modularity. Trends Cogn Sci 4:233–246.

Hämäläinen MS, Ilmoniemi RJ (1984) Interpreting measured magnetic fields of the brain: Estimates of current distributions. Helsinki: Helsinki University of Technology, Finland, Technical Report TKK-F-A620.

Hämäläinen MS, Hari R, Ilmoniemi RJ, Knuutila JE, Lounasmaa OV (1993) Magnetoencephalography-theory, instrumentation, and applications to noninvasive studies of the working human brain. Rev Mod Phys 65:413–497.

Hanslmayr S, Aslan A, Staudigl T, Klimesch W, Herrmann CS, Bauml KH (2007) Prestimulus oscillations predict visual perception performance between and within subjects. Neuroimage 37:1465–1473.

Hari R, Salmelin R (1997) Human cortical oscillations: a neuromagnetic view through the skull. Trends Neurosci 20:44–49.

He B, Lian J (2002) High-resolution spatio-temporal functional neuroimaging of brain activity. Crit Rev Biomed Eng 30:283–306.

He B, Lian J (2005) Electrophysiological Neuroimaging: solving the EEG inverse problem. In: Neuroal engineering (He B, ed), pp. 221–261. Norwell, MA: Kluwer Academic Publishers.

Henze DA, Borhegyi Z, Csicsvari J, Mamiya A, Harris KD, Buzsaki G (2000) Intracellular features predicted by extracellular recordings in the hippocampus in vivo. J Neurophysiol 84:390–400.

Holmes MD, Brown M, Tucker DM (2004) Are "generalized" seizures truly generalized? Evidence of localized mesial frontal and frontopolar discharges in absence. Epilepsia 45:1568–1579.

IFSECN (1974) A glossary of terms most commonly used by clinical electroencephalographers. Electroencephalogr Clin Neurophysiol 37:538–548.

Ioannides AA, Fenwick PBC (2004) Imaging cerebellum activity in real time with magnetoencephalographic data. Prog Brain Res 148:139–150.

James CE, Britz J, Vuilleumier P, Hauert CA, Michel CM (2008) Plasticity in right limbic structures mediates harmony incongruity processing in musical experts. Neuroimage 42:1597–1608.

Jensen O, Gelfand J, Kounios J, Lisman JE (2002) Oscillations in the alpha band (9-12 Hz) increase with memory load during retention in a short-term memory task. Cereb Cortex 12:877–882.

Jokisch D, Jensen O (2007) Modulation of gamma and alpha activity during a working memory task engaging the dorsal or ventral stream. J Neurosci 27:3244–3251.

Kaufmann C, Wehrle R, Wetter TC, Holsboer F, Auer DP, Pollmacher T, Czisch M (2006) Brain activation and hypothalamic functional connectivity during human non-rapid eye movement sleep: an EEG/fMRI study. Brain 129:655–667.

Kelly SP, Lalor EC, Reilly RB, Foxe JJ (2006) Increases in alpha oscillatory power reflect an active retinotopic mechanism for distracter suppression during sustained visuo-spatial attention. J Neurophysiol 95:3844–3851.

Kinoshita T, Strik WK, Michel CM, Yagyu T, Saito M, Lehmann D (1995) Microstate segmentation of spontaneous multichannel

EEG map series under diazepam and sulpiride. Pharmaco-psychiatry 28:51–55.

Klimesch W (1999) EEG alpha and theta oscillations reflect cognitive and memory performance: a review and analysis. Brain Res Brain Res Rev 29:169–195.

Klimesch W, Schack B, Sauseng P (2005) The functional significance of theta and upper alpha oscillations. Exp Psychol 52:99–108.

Klimesch W, Sauseng P, Hanslmayr S (2007) EEG alpha oscillations: the inhibition-timing hypothesis. Brain Res Rev 53:63–88.

Kobayashi K, Akiyama T, Nakahori T, Yoshinaga H, Gotman J (2002) Systematic source estimation of spikes by a combination of independent component analysis and RAP-MUSIC. I. Principles and simulation study. Clin Neurophysiol 113:713–724.

Kobayashi K, Yoshinaga H, Ohtsuka Y, Gotman J (2005) Dipole modeling of epileptic spikes can be accurate or misleading. Epilepsia 46:397–408.

Koenig T, Lehmann D, Merlo MC, Kochi K, Hell D, Koukkou M (1999) A deviant EEG brain microstate in acute, neuroleptic-naive schizophrenics at rest. Eur Arch Psychiatry Clin Neurosci 249:205–211.

Koenig T, Marti-Lopez F, Valdes-Sosa P (2001) Topographic time-frequency decomposition of the EEG. Neuroimage 14:383–390.

Koenig T, Prichep L, Lehmann D, Sosa PV, Braeker E, Kleinlogel H, Isenhart R, John ER (2002) Millisecond by millisecond, year by year: normative EEG microstates and developmental stages. Neuroimage 16:41–48.

Koenig T, Studer D, Hubl D, Melie L, Strik WK (2005a) Brain connectivity at different time-scales measured with EEG. Philos T Roy Soc B 360:1015–1023.

Koenig T, Prichep L, Dierks T, Hubl D, Wahlund LO, John ER, Jelic V (2005b) Decreased EEG synchronization in Alzheimer's disease and mild cognitive impairment. Neurobiol Aging 26:165–171.

Koles ZJ, Soong AC (1998) EEG source localization: implementing the spatio-temporal decomposition approach. Electroencephalogr Clin Neurophysiol 107:343–352.

Korvenoja A, Huttunen J, Salli E, Pohjonen H, Martinkauppi S, Palva JM, Lauronen L, Virtanen J, Ilmoniemi RJ, Aronen HJ (1999) Activation of multiple cortical areas in response to somatosensory stimulation: combined magnetoencephalographic and functional magnetic resonance imaging. Hum Brain Mapp 8:13–27.

Lai Y, van Drongelen W, Ding L, Hecox KE, Towle VL, Frim DM, He B (2005) Estimation of in vivo human brain-to-skull conductivity ratio from simultaneous extra- and intra-cranial electrical potential recordings. Clin Neurophysiol 116:456–465.

Lakatos P, Shah AS, Knuth KH, Ulbert I, Karmos G, Schroeder CE (2005) An oscillatory hierarchy controlling neuronal excitability and stimulus processing in the auditory cortex. J Neurophysiol 94:1904–1911.

Lantz G, Holub M, Ryding E, Rosen I (1996) Simultaneous intracranial and extracranial recording of interictal epileptiform activity in patients with drug resistant partial epilepsy: patterns of conduction and results from dipole reconstructions. Electroencephalogr Clin Neurophysiol 99:69–78.

Lantz G, Grave de Peralta R, Gonzalez S, Michel CM (2001a) Noninvasive localization of electromagnetic epileptic activity. II. Demonstration of sublobar accuracy in patients with simultaneous surface and depth recordings. Brain Topogr 14:139–147.

Lantz G, Michel CM, Seeck M, Blanke O, Spinelli L, Thut G, Landis T, Rosen I (2001b) Space-oriented segmentation and 3-dimensional source reconstruction of ictal EEG patterns. Clin Neurophysiol 112:688–697.

Lantz G, Grave de Peralta R, Spinelli L, Seeck M, Michel CM (2003a) Epileptic source localization with high density EEG: how many electrodes are needed? Clin Neurophysiol 114:63–69.

Lantz G, Spinelli L, Seeck M, Grave de Peralta Menendez R, Sottas C, Michel C (2003b) Propagation of interictal epileptiform activity can lead to erroneous source localizations: A 128 channel EEG mapping study. J Clin Neurophysiol 20:311–319.

Laufs H, Kleinschmidt A, Beyerle A, Eger E, Salek-Haddadi A, Preibisch C, Krakow K (2003a) EEG-correlated fMRI of human alpha activity. Neuroimage 19:1463–1476.

Laufs H, Krakow K, Sterzer P, Eger E, Beyerle A, Salek-Haddadi A, Kleinschmidt A (2003b) Electroencephalographic signatures of attentional and cognitive default modes in spontaneous brain activity fluctuations at rest. Proc Natl Acad Sci U S A 100:11053–11058.

Laufs H, Holt JL, Elfont R, Krams M, Paul JS, Krakow K, Kleinschmidt A (2006) Where the BOLD signal goes when alpha EEG leaves. Neuroimage 31:1408–1418.

Lehmann D (1971) Multichannel topography of human alpha EEG fields. Electroencephalogr Clin Neurophysiol 31:439–449.

Lehmann D (1992) Brain electric fields and brain functional states. In: Evolution of dynamical structures in complex systems (Friedrich R, Wunderlin A, eds), pp 235–248. Berlin: Springer.

Lehmann D, Ozaki H, Pal I (1987) EEG alpha map series: brain micro-states by space-oriented adaptive segmentation. Electroencephalogr Clin Neurophysiol 67:271–288.

Lehmann D, Wackermann J, Michel CM, Koenig T (1993) Space-oriented EEG segmentation reveals changes in brain electric field maps under the influence of a nootropic drug. Psychiatry Res 50:275–282.

Lehmann D, Strik WK, Henggeler B, Koenig T, Koukkou M (1998) Brain electric microstates and momentary conscious mind states as building blocks of spontaneous thinking: I. Visual imagery and abstract thoughts. Int J Psychophysiol 29:1–11.

Lehmann D, Faber PL, Galderisi S, Herrmann WM, Kinoshita T, Koukkou M, Mucci A, Pascual-Marqui RD, Saito N, Wackermann J, Winterer G, Koenig T (2005) EEG microstate duration and syntax in acute, medication-naive, first-episode schizophrenia: a multi-center study. Psychiatry Res 138:141–156.

Lehmann D, Pascual-Marqui R, Michel CM (2009) EEG microstates. Scholarpedia 4:7632. (http://www.scholarpedia.org/article/EEG_microstates).

Leresche N, Jassik-Gerschenfeld D, Haby M, Soltesz I, Crunelli V (1990) Pacemaker-like and other types of spontaneous membrane potential oscillations of thalamocortical cells. Neurosci Lett 113:72–77.

Logothetis NK, Pauls J, Augath M, Trinath T, Oeltermann A (2001) Neurophysiological investigation of the basis of the fMRI signal. Nature 412:150–157.

Lopes da Silva F (1991) Neural mechanisms underlying brain waves: from neural membranes to networks. Electroencephalogr Clin Neurophysiol 79:81–93.

Lopes da Silva FH, Vos JE, Mooibroek J, Van Rotterdam A (1980) Relative contributions of intracortical and thalamo-cortical processes in the generation of alpha rhythms, revealed by partial coherence analysis. Electroencephalogr Clin Neurophysiol 50:449–456.

Martin T, Houck JM, Pearson Bish J, Dubravko K, Woodruff CC, Moses SN, Lee DC, Tesche CD (2006) MEG reveals different contributions of somatomotor cortex and cerebellum to simple reaction time after temporally structured cues. Hum Brain Mapp 27:552–561.

Martuzzi R, Murray MM, Meuli RA, Thiran JP, Maeder PP, Michel CM, Grave de Peralta Menendez R, Gonzalez Andino S (2008) Methods for determining frequency- and region- dependant relationships between estimated LFPs and BOLD responses in humans. J Neurophysiol 12:12.

Massimini M, Rosanova M, Mariotti M (2003) EEG slow (approximately 1 Hz) waves are associated with nonstationarity of thalamo-cortical sensory processing in the sleeping human. J Neurophysiol 89:1205–1213.

McCormick DA, Pape HC (1990) Noradrenergic and serotonergic modulation of a hyperpolarization-activated cation current in thalamic relay neurones. J Physiol 431:319–342.

Megevand P, Quairiaux C, Lascano AM, Kiss JZ, Michel CM (2008) A mouse model for studying large-scale neuronal networks using EEG mapping techniques. Neuroimage 42:591–602.

Meltzer JA, Negishi M, Mayes LC, Constable RT (2007) Individual differences in EEG theta and alpha dynamics during working memory correlate with fMRI responses across subjects. Clin Neurophysiol 118:2419–2436.

Meltzer JA, Zaveri HP, Goncharova II, Distasio MM, Papademetris X, Spencer SS, Spencer DD, Constable RT (2008) Effects of working memory load on oscillatory power in human intracranial EEG. Cereb Cortex 18:1843–1855.

Menon V, Ford JM, Lim KO, Glover GH, Pfefferbaum A (1997) Combined event-related fMRI and EEG evidence for temporal-parietal cortex activation during target detection. Neuroreport 8:3029–3037.

Michel CM, Grave de Peralta R, Lantz G, Gonzalez Andino S, Spinelli L, Blanke O, Landis T, Seeck M (1999) Spatio-temporal EEG analysis and distributed source estimation in presurgical epilepsy evaluation. J Clin Neurophysiol 16:225–238.

Michel CM, Thut G, Morand S, Khateb A, Pegna AJ, Grave de Peralta R, Gonzalez S, Seeck M, Landis T (2001) Electric source imaging of human brain functions. Brain Res Brain Res Rev 36:108–118.

Michel CM, Lantz G, Spinelli L, De Peralta RG, Landis T, Seeck M (2004a) 128-channel EEG source imaging in epilepsy: clinical yield and localization precision. J Clin Neurophysiol 21:71–83.

Michel CM, Murray MM, Lantz G, Gonzalez S, Spinelli L, Grave de Peralta R (2004b) EEG source imaging. Clin Neurophysiol 115:2195–2222.

Michel CM, Brandeis D, Koenig T (2009) Electrical neuroimaging in the time domain. In: Electrical neuroimaging (Michel CM, Koenig T, Brandeis D, Gianotti LRR, Wackermann J, eds), pp. 111-143. Cambridge: Cambridge University Press.

Michels L, Moazami-Goudarzi M, Jeanmonod D, Sarnthein J (2008) EEG alpha distinguishes between cuneal and precuneal activation in working memory. Neuroimage 40:1296–1310.

Mitchell DJ, McNaughton N, Flanagan D, Kirk IJ (2008) Frontal-midline theta from the perspective of hippocampal "theta." Prog Neurobiol 86:156–185.

Mitzdorf U (1985) Current source-density method and application in cat cerebral cortex: investigation of evoked potentials and EEG phenomena. Physiol Rev 65:37–100.

Molle M, Marshall L, Gais S, Born J (2002) Grouping of spindle activity during slow oscillations in human non-rapid eye movement sleep. J Neurosci 22:10941–10947.

Mosher JC, Leahy RM (1998) Recursive MUSIC: a framework for EEG and MEG source localization. IEEE Trans Biomed Eng 45:1342–1354.

Murakami S, Okada Y (2006) Contributions of principal neocortical neurons to magnetoencephalography and electroencephalography signals. J Physiol-London 575:925–936.

Murphy M, Riedner BA, Huber R, Massimini M, Ferrarelli F, Tononi G (2009) Source modeling sleep slow waves. Proc Natl Acad Sci U S A 106:1608–1613.

Murray MM, Wylie GR, Higgins BA, Javitt DC, Schroeder CE, Foxe JJ (2002) The spatiotemporal dynamics of illusory contour processing: combined high-density electrical mapping, source analysis, and functional magnetic resonance imaging. J Neurosci 22:5055–5073.

Murray MM, Camen C, Gonzalez Andino SL, Bovet P, Clarke S (2006) Rapid brain discrimination of sounds of objects. J Neurosci 26:1293–1302.

Murray MM, Camen C, Spierer L, Clarke S (2008) Plasticity in representations of environmental sounds revealed by electrical neuroimaging. Neuroimage 39:847–856.

Napflin M, Wildi M, Sarnthein J (2007) Test-retest reliability of resting EEG spectra validates a statistical signature of persons. Clin Neurophysiol 118:2519–2524.

Nayak D, Valentin A, Alarcon G, Garcia Seoane JJ, Brunnhuber F, Juler J, Polkey CE, Binnie CD (2004) Characteristics of scalp electrical fields associated with deep medial temporal epileptiform discharges. Clin Neurophysiol 115:1423–1435.

Nita DA, Steriade M, Amzica F (2003) Hyperpolarisation rectification in cat lateral geniculate neurons modulated by intact corticothalamic projections. J Physiol 552:325–332.

Onton J, Delorme A, Makeig S (2005) Frontal midline EEG dynamics during working memory. Neuroimage 27:341–356.

Pascual-Marqui RD (1999) Review of methods for solving the EEG inverse problem. International Journal of Bioelectromagnetism 1:75–86.

Pascual-Marqui RD, Michel CM, Lehmann D (1994) Low resolution electromagnetic tomography: a new method for localizing electrical activity in the brain. Int J Psychophysiol 18:49–65.

Pascual-Marqui RD, Michel CM, Lehmann D (1995) Segmentation of brain electrical activity into microstates: model estimation and validation. IEEE Trans Biomed Eng 42:658–665.

Perez-Borja C, Chatrian GE, Tyce FA, Rivers MH (1962) Electrographic patterns of the occipital lobe in man: a topographic study based on use of implanted electrodes. Electroencephalogr Clin Neurophysiol 14:171–182.

Pfurtscheller G (1992) Event-related synchronization (ERS): an electrophysiological correlate of cortical areas at rest. Electroencephalogr Clin Neurophysiol 83:62–69.

Pfurtscheller G, Andrew C (1999) Event-Related changes of band power and coherence: methodology and interpretation. J Clin Neurophysiol 16:512–519.

Pfurtscheller G, Lopes da Silva FH (1999) Event-related EEG/MEG synchronization and desynchronization: basic principles. Clin Neurophysiol 110:1842–1857.

Pfurtscheller G, Neuper C, Flotzinger D, Pregenzer M (1997) EEG-based discrimination between imagination of right and left hand movement. Electroencephalogr Clin Neurophysiol 103:642–651.

Raichle ME, Snyder AZ (2007) A default mode of brain function: a brief history of an evolving idea. Neuroimage 37:1083–1090; discussion 1097–1099.

Raichle ME, MacLeod AM, Snyder AZ, Powers WJ, Gusnard DA, Shulman GL (2001) A default mode of brain function. Proc Natl Acad Sci U S A 98:676–682.

Rihs TA, Michel CM, Thut G (2007) Mechanisms of selective inhibition in visual spatial attention are indexed by alpha-band EEG synchronization. Eur J Neurosci 25:603–610.

Rihs TA, Michel CM, Thut G (2009) A bias for posterior alpha-band power suppression versus enhancement during shifting versus maintenance of spatial attention. Neuroimage 44:190–199.

Romei V, Brodbeck V, Michel C, Amedi A, Pascual-Leone A, Thut G (2007) Spontaneous fluctuations in posterior {alpha}-Band EEG activity reflect variability in excitability of human visual areas. Cereb Cortex 18: 2010–2018. Sammer G, Blecker C, Gebhardt H, Bischoff M, Stark R, Morgen K, Vaitl D (2007) Relationship between regional hemodynamic activity and simultaneously recorded EEG-theta associated with mental arithmetic-induced workload. Hum Brain Mapp 28:793–803.

Sanchez-Vives MV, McCormick DA (2000) Cellular and network mechanisms of rhythmic recurrent activity in neocortex. Nat Neurosci 3:1027–1034.

Sauseng P, Klimesch W, Gruber W, Doppelmayr M, Stadler W, Schabus M (2002) The interplay between theta and alpha oscillations in the human electroencephalogram reflects the transfer of information between memory systems. Neurosci Lett 324:121–124.

Sauseng P, Klimesch W, Doppelmayr M, Pecherstorfer T, Freunberger R, Hanslmayr S (2005) EEG alpha synchronization and functional coupling during top-down processing in a working memory task. Hum Brain Mapp:148–155.

Scheeringa R, Bastiaansen MC, Petersson KM, Oostenveld R, Norris DG, Hagoort P (2008a) Frontal theta EEG activity correlates negatively with the default mode network in resting state. Int J Psychophysiol 67:242–251.

Scheeringa R, Petersson KM, Oostenveld R, Norris DG, Hagoort P, Bastiaansen MC (2008b) Trial-by-trial coupling between EEG and BOLD identifies networks related to alpha and theta EEG power increases during working memory maintenance. Neuroimage 44:1224–1238.

Scherg M, Vajsar J, Picton TW (1989) A source analysis of the late human auditory evoked potential. J Cognitive Neurosci 1:336–355.

Schevon CA, Cappell J, Emerson R, Isler J, Grieve P, Goodman R, McKhann G, Jr., Weiner H, Doyle W (2007) Cortical abnormalities in epilepsy revealed by local EEG synchrony. NeuroImage 35:140–148.

Schroeder C, Mehta A, Givre S (1998) A spatiotemporal profile of visual system activation revealed by current source density analysis in the awake macaque. Cereb Cortex 8:575–592.

Schulz E, Maurer U, van der Mark S, Bucher K, Brem S, Martin E, Brandeis D (2008) Impaired semantic processing during sentence reading in children with dyslexia: Combined fMRI and ERP evidence. Neuroimage 41:153–168.

Shah AS, Bressler SL, Knuth KH, Ding M, Mehta AD, Ulbert I, Schroeder CE (2004) Neural dynamics and the fundamental mechanisms of event-related brain potentials. Cereb Cortex 14:476–483.

Simon NR, Manshanden I, Lopes da Silva FH (2000) A MEG study of sleep. Brain Res 860:64–76.

Singer W (1999) Neuronal synchrony: a versatile code for the definition of relations? Neuron 24:49–65, 111–125.

Smith DB, Sidman RD, Henke JS, Flanigan H, Labiner D, Evans CN (1983) Scalp and depth recordings of induced deep cerebral potentials. Electroencephalogr Clin Neurophysiol 55:145–150.

Sperli F, Spinelli L, Seeck M, Kurian M, Michel CM, Lantz G (2006) EEG source imaging in paediatric epilepsy surgery: a new perspective in presurgical workup. Epilepsia 47:981–990.

Stein M, Dierks T, Brandeis D, Wirth M, Strik W, Koenig T (2006) Plasticity in the adult language system: a longitudinal electrophysiological study on second language learning. Neuroimage 33:774–783.

Steinschneider M, Tenke CE, Schroeder CE, Javitt DC, Simpson GV, Arezzo JC, Vaughan HG, Jr. (1992) Cellular generators of the cortical auditory evoked potential initial component. Electroencephalogr Clin Neurophysiol 84:196–200.

Steriade M (2001) Impact of network activities on neuronal properties in corticothalamic systems. J Neurophysiol 86:1–39.

Steriade M, Amzica F (1996) Intracortical and corticothalamic coherency of fast spontaneous oscillations. Proc Natl Acad Sci U S A 93:2533–2538.

Steriade M, Amzica F, Contreras D (1996) Synchronization of fast (30–40 Hz) spontaneous cortical rhythms during brain activation. J Neurosci 16:392–417.

Strik WK, Lehmann D (1993) Data determined window size and space-oriented segmentation of spontaneous EEG map series. Electroencephalogr Clin Neurophysiol 87:169–174.

Strik WK, Dierks T, Becker T, Lehmann D (1995) Larger topographical variance and decreased duration of brain electric microstates in depression. J Neural Transm 99:213–222.

Strik WK, Chiaramonti R, Muscas GC, Paganini M, Mueller TJ, Fallgatter AJ, Versari A, Zappoli R (1997) Decreased EEG microstate duration and anteriorisation of the brain electrical fields in mild and moderate dementia of the Alzheimer type. Psychiat Res 75:183–191.

Suffczynski P, Kalitzin S, Pfurtscheller G, Lopes da Silva FH (2001) Computational model of thalamo-cortical networks: dynamical control of alpha rhythms in relation to focal attention. Int J Psychophysiol 43:25–40.

Tao JX, Ray A, Hawes-Ebersole S, Ebersole JS (2005) Intracranial EEG substrates of scalp EEG interictal spikes. Epilepsia 46:669–676.

Tenke CE, Schroeder CE, Arezzo JC, Vaughan HG, Jr. (1993) Interpretation of high-resolution current source density profiles: a simulation of sublaminar contributions to the visual evoked potential. Exp Brain Res 94:183–192.

Thut G, Nietzel A, Brandt SA, Pascual-Leone A (2006) Alpha-band electroencephalographic activity over occipital cortex indexes visuospatial attention bias and predicts visual target detection. J Neurosci 26:9494–9502.

Timmermann L, Gross J, Dirks M, Volkmann J, Freund H-J, Schnitzler A (2002) The cerebral oscillatory network of parkinsonian resting tremor. Brain 126:199–212.

Timofeev I, Contreras D, Steriade M (1996) Synaptic responsiveness of cortical and thalamic neurones during various phases of slow sleep oscillation in cat. J Physiol 494 (Pt 1):265–278.

Tyvaert L, Levan P, Grova C, Dubeau F, Gotman J (2008) Effects of fluctuating physiological rhythms during prolonged EEG-fMRI studies. Clin Neurophysiol 119:2762–2774.

Ulbert I, Heit G, Madsen J, Karmos G, Halgren E (2004) Laminar analysis of human neocortical interictal spike generation and propagation: current source density and multiunit analysis in vivo. Epilepsia 45 (Suppl 4):48–56.

Vitacco D, Brandeis D, Pascual-Marqui RD, Martin E (2002) Correspondence of event-related potential tomography and functional magnetic resonance imaging during language processing. Hum Brain Mapp 17:4–12.

von der Malsburg C, Schneider W (1986) A neural cocktail-party processor. Biol Cybern 54:29–40.

Vulliemoz S, Thornton R, Rodionov R, Carmichael DW, Guye M, Lhatoo SA, McEvoy AW, Spinelli L, Michel CM, Duncan JS, Lemieux L (2009) The spatio-temporal mapping of epileptic networks: combination of EEG-fMRI and EEG source imaging. Neuroimage 46:834–843.Wackerman J, Lehmann D, Michel CM, Strik WK (1993) Adaptive segmentation of spontaneous EEG map series into spatially defined microstates. Int J Psychophysiol 14:269–283.

Whitham EM, Lewis T, Pope KJ, Fitzgibbon SP, Clark CR, Loveless S, DeLosAngeles D, Wallace AK, Broberg M, Willoughby JO (2008) Thinking activates EMG in scalp electrical recordings. Clin Neurophysiol 119:1166–1175.

Worden MS, Foxe JJ, Wang N, Simpson GV (2000) Anticipatory biasing of visuospatial attention indexed by retinotopically specific alpha-band electroencephalography increases over occipital cortex. J Neurosci 20:RC63.

Yamagishi N, Goda N, Callan DE, Anderson SJ, Kawato M (2005) Attentional shifts towards an expected visual target alter the level of alpha-band oscillatory activity in the human calcarine cortex. Brain Res Cogn Brain Res. 25:799–809.

Yuval-Greenberg S, Tomer O, Keren AS, Nelken I, Deouell LY (2008) Transient induced gamma-band response in EEG as a manifestation of miniature saccades. Neuron 58:429–441.

Zhang Y, Ding L, van Drongelen W, Hecox K, Frim DM, He B (2006) A cortical potential imaging study from simultaneous extra- and intracranial electrical recordings by means of the finite element method. NeuroImage 31:1513–1524.

Zumsteg D, Friedman A, Wennberg RA, Wieser HG (2005) Source localization of mesial temporal interictal epileptiform discharges: correlation with intracranial foramen ovale electrode recordings. Clin Neurophysiol 116:2810–2818.

Zumsteg D, Friedman A, Wieser HG, Wennberg RA (2006) Source localization of interictal epileptiform discharges: comparison of three different techniques to improve signal to noise ratio. Clin Neurophysiol 117:562–571

Physiological Basis of the BOLD Signal

Introduction

fMRI and other non-invasive imaging methods have greatly expanded our knowledge of human brain function. Although MRI was invented in the early 1970s (Lauterbur, 1973) and has been used clinically since the mid–1980s, its use in cognitive neuroscience expanded greatly with the advent of blood oxygenation level dependent (BOLD) functional imaging, and by now fMRI is a mainstay of neuroscience research. The BOLD contrast is based on an increase in blood oxygenation and flow to activated regions. In the late 1800s Mosso first observed that neural activation increases blood flow to the activated brain region (see Iadecola, 2004, Zago et al., 2009, or Raichle, 2000, for review). Ogawa et al. (1990) and Belliveau et al. (1990) first used MRI to measure such changes in cerebral flow and oxygenation in rats. Belliveau et al. (1990) used an exogenous contrast agent to measure changes in blood volume, but Ogawa et al. (1990) showed that deoxyhemoglobin acts as an endogenous contrast agent. By manipulating O_2 and CO_2 levels, they showed that excess deoxygenated blood leads to signal loss near vessels, which could be reversed by increasing the flow of freshly oxygenated blood. Soon thereafter it was shown in humans that changes in normal brain function lead to changes in blood oxygenation and flow that can be measured with MRI (Belliveau et al., 1991; Kwong et al., 1992; Ogawa et al., 1992). The origin of the functional BOLD contrast is actually an oversupply of freshly oxygenated blood that leads to a signal increase in the activated areas. Compared to other functional imaging methods, fMRI offers much higher spatial resolution and it is entirely non-invasive, which has allowed us to improve the mapping of the functional parcellation in human brain.

fMRI activation is usually without much question interpreted as a marker of neural function. But as the fMRI signal is a hemodynamic signal, it is only an indirect marker, and our ability to interpret fMRI in terms of neural function depends on how well the fMRI signal reflects the neural activation. For example, it is not known if the different neural processes are all represented equally in the fMRI signal, or whether some are overrepresented or underrepresented. This is still relatively unknown territory that many different groups are currently trying to address with multidisciplinary approaches.

There has been over 50 years of neurophysiological work in nonhuman primates and other animals, often painstakingly mapping the functional properties of isolated neurons. And although this has offered a wealth of knowledge about brain function, for obvious reasons a direct extrapolation to human brain function is difficult. In recent years there has been an increasing amount of work aimed at elucidating how the neural signals that are measured invasively with intracortical microelectrodes in animals relate to the non-invasive measures of brain function that can be researched in humans, like fMRI, electroencephalography (EEG) and magnetoencephalography (MEG). The goal would be to arrive at measures for non-invasively interpreting neural functioning at high resolution in humans. Clearly, fMRI is an excellent candidate for such an endeavor, but because fMRI measures blood-flow, it can only be used as a surrogate measure of neural activation. To allow us to better relate the body of fMRI work in humans to the bulk of neurophysiological work done in animals, it is necessary to determine how fMRI signals relate to neural activity. This can be done by combining invasive methods with fMRI in monkeys or other animals, either simultaneously (Goense and Logothetis, 2008; Logothetis et al., 2001) or consecutively (Maandag et al., 2007; Disbrow et al., 2000; Lipton et al., 2006; Tsao et al., 2006; Smith et al., 2002; Lu et al., 2007). Neurophysiological recording in humans also offers opportunities to study directly the relationship between neural signals and fMRI (Privman et al., 2007; Mukamel et al., 2005). However, most invasive neurophysiology in humans is limited to specialized areas and cases, such as seizure-prone areas like the temporal lobe, and is usually conducted in a surgical or presurgical context (Engel et al., 2005; Privman et al., 2007; Mukamel et al., 2005). Another approach to a better understanding and interpretation of the human fMRI studies is to perform comparative fMRI in humans and monkeys, which allows us to look at homology questions and provides a better basis for extrapolating animal work to human work (Nakahara et al., 2002; Koyama et al., 2004; VanDuffel et al., 2002; Tsao et al., 2003; Sawamura et al., 2005; Rajimehr et al., 2009; Tsao et al., 2008; Denys et al., 2004).

As both electrophysiological and imaging methods have their strengths and limitations and measure only particular aspects of brain function, the integrative approach allows us to obtain a more complete picture. This is expected to improve our interpretation of both methods. The most obvious limitation of intracortical microelectrodes is its highly restricted spatial sampling; for EEG it is the limited spatial resolution of its reconstructed sources (which is an ill-posed inverse problem; cf. Chapters 1.1 and 3.8) and for fMRI its limited temporal resolution, which also stems from the fact that it is a hemodynamic signal and does not measure the neural events themselves.

The goal of this chapter is to give an overview of the relation between the BOLD signal and the underlying neural signals. Our focus is mainly on intracortically recorded neural signals, recorded with microelectrodes. Neural signals that are recorded are spikes, or single- and multi-unit activity (SUA and MUA) and local field potentials (LFP). The increases in local neural activity upon stimulus presentation, and the concomitant increased energy demands of neurotransmission and spiking, lead to an increase in blood flow to the activated area, which ultimately drives the BOLD response. Logothetis et al. (2001) showed that the BOLD signal is not as well correlated to single-unit activity, but correlates better with the LFP, a mesoscopic signal that includes membrane potential fluctuations, oscillations, and postsynaptic and presynaptic events. This raises questions about whether all aspects of neural activity drive the BOLD response equally, and if not, which ones are more important—for instance, the input versus the output from an area, or inhibition versus excitation, or stimulus-driven or neuromodulatory activity. Answers to such questions will directly affect our interpretation of fMRI results and help us to better understand results obtained with fMRI. We will discuss which neural events are thought to drive the hemodynamic response, but to get some insight in the coupling between neural activity and BOLD, we will also discuss neurovascular coupling and the specificity of the BOLD response, as these issues have direct bearing on our understanding of the coupling between BOLD and neurophysiological signals.

BOLD Contrast Mechanism

Ogawa et al. (1990) first discovered the BOLD contrast in rats, when they observed that the intensity of the vascular signal in gradient-echo (GE) images decreased when blood was deoxygenated, and increased when the flow of freshly oxygenated blood increased. Soon after, it was shown that that the BOLD contrast could be used to detect functional activation in humans (Kwong et al., 1992; Ogawa et al., 1992). When neural activity in a given brain area increases, via stimulation or task performance, this triggers an increase in the flow of fresh blood to the activated area in order to meet the increased metabolic demands. The BOLD contrast is based on the concentration of deoxyhemoglobin in the blood, since deoxyhemoglobin is paramagnetic and acts as a contrast agent: an increase in its concentration decreases the relaxation time (T_2^*). The increase in oxygen supply to the active tissue is more than the oxygen that is used by the neurons, and hence there is a relative increase in the oxyhemoglobin concentration, and a decrease in the deoxyhemoglobin concentration. This increases T_2^* and leads to a signal increase in the GE images (Kwong et al., 1992; Ogawa et al., 1992). Belliveau et al. (1990; 1991) showed functional MRI based on similar principles but using an exogenous contrast agent that is sensitive to changes in blood volume.

Although the first fMRI experiments were performed in early 1990s, what exactly the BOLD signal represents is still unclear. Questions remain not only about which neural or metabolic changes exactly trigger the BOLD signal, but also about the relative contributions of flow increases versus oxygen extraction, or which parts of the vascular tree contribute most to the BOLD signal. And given these uncertainties, the BOLD signal is not (yet) suitable as a quantitative metric for brain function.

Properties of the BOLD Signal

The presence of paramagnetic deoxyhemoglobin (dHb) in the blood leads to susceptibility gradients, which are local variations in the magnetic field. These gradients exist near vessels because of their high dHb content, and their size depends on the vessel size and dHb concentration among other things. Spins within these gradients experience dephasing, which leads to T_2^*-based signal loss. Based on theory and simulations (Boxerman et al., 1995; Kennan et al., 1994; Weisskoff et al., 1994) it has been determined that with the typically used GE-based sequences, one observes BOLD signal arising from different vessel sizes ranging from capillaries to large veins. Large draining veins can have very strong BOLD signals, but they are downstream from the neural activation and can be quite remote from the activated area. However, the relative contribution of large and small vessels to the BOLD signal is still debated. One of the reasons why there is still debate about this is that the properties of the BOLD signal depend strongly on MR-hardware (most obviously field strength) and acquisition parameters (Duong et al., 2003; Goense and Logothetis, 2006; Jin et al., 2006; Yacoub et al., 2001), which complicates the comparison of results across labs or studies. For example, it is well established that at low magnetic field (e.g., 1.5T) the BOLD signal is very sensitive to large vessels. This sensitivity progressively decreases at higher field (Yacoub et al., 2001). But although the vessel-fraction is decreased at high field, high-resolution studies show that also at high field there can still be a substantial large vessel contribution (Harel et al., 2006; Jin et al., 2006; Zhao et al., 2004). Because large-vessel BOLD signals decrease the accuracy with which functional activity can be localized, it is important to decrease the sensitivity to large-vessel signal as much as possible.

Figure 1.2.1 shows the BOLD signal elicited by visual stimulation in monkey visual cortex acquired at 7T. Functional activation is seen in the entire early visual cortex (V1–V5) and at

this resolution it can easily be seen that the BOLD signal occurs at both the cortical surface and in gray matter, with the strongest BOLD signals at the cortical surface and in the calcarine sulcus. This is the large-vessel contribution, which can be more easily distinguished at high resolution. Note that often statistical maps (instead of percentage change maps) are used to display activation, and they depict correlation with the stimulus. These do not necessarily show the highest p-values at the surface, because although vessels typically have larger signals they also tend to have higher noise (Goense and Logothetis, 2006). The sensitivity to large vessels has the drawback that an area of activation

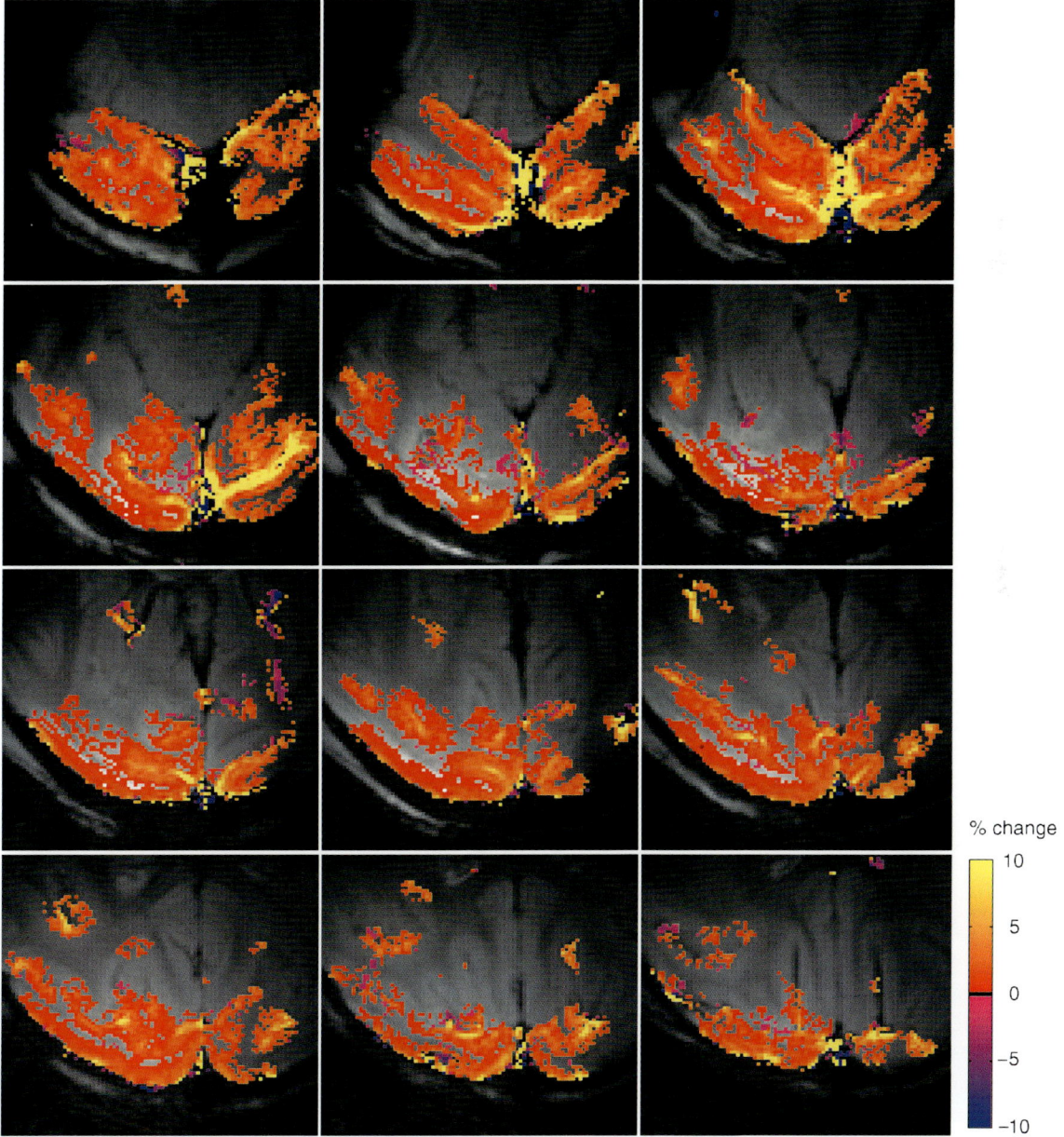

% change
10
5
0
−5
−10

Figure 1.2.1. Functional activation acquired in visual cortex of an anesthetized monkey at 7T at a spatial resolution of 500x500x 2000 μm^3. The map shows the percent signal change in response to a full-field (30°) black-and-white rotating checkerboard presented to both eyes. Functional activation is seen in visual areas V1-V5. The scanner and anesthesia procedures have been described previously (Logothetis et al., 1999; Pfeuffer et al., 2004), volume transmit coil, 30 mm receive coil, 8-segment GE-EPI, TE 20 ms, TR 750 ms.

identified in a functional map could in fact be a vessel remote from the area of neural activity. Also, when a blood vessel in a sulcus shows activation, at low resolution it could lead to ambiguity about the exact location of the activated tissue.

Many details of the BOLD signal are still poorly understood, in particular the relative contributions of venous, arterial, and capillary fractions to the BOLD signal, and the relative contributions of blood flow increases and oxygen consumption (Haacke et al., 2001; Buxton et al., 2004; Uludag et al., 2009). This is the case for the positive BOLD response, for the initial dip (the existence of which is still debated), the poststimulus undershoot, as well as for fMRI signals recorded with different methods (Zhao et al., 2007; Yacoub et al., 2006; Ugurbil et al., 2006; Kim et al., 2007). A discussion of the different fMRI methods and their properties is beyond the scope of this chapter. Here we note only that the general consensus is that GE-BOLD represents mostly a venous signal, which becomes more strongly weighted toward smaller venules and capillaries as the field strength increases, spin-echo (SE) BOLD represents mostly a capillary signal, the cerebral blood volume (CBV) signal is thought to represent smaller vessels (arteries and veins) and capillaries, and the cerebral blood flow (CBF) signal is thought to represent mostly arterioles and capillaries.

Spatial Resolution and Specificity of fMRI

How well the functional activation is localized to the actual place of neural activation depends on the achievable fMRI resolution and the specificity of the hemodynamic signal.

The achievable spatial resolution is determined by scanner hardware and the signal-to-noise ratio (SNR). The specificity is determined by the fMRI method that is used and how closely the hemodynamic response reflects the actual neural activity. BOLD signal originating from large vessels may be remote from the site of activation, but BOLD signal from capillaries can reasonably be assumed to be closely related to the neural activity in that area. Hence, the specificity is not only determined by biological factors, but also by the choice of fMRI method, hardware, and sequence parameters (Harel et al., 2006b; Ugurbil et al., 2003).

With advanced scanner hardware the spatial resolution achievable for structural imaging in vivo is of the order of 200–300 μm in-plane for whole-head imaging in humans (Wald et al., 2006; Ugurbil et al., 2006) and ~100 μm for localized imaging (Nakada et al., 2005). In animals, resolutions of 70–100 μm have been achieved in macaques (Logothetis et al., 2002) (Figure 1.2.2), a few tens of μm in rodents, and even higher resolutions in vitro (Ciobanu and Pennington, 2004; Fu et al., 2005). In principle fMRI can also be done at such resolutions, although it is constrained by the relatively low contrast-to-noise ratio (CNR) of the functional activation and the limited amount of time available for the acquisition of each image. Because of its speed, echo-planar imaging (EPI) (Mansfield, 1977) is typically used for fMRI (it can collect one image per excitation or repetition time TR). However, EPI requires high-performance hardware, and the limitations of the gradients often restrict the maximally achievable resolution. Despite this, by using segmented EPI

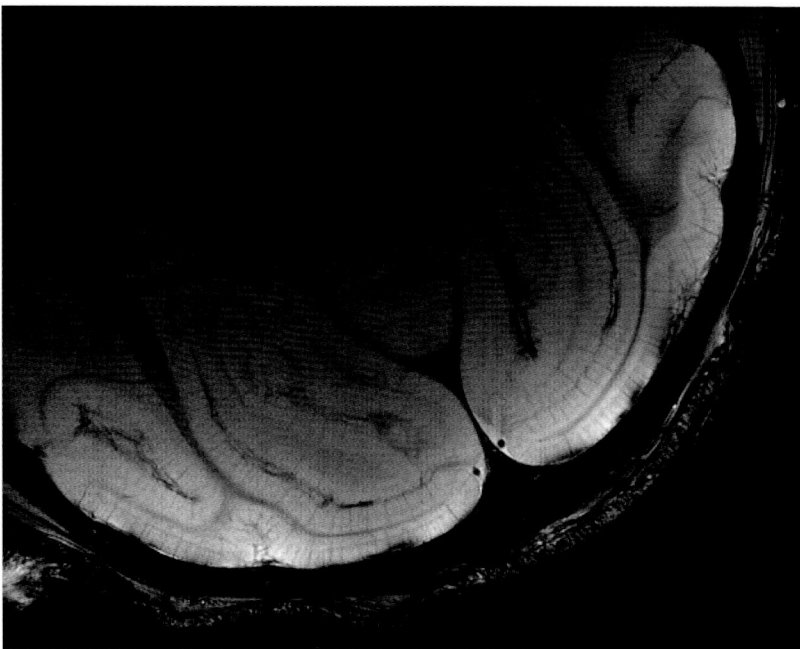

Figure 1.2.2. Anatomical image of macaque V1. The high-resolution GE image at a resolution of 100x100x1000 μm^3 and volume of 0.01 μl shows the small perpendicular intracortical veins and layer IV, which is indicated by the Gennari line. The Gennari line has a higher myelin content than the rest of the cortex. Technical data: vertical 4.7T scanner, described in Logothetis et al. (1999), volume transmit coil with 4-channel receive array, matrix 768x512x22, TE 23.5 ms, TR 2000 ms.

or parallel imaging, high resolution fMRI can be done, and in monkeys functional maps at 125 μm in-plane resolution have been shown (Logothetis et al., 2002), while in rats, maps with 50–100 μm have been demonstrated (Silva and Koretsky, 2002; Xu et al., 2003). In human fMRI studies, typical resolution is ~3x3x3 mm^3, and currently the highest resolution achieved is about 500 μm in-plane (Pfeuffer et al., 2002; Yacoub et al., 2005). The magnitude of the functional activation in gray-matter is only a few percent, and although image SNR decreases for smaller voxels, the functional signal tends to actually increase as the voxel size decreases, due to a decrease in partial volume effects. At a few hundred μm or less, the fMRI resolution can be higher than the point spread function (PSF) of the activation. Hence, the theoretically achievable spatial resolution is probably limited by the spatial extent of the neural signals and the hemodynamic regulation.

At high resolution specificity is important to be able to visualize structures like patches, columns, or layers. But also at low resolution increasing the specificity of the functional signal is important to eliminate the effect of draining veins and thus to increase the accuracy of the mapping. Specificity depends on *(1)* the anatomy of the capillary bed, *(2)* which fMRI method is used, and *(3)* neurovascular coupling and the spatial scale of the regulation of blood flow.

Anatomy of the Cortical Vascular System

Since the fMRI signal is a blood-flow-dependent signal, its specificity ultimately depends on the anatomy of the vascular bed and the spatial scale of blood-flow regulation. Figure 1.2.3 shows a corrosion cast of the cortical vasculature in macaque V1. The cortical blood supply is characterized by large arteries that run along the surface of the cortex, branch into smaller pial arteries, and branch finally into intracortical arterioles (100–200 μm) that enter the cortical gray matter perpendicular to the surface. These intracortical vessels eventually branch into capillaries, and blood is collected in intracortical venules of 100–200 μm, which form larger venules and veins on the surface of the cortex (Duvernoy et al., 1981). The distance between capillaries at any place in the gray matter of the cortex is about 40 μm (Weber et al., 2008). Gray matter is more highly vascularized than white matter, and there are differences in vascular density between different cortical areas; areas with higher vascularization, like primary sensory cortex, typically also show higher fMRI responses.

The differences in cerebral blood volume in vivo are shown in Figure 1.2.4. The steady-state CBV image shows the change in relaxivity ΔR_2^* induced upon injection of the intravascular iron-based contrast agent MION (monocrystalline iron oxide nanocolloid), which is a function of blood

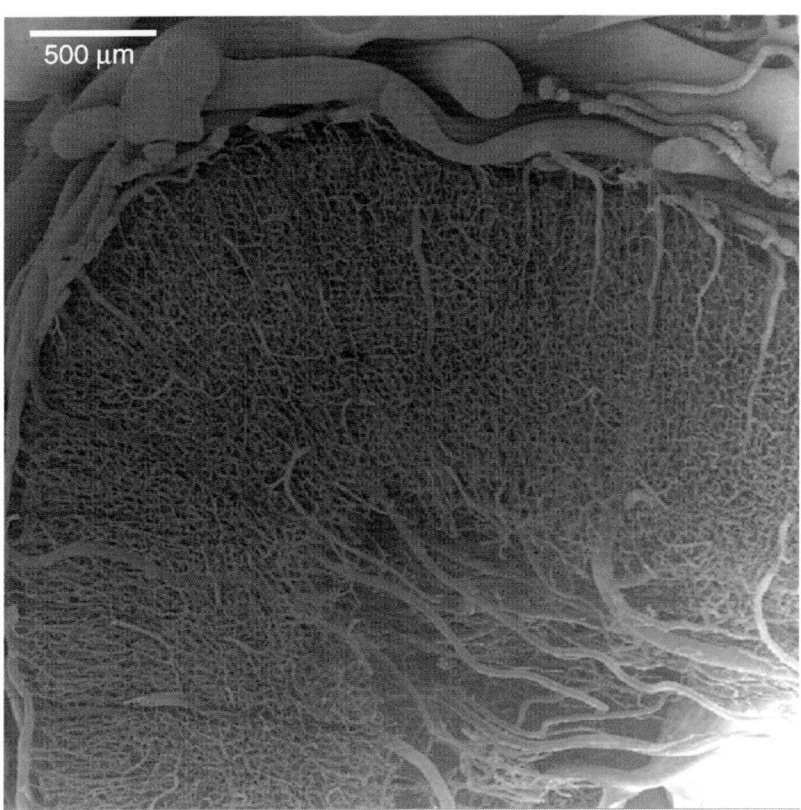

Figure 1.2.3. Corrosion cast of monkey V1 showing the microvasculature of the cortex (from Weber et al. [2008], with permission). Arteries and large draining veins are located in the pial layer. Penetrating arterioles and venules can be seen in addition to the capillary network. Intracortical arteries are shown in red and intracortical veins in blue. The vascular density in white matter is lower than in the gray matter.

A   B

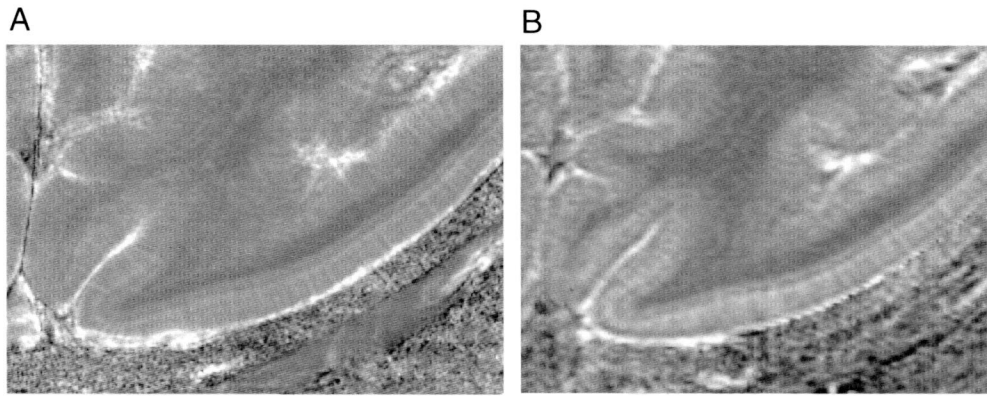

Figure 1.2.4. High-resolution steady-state GE-CBV image of macaque V1 showing the relaxivity changes induced by MION-injection (A). CBV is higher in gray matter than in white matter and it is high in the pial layers where the large vessels are located. In addition, differences in CBV can be observed within the cortex with layer IV having a higher blood volume. Intracortical vessels can also be seen. The SE-CBV map (B) is more sensitive to the microvascular fraction and also shows a maximum at the level of the Gennari line. Technical data: 4.7T, volume transmit coil, 28 mm surface receive coil, (A) FLASH, resolution 100x100x2000 μm^3, TE 20 ms, TR 2000 ms, (B) 16-segment SE-EPI, resolution 250x188x2000 μm^3, TE 70 ms, TR 3000 ms. 8 mg/kg MION. MION was obtained from the Center for Molecular Imaging Research, Massachusetts General Hospital, Boston, USA.

volume (Dennie et al., 1998; Wu et al., 2004). The figure shows the higher blood volume in gray matter than in white matter as well as the high blood volume at the surface of the cortex. But there are also differences in capillary density within the cortex, for instance laminar differences (Lauwers et al., 2008; Weber et al., 2008), which are reflected in differences in perfusion. Figure 1.2.4 shows these differences in macaque V1, indicating that the middle cortical layers have higher blood volume (Goense et al., 2007).

Regulation of Cortical Blood Flow

Because the brain has high energy demands, it needs a relatively constant supply of nutrients and oxygen and is sensitive to blood-flow changes. To protect the brain from injury, cerebral blood flow is tightly regulated at multiple levels, from macroscopic to microscopic (Faraci and Heistad, 1998; Hamel, 2006; Iadecola, 2004). An important aspect of cerebrovascular regulation is its autoregulation, whereby cerebral blood flow is kept within the normal range despite changes in systemic blood pressure.

Cerebral blood flow is coupled to neural metabolism, meaning that changes in neural activity produce concomitant changes in blood flow. There are multiple mechanisms whereby changes in neural activity and metabolism lead to a change in blood flow. Events triggering changes in perfusion can be the partial pressure of CO_2 and oxygen, the pH, or tissue concentrations of metabolites (Faraci and Heistad, 1998). There are also multiple signaling molecules and pathways involved in the neurovascular coupling, for instance, NO, prostaglandins, etc. (Hamel, 2006; Iadecola, 2004).

The specificity of the BOLD response to localized neural activation depends on the spatial scale of the blood flow regulation. Changes in blood flow are mediated by dilation and constriction of arteries and arterioles, while venules and veins have no smooth muscle and are mostly kept open in the brain. The neurovascular response can be quite localized as evidenced by optical imaging and two-photon microscopy experiments. For instance, ocular dominance columns and blobs in macaque V1, which are of the order of a few 100 μm, have been shown with optical imaging (Ts'o et al., 1990). Chaigneau et al. (2003) showed that blood flow in the rat olfactory system in vivo is regulated at the level of individual glomeruli, and with two-photon microscopy it has been shown that blood flow is regulated at the level of individual arterioles or even capillaries. Neurons and associated astrocytes form the so-called neurovascular units, and astrocytes are thought to play an important role in mediating the blood-flow response (Schummers et al., 2008). Constriction and dilation of individual arterioles were observed to be mediated by astrocytes by inducing local Ca^{2+} increases (Metea and Newman, 2006; Mulligan and Macvicar, 2004; Zonta et al., 2003; Takano et al., 2006). Dilation and constriction of capillaries by specialized structures called pericytes have been shown in the retina (Peppiatt and Attwell, 2004) and pericytes may perform similar functions in the brain, although this is still unclear (Hirase et al., 2004).

Specificity of Different fMRI Methods

Based on the above, the expectation is that the scale of the hemodynamic regulation is currently not the limiting factor for most fMRI applications except possibly for ultra–high resolution fMRI. The specificity of the fMRI signal further depends on the fMRI method that is used, scanner hardware (for instance field strength), and acquisition parameters. Different fMRI methods have different specificity (Weisskoff et al., 1994; Boxerman et al., 1995;

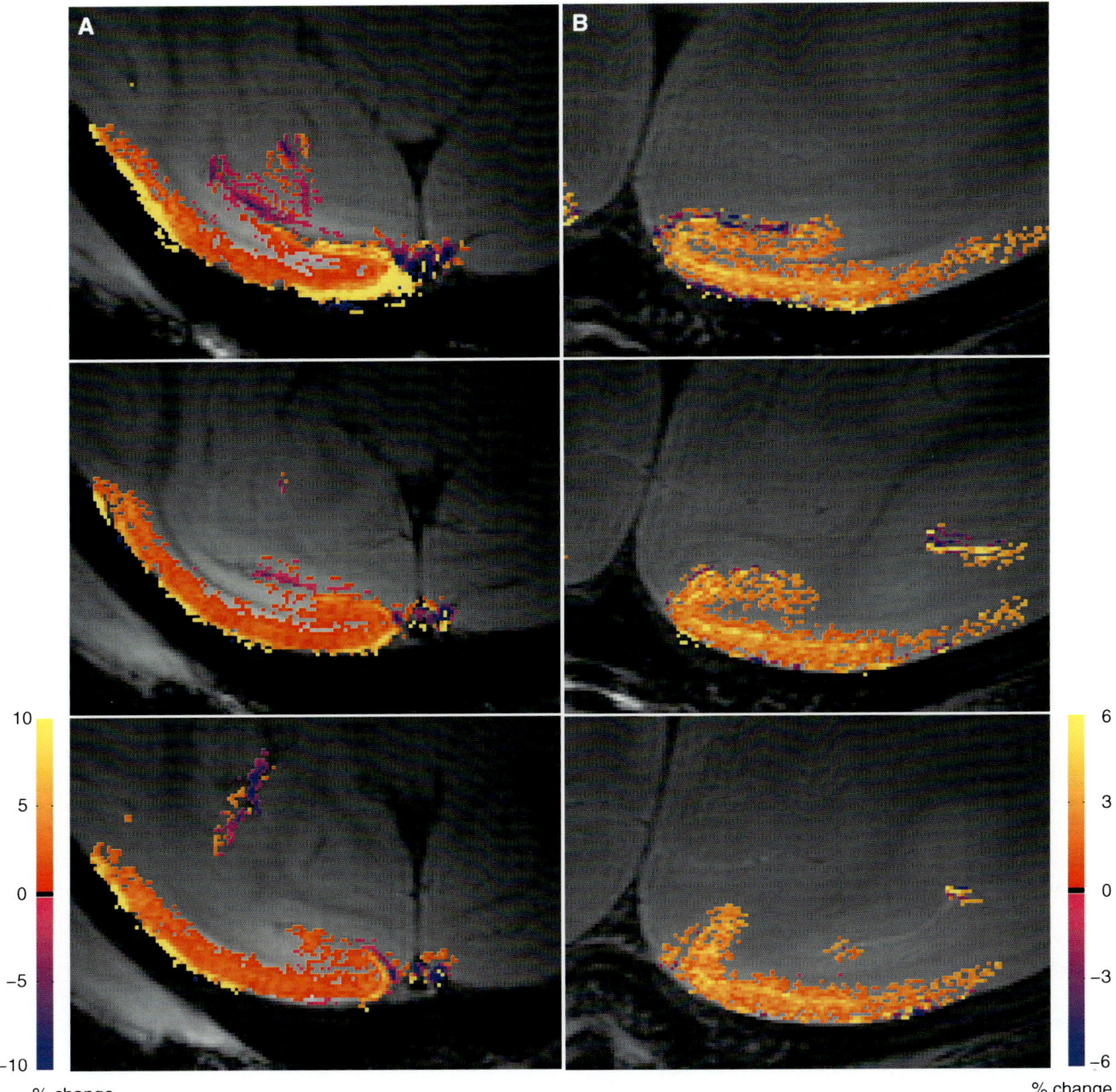

Figure 1.2.5. Specificity of GE- and SE-BOLD fMRI acquired at 4.7T. The GE-BOLD map (A) at a resolution of 333x333x2000 μm³ shows highest activity at the cortical surface and near vessels in the sulcus (Goense et al., 2007; Logothetis, 2008), whereas the SE-BOLD map (B) at a resolution of 250x175x2000 μm³ shows a BOLD signal that is better confined to the gray matter. Laminar structure can be seen in the SE-fMRI signal. Partial volume effects in the slice direction were not detrimental due to the anatomy of monkey V1 and a slice angle that was perpendicular to the cortical surface.

Kennan et al., 1994). We already mentioned that for instance GE-BOLD although sensitive to both vessels and capillaries, at low field is dominated by large vessels, and the contribution of the capillary signal increases at high field. SE-BOLD, CBV, and CBF methods are less sensitive to large vessels (Harel et al., 2006b). The GE signal is sensitive to the phase dispersal near large vessels, i.e., water-protons in voxels near large vessels

exhibit a range of phases due to the susceptibility gradients, and the phase dispersal in a voxel causes signal within a voxel to cancel out (called static dephasing). SE is not sensitive to static dephasing because the accumulated phase dispersal is refocused by the 180 degree pulse. However, near capillaries a dynamic effect is dominant which gives rise to the SE-BOLD signal, that is, spins that move within the field gradients accrue phase dispersal, and the change in phase due to this movement cannot be refocused. This is called dynamic averaging, characterized by the "apparent T_2" or T_2' (Ugurbil et al., 2000). In addition, there is a T_2-effect that arises from intravascular protons. This is at fields up to 3T the dominant contributor to the SE-BOLD signal (Duong et al., 2003). At higher field, T_2 of blood is short and the T_2-effect becomes less dominant.

Differences in specificity between the different methods can most easily be seen in high resolution fMRI. Figure 1.2.3 shows that large vessels are only located on the surface of the cortex and that vessels within gray matter are up to ~200 μm in monkeys. In high-resolution GE-EPI fMRI, the largest functional changes occur at the surface and near large vessels (Figure 1.2.5). In contrast, the largest SE-BOLD functional changes occur within the gray matter, approximately in layer IV, and not much functional activation is seen near large vessels, illustrating the improved specificity of SE-BOLD over GE-BOLD. However, if the spatial resolution is 1 mm or lower, signals cannot be clearly differentiated as originating from the surface or from within gray matter because of partial volume effects.

The specificity of the different fMRI methods can also be demonstrated by visualizing cortical columns. Ocular dominance columns (ODCs) in humans (~1 mm in diameter; Adams et al., 2007) are often used, or orientation columns in cats (also ~1 mm in diameter; Lowel et al., 1987). Columnar resolution was successfully demonstrated in humans and cats using GE-EPI (Moon et al., 2007; Cheng et al., 2001; Menon and Goodyear, 1999; Dechent and Frahm, 2000; Yacoub et al., 2008). When GE-BOLD is used, typically subtraction paradigms are used that subtract out the signals common to both stimuli, and hence it removes the nonspecific vessel signals, or alternatively vessel signals are thresholded to ameliorate the predominance of vessel signal in GE-BOLD (Moon et al., 2007; Cheng et al., 2001; Logothetis et al., 2002). The drawback of subtraction paradigms is that orthogonal stimuli are needed, which for many stimuli are not available. With SE-EPI, ocular dominance columns have been shown in humans (Yacoub et al., 2007; Yacoub et al., 2008), and using CBV and CBF methods, single-condition maps of orientation columns were demonstrated in cat V1 (Duong et al., 2001; Zhao et al., 2005). These more specific methods also allow functional mapping of laminar differences within the cortex, as demonstrated in V1 of cats and monkeys (Goense et al., 2007; Harel et al., 2006a; Zhao et al., 2006; Zappe et al., 2008).

BOLD Temporal Resolution

The temporal resolution of the BOLD signal is determined by the hemodynamic response, which is relatively slow, and hence fMRI cannot capture quick neuronal changes. The hemodynamic response takes a few seconds to develop and reaches its peak between 5 and 10 s after stimulus onset. Unless special paradigms are used, for instance, making use of the prolonged hemodynamic response to brief and strong stimuli (Ogawa et al., 2000) the useful temporal resolution of fMRI is in the second-range.

The Neural Signals

To be able to answer the question how BOLD relates to the neural signals and what aspects of the neural signals are best represented by the fMRI signals, we need to take a closer look at what we actually mean when we talk about "the neural signals." Usually the assumption is that they represent signals measured by intracortical electrodes or microelectrodes with standard extracellular methods. And we do wish to compare the BOLD signal to such electrophysiological recordings because a large amount of our knowledge about neural and brain function is based on these extracellular techniques. Typically single- or multiple-unit activity is recorded with microelectrodes, and we look at the specificity and spatial extent of these signals, for example, what types of neurons are recorded and how large is the area that is sampled. However, what is recorded by an electrode is not always fully representative of all the processes that occur in the brain because electrodes measure only a subset of the neural processes.

The signal measured by an electrode placed at a neural site is the mean extracellular field potential (mEFP) from the weighted sum of the electrical sinks and sources along multiple cells. Its waveform is characterized by fast action potentials superimposed on relatively slowly varying field potentials. Different signals are recorded depending on the impedance of the electrode. If a microelectrode with a small tip is placed close to the soma or axon of a neuron, then the measured mEFP directly reports the spiking of that neuron and frequently also that of its immediate neighbors. With electrodes of the order of several 100s of kΩ, single spikes or single-unit activity (SUA), multi-unit activity (MUA), and local field potentials (LFP) are recorded. Low impedance electrodes record predominantly LFP, while sharp electrodes/pipettes are typically used to record single units, and not much LFP is observed.

Single- and Multi-Unit Activity

The standard technique in neurophysiological research has been the recording of single spikes. Single spike monitoring has the best possible spatial and temporal resolution and it has been and it will continue to be the method of choice when single cell properties are the subject of investigation. It provides information of the spike output of the isolated cell and its response properties, for instance its receptive field or its tuning to different stimuli. Depending on the location and impedance of the electrode, often multiple neurons are recorded simultaneously. If MUA is recorded, the spikes generated by different neurons can be sorted based on their

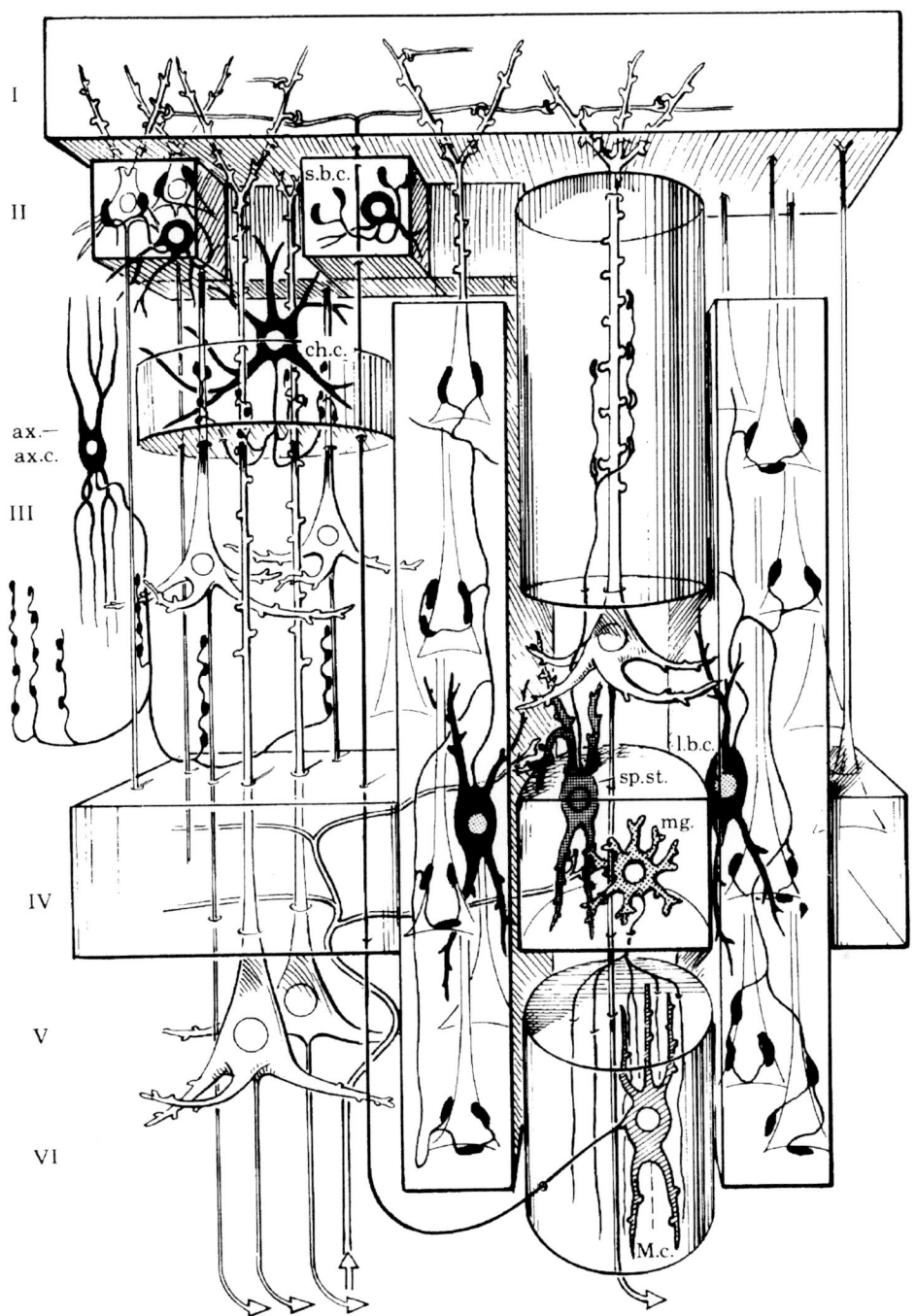

Figure 1.2.6. Schematic of the modular arrangement of cortical cells and connections (reproduced from Szentagothai [1978], with permission). The cortex has a columnar and well-ordered parallel structure. The drawing shows the different types of neurons and connections. Pyramidal cells, spiny stellate (sp.st.), small and large basket cells (s.b.c. and l.b.c.), microgliform cells (m.g.), chandelier cells (ch.c.), Martinotti cells.

shape. The spike shape that is recorded can vary depending on the location of the electrode with respect to the neuron. However, for accurate sorting, tetrodes (4-contact electrodes) or multicontact electrodes are advantageous or often necessary, particularly when the spike shapes of the neurons are similar.

A drawback of single- and multi-unit recordings is that they suffer from an element of bias toward certain cell types and sizes (Stone, 1973; Towe and Harding, 1970). Figure 1.2.6 shows a drawing of the cortical circuit and illustrates the variation in size and morphology of neurons within the cortical sheet. The measured spikes however mostly represent only very small neural populations of large cells, which are by and large the pyramidal cells in cerebral cortex and Purkinje neurons in cerebellar cortex. The magnitude of EFPs in the MUA range, for example, was shown to be a function of cell- and axon size (Gur et al., 1999). Combined physiology-histology experiments also demonstrated that the magnitude of MUA is site- (Buchwald and Grover, 1970) and cell-size specific (Nelson, 1966), varying considerably from one brain region to another (e.g., neocortex vs. hippocampus) but remaining relatively constant within a particular region. Homogeneous populations of large cells were found to systematically occur at sites of large-amplitude fast activity and vice versa (Grover and Buchwald, 1970). Similarly, the magnitude of axonal spikes is directly correlated with the size of the transmitting axon (Hunt, 1951; Gasser and Grundfest, 1939).

Recording from nonpyramidal cell types, for instance interneurons, is often difficult both because of their small size and because their response is often uncorrelated to the stimulus or to the behavioral state of the animal. Since response to a stimulus is often the criterion for successful isolation of a neuron or cluster of neurons, this can lead to a bias against certain neurons, for instance inhibitory neurons, against neuromodulatory neurons, or against neurons that have very low firing rates. This could introduce a substantial bias because there is reason to believe that neurons with very low firing rates may actually be very common in the cortex (Henze et al., 2000; Shoham et al., 2006).

Local Field Potentials

The obvious drawback of single-unit recording is that it provides information mainly on the output of the recorded single neuron with no access to its subthreshold integrative processes or the associational operations taking place. To this end, we also record the LFP, to which these processes do contribute. LFPs are recorded when the impedance of the microelectrode is sufficiently low and its exposed tip is a bit farther from the spike generating sources, so that action potentials do not dominate the neural signal. The electrode then monitors the totality of the potentials. LFPs are related both to integrative processes (dendritic events) and to spikes generated by several hundreds of neurons (Lorente de Nœ, 1947) and they represent mostly slow events reflecting cooperative activity in neural populations. They rather reflect the input of a given cortical area as well as its local intracortical processing, including the activity of excitatory and inhibitory interneurons. Based on current-source density (CSD) analysis and combined field potential and intracellular recordings, Mitzdorf (1985; 1987) suggested that LFPs reflect a weighted average of synchronized dendro-somatic components of the synaptic signals of a neural population near the electrode tip. Studies of inhibitory networks in the hippocampus (Buzsaki and Chrobak, 1995; Kandel and Buzsaki, 1997; Kocsis et al., 1999) have shown that other types of slow activity, including voltage-dependent membrane oscillations (Kamondi et al., 1998) and spike afterpotentials, also contribute to the LFP

(Buzsaki et al., 1988). The soma-dendritic spikes in neurons of the CNS are generally followed by afterpotentials, a brief delayed *afterdepolarization*, and a longer lasting *afterhyperpolarization* (Granit et al., 1963; Gustafsson, 1984), which have a duration on the order of tens of ms (Kobayashi et al., 1997; Harada and Takahashi, 1983; Higashi et al., 1993).

Another finding in studies combining EEG and intracortical recording was that unlike MUA, the magnitude of the slow fluctuations was not correlated with cell size, but instead reflected the extent and geometry of dendrites at the recording site (Buchwald et al., 1965; Fromm and Bond, 1964, 1967) Cells in a so-called *open field* geometrical arrangement, in which dendrites extend in one direction and somata in another produce strong dendrite-to-soma dipoles when they are activated by synchronous synaptic input. The pyramidal cells with their apical dendrites running parallel to each other and perpendicular to the pial surface (Figure 1.2.6) form an ideal open field arrangement, and contribute maximally to both the macroscopically measured EEG and the LFP. But the dependence on geometry also implies that neurons that are oriented horizontally or have spherical symmetric dendritic fields (closed field arrangement) contribute less efficiently or not at all to the sum of potentials. Because of this large contributions arise from pyramidal/Purkinje neurons with interneurons often contributing less (cf. Chapter 1.1).

LFP and MUA signals can be separated by filtering; a high-pass filter with cutoff of approximately 500 Hz is typically used to obtain MUA and a low-pass filter cutoff of ~300 Hz to obtain the LFP. The modulations in the LFP are classified in a number of specific frequency bands initially introduced in the EEG literature. EEG is subdivided into frequency bands known as **delta** (DC–4 Hz), **theta** (4–8 Hz), *alpha* (8–12 Hz), **beta** (12–24 Hz) and **gamma** (24–40/80 Hz) (Lindsley and Wicke, 1974; Basar, 1980; Steriade, 1991; Steriade and Hobson, 1976). The classification is based on the strong correlation of each band with a distinct behavioral state. An alternative band separation is based on information theory, where the information carried by the different bands in the LFP or MUA range was calculated in recordings from monkeys that were viewing movies with natural images (Belitski et al., 2008). The most informative LFP frequency ranges were 1–8 Hz and 60–100 Hz. Positive signal correlations were found between LFPs (60–100 Hz) and spikes, and between the frequencies within the 60–100 Hz LFP range, suggesting that the 60–100 Hz LFP range and spikes are possibly generated within the same network. LFPs in the range of 20–60 Hz carried very little information about the stimulus, although they shared strong trial-to-trial correlations, indicating that they might be influenced by a common source such as diffuse neuromodulatory input.

Spatial extent and propagation of neural signals

The volume from which electrical signals are measured by a recording electrode depends on the properties of the

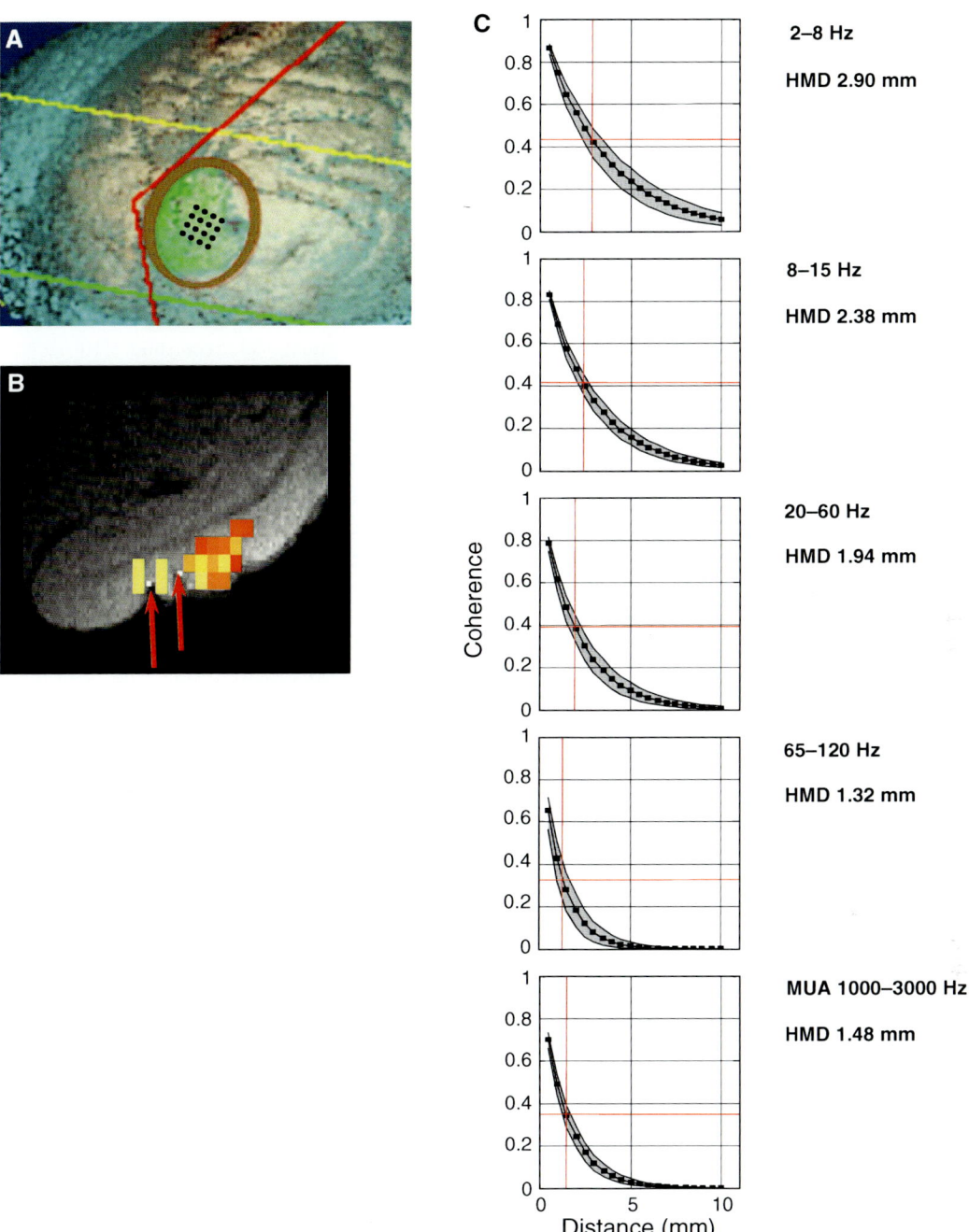

Figure 1.2.7. Coherence between signal recorded at different electrodes as a function of electrode distance for the different neural signals. (A): diagram of the electrode array used in physiological experiments, a 4x4 electrode array with inter-electrode distance of 1 mm was used. (B): position of two electrodes (arrows) in combined MRI and physiology experiments. (C): Average of all fits to the coherence-over-distance data for the different neural signals. The plots show the drop-off of coherence with inter-electrode distance. The gray shading indicates the 1–99% confidence intervals. The distance at which the coherence is halved is marked by the red lines and shown next to the panels. The loss of coherence with distance was comparable for all neural frequency bands (1–3 mm). Adapted from Goense and Logothetis (2008), with permission.

electrode. The activity from each point within the volume is weighted by a factor depending on the distance from the tip of the electrode. Single-unit activity or separable spikes are typically recorded from areas close to the electrode, for instance, Henze et al. (2000) and Gray et al. (1995) measured spikes within 50–150 µm from a tetrode. Electrodes with

exposed tips of approximately 100 µm (impedance from 40–120 kΩ) were estimated to record from a sphere with a radius of 50–350 µm (Grover and Buchwald, 1970; Legatt et al., 1980; Nicholson and Llinas, 1971). The volume from which LFP signals arise is larger, and the spatial extent of LFP summation can be calculated by computing the coherence of

LFP as a function of inter-electrode distance in experiments using simultaneous multi-electrode recordings (Juergens et al., 1996). The volume from which LFP signals arise is estimated to range from 0.25 to 3 mm distance from the electrode tip (Juergens et al., 1999; Katzner et al., 2009; Nauhaus et al., 2009; Mitzdorf, 1987).

The electrical properties of the conductive medium through which the current travels will obviously affect the voltages that are recorded. Within the physiological frequency range a current source can be described as a simple static point source. The description of the volume conductor is further simplified by the fact that the propagation of signals in gray matter is independent of their frequency. Intracranial measurements showed that the tissue impedance is actually frequency-independent and isotropic, allowing the description of the cortex as an ohmic resistor (Logothetis et al., 2007). Hence, this implies that the distance over which the signals can be measured is not dependent on the frequency of the signals but is determined by the relative size of the electrical sources.

The spatial extent of the different neural signals can be estimated by coherence analysis. The coherence between two electrodes is measured as a function of the distance between the electrodes for the different neural signals (Figure 1.2.7). This showed that the half-maximum of the coherence-to-distance functions was 2.9 mm for the 2–8 Hz LFP range, 2.4 mm for the 8–15 Hz range, 1.9 mm for the 20–60 Hz range, and 1.5 mm for MUA (Goense and Logothetis, 2008). Comparable distance-ranges were found for the LFP in V1/V2 (Juergens et al., 1999) and for the similarity of object preferences encoded by MUA and LFP in macaque IT (Kreiman et al., 2006). These findings suggest that the range over which the neural signals are measured in V1 are similar, and in the range of the typical voxel sizes in fMRI, and that this holds for the LFP band as well as for the MUA.

Combined MRI and Physiology

To address some of the questions raised earlier, we simultaneously measured fMRI and neurophysiological signals. Measurement of BOLD and neural signals is ideally done simultaneously; an important reason for this is that nonsimultaneous fMRI/electrophysiology increases experimental variability, making subtle or not so subtle effects harder to discriminate. For instance, in anesthetized animals the response of the animal to anesthesia can be different from one animal to the next or from one experiment to the next. In awake subjects also, the magnitude of the BOLD response is different for different individuals and different sessions, and variability can also arise due to factors relating to the behavioral state of the animal, like attention, arousal, etc. Given that the method of analysis is based on finding trends or correlations between phenomena that often yield weak signals, like the BOLD signal, or are highly correlated, like different neural signals, the added variance of nonsimultaneous

measurement may further complicate interpretation of data. That said, to record BOLD and intracortical electrophysiological signals simultaneously some formidable hurdles need to be overcome. These are the interference of the scanner on the electrophysiological recordings and measuring equipment, and the possible degrading effect of the recording hardware on MR image quality. The scanner introduces electrical and mechanical interference on the electrophysiological signal due to the switching of the gradients (driven by 100–1000 V for our systems for example) and strong RF-signals for excitation (output of the amplifier in the kW-range) that interfere with the neurophysiological recording (10–100s of μV). The recording hardware can cause susceptibility artifacts in the images wherever metal is used, and any conducting leads into the magnet bore act as an antenna and can drag in noise. This is a problem because the received MR signal is a low voltage signal (μV-range) and hence image quality is sensitive to RF interference. In addition, all equipment that enters the bore needs to be nonmagnetic, and it should function in strong magnetic fields. The latter is a problem for equipment that enters the magnet bore, and for equipment that stays outside the bore it can be a problem if the magnet is not shielded, as is the case for instance for ultra-high-field magnets (Thulborn, 2006).

Methodology and Practical Aspects

We present a brief overview of our methodology for simultaneous fMRI and electrophysiological recordings. For details on the setup and experimental procedures we refer to the relevant publications (Goense and Logothetis, 2008; Keliris et al., 2007; Logothetis et al., 1999; Logothetis et al., 2001; Logothetis et al., 2002; Oeltermann et al., 2007; Pfeuffer et al., 2004). fMRI-electrophysiology experiments are performed on vertical scanners (4.7T and 7T with 40 and 60 cm diameter bore respectively, BioSpec 47/40v and 70/60v, Bruker BioSpin, Ettlingen, Germany). These setups further consist of custom-built primate chairs and devices to fixate the monkey's head, equipment to display the stimulus, and anesthesia monitoring equipment for anesthetized monkeys, and for awake monkeys: sensors to record the animal's movement and track its eye-movements and a juice-delivery system.

Prior to experiments animals are implanted stereotaxically under general anesthesia with a custom-made headpost to fixate the animal's head to the primate chair and a recording chamber (Logothetis et al., 2001; Logothetis et al., 2002). Animals used in awake experiments are extensively trained using operant conditioning methods on the behavioral task and to remain motionless for the duration of the experimental trial.

Electrophysiological Recording

For electrophysiological recording a small trepanation is made through which the electrode is introduced into the brain, and the electrode drive-assembly is fastened on the chamber with the electrode positioned above the craniotomy. The drive-assembly consists of an electrode holder, a mechanism for manually advancing the electrode, and the magnetic-field sensor for the "near" interference circuit (see below) mounted on the microdrive (Figure 1.2.8). The electrode holder is composed of a glass-coated platinum-iridium electrode, the sensor for the "far" interference circuit (see below), and the

ground contact. The holder consists of three concentric metallic cylinders: the inner cylinder is the contact point for the electrode, the middle the far-interference sensor, and the outer layer serves as the amplifier ground. These cylinders, in particular the outer cylinder, are a rotation-symmetric shield for the electrode, permitting optimal ground contact to the animal and avoiding loops susceptible to induction. Ground contact is provided by filling the chamber with deuterium saline and agar, which also reduces susceptibility artifacts in the MR images from air in the chamber.

The animal has a gold wire implanted (awake monkey) or a silver mouth electrode (anesthetized monkey) that acts as a "feedback" electrode. This electrode is part of the "far" interference compensation circuit and delivers the calculated counterinterference signal to the animal. The three-coil magnetic field sensor, necessary for the "near" interference compensation circuit, is positioned on or near the electrode-drive. Prior to the first functional scan the interference compensation is manually adjusted such that gradient interference on the electrode signal is minimal.

Signal Acquisition and Interference Compensation

The main problems arising when doing electrophysiology in the scanner are interference due to gradient switching and the fact that the preamplifier needs to be moved outside the magnet, which requires use of long cables that lead to large signal losses due to cable capacitance. To avoid signal loss, current is measured instead of voltage and prior to amplification the current is converted to voltage (see Oeltermann et al., 2007). The problem of interference was solved by using two separate interference compensation circuits (Logothetis et al., 2001; Oeltermann et al., 2007): a circuit to compensate for far interference arising from a distance larger than the distance from electrode tip to electrode ground and a circuit that compensates for near interference originating from the immediate vicinity of the electrode tip (Figure 1.2.9). Far interference arises due to capacitive coupling of the animal to metal resulting from the metal-to-electrolyte interface of the electrode. This allows interference currents to flow from, for example, ECG lines to the animal. By placing a sensor around the electrode and feeding an inverted copy of all interfering signals through it interference currents flowing to the animal can be eliminated (Logothetis et al., 2001; Oelter-mann et al., 2007).

Because of the finite distance between the above sensor and electrode, interference originating from areas within this distance cannot be compensated for by the far-interference circuit. This interference is large enough to be problematic and hence it was compensated for by a near-interference circuit. Magnetic field changes due to the gradients were monitored by three small, orthogonally oriented coils positioned near the electrode, and the measured signal was added to the "ground" of the current-to-voltage converter to neutralize the interference. Because the

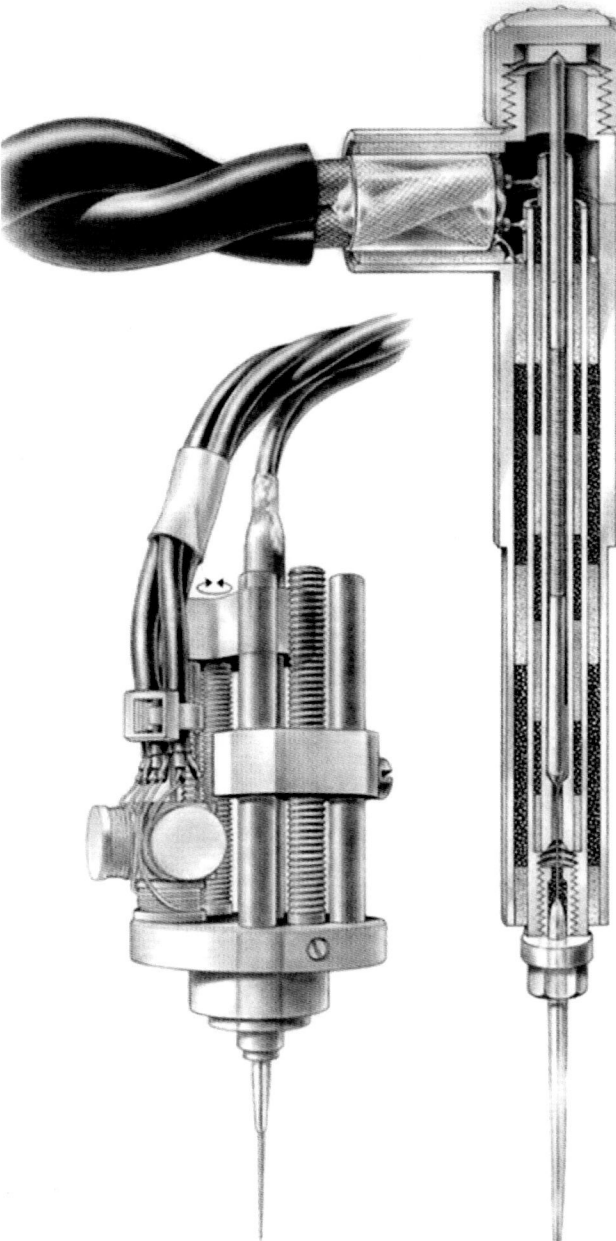

Figure 1.2.8. Intracortical electrode (right) and electrode drive (left). The right panel shows the electrode with holder; the cutout shows the concentric cylinders that are part of the far interference compensation and shield of the electrode. Left: the mechanical electrode drive with the sensor for the near interference circuit mounted on the drive. Adapted from Logothetis et al. (2001), with permission.

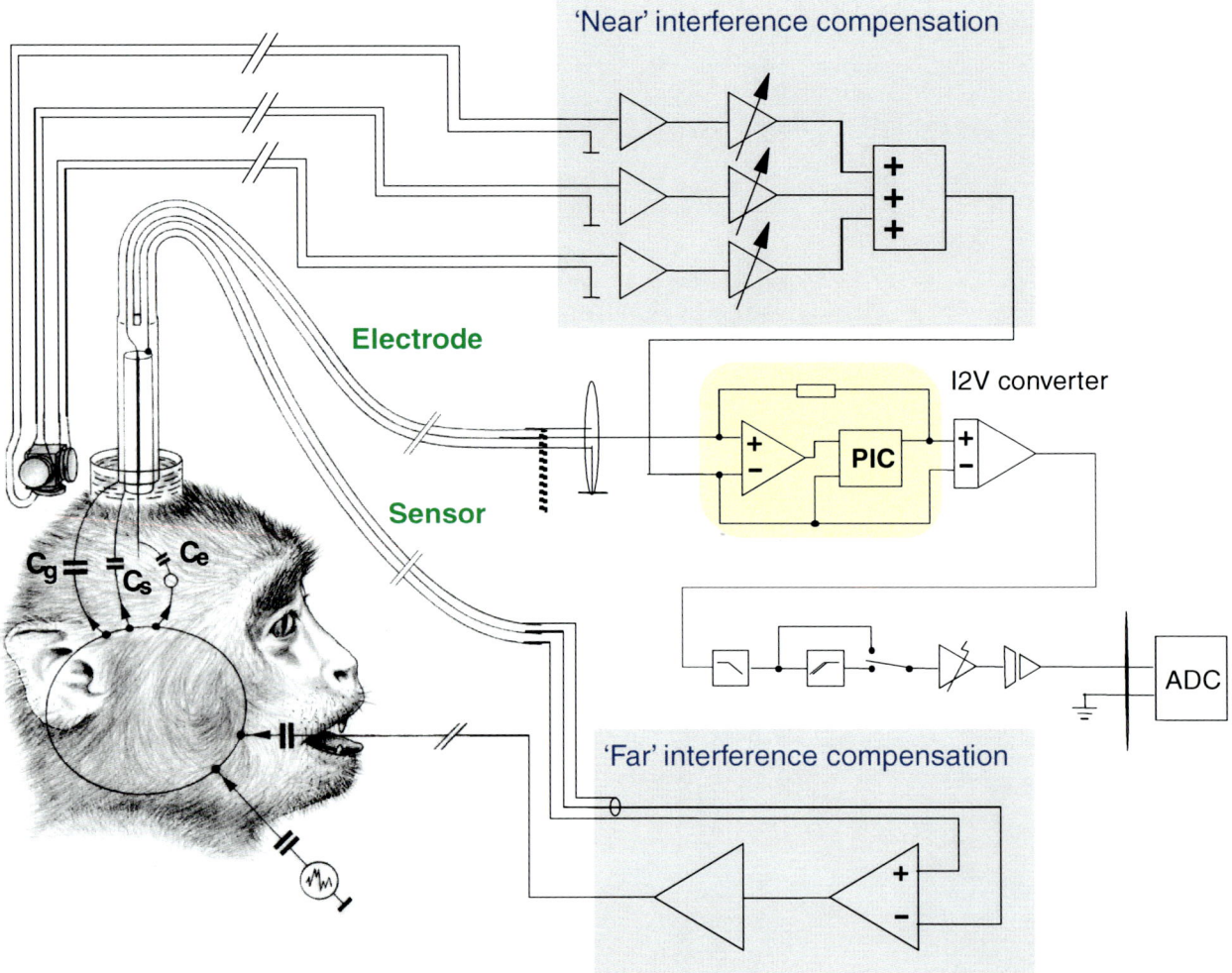

Figure 1.2.9. Schematic of the electronic circuits to compensate for interference of the electrophysiological signals by the RF- and gradient switching of the scanner. The diagram shows two types of interference that need to be compensated for, the "near" and "far" interference (see text). Adapted from Logothetis et al. (2001), with permission.

small coils are oriented orthogonally and the gain and sign of the signals is manually adjustable, it is possible to simulate the induction voltage in a wire loop of any diameter and orientation. In this way a virtual wire loop that has opposite direction of winding can be adjusted such that the loops caused by asymmetries in the electrode holder and cable are effectively compensated (Logothetis et al., 2001; Oeltermann et al., 2007).

The above interference reduction techniques yield a non-saturated, measurable signal that, however, still contains some gradient interference. This residual interference is eliminated by principal component analysis (PCA) and elimination of those principal components that strongly correlate with the interference directly recorded from the gradient amplifiers results in a "clean" signal (Logothetis et al., 2001).

Neural Basis of the BOLD Response

To investigate the neural origins of the fMRI response and the coupling between neural and BOLD signals, simultaneous fMRI and electrophysiology were performed in anesthetized (Logothetis et al., 2001; Rauch et al., 2008; Shmuel et al., 2006) and awake monkeys (Goense and Logothetis, 2008). In the well-known 2001 study it was shown that the LFP is generally a better predictor of the BOLD response than the MUA (Logothetis et al., 2001). Figure 1.2.10 shows an example of a comparison of the time course of the BOLD signal and the neural signals in the MUA- and LFP bands in an awake monkey.

The figure shows time courses of seven band-limited power (BLP) signals extracted from the comprehensive neurophysiological signal following removal of gradient interference, band separation, and rectification. The first

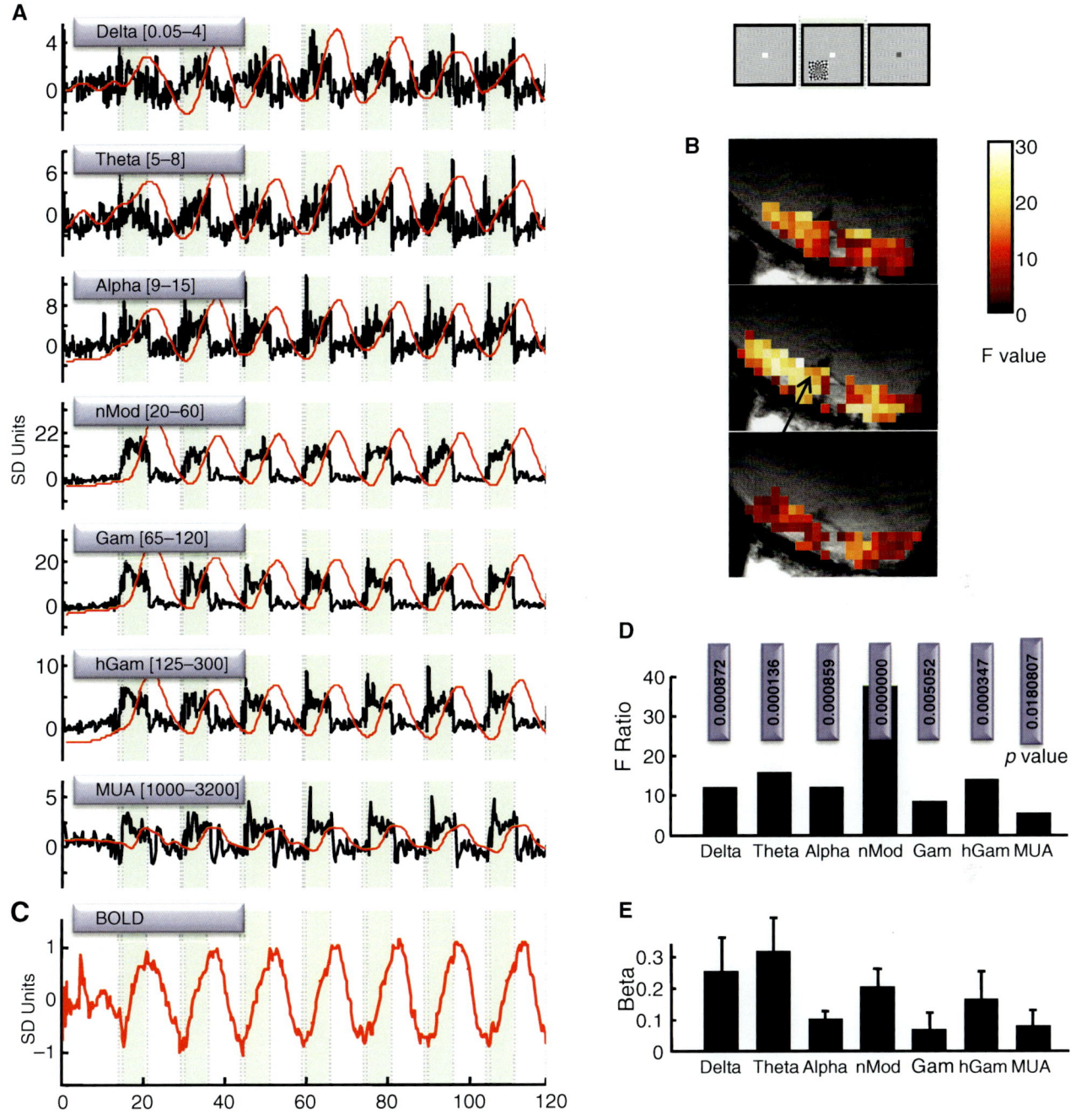

Figure 1.2.10. Dependencies between BOLD and neural signals in V1 in awake monkeys. (A) Band-separated neural signals (black) in response to a 6° visual stimulus (top right). The band-limited power (BLP) signals were convolved with a theoretical hemodynamic response (HRF) and used as regressors for each band (red). Green shading indicates the times the stimulus was presented. The response to the stimulus is especially pronounced in the neuromodulatory and gamma bands. (B) Functional activation map superimposed on anatomical images. The location of the electrode is shown by the arrow. (C) The BOLD time course acquired at a temporal resolution of 250 ms shows obvious modulation to the stimulus. The output of the GLM analysis and F-test yielded significant *p*-values for all neural bands (D) indicating that all bands contributed significantly to the BOLD response. (E) Beta values lacked dramatic differences across bands. Adapted from Goense and Logothetis (2008), with permission.

three bands are known from the EEG literature, while the other bands were defined based on recent work (Belitski et al., 2008). There the relationship between visual information carried by different frequency bands of LFP and spikes was investigated in recordings while the monkey was viewing five-minute color movie clips. This ensured that the stimulation was diverse and likely stimulated all visual cortices not affected by anesthesia.

In Figure 1.2.10, however, the stimuli were simple geometrical shapes that optimally drive V1. Moreover, due to the limitations imposed by the behavioral task, the stimuli could only be shown for short periods of time in sequential trials. It is therefore not surprising that the time courses of the signals in all bands are relatively similar to each other due to the presence of onset responses. Nonetheless, analysis using the general linear model (GLM)(Friston et al., 1995) revealed a differential contribution of the different neural signals to the BOLD response. Whether a frequency band has a unique contribution to the BOLD signal can be assessed by calculating the F-ratio, which showed that all frequency bands contributed significantly to the BOLD signal, and significant F-ratios for all bands indicates that each band explains a component of the BOLD response that cannot be explained by any of the other bands (Goense and Logothetis, 2008). The average beta values were comparable across frequency bands, suggesting that under these stimulus conditions no one single band especially determines the BOLD response.

Studies in awake and anesthetized monkeys have shown higher correlation coefficients between LFP and the BOLD signal than between MUA and the BOLD signal (Goense and Logothetis, 2008; Logothetis et al., 2001). This implies that the overall synaptic activity or the input of an area is a stronger generator of the BOLD signal than its output. But although the correlation of the LFP to the BOLD signal is consistently higher than the correlation of the MUA to the BOLD signal, MUA is also positively correlated, and is also significant. High correlations of spiking with the BOLD response were also found in humans (Mukamel et al., 2005). This is not surprising given that in most cases the MUA is correlated to the LFP, and in most cases a positive correlation exists between the input and the output of a neural system. Thus, based on differences in correlation coefficients we cannot unambiguously determine which signal better drives the BOLD response. This is further complicated by the fact that the neural and BOLD responses are often noisy. Because of the correlation between MUA and the BOLD signal, one needs to find circuits or stimulus conditions where

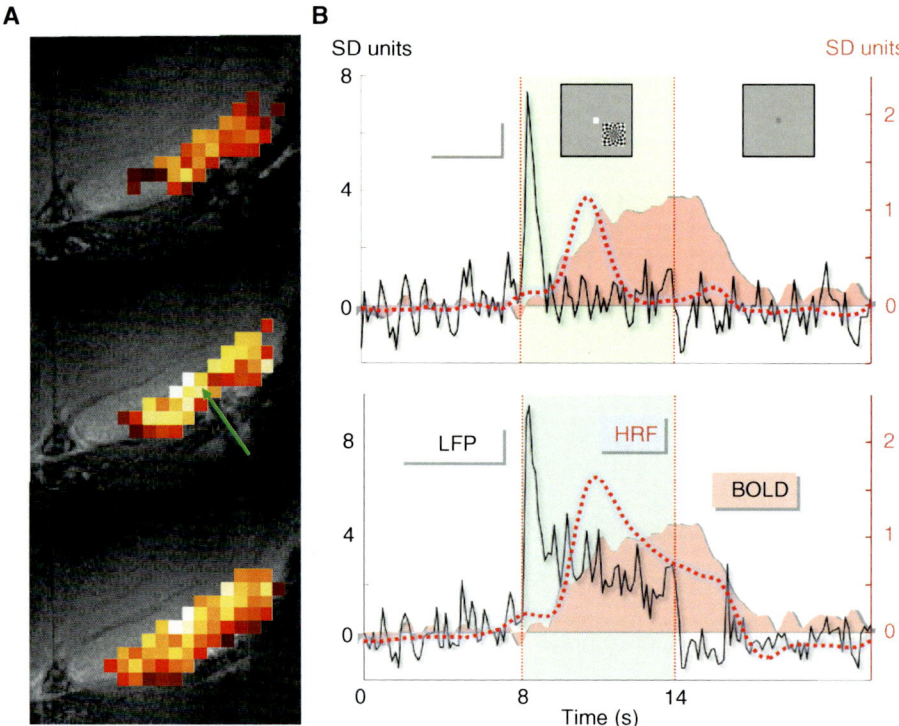

Figure 1.2.11. Dissociation between the MUA and BOLD response. (A) Functional activation maps in response to a 6° peripheral rotating checkerboard stimulus centered at 6.5° (inset in B). The arrow indicates the location of the electrode. (B) The average MUA, LFP in the 20–60 Hz range and BOLD time courses show that while the neuromodulatory component of the LFP stayed elevated for the duration of the stimulus, the MUA rapidly returned to baseline after a transient onset response. The prolonged time course of the BOLD response suggests a more sustained driving mechanism of the BOLD response as opposed to the transient MUA signal. The dotted line shows the regressor, i.e., the neural signal convolved with the theoretical HRF, which indicates that the MUA-derived regressor cannot capture the sustained part of the BOLD response. Adapted from Goense and Logothetis (2008), with permission.

there is dissociation to obtain more conclusive evidence. In other words, conditions where the LFP is not or only weakly correlated with the MUA.

An example of such a case in the awake monkey is shown in Figure 1.2.11. Dissociation of the LFP and MUA can occur when there is strong adaptation and the LFP stays elevated long after the MUA has returned to baseline (Logothetis et al., 2001). In these cases the BOLD response also stayed elevated and this clearly shows the better correlation between BOLD and LFP than between BOLD and MUA. Similar results, i.e., better coupling of the hemodynamic response to the LFP in cases of dissociation, were observed by other groups, for instance in V1 of cats using optical imaging (Niessing et al., 2005). Another way to induce dissociation was demonstrated by Viswanathan and Freeman (2007), who used high temporal frequency stimuli that did not elicit spikes in V1 and who observed that LFP activity elicits changes in tissue oxygen in the absence of spiking.

Dissociation of LFP and MUA can also be induced by pharmacological intervention. For example intracortical injection of serotonin or a 5-HT1A serotonin receptor agonist abolishes spiking of the output neurons that are typically recorded in the MUA (Logothetis, 2003; Rauch et al., 2008). The LFP on the other hand did not change substantially, and similarly the BOLD response did not show changes. Such cases indicate that the signals recorded in the LFP and representing the input in an area are more likely driving the BOLD signal than the MUA signal, which mostly represents the output of large pyramidal neurons.

Other cases of dissociation of neural activity and metabolism or blood flow have been observed in structures where the anatomical and functional properties of the neural circuit allow a clear segregation between input and output. For instance, in the lateral superior olive (LSO) of the cat auditory system Nudo and Masterton (1986) observed that inhibitory synaptic activity increased 2-DG labeling although postsynaptic spiking is suppressed. In the cerebellum, Mathiesen et al. (1998) observed that stimulation of the parallel fiber system provides inhibitory synaptic input and inhibits Purkinje cell firing but that the CBF response remained.

Given the similar volumes from which the neural signals are recorded (see above) the stronger coupling of LFP to BOLD (Goense and Logothetis, 2008; Logothetis et al., 2001) can not be explained by differences in spatial summation of the neural signals. Also the spatial area from which the neural signals are sampled provides justification to use fMRI resolutions of 1–2 mm to determine the correlation between MR- and neural signals.

LFP, Spikes, Metabolism, and Blood Flow

The results above show that the BOLD response is better correlated with LFP than with MUA, implying that the BOLD response is better correlated with the input and local processing of the neurons in an area than with the output of the large pyramidal cells. Note that "synaptic input" does not necessarily imply input from another cortical or subcortical area, but it also refers to local (intrinsic) connections. Like the positive BOLD response, negative BOLD responses were also associated with decreases in LFP and MUA (Shmuel et al., 2006).

The energy demands of neurotransmission and spiking determine the blood flow to an activated area. Ultimately, the function of perfusion is the supply of nutrients and O_2, removal of waste products, and removal of heat. This raises questions about which processes have the highest metabolic demands (synaptic processes vs. spiking) and whether the neurovascular response is driven by the processes that have the highest metabolic demands or if there is some kind of anticipatory or feedforward process.

The brain consumes 20% of the body's total energy (Sokoloff, 1960), and it is oxidative phosphorylation that feeds the brain. Most of the energy (50–80%) is used for neural signaling, while cellular maintenance processes like protein synthesis use a minor (5–15%) fraction of the energy budget (Ames III, 2000; Raichle and Mintun, 2006; Shulman et al., 2004; Riera et al., 2008). Because the sodium-potassium pump or Na^+/K^+-ATPase maintains the transmembrane electrochemical gradients that are the driving force for most signaling processes, the main energy consumer in the brain is the Na^+/K^+-ATPase (Sokoloff, 1999). The pump depends on oxidative phosphorylation for its energy needs (Erecinska and Silver, 1994) and high concentrations of Na^+/K^+-ATPase co-localize with high levels of cytochrome oxidase (CytOx) reactivity (Hevner et al., 1992; Wong-Riley, 1989). Cytochrome oxidase is the enzyme in the electron transport chain that catalyzes the reduction of O_2 to H_2O and hence is a marker for oxidative metabolism. The vascularization of the cortex also reflects its energy use: areas that have high energy needs have denser vascularization. For instance, in V1 energy use is highest in layer IV and it is higher in blobs than in interblobs. This is evidenced by higher CytOx-reactivity (Wong-Riley, 1989) and higher ^{14}C-deoxyglucose (2-[^{14}C]-DG) uptake (Kennedy et al., 1976), and is reflected in the higher vascularization of these areas (Weber et al., 2008).

At the cellular level, we can also ask which signaling processes use the most energy, for instance, spiking, synaptic transmission, neurotransmitter recycling, or the maintenance of transmembrane gradients (Ames III, 2000; Attwell and Laughlin, 2001). It is generally believed that synaptic transmission and associated processes use more energy (Ames III, 2000; Shulman et al., 2004), although the relative contribution of spiking is still debated (Attwell and Laughlin, 2001; Lennie, 2003). The higher presence of cytochrome oxidase and mitochondria in dendrites (especially in postsynaptic areas) compared to cell bodies and axons indicates that these are the more metabolically active sites (Wong-Riley, 1989). Similarly, Schwartz et al. (1979) also found that nerve terminals have a higher uptake of radiolabeled glucose than areas with cell bodies.

Despite these energy needs however, the cerebral metabolic rate of oxygen consumption, or $CMRO_2$, measured with PET showed little increase under visual stimulation, while blood flow and glucose consumption did increase, indicating an uncoupling between blood flow and oxidative metabolism (Fox and Raichle, 1986; Fox et al., 1988; Raichle and Mintun, 2006). These observations have incited the debate about the importance of glycolytic versus oxidative metabolism in brain function (Pellerin and Magistretti, 2003; Pellerin et al., 2007; Chih and Roberts Jr., 2003; Shulman et al., 2004; Gladden, 2004) as it was also found with MR spectroscopy that excess lactate is produced during functional activation (Mangia et al., 2007; Prichard et al., 1991; Sappey-Marinier et al., 1992).

Pellerin and Magistretti (1994; Pellerin et al., 2007) put forward the hypothesis that glutamate released at the synapse is taken up into astrocytes, where it induces glycolysis leading to the production of lactate, which is then released and taken up by neurons to be used as an energy substrate. This is also called the astrocyte-neuron lactate shuttle hypothesis (ANLSH). The competing view holds that both neurons and astrocytes use glucose as their main substrate, and lactate is produced when glycolysis exceeds the rate of oxidative metabolism, a situation that is both transient and potentially detrimental (Chih and Roberts Jr., 2003). Hence the debate focuses on the compartimentalization of glycolysis versus oxidative metabolism, with one side arguing that astrocyte metabolism is predominantly glycolytic and neural metabolism mostly oxidative and the other side that both oxidative and glycolytic metabolism occur in neurons *and* astrocytes. Astrocytes have many different functions in the brain and play an important role in neurovascular coupling and metabolism. They are a subtype of glial cells characterized by their star shape and until quite recently they were mostly considered filler material. They are involved in regulating homeostasis in the brain (Simard and Nedergaard, 2004) and providing energy to the neurons by supplying nutrients to the neurons. Another function of astrocytes is the uptake of neurotransmitters released from nerve terminals, however, they can also release neuroactive agents themselves, for instance glutamate (Newman, 2003).

During activation, most of the energy used also seems to be accounted for by the needs of the Na^+/K^+-ATPase; Mata et al. (1980) found that glucose uptake induced by stimulation is due to activity of the Na^+/K^+-ATPase. The pump is linked to glycolysis in different tissues and may be in brain (see Ames III [2000] for review) but glycolysis by itself is insufficient to feed the pump. However, it is possible that for fast and/or small increases like activation, neurons rely more on glycolysis while for sustained activity they rely on oxidative metabolism (Raichle and Mintun, 2006; Erecinska and Silver, 1994; Wong-Riley, 1989). In experiments by Fox et al. (1986; Fox et al., 1988) and others (Ito et al., 2005) $CMRO_2$ was not much elevated by functional activity, but it was observed that $CMRO_2$ increased with prolonged stimulation (Gjedde and Marrett, 2001; Mintun et al., 2002; Vlassenko

et al., 2006b). Hence there may be a shift from initially more glycolytic metabolism toward more oxidative metabolism under sustained stimulation (Gjedde and Marrett, 2001; Mintun et al., 2002; Raichle and Mintun, 2006; Vlassenko et al., 2006a). However, further studies are needed to clarify the contributions of glycolysis and oxidative metabolism during both baseline and activation.

But whether metabolism under activation is primarily oxidative or glycolytic, or whether the nutrient that needs to be supplied is glucose or O_2 may not be the main factor in understanding the BOLD response. What matters for the BOLD signal is what drives the signaling cascade that leads to the increase in blood flow, given that it is the blood flow response that is taken as an indicator of increased neural activity. Hence, to understand the BOLD signal, we need to look at neurovascular coupling and ask what is the trigger for the neurovascular response. Again, the processes related to synaptic function—synaptic transmission, restoration of electrical gradients, and neurotransmitter recycling—elicit the functional blood flow increases (Wang et al., 2005; Lauritzen, 2005; Hoffmeyer et al., 2007; Iadecola and Nedergaard, 2007). Especially glutamatergic neurotransmission leads to an increase in blood flow (Li and Iadecola, 1994; Hoffmeyer et al., 2007; Gsell et al., 2006; Yang et al., 2003; Mathiesen et al., 1998) although there are numerous vasoactive signaling molecules and multiple vasodilatory and constrictive mechanisms (Cauli et al., 2004; Iadecola and Nedergaard, 2007; Iadecola, 2004). Molecules involved in signaling pathways leading to vasodilation during functional activation are also associated more with synaptic signaling (Zhang and Wong-Riley, 1996; Hoffmeyer et al., 2007; Yang et al., 2003) than with action potentials or metabolic signals (Attwell and Iadecola, 2002; Iadecola, 2004) although the redox state during activation possibly plays a role through the cytosolic $NADH/NAD^+$ in astrocytes (Ido et al., 2001; Ido et al., 2004; Raichle and Mintun, 2006; Vlassenko et al., 2006b). Many of these neurovascular coupling processes are also mediated by astrocytes, because of their key location between vasculature and neurons (Nedergaard et al., 2003). Their numerous processes contact the blood vessels and envelope synapses, and they are involved in the regulation of local blood flow, and hence are an important mediator of the BOLD signal. Their effect on the blood flow responses are again often triggered by neuronal glutamate release (Zonta et al., 2003; Takano et al., 2006; Schummers et al., 2008; Metea and Newman, 2006; Koehler et al., 2006; Petzold et al., 2008).

The Cortical Circuit and the BOLD Response

The BOLD response is associated more with input and local processing of cortical neurons than with their spiking output. But this opens further questions about what specific cortical processes and what properties of the cortical circuitry determine the BOLD response. For a better interpretation of fMRI it is essential that we understand which processes are represented in the BOLD response, and which less, or not at all

(Logothetis, 2008). In essence this boils down to a question about the transfer function: Do all neural events contribute equally to the BOLD response, or do some events contribute more than others? The same questions can be asked for the LFP and metabolic signals.

Different cortical processes can and without much doubt do have different contributions to the BOLD, LFP, and MUA signals. The fMRI signal may also reflect different aspects of neural processing that are not always observed with single-unit recording. For instance, a binocular rivalry stimulus showed robust functional activation in V1, while only a small fraction of the single neuron's responses were modulated by the percept (Blake and Logothetis, 2002). Different processes, like feedforward vs. feedback processes, or stimulus driven or neuromodulatory processes, or for instance subcortical input vs. cortico-cortical input or recurrent intracortical input, may affect these signals differently. If we look at connectivity we find that most cortical connections are highly local. In contrast, subcortical input is rather weak in terms of number of synapses (Douglas and Martin, 2007; Peters and Payne, 1993; Peters et al., 1994), for instance thalamocortical input typically comprises only about 10–20% of synapses (Douglas and Martin, 2007), and in V1 only ~5% (Peters and Payne, 1993; Peters et al., 1994). It is not known whether the BOLD signal is more or less strongly weighted toward intracortical processing or cortico-cortical or thalamocortical processing.

Furthermore, different types of neurons may have different contributions to the BOLD signals than they do to the neural signals. For instance, interneurons are less visible in LFP and MUA signals than pyramidal neurons, but because they can have high firing rates they could possibly have substantial metabolic demands (Buzsaki et al., 2007) and a considerable effect on the BOLD response. Interneurons also have been shown to cause dilation and constriction of microvessels (Cauli et al., 2004). Another example is smaller cells that can also have higher firing rates and are more easily stimulated than large cells (Gur et al., 1999) and hence may have a substantial contribution to the BOLD response, although their contribution to the recorded MUA and LFP will be less.

Another question is how excitation and inhibition contribute to the fMRI responses (Logothetis, 2008; Buzsaki et al., 2007) and whether the BOLD signal is mediated by specific neurotransmitters or receptors. We can ask the same question about the LFP and MUA because different types of neurotransmission may also not be equally represented in the recorded neural signals. Glutamatergic excitatory neurotransmission is commonly associated with BOLD and CBF responses (Gsell et al., 2006; Hoffmeyer et al., 2007). One reason is that these are the most common synapses in the cortex and they outnumber inhibitory synapses by about five to one (Braitenberg and Schüz, 1998). Glutamatergic excitatory synapses are also correlated with high cytochrome oxidase levels (Wong-Riley, 1989). However, although N-methyl-D-aspartate (NMDA) and α-amino-3-hydroxy-5-methyl-4-isoxazole propionate (AMPA) receptor activity were both shown to contribute to the CBF and BOLD responses, in contrast to AMPA receptor activity, NMDA receptor activity did not contribute to the LFP (Mathiesen et al., 1998; Gsell et al., 2006; Hoffmeyer et al., 2007). NMDA receptor activity is linked to increased blood flow through the nitric oxide (NO) signaling pathway (Li and Iadecola, 1994; Akgoren et al., 1994) which mediates glutamate induced blood flow increases. For instance nitric oxide synthase (NOS) knockout mice showed decreased activation-induced blood flow responses in the cerebellum (Yang et al., 2003). The effect of inhibitory neurotransmission on the blood flow responses is much less clear (Logothetis, 2008; Buzsaki et al., 2007) and may be small (Waldvogel et al., 2000), which could be due to the lower number of inhibitory synapses. However a contribution of inhibitory neurotransmission to the BOLD signal in the cortex is not unlikely because gamma aminobutyric acid (GABA)ergic neurotransmission has been shown to account for ~15% of the energy consumption (Patel et al., 2005; Hyder et al., 2006). Furthermore, inhibitory neurons can have high firing rates, and their synapses are also associated with mitochondria and high CytOx levels (Wong-Riley, 1989). Inhibition has also been shown to increase 2-DG uptake (McCasland and Hibbard, 1997; Nudo and Masterton, 1986; Ackermann et al., 1984), and GABA was shown to induce vasodilation in hippocampal microvessels (Fergus and Lee, 1997). Finally, other neurotransmitters and neuromodulators are known to be vasoactive and may play a role in the BOLD response, for example acetylcholine, serotonin, dopamine, noradrenaline (Attwell and Iadecola, 2002).

Hence, although it is without doubt true that the BOLD signal is related to neural processing, what cortical processes exactly it does and does not represent is still far from clear. For many studies, knowing that activation is due to neural activity may be all that one needs to know. But if we want to go beyond that and interpret the BOLD findings in the context of these different neural processes it becomes increasingly important to better understand the neurovascular response and its relation to the underlying neural processes.

Conclusion

The finding that the fMRI response is better correlated with the LFP, which represents the input and local processing of a neural circuit, than to the MUA, representing the output, has important implications for the interpretation of the BOLD signal. Especially when BOLD signals are compared to, or interpreted in terms of, the results obtained in electrophysiological (typically single-unit) recordings. Although in most cases spiking output is correlated with synaptic input, and hence in most cases the spiking activity and BOLD are well correlated, there may be cortical processes where the relationship and thus the interpretation of the BOLD signal is not so straightforward.

Although we now have a clearer picture of the origins of the fMRI responses, we still do not fully understand the details of the processes underlying the BOLD response, and many issues are still unresolved. Hence the obvious conclusion is that further experiments are needed to elucidate the exact nature of the functional responses. This of course needs a better understanding of the metabolic and neurovascular processes that take place during functional activation, regardless of whether these are measured by MRI, PET, or optical methods. And although the neurophysiological methods like single- and multi-unit recording and EEG have been around for decades, many questions of what exactly is being measured are still unresolved. Progress can be made by improving current functional imaging methods or development of new functional imaging methodology, the combination of multisite or array electrode recordings with functional imaging, or intervention by for instance pharmacological injections (Kida et al., 2006; Stefanovic et al., 2007; Rauch et al., 2008) or electrical stimulation (Tolias et al., 2005). Many insights in recent years have come from a combination of methods, not only fMRI or spectroscopy and neurophysiology (Logothetis et al., 2001; Mukamel et al., 2005; Smith et al., 2002), but also from combining optical methods with electrophysiology (Lauritzen and Gold, 2003; Arieli and Grinvald, 2002; Arieli et al., 1996) or fMRI (Kennerley et al., 2005). Because the different methods have different strengths and weaknesses, they provide complementary information, underscoring the importance of multidisciplinary work.

ACKNOWLEDGMENTS

We wish to thank Dr. Alexander Rauch and Dr. Kevin Whittingstall for comments on an earlier version of the manuscript. Supported by the Max-Planck Society.

REFERENCES

Ackermann RF, Finch DM, Babb TL, Engel J, Jr. (1984) Increased glucose metabolism during long-duration recurrent inhibition of hippocampal pyramidal cells. J Neurosci 4:251–264.

Adams DL, Sincich LC, Horton JC (2007) Complete pattern of ocular dominance columns in human primary visual cortex. J Neurosci 27:10391–10403.

Akgoren N, Fabricius M, Lauritzen M (1994) Importance of nitric oxide for local increases of blood flow in rat cerebellar cortex during electrical stimulation. Proc Natl Acad Sci U S A 91:5903–5907.

Ames A, III (2000) CNS energy metabolism as related to function. Brain Res Brain Res Rev 34:42–68.

Arieli A, Grinvald A (2002) Optical imaging combined with targeted electrical recordings, microstimulation, or tracer injections. J Neurosci Methods 116:15–28.

Arieli A, Sterkin A, Grinvald A, Aertsen A (1996) Dynamics of ongoing activity: explanation of the large variability in evoked cortical responses. Science 273:1868–1871.

Attwell D, Iadecola C (2002) The neural basis of functional brain imaging signals. Trends Neurosci 25:621–625.

Attwell D, Laughlin SB (2001) An energy budget for signaling in the grey matter of the brain. J Cereb Blood Flow Metab 21:1133–1145.

Basar E (1980) EEG-Brain dynamics: relation between EEG and brain evoked potentials. Amsterdam, New York, Oxford: Elsevier/North Holland Biomedical Press.

Belitski A, Gretton A, Magri C, Murayama Y, Montemurro MA, Logothetis NK, Panzeri S (2008) Low-frequency local field potentials and spikes in primary visual cortex convey independent visual information. J Neurosci 28:5696–5709.

Belliveau JW, Rosen BR, Kantor HL, Rzedzian RR, Kennedy DN, McKinstry RC, Vevea JM, Cohen MS, Pykett IL, Brady TJ (1990) Functional cerebral imaging by susceptibility-contrast NMR. Magn Reson Med 14:538–546.

Belliveau JW, Kennedy DN, Jr., McKinstry RC, Buchbinder BR, Weisskoff RM, Cohen MS, Vevea JM, Brady TJ, Rosen BR (1991) Functional mapping of the human visual cortex by magnetic resonance imaging. Science 254:716–719.

Blake R, Logothetis NK (2002) Visual competition. Nat Rev Neurosci 3:13–23.

Boxerman JL, Hamberg LM, Rosen BR, Weisskoff RM (1995) MR contrast due to intravascular magnetic susceptibility perturbations. Magn Reson Med 34:555–566.

Braitenberg V, Schüz A (1998) Cortex: statistics and geometry of neuronal connectivity. Berlin: Springer.

Buchwald JS, Grover FS (1970) Amplitudes of background fast activity characteristic of specific brain sites. J Neurophysiol 33:148–159.

Buchwald JS, Hala ES, Schramm S (1965) A comparison of multi-unit activity and EEG activity recorded from the same brain site in chronic cats during behavioral conditioning. Nature 205:1012–1014.

Buxton RB, Uludag K, Dubowitz DJ, Liu TT (2004) Modeling the hemodynamic response to brain activation. Neuroimage 23 (Suppl 1):S220-S233.

Buzsaki G, Chrobak JJ (1995) Temporal structure in spatially organized neuronal ensembles: a role for interneuronal networks. Curr Opin Neurobiol 5:504–510.

Buzsaki G, Bickford RG, Ponomareff G, Thal LJ, Mandel R, Gage FH (1988) Nucleus basalis and thalamic control of neocortical activity in the freely moving rat. J Neurosci 8:4007–4026.

Buzsaki G, Kaila K, Raichle M (2007) Inhibition and brain work. Neuron 56:771–783.

Cauli B, Tong XK, Rancillac A, Serluca N, Lambolez B, Rossier J, Hamel E (2004) Cortical GABA interneurons in neurovascular coupling: relays for subcortical vasoactive pathways. J Neurosci 24:8940–8949.

Chaigneau E, Oheim M, Audinat E, Charpak S (2003) Two-photon imaging of capillary blood flow in olfactory bulb glomeruli. Proc Natl Acad Sci U S A 100:13081–13086.

Cheng K, Waggoner RA, Tanaka K (2001) Human ocular dominance columns as revealed by high-field functional magnetic resonance imaging. Neuron 32:359–374.

Chih CP, Roberts EL, Jr. (2003) Energy substrates for neurons during neural activity: a critical review of the astrocyte-neuron lactate shuttle hypothesis. J Cereb Blood Flow Metab 23:1263–1281.

Ciobanu L, Pennington CH (2004) 3D micron-scale MRI of single biological cells. Solid State Nucl Magn Reson 25:138–141.

Dechent P, Frahm J (2000) Direct mapping of ocular dominance columns in human primary visual cortex. Neuroreport 11:3247–3249.

Dennie J, Mandeville JB, Boxerman JL, Packard SD, Rosen BR, Weisskoff RM (1998) NMR imaging of changes in vascular morphology due to tumor angiogenesis. Magn Reson Med 40:793–799.

Denys K, VanDuffel W, Fize D, Nelissen K, Peuskens H, Van ED, Orban GA (2004) The processing of visual shape in the cerebral cortex of human and nonhuman primates: a functional magnetic resonance imaging study. J Neurosci 24:2551–2565.

Disbrow EA, Slutsky DA, Roberts TP, Krubitzer LA (2000) Functional MRI at 1.5 Tesla: a comparison of the blood oxygenation level-dependent signal and electrophysiology. Proc Natl Acad Sci U S A 97:9718–9723.

Douglas RJ, Martin KA (2007) Mapping the matrix: the ways of neocortex. Neuron 56:226–238.

Duong TQ, Kim DS, Ugurbil K, Kim SG (2001) Localized cerebral blood flow response at submillimeter columnar resolution. Proc Natl Acad Sci U S A 98:10904–10909.

Duong TQ, Yacoub E, Adriany G, Hu XP, Ugurbil K, Kim SG (2003) Microvascular BOLD contribution at 4 and 7T in the human brain: Gradient-echo and spin-echo fMRI with suppression of blood effects. Magn Reson Med 49:1019–1027.

Duvernoy HM, Delon S, Vannson JL (1981) Cortical blood vessels of the human brain. Brain Res Bull 7:519–579.

Engel AK, Moll CK, Fried I, Ojemann GA (2005) Invasive recordings from the human brain: clinical insights and beyond. Nat Rev Neurosci 6:35–47.

Erecinska M, Silver IA (1994) Ions and energy in mammalian brain. Prog Neurobiol 43:37–71.

Faraci FM, Heistad DD (1998) Regulation of the cerebral circulation: role of endothelium and potassium channels. Physiol Rev 78:53–97.

Fergus A, Lee KS (1997) GABAergic regulation of cerebral microvascular tone in the rat. J Cereb Blood Flow Metab 17:992–1003.

Fox PT, Raichle ME (1986) Focal physiological uncoupling of cerebral blood-flow and oxidative-metabolism during somatosensory stimulation in human-subjects. Proc Natl Acad Sci U S A 83:1140–1144.

Fox PT, Raichle ME, Mintun MA, Dence C (1988) Nonoxidative glucose consumption during focal physiologic neural activity. Science 241:462–464.

Friston KJ, Holmes AP, Poline JB, Grasby PJ, Williams SC, Frackowiak RS, Turner R (1995) Analysis of fMRI time-series revisited. Neuroimage 2:45–53.

Fromm GH, Bond HW (1964) Slow changes in the electrocorticogram and the activity of cortical neurons. Electroencephalogr Clin Neurophysiol 17:520–523.

Fromm GH, Bond HW (1967) The relationship between neuron activity and cortical steady potentials. Electroen Clin Neuro 22:159–166.

Fu R, Brey WW, Shetty K, Gor'kov P, Saha S, Long JR, Grant SC, Chekmenev EY, Hu J, Gan Z, Sharma M, Zhang F, Logan TM, Bruschweller R, Edison A, Blue A, Dixon IR, Markiewicz WD, Cross TA (2005) Ultra-wide bore 900 MHz high-resolution NMR at the National High Magnetic Field Laboratory. J Magn Reson 177:1–8.

Gasser HS, Grundfest H (1939) Axon diameters in relation to the spike dimensions and the conduction velocity in mammalian A fibers. Am J Physiol 127:393–414. Gjedde A, Marrett S (2001) Glycolysis in neurons, not astrocytes, delays oxidative metabolism of human visual cortex during sustained checkerboard stimulation in vivo. J Cereb Blood Flow Metab 21:1384–1392.

Gladden LB (2004) Lactate metabolism: a new paradigm for the third millennium. J Physiol 558:5–30.

Goense JB, Logothetis NK (2006) Laminar specificity in monkey V1 using high-resolution SE-fMRI. Magn Reson Imaging 24:381–392.

Goense JB, Logothetis NK (2008) Neurophysiology of the BOLD fMRI signal in awake monkeys. Curr Biol 18:631–640.

Goense JB, Zappe AC, Logothetis NK (2007) High-resolution fMRI of macaque V1. Magn Reson Imaging 25:740–747.

Granit R, Kernell D, Smith RS (1963) Delayed depolarization and the repetitive response to intracellular stimulation of mammalian motoneurones. J Physiol 168:890–910.

Gray CM, Maldonado PE, Wilson M, McNaughton B (1995) Tetrodes markedly improve the reliability and yield of multiple single-unit isolation from multi-unit recordings in cat striate cortex. J Neurosci Methods 63:43–54.

Grover FS, Buchwald JS (1970) Correlation of cell size with amplitude of background fast activity in specific brain nuclei. Journal of Neurophysiology 33:160–171.

Gsell W, Burke M, Wiedermann D, Bonvento G, Silva AC, Dauphin F, Buhrle C, Hoehn M, Schwindt W (2006) Differential effects of NMDA and AMPA glutamate receptors on functional magnetic resonance imaging signals and evoked neuronal activity during forepaw stimulation of the rat. J Neurosci 26:8409–8416.

Gur M, Beylin A, Snodderly DM (1999) Physiological properties of macaque V1 neurons are correlated with extracellular spike amplitude, duration, and polarity. J Neurophysiol 82:1451–1464.

Gustafsson B (1984) Afterpotentials and transduction properties in different types of central neurones. Arch Ital Biol 122:17–30.

Haacke EM, Lin WL, Hu XP, Thulborn K (2001) A current perspective of the status of understanding BOLD imaging and its use in studying brain function: a summary of the workshop at the University of North Carolina in Chapel Hill, 26–28 October, 2000. NMR in Biomedicine 14:384–388.

Hamel E (2006) Perivascular nerves and the regulation of cerebrovascular tone. J Appl Physiol 100:1059–1064.

Harada Y, Takahashi T (1983) The calcium component of the action potential in spinal motoneurones of the rat. J Physiol 335:89–100.

Harel N, Lin J, Moeller S, Ugurbil K, Yacoub E (2006a) Combined imaging-histological study of cortical laminar specificity of fMRI signals. Neuroimage 29:879–887.

Harel N, Ugurbil K, Uludag K, Yacoub E (2006b) Frontiers of brain mapping using MRI. J Magn Reson Imaging 23:945–957.

Henze DA, Borhegyi Z, Csicsvari J, Mamiya A, Harris KD, Buzsaki G (2000) Intracellular features predicted by extracellular recordings in the hippocampus in vivo. J Neurophysiol 84:390–400.

Hevner RF, Duff RS, Wong-Riley MT (1992) Coordination of ATP production and consumption in brain: parallel regulation of cytochrome oxidase and Na+, K(+)-ATPase. Neurosci Lett 138:188–192.

Higashi H, Tanaka E, Inokuchi H, Nishi S (1993) Ionic mechanisms underlying the depolarizing and hyperpolarizing afterpotentials of single spike in guinea-pig cingulate cortical neurons. Neuroscience 55:129–138.

Hirase H, Creso J, Singleton M, Bartho P, Buzsaki G (2004) Two-photon imaging of brain pericytes in vivo using dextran-conjugated dyes. Glia 46:95–100.

Hoffmeyer HW, Enager P, Thomsen KJ, Lauritzen MJ (2007) Nonlinear neurovascular coupling in rat sensory cortex by activation of transcallosal fibers. J Cereb Blood Flow Metab 27:575–587.

Hunt C (1951) The reflex activity of mammalian small-nerve fibers. J Physiol (Lond) 115:456–469.

Hyder F, Patel AB, Gjedde A, Rothman DL, Behar KL, Shulman RG (2006) Neuronal-glial glucose oxidation and glutamatergic-GABAergic function. J Cereb Blood Flow Metab 26:865–877.

Iadecola C (2004) Neurovascular regulation in the normal brain and in Alzheimer's disease. Nat Rev Neurosci 5:347–360.

Iadecola C, Nedergaard M (2007) Glial regulation of the cerebral microvasculature. Nat Neurosci 10:1369–1376.

Ido Y, Chang K, Woolsey TA, Williamson JR (2001) NADH: sensor of blood flow need in brain, muscle, and other tissues. FASEB J 15:1419–1421.

Ido Y, Chang K, Williamson JR (2004) NADH augments blood flow in physiologically activated retina and visual cortex. Proc Natl Acad Sci U S A 101:653–658.

Ito H, Ibaraki M, Kanno I, Fukuda H, Miura S (2005) Changes in the arterial fraction of human cerebral blood volume during hypercapnia and hypocapnia measured by positron emission tomography. J Cereb Blood Flow Metab 25:852–857.

Jin T, Zhao F, Kim SG (2006) Sources of functional apparent diffusion coefficient changes investigated by diffusion-weighted spin-echo fMRI. Magn Reson Med 56:1283–1292.

Juergens E, Eckhorn R, Frien A, Woelbern T (1996) Restricted coupling range of fast oscillations in striate cortex of awake monkey. In: Brain and evolution (Elsner N, Schnitzler, H-U, eds), pp 418. Berlin, New York: Thieme.

Juergens E, Guettler A, Eckhorn R (1999) Visual stimulation elicits locked and induced gamma oscillations in monkey intracortical- and EEG-potentials, but not in human EEG. Exp Brain Res 129:247–259.

Kamondi A, Acsady L, Wang XJ, Buzsaki G (1998) Theta oscillations in somata and dendrites of hippocampal pyramidal cells in vivo: activity-dependent phase-precession of action potentials. Hippocampus 8:244–261.

Kandel A, Buzsaki G (1997) Cellular-synaptic generation of sleep spindles, spike-and-wave discharges, and evoked thalamocortical responses in the neocortex of the rat. J Neurosci 17:6783–6797.

Katzner S, Nauhaus I, Benucci A, Bonin V, Ringach DL, Carandini M (2009) Local origin of field potentials in visual cortex. Neuron 61:35–41.

Keliris GA, Shmuel A, Ku SP, Pfeuffer J, Oeltermann A, Steudel T, Logothetis NK (2007) Robust controlled functional MRI in alert monkeys at high magnetic field: effects of jaw and body movements. Neuroimage 36:550–570.

Kennan RP, Zhong J, Gore JC (1994) Intravascular susceptibility contrast mechanisms in tissues. Magn Reson Med 31:9–21.

Kennedy C, Des Rosiers MH, Sakurada O, Shinohara M, Reivich M, Jehle JW, Sokoloff L (1976) Metabolic mapping of the primary visual system of the monkey by means of the autoradiographic [14C]deoxyglucose technique. Proc Natl Acad Sci U S A 73:4230–4234.

Kennerley AJ, Berwick J, Martindale J, Johnston D, Papadakis N, Mayhew JE (2005) Concurrent fMRI and optical measures for the investigation of the hemodynamic response function. Magn Reson Med 54:354–365.

Kida I, Smith AJ, Blumenfeld H, Behar KL, Hyder F (2006) Lamotrigine suppresses neurophysiological responses to somatosensory stimulation in the rodent. Neuroimage 29:216–224.

Kim T, Hendrich KS, Masamoto K, Kim SG (2007) Arterial versus total blood volume changes during neural activity-induced cerebral blood flow change: implication for BOLD fMRI. J Cereb Blood Flow Metab 27:1235–1247.

Kobayashi M, Inoue T, Matsuo R, Masuda Y, Hidaka O, Kang Y, Morimoto T (1997) Role of calcium conductances on spike afterpotentials in rat trigeminal motoneurons. J Neurophysiol 77:3273–3283.

Kocsis B, Bragin A, Buzsaki G (1999) Interdependence of multiple theta generators in the hippocampus: a partial coherence analysis. J Neurosci 19:6200–6212.

Koehler RC, Gebremedhin D, Harder DR (2006) Role of astrocytes in cerebrovascular regulation. J Appl Physiol 100:307–317.

Koyama M, Hasegawa I, Osada T, Adachi Y, Nakahara K, Miyashita Y (2004) Functional magnetic resonance imaging of macaque monkeys performing visually guided saccade tasks: comparison of cortical eye fields with humans. Neuron 41:795–807.

Kreiman G, Hung CP, Kraskov A, Quiroga RQ, Poggio T, DiCarlo JJ (2006) Object selectivity of local field potentials and spikes in the macaque inferior temporal cortex. Neuron 49:433–445.

Kwong KK, Belliveau JW, Chesler DA, Goldberg IE, Weisskoff RM, Poncelet BP, Kennedy DN, Hoppel BE, Cohen MS, Turner R (1992) Dynamic magnetic resonance imaging of human brain activity during primary sensory stimulation. Proc Natl Acad Sci U S A 89:5675–5679.

Lauritzen M (2005) Reading vascular changes in brain imaging: is dendritic calcium the key? Nat Rev Neurosci 6:77–85.

Lauritzen M, Gold L (2003) Brain function and neurophysiological correlates of signals used in functional neuroimaging. J Neurosci 23:3972–3980.

Lauterbur PC (1973) Image formation by induced local interactions—examples employing nuclear magnetic-resonance. Nature 242:190–191.

Lauwers F, Cassot F, Lauwers-Cances V, Puwanarajah P, Duvernoy H (2008) Morphometry of the human cerebral cortex microcirculation: general characteristics and space-related profiles. Neuroimage 39:936–948.

Legatt AD, Arezzo J, Vaughan HGJ (1980) Averaged multiple unit activity as an estimate of phasic changes in local neuronal activity: effects of volume-conducted potentials. J Neurosci Meth 2:203–217.

Lennie P (2003) The cost of cortical computation. Curr Biol 13:493–497.

Li J, Iadecola C (1994) Nitric oxide and adenosine mediate vasodilation during functional activation in cerebellar cortex. Neuropharmacology 33:1453–1461.

Lindsley DB, Wicke JD (1974) The electroencephalogram: autonomous electrical activity in man and animals. In: Electroencephalography and human brain potentials (Thomson RF, Patterson MM, eds), pp 3–83. New York: Academic Press.

Lipton ML, Fu KMG, Branch CA, Schroeder CE (2006) Ipsilateral hand input to area 3b revealed by converging hemodynamic and electrophysiological analyses in macaque monkeys. J Neurosci 26:180–185.

Logothetis NK (2003) MR imaging in the non-human primate: studies of function and of dynamic connectivity. Curr Opin Neurobiol 13:630–642.

Logothetis NK (2008) What we can do and what we cannot do with fMRI. Nature 453:869–878.

Logothetis NK, Guggenberger H, Peled S, Pauls J (1999) Functional imaging of the monkey brain. Nat Neurosci 2:555–562.

Logothetis NK, Pauls J, Augath M, Trinath T, Oeltermann A (2001) Neurophysiological investigation of the basis of the fMRI signal. Nature 412:150–157.

Logothetis NK, Merkle H, Augath M, Trinath T, Ugurbil K (2002) Ultra high-resolution fMRI in monkeys with implanted RF coils. Neuron 35:227–242.

Logothetis NK, Kayser C, Oeltermann A (2007) In vivo measurement of cortical impedance spectrum in monkeys: implications for signal propagation. Neuron 55:809–823.

Lorente de Nó (1947) A study of nerve physiology. Part I and II. Studies from the Rockefeller Institute for medical Research 131 and 132.

Lowel S, Freeman B, Singer W (1987) Topographic organization of the orientation column system in large flat-mounts of the cat visual cortex: a 2-deoxyglucose study. J Comp Neurol 255:401–415.

Lu H, Zuo Y, Gu H, Waltz JA, Zhan W, Scholl CA, Rea W, Yang Y, Stein EA (2007) Synchronized delta oscillations correlate with the resting-state functional MRI signal. Proc Natl Acad Sci U S A 104:18265–18269.

Maandag NJ, Coman D, Sanganahalli BG, Herman P, Smith AJ, Blumenfeld H, Shulman RG, Hyder F (2007) Energetics of neuronal signaling and fMRI activity. Proc Natl Acad Sci U S A 104:20546–20551.

Mangia S, Tkac I, Gruetter R, Van de Moortele PF, Maraviglia B, Ugurbil K (2007) Sustained neuronal activation raises oxidative metabolism to a new steady-state level: evidence from 1H NMR spectroscopy in the human visual cortex. J Cereb Blood Flow Metab 27:1055–1063.

Mansfield P (1977) Multi-planar image-formation using NMR spin echoes. J Phys C Solid State 10:L55–L58.

Mata M, Fink DJ, Gainer H, Smith CB, Davidsen L, Savaki H, Schwartz WJ, Sokoloff L (1980) Activity-dependent energy metabolism in rat posterior pituitary primarily reflects sodium pump activity. J Neurochem 34:213–215.

Mathiesen C, Caesar K, Akgoren N, Lauritzen M (1998) Modification of activity-dependent increases of cerebral blood flow by excitatory synaptic activity and spikes in rat cerebellar cortex. J Physiol 512 (Pt 2):555–566.

McCasland JS, Hibbard LS (1997) GABAergic neurons in barrel cortex show strong, whisker-dependent metabolic activation during normal behavior. J Neurosci 17:5509–5527.

Menon RS, Goodyear BG (1999) Submillimeter functional localization in human striate cortex using BOLD contrast at 4 Tesla: implications for the vascular point-spread function. Magn Reson Med 41:230–235.

Metea MR, Newman EA (2006) Glial cells dilate and constrict blood vessels: a mechanism of neurovascular coupling. J Neurosci 26:2862–2870.

Mintun MA, Vlassenko AG, Shulman GL, Snyder AZ (2002) Time-related increase of oxygen utilization in continuously activated human visual cortex. Neuroimage 16:531–537.

Mitzdorf U (1985) Current source-density method and application in cat cerebral cortex: investigation of evoked potentials and EEG phenomena. Physiol Rev 65:37–100.

Mitzdorf U (1987) Properties of the evoked potential generators: current source-density analysis of visually evoked potentials in the cat cortex. Int J Neurosci 33:33–59.

Moon CH, Fukuda M, Park SH, Kim SG (2007) Neural interpretation of blood oxygenation level-dependent fMRI maps at submillimeter columnar resolution. J Neurosci 27:6892–6902.

Mukamel R, Gelbard H, Arieli A, Hasson U, Fried I, Malach R (2005) Coupling between neuronal firing, field potentials, and fMRI in human auditory cortex. Science 309:951–954.

Mulligan SJ, Macvicar BA (2004) Calcium transients in astrocyte endfeet cause cerebrovascular constrictions. Nature 431:195–199.

Nakada T, Nabetani A, Kabasawa H, Nozaki A, Matsuzawa H (2005) The passage to human MR microscopy: a progress report from Niigata on April 2005. Magn Reson Med Sci 4:83–87.

Nakahara K, Hayashi T, Konishi S, Miyashita Y (2002) Functional MRI of macaque monkeys performing a cognitive set-shifting task. Science 295:1532–1536.

Nauhaus I, Busse L, Carandini M, Ringach DL (2009) Stimulus contrast modulates functional connectivity in visual cortex. Nat Neurosci 12:70–76.

Nedergaard M, Ransom B, Goldman SA (2003) New roles for astrocytes: redefining the functional architecture of the brain. Trends Neurosci 26:523–530.

Nelson PG (1966) Interaction between spinal motoneurons of the cat. J Neurophysiol 29:275–287.

Newman EA (2003) New roles for astrocytes: regulation of synaptic transmission. Trends Neurosci 26:536–542.

Nicholson C, Llinas R (1971) Field potentials in the alligator cerebellum and theory of their relationship to Purkinje cell dendritic spikes. J Neurophysiol 34:509–531.

Niessing J, Ebisch B, Schmidt KE, Niessing M, Singer W, Galuske RA (2005) Hemodynamic signals correlate tightly with synchronized gamma oscillations. Science 309:948–951.

Nudo RJ, Masterton RB (1986) Stimulation-induced [14C]2-Deoxyglucose labeling of synaptic activity in the central auditory system. J Comp Neurol 245:553–565.

Oeltermann A, Augath MA, Logothetis NK (2007) Simultaneous recording of neuronal signals and functional NMR imaging. Magn Reson Imaging 25:760–774.

Ogawa S, Lee TM, Kay AR, Tank DW (1990) Brain magnetic resonance imaging with contrast dependent on blood oxygenation. Proc Natl Acad Sci U S A 87:9868–9872.

Ogawa S, Tank DW, Menon R, Ellermann JM, Kim SG, Merkle H, Ugurbil K (1992) Intrinsic signal changes accompanying sensory stimulation—functional brain mapping with magnetic-resonance-imaging. Proc Natl Acad Sci U S A 89:5951–5955.

Ogawa S, Lee TM, Stepnoski R, Chen W, Zhuo XH, Ugurbil K (2000) An approach to probe some neural systems interaction by functional MRI at neural time scale down to milliseconds. Proc Natl Acad Sci U S A 97:11026–11031.

Patel AB, de Graaf RA, Mason GF, Rothman DL, Shulman RG, Behar KL (2005) The contribution of GABA to glutamate/glutamine cycling and energy metabolism in the rat cortex in vivo. Proc Natl Acad Sci U S A 102:5588–5593.

Pellerin L, Magistretti PJ (1994) Glutamate uptake into astrocytes stimulates aerobic glycolysis: a mechanism coupling neuronal activity to glucose utilization. Proc Natl Acad Sci U S A 91:10625–10629.

Pellerin L, Magistretti PJ (2003) Food for thought: challenging the dogmas. J Cereb Blood Flow Metab 23:1282–1286.

Pellerin L, Bouzier-Sore AK, Aubert A, Serres S, Merle M, Costalat R, Magistretti PJ (2007) Activity-dependent regulation of energy metabolism by astrocytes: an update. Glia 55:1251–1262.

Peppiatt C, Attwell D (2004) Neurobiology: feeding the brain. Nature 431:137–138.

Peters A, Payne BR (1993) Numerical relationships between geniculocortical afferents and pyramidal cell modules in cat primary visual cortex. Cereb Cortex 3:69–78.

Peters A, Payne BR, Budd J (1994) A numerical analysis of the geniculocortical input to striate cortex in the monkey. Cereb Cortex 4:215–229.

Petzold GC, Albeanu DF, Sato TF, Murthy VN (2008) Coupling of neural activity to blood flow in olfactory glomeruli is mediated by astrocytic pathways. Neuron 58:897–910.

Pfeuffer J, Van de Moortele PF, Yacoub E, Shmuel A, Adriany G, Andersen P, Merkle H, Garwood M, Ugurbil K, Hu XP (2002) Zoomed functional imaging in the human brain at 7 Tesla with simultaneous high spatial and high temporal resolution. Neuroimage 17:272–286.

Pfeuffer J, Merkle H, Beyerlein M, Steudel T, Logothetis NK (2004) Anatomical and functional MR imaging in the macaque monkey using a vertical large-bore 7 Tesla setup. Magn Reson Imaging 22:1343–1359.

Prichard J, Rothman D, Novotny E, Petroff O, Kuwabara T, Avison M, Howseman A, Hanstock C, Shulman R (1991) Lactate rise detected by 1H NMR in human visual cortex during physiologic stimulation. Proc Natl Acad Sci U S A 88:5829–5831.

Privman E, Nir Y, Kramer U, Kipervasser S, Andelman F, Neufeld MY, Mukamel R, Yeshurun Y, Fried I, Malach R (2007) Enhanced category tuning revealed by intracranial electroencephalograms in high-order human visual areas. J Neurosci 27:6234–6242.

Raichle ME (2000) A brief history of human functional brain mapping. In: Brain mapping: the systems (Toga AW, Mazziotta JC, eds), pp 33–75. San Diego: Academic Press.

Raichle ME, Mintun MA (2006) Brain work and brain imaging. Annu Rev Neurosci 29:449–476.

Rajimehr R, Young JC, Tootell RB (2009) An anterior temporal face patch in human cortex, predicted by macaque maps. Proc Natl Acad Sci U S A 106:1995–2000.

Rauch A, Rainer G, Logothetis NK (2008) The effect of a serotonin-induced dissociation between spiking and perisynaptic activity on BOLD functional MRI. Proc Natl Acad Sci U S A 105:6759–6764.

Riera JJ, Schousboe A, Waagepetersen HS, Howarth C, Hyder F (2008) The micro-architecture of the cerebral cortex: functional neuroimaging models and metabolism. Neuroimage 40:1436–1459.

Sappey-Marinier D, Calabrese G, Fein G, Hugg JW, Biggins C, Weiner MW (1992) Effect of photic stimulation on human visual cortex lactate and phosphates using 1H and 31P magnetic resonance spectroscopy. J Cereb Blood Flow Metab 12:584–592.

Sawamura H, Georgieva S, Vogels R, VanDuffel W, Orban GA (2005) Using functional magnetic resonance imaging to assess adaptation and size invariance of shape processing by humans and monkeys. J Neurosci 25:4294–4306.

Schummers J, Yu H, Sur M (2008) Tuned responses of astrocytes and their influence on hemodynamic signals in the visual cortex. Science 320:1638–1643.

Schwartz WJ, Smith CB, Davidsen L, Savaki H, Sokoloff L, Mata M, Fink DJ, Gainer H (1979) Metabolic mapping of functional activity in the hypothalamo-neurohypophysial system of the rat. Science 205:723–725.

Shmuel A, Augath M, Oeltermann A, Logothetis NK (2006) Negative functional MRI response correlates with decreases in neuronal activity in monkey visual area V1. Nat Neurosci 9:569–577.

Shoham S, O'Connor DH, Segev R (2006) How silent is the brain: is there a "dark matter" problem in neuroscience? J Comp Physiol A 192:777–784.

Shulman RG, Rothman DL, Behar KL, Hyder F (2004) Energetic basis of brain activity: implications for neuroimaging. Trends Neurosci 27:489–495.

Silva AC, Koretsky AP (2002) Laminar specificity of functional MRI onset times during somatosensory stimulation in rat. Proc Natl Acad Sci U S A 99:15182–15187.

Simard M, Nedergaard M (2004) The neurobiology of glia in the context of water and ion homeostasis. Neuroscience 129:877–896.

Smith AJ, Blumenfeld H, Behar KL, Rothman DL, Shulman RG, Hyder F (2002) Cerebral energetics and spiking frequency: the neurophysiological basis of fMRI. Proc Natl Acad Sci U S A 99:10765–10770.

Sokoloff L (1960) The metabolism of the central nervous system in vivo. In: Handbook of physiology-neurophysiology (Field J, Magoun HW, Hall VE, eds), pp 1843–1864. Washington DC: American Physiological Society.

Sokoloff L (1999) Energetics of functional activation in neural tissues. Neurochem Res 24:321–329.

Stefanovic B, Schwindt W, Hoehn M, Silva AC (2007) Functional uncoupling of hemodynamic from neuronal response by inhibition of neuronal nitric oxide synthase. J Cereb Blood Flow Metab 27:741–754.

Steriade M (1991) Alertness, quiet sleep, dreaming. In: Cerebral Cortex Vol 9 (Peters A, ed), pp 279–357. New York, London: Plenum Press.

Steriade M, Hobson J (1976) Neuronal activity during the sleep-waking cycle. Prog Neurobiol 6:155–376.

Stone J (1973) Sampling properties of microelectrodes assessed in the cat's retina. J Neurophysiol 36:1071–1079.

Szentagothai J (1978) The Ferrier Lecture, 1977. The neuron network of the cerebral cortex: a functional interpretation. Proc R Soc Lond B Biol Sci 201:219–248.

Takano T, Tian GF, Peng W, Lou N, Libionka W, Han X, Nedergaard M (2006) Astrocyte-mediated control of cerebral blood flow. Nat Neurosci 9:260–267.

Thulborn KR (2006) The challenges of integrating a 9.4T MR scanner for human brain imaging. In: Ultra high magnetic field resonance imaging (Robitaille PM, Berliner LJ, eds), pp 105–126. New York: Springer.

Tolias AS, Sultan F, Augath M, Oeltermann A, Tehovnik EJ, Schiller PH, Logothetis NK (2005) Mapping cortical activity elicited with electrical microstimulation using FMRI in the macaque. Neuron 48:901–911.

Towe AL, Harding GW (1970) Extracellular microelectrode sampling bias. Exp Neurol 29:366–381.

Ts'o DY, Frostig RD, Lieke EE, Grinvald A (1990) Functional organization of primate visual cortex revealed by high resolution optical imaging. Science 249:417–420.

Tsao DY, VanDuffel W, Sasaki Y, Fize D, Knutsen TA, Mandeville JB, Wald LL, Dale AM, Rosen BR, Van Essen DC, Livingstone MS, Orban GA, Tootell RB (2003) Stereopsis activates V3A and caudal intraparietal areas in macaques and humans. Neuron 39:555–568.

Tsao DY, Freiwald WA, Tootell RB, Livingstone MS (2006) A cortical region consisting entirely of face-selective cells. Science 311:670–674.

Tsao DY, Moeller S, Freiwald WA (2008) Comparing face patch systems in macaques and humans. Proc Natl Acad Sci U S A 105:19514–19519.

Ugurbil K, Adriany G, Andersen P, Chen W, Gruetter R, Hu XP, Merkle H, Kim DS, Kim SG, Strupp J, Zhu XH, Ogawa S (2000) Magnetic resonance studies of brain function and neurochemistry. Annu Rev Biomed Eng 2:633–660.

Ugurbil K, Toth L, Kim DS (2003) How accurate is magnetic resonance imaging of brain function? Trends Neurosci 26:108–114.

Ugurbil K, Adriany G, Akgun C, Andersen P, Chen W, Garwood M, Gruetter R, Henry PG, Marjanska M, Moeller S, Van de Moortele PF, Pruessmann KP, Tkac I, Vaughan JT, Wiesinger F, Yacoub E, Zhu XH (2006) High magnetic fields for imaging cerebral morphology, function, and biochemistry. In: Ultra high field magnetic resonance imaging (Robitaille PM, Berliner LJ, eds), pp 285–342. New York: Springer.

Uludag K, Müller-Bierl B, Ugurbil K (2009) An Integrative model for neuronal activity-induced signal changes for gradient and spin echo functional imaging. Neuroimage 48:150–165.

VanDuffel W, Fize D, Peuskens H, Denys K, Sunaert S, Todd JT, Orban GA (2002) Extracting 3D from motion: differences in human and monkey intraparietal cortex. Science 298:413–415.

Viswanathan A, Freeman RD (2007) Neurometabolic coupling in cerebral cortex reflects synaptic more than spiking activity. Nat Neurosci 10:1308–1312.

Vlassenko AG, Rundle MM, Mintun MA (2006a) Human brain glucose metabolism may evolve during activation: findings from a modified FDG PET paradigm. Neuroimage 33:1036–1041.

Vlassenko AG, Rundle MM, Raichle ME, Mintun MA (2006b) Regulation of blood flow in activated human brain by cytosolic NADH/NAD+ ratio. Proc Natl Acad Sci U S A 103: 1964–1969.

Wald LL, Fischl B, Rosen BR (2006) High-resolution and microscopic imaging at high field. In: Ultra high field magnetic resonance imaging (Robitaille PM, Berliner LJ, eds), pp. 343–371. New York: Springer.

Waldvogel D, van GP, Muellbacher W, Ziemann U, Immisch I, Hallett M (2000) The relative metabolic demand of inhibition and excitation. Nature 406:995–998.

Wang H, Hitron IM, Iadecola C, Pickel VM (2005) Synaptic and vascular associations of neurons containing cyclooxygenase-2 and nitric oxide synthase in rat somatosensory cortex. Cereb Cortex 15:1250–1260.

Weber B, Keller AL, Reichold J, Logothetis NK (2008) The microvascular system of the striate and extrastriate visual cortex of the macaque. Cereb Cortex 18:2318–2330.

Weisskoff RM, Zuo CS, Boxerman JL, Rosen BR (1994) Microscopic susceptibility variation and transverse relaxation: theory and experiment. Magn Reson Med 31:601–610.

Wong-Riley MT (1989) Cytochrome oxidase: an endogenous metabolic marker for neuronal activity. Trends Neurosci 12:94–101.

Wu EX, Tang H, Jensen JH (2004) Applications of ultrasmall superparamagnetic iron oxide contrast agents in the MR study of animal models. NMR Biomed 17:478–483.

Xu F, Liu N, Kida I, Rothman DL, Hyder F, Shepherd GM (2003) Odor maps of aldehydes and esters revealed by functional MRI in the glomerular layer of the mouse olfactory bulb. Proc Natl Acad Sci U S A 100:11029–11034.

Yacoub E, Shmuel A, Pfeuffer J, Van de Moortele PF, Adriany G, Andersen P, Vaughan JT, Merkle H, Ugurbil K, Hu XP (2001) Imaging brain function in humans at 7 Tesla. Magn Reson Med 45:588–594.

Yacoub E, Van de Moortele PF, Shmuel A, Ugurbil K (2005) Signal and noise characteristics of Hahn SE and GE BOLD fMRI at 7T in humans. Neuroimage 24:738–750.

Yacoub E, Ugurbil K, Harel N (2006) The spatial dependence of the poststimulus undershoot as revealed by high-resolution BOLD- and CBV-weighted fMRI. J Cereb Blood Flow Metab 26:634–644.

Yacoub E, Shmuel A, Logothetis N, Ugurbil K (2007) Robust detection of ocular dominance columns in humans using Hahn Spin Echo BOLD functional MRI at 7 Tesla. Neuroimage 37:1161–1177.

Yacoub E, Harel N, Ugurbil K (2008) High-field fMRI unveils orientation columns in humans. Proc Natl Acad Sci U S A 105:10607–10612.

Yang G, Zhang Y, Ross ME, Iadecola C (2003) Attenuation of activity-induced increases in cerebellar blood flow in mice lacking neuronal nitric oxide synthase. Am J Physiol Heart Circ Physiol 285:H298-H304.

Zago S, Ferrucci R, Marceglia S, Priori A (2009) The Mosso method for recording brain pulsation: the forerunner of functional neuroimaging. Neuroimage 48:652-656

Zappe AC, Pfeuffer J, Merkle H, Logothetis NK, Goense JB (2008) The effect of labeling parameters on perfusion-based fMRI in nonhuman primates. J Cereb Blood Flow Metab 28:640–652.

Zhang C, Wong-Riley MT (1996) Do nitric oxide synthase, NMDA receptor subunit R1 and cytochrome oxidase co-localize in the rat central nervous system? Brain Res 729:205–215.

Zhao F, Wang P, Kim SG (2004) Cortical depth-dependent gradient-echo and spin-echo BOLD fMRI at 9.4T. Magn Reson Med 51:518–524.

Zhao F, Wang P, Hendrich K, Kim SG (2005) Spatial specificity of cerebral blood volume-weighted fMRI responses at columnar resolution. Neuroimage 27:416–424.

Zhao F, Wang P, Hendrich K, Ugurbil K, Kim SG (2006) Cortical layer-dependent BOLD and CBV responses measured by spin-echo and gradient-echo fMRI: insights into hemodynamic regulation. Neuroimage 30:1149–1160.

Zhao F, Jin T, Wang P, Kim SG (2007) Improved spatial localization of post-stimulus BOLD undershoot relative to positive BOLD. Neuroimage 34:1084–1092.

Zonta M, Angulo MC, Gobbo S, Rosengarten B, Hossmann KA, Pozzan T, Carmignoto G (2003) Neuron-to-astrocyte signaling is central to the dynamic control of brain microcirculation. Nat Neurosci 6:43–50.

1.3

Abraham Z. Snyder and Marcus E. Raichle

Studies of the Human Brain Combining Functional Neuroimaging and Electrophysiological Methods

Introduction

If it is accepted that the brain implements logic via dendritic currents, action potentials, and synaptic signaling, it follows that the operations of the brain can be directly observed by electrophysiological recording. Electrophysiological techniques that are generally applicable to the human brain include gross potential recording directly over the cortical surface (electrocorticography, or ECoG), magnetoencephalography (MEG) and electroencephalography (scalp recording, or EEG). While these techniques provide essentially unlimited sampling of high temporal frequencies, they provide only limited spatial sampling, and none are capable of recording from the whole brain at once. Awareness of this spatial limitation and the availability of functional neuroimaging (FNI) techniques such as positron emission tomography (PET) and functional magnetic resonance imaging (fMRI) have led to efforts to combine techniques, particularly in studies of the human brain.

FNI techniques such as PET and fMRI gain access to the activity of the brain through changes in blood flow and metabolism that accompany with remarkable fidelity regional changes in the activity of the brain (Raichle and Mintun, 2006). While the temporal resolution of these techniques falls far below that of the electrophysiological techniques (Table 1.3.1) they do offer full 3D coverage of the human brain at subcentimeter resolution. For example, fMRI voxel dimensions typically are on the order of 2 to 4 mm and, thus, far superior to electrophysiological techniques available for the study of normal humans. Because fMRI BOLD imaging is now the dominant FNI technique it will be the focus of this review.

Because of their complementarity with regard to spatial and temporal resolution, research combining the EEG with fMRI has been advocated. However, combining electrophysiology with neuroimaging does not necessarily yield a hybrid technique with good sampling properties in both the temporal and spatial domains (see Figure 1.3.1).

Nevertheless, combined methodology studies, mostly using EEG and BOLD fMRI, have produced significant advances in systems neuroscience. Before reviewing what has been accomplished with combined methodology, we briefly review what is known about the underlying physiology with a view to understanding potential points of connection between FNI and electrophysiology.

A Brief Physiological Review

The electrophysiological correlates of fMRI have been elucidated in considerable detail during the past several years (Logothetis and Pfeuffer, 2004; see also Chapter 1.2 in this volume). Arguably, the most remarkable physiological finding of the past decade is that BOLD modulations are more tightly coupled to local field potentials (LFPs), which reflect dendritic activity, than to single-unit discharge (Logothetis et al., 2001). This result expands one's view of what is important in neurophysiology, a field that has since the 1950s attached importance primarily if not exclusively to action potentials recorded from single neurons. Thus, it makes sense to formulate the level of activity within brain areas as a state variable that can be both imaged as the BOLD signal and electrophysiologically measured as LFP power. This notion applies to activity decreases as well as increases (Shmuel et al., 2006). Power over a broad range of LFP temporal frequencies exhibits tight linkage to the task-evoked fMRI BOLD signal; this coupling is strongest at 20–60 Hz (Goense and Logothetis, 2008), that is, frequencies spanning the beta (13–30 Hz) and lower end gamma bands (30–80 Hz).

The importance of the LFP-BOLD coupling in the study of cognition is magnified by evidence that synchronous

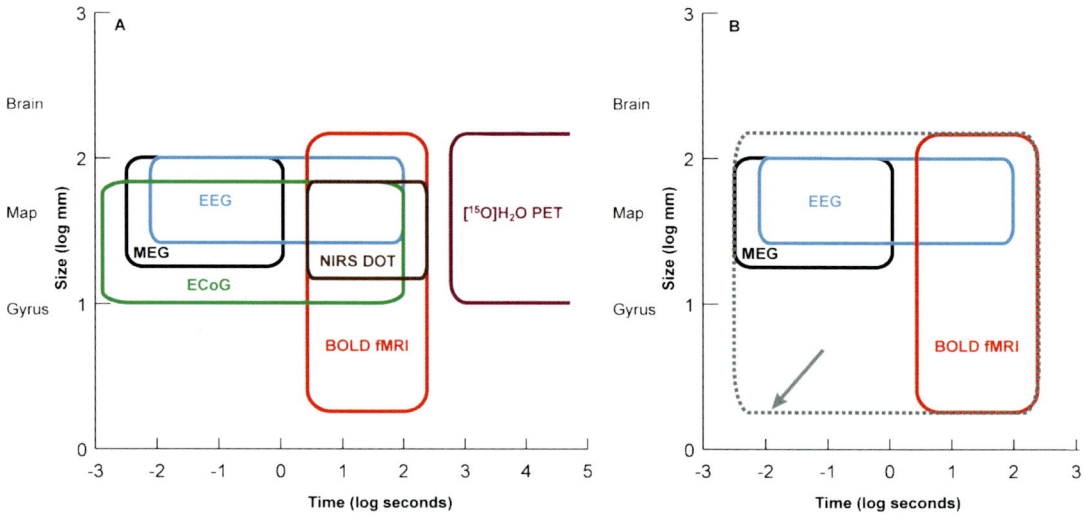

Figure 1.3.1. A: Spatiotemporal sampling characteristics of the techniques listed in Table 1.3.1 (after Churchland and Sejnowski, 1988). Each technique is represented as a closed region. The left edge of each region indicates the reciprocal of the highest physiologically meaningful temporal frequency accessible to each technique. The right edge indicates the longest practical period of continuous observation. The lower edge indicates the smallest practical distance between independent samples. The upper edge indicates the spatial range of contiguous recording. Note: Electrophysiological and imaging techniques provide, respectively, faster and slower sampling (appear on the left and right portions of the Time axis). NIRS DOT and BOLD fMRI have identical temporal (but not spatial) sampling characteristics. The gap between BOLD fMRI and [^{15}O]H$_2$O PET corresponds to the fact that drift in the BOLD signal limits meaningful comparison of physiological responses to intervals shorter than ~5 minutes, whereas successive PET scans must be separated by at least 12 minutes (~6 half-lives of ^{15}O). The open right edge of the [^{15}O]H$_2$O PET figure corresponds to the fact that it is theoretically possible to measure changes in absolute regional cerebral blood flow (rCBF) over arbitrarily long intervals. B: Techniques used in combined electrophysiology-functional neuroimaging experiments. The dotted outline represents the sampling characteristics of the nonexistent technique suggested by the phrase, "combine the temporal resolution of EEG recording with the spatial resolution of fMRI." In fact, a substantial fraction of the abstract space containing all possible electrophysiological records is inaccessible by non-invasive means. Thus, it is not possible to sample at 100 Hz with 2 mm voxels (arrow).

neuronal activity, especially in the gamma frequency range, is central to the genesis of behavior (Engel et al., 2001; Engel and Singer, 2001). A wealth of evidence indicates that the central nervous system (CNS) coordinates the machinery responsible for behavior by means of transient synchronization of activity, principally in the beta and gamma bands (Ohara et al., 2001; Buzsaki and Draguhn, 2004; Linkenkaer-Hansen et al., 2004; Fries, 2005; Knight, 2007). The close connection between gamma-band LFP power (γ-BLP) and the BOLD signals is now well established in animals (Niessing et al., 2005) and humans (Lachaux et al., 2007). Indeed, ECoG studies have demonstrated task-related γ-BLP "activation" maps resembling task-evoked fMRI BOLD responses (Crone et al., 2006; Miller et al., 2006; Towle et al., 2008).

A very different connection between electrophysiology and behavior has its origins in the observation that voluntary movements are preceded by slow negative shifts in the scalp potentials recorded over the motor cortex of the contralateral hemisphere (Kornhuber and Deecke, 1965). The readiness potential (bereitschaftspotential) was originally associated with voluntary movement, but essentially the same phenomenon (the contingent negative variation, or CNV) has been observed with a wide variety of cognitive paradigms (Birbaumer et al., 1990; Rosler

et al., 1997; Brunia and van Boxtel, 2001). Depolarization of the apical dendrites of large pyramidal cells, for example, by excitatory input from nonspecific thalamic afferents, is a likely neuronal mechanisms underlying cortical surface negativity (Mitzdorf, 1985). This view is strongly supported by the recent report of Lakatos et al. (2008), in which it was shown that increased attention to the auditory or visual sensorium is attended by depolarization (current sinks) within the upper layers in the respective primary sensory cortical area. The sustained character of slow cortical potentials (SCPs) and the behavioral paradigms used to evoke them (e.g., "concept formation task," M Lang et al., 1987) suggest a close relation to functional neuroimaging. Indeed, it is now clear that such a relation exists (see below). Thus, it is reasonable to propose that cortical surface negativity and LFP γ-band power both are correlates of a local cortical state variable (the "activation" level) as imaged by BOLD fMRI. Invasive gross potential recordings in humans suggest that *desynchronization* (reduced power) in the alpha band also is a correlate of task-evoked increases in cortical activity (Pfurtscheller, 2006; Rektor et al., 2006).

What are the implications of the above considerations for combining EEG and fMRI in the study of human cognition? The major determinant of gross potentials (ECoG and EEG) is synchronous synaptic activity over some spatial scale. It is empirically observed that the spatial scale of synchronous activity tends to be inversely proportional to its temporal frequency (Bullock et al., 1995; Varela et al., 2001; Leopold et al., 2003). Thus, phase coherence in the gamma frequency range characteristically is observed on a scale measured in millimeters, while slow cortical potentials (nominally, frequencies less than 1 Hz) may be synchronous over many cm. This basic electrophysiological principle governs the degree to which brain electrophysiology is accessible to various recording techniques (Table 1.3.1). Behavioral engagement, e.g., in response to stimuli, characteristically increases the spatial range of phase coherent activity; this effect is primarily local (within 1–5 mm) in the gamma frequency range (Nir et al., 2007) but widely distributed at lower frequencies (Gross et al., 2004; Kahana, 2006; Saalmann et al., 2007). Thus, event-related increases in neuronal synchronization likely account at least in part for the changes we observe in the fMRI BOLD signal during task performance.

To summarize the methodology relevant to human neuroscience, functional neuroimaging (FNI) techniques (at present predominantly fMRI BOLD imaging) and three electrophysiological techniques (ECoG, MEG, EEG) are available for use singly and in combination. The principal application of FNI is to localize the representation of behavior by detecting focal metabolic and hemodynamic correlates of neuronal responses to controlled task paradigms. Of the three electrophysiological techniques listed in Table 1.3.1, only ECoG is based on close contact with the brain and hence, relatively secure generator localization. However ECoG can be used only in patients undergoing surgical treatment for intractable epilepsy. Localization of current sources within the brain is insecure with both MEG and EEG because of the fundamentally ill-posed nature of the inverse problem (see below). MEG offers somewhat better spatial and temporal resolution in comparison to EEG but is effectively blind to radial current sources (Pizzella and Romani, 1990). Thus, radial current generated by transcortical dipoles on gyral crowns is not (or almost not) detected. Special techniques are required to record MEG at frequencies less than ~1 Hz (Leistner et al., 2007). EEG is capable of sensing currents flowing in any direction throughout the brain; however, the poor conductivity of the skull severely reduces the achievable spatial specificity of scalp recording (Nunez and Silberstein, 2000). Thus, behaviorally induced

Table 1.3.1.
Spatial and temporal sampling properties of techniques used in human neuroscience.

Technique	Invasive?	Temporal resolution		Spatial resolution	Spatial coverage
[^{15}O]H$_2$O PET	No♣	20 min		15 mm	complete
BOLD fMRI	No	3 sec♥		6 mm♦	complete
NIRS DOT	No	3 sec		3 cm	brain surface†
ECoG	Yes	0.004 sec	0.01♠–250 Hz	2 cm*	brain surface
MEG	No	0.05 sec	1–200 Hz	2–3 cm¶	brain surface§
EEG	No	0.02 sec	0.01♠–50 Hz	3–5 cm¶	complete

The tabulated quantities are necessarily approximate and are intended primarily to convey relative scale. Resolution is defined as the minimum separation at which discrete events/sources can be distinguished. Presently tabulated temporal resolution generally has been computed as the reciprocal of the highest temporal frequency carrying neurophysiological information. Only in the case of PET, the tabulated value reflects the instrumental sampling frequency. Localization precision can be considerably finer than spatial resolution (see Fox et al., 1987, for discussion). Thus, ERP generator localization errors may be as low as a 5–10 mm for superficial sources (Bai et al., 2007).

♣ [^{15}O]H$_2$O PET is non-invasive apart from intravenous injection of radio-tracer. However, radiation safety concerns significantly limit the quantity of tracer that can be administered. Hence, the obtainable spatial resolution in practice is limited by statistical image quality, which is dose-related. In addition, the inherent physics of positron annihilation fundamentally limit human PET spatial resolution to ~5 mm.

♥ In comparing electrophysiology to functional neuroimaging, the temporal sampling property of BOLD fMRI that seems most limiting is the upper frequency limit. However, slow drifts that almost certainly are of non-neuronal origin contaminate fMRI and impose practical limits also at low temporal frequencies, nominally <0.01 Hz.

♠ The practical lower temporal frequency limit of "DC" recording is uncertain. The tabulated value reflects the fact that interpretation of recorded potential differences at intervals >100 sec is rarely attempted.

* The spatial resolution of ECoG is determined by contact dimensions and inter-electrode spacing. The presently tabulated value reflects the fact that grids with 1 cm center-to-center spacing are standard in clinical electrocorticography. Coverage is limited to areas of cortex selected for recording, which selection is determined strictly on the basis of clinical considerations.

♦ The tabulated value reflects currently available human MRI scanners. High-field animal fMRI is capable of considerably finer spatial sampling (e.g., 0.68 × 0.86 × 0.86 mm voxels; Moon et al., 2007).

† DOT is fundamentally limited by the scattering properties of light in tissue (Yodh and Boas, 2003). Signal-to-noise ratios limit currently available DOT systems to operating within several mm of the brain surface and provide only partial head coverage owing to the high cost of optodes.

§ Although MEG generators can theoretically be modeled at any depth, MEG source localization is reliable only to a depth of ~3–4 cm. MEG resolution depends on dipole orientation, depth, and signal-to-noise ratio (Hari et al., 1988; Mosher et al., 1993). Strictly speaking, the notion of "resolution" does not rigorously apply to inverse dipole localization in the same sense as it does in imaging, where the signal is independently reconstructed at voxels on a regular grid.

¶ The tabulated values refer to unconstrained inverse current source localization (Pascual-Marqui, 1999). Achievable resolution depends on depth and is greatest at the brain surface. The spatial specificity of EEG and MEG can be considerably improved by adding inverse modeling constraints derived from anatomical and functional imaging (Dale and Sereno, 1993; Dale et al., 2000).

focal gamma-band activity is often seen with MEG (e.g., Schoffelen et al., 2005; Siegel et al., 2007) but sometimes not with EEG (Juergens et al., 1999). Since it has recently been shown that event-related EEG gamma-band activity can be generated by the extraocular muscles (Yuval-Greenberg et al., 2008), the reliability of scalp potential recording in this domain currently is open to question. On the other hand, EEG but not conventional MEG is capable of recording very slow activity ("DC" potentials), which may represent a critical link between electrophysiology and FNI.

Analysis of Combined FNI-Electrophysiology Data

Combined electrophysiology-FNI studies have used a wide range of analysis strategies. A major criterion for categorizing these strategies is in the approach taken to defining the spatial specificity of the electrophysiological data:

(I) Analysis in data space without inverse modeling. Results may be reported in terms of specific EEG electrodes or MEG channels. Interpolation over electrodes or channels can be used to generate continuous scalp topography maps (Perrin et al., 1987). The spatial specificity of EEG may be improved by application of the Laplacian operator, which isolates vertical current (Nunez and Pilgreen, 1991). Type I analyses involve no generator or conductivity models. However, the only basis for associating electrophysiological results with brain structure is proximity (Nunez and Silberstein, 2000).

(II) Unconstrained inverse current source (generator) localization. The locations of generators within the brain are deduced by finding a best-fitting model. Brain electrical source analysis (BESA; Scherg and Picton, 1991) finds one or more dipoles at discrete points within the brain. Dipole models are inherently signed (that is, specify the direction of current flow). In practice, BESA is not strictly unconstrained as the procedure typically is "seeded" at user-selected loci. Low resolution brain electromagnetic tomography (LORETA; Pascual-Marqui et al., 1994) models the generator as a continuous current density distribution over the brain volume. Response sign (direction of current flow) is lost in conventional LORETA current source density maps. All inverse source modeling depends on the availability of a head conductivity model, which may be simple (Rush and Driscoll, 1968) or elaborate (e.g., Darvas et al., 2006). Total model adequacy conventionally is evaluated in terms of goodness of fit, i.e., by how well the model accounts for the recorded data. However, even perfect goodness of fit is a very poor indicator of model correctness (Snyder, 1991).

(III)Location-constrained inverse dipole localization. The location of current sources but not their orientation is restricted to known response foci. In practice, such foci are used to "seed" BESA, which finds the best fitting dipole orientations.

(IV) Cortical surface constrained inverse generator localization (Dale and Sereno, 1993). This technique requires prior knowledge of the location of the cortical surface, which must be obtained by segmentation of structural images (Dale et al., 1999). The orientation of current flow optionally may be constrained to be perpendicular to the cortical surface. This constraint is sensible as the generators of gross potentials are reasonably well represented as net transcortical dipoles or dipole sheets (Nunez and Silberstein, 2000).

(V) Completely a priori defined generator geometry. The geometry (location and orientation) of all current generators is determined by a combination of anatomical and functional neuroimaging (combined analysis strategies III+IV). Once this geometry is known, the electrical state of the system is completely specified by the head conductivity model and the instantaneous generator strengths (the forward model). Generator time courses then are directly computable from the recorded data by application of the inverted forward model.

(VI) Temporal independent component analysis (temporal ICA). The entire EEG (or MEG) record is decomposed into the sum of components, each component being the product of a fixed spatial distribution (channel weights) and a time course. Temporal ICA maximizes the independence of component time courses. It has been empirically observed that component spatial weights characteristically exhibit scalp distributions approximately attributable to single dipoles within the brain. Moreover, components often can be clustered, and these clusters can then be efficiently represented in terms of equivalent dipolar generators (Makeig et al., 2004). A major advantage of ICA is that sources of spurious variance (e.g., the eyes) generally can be easily identified and excluded from subsequent analyses. ICA is data driven, whereas analysis strategies II–V are model-based. However, both temporal ICA and analysis strategy type V transform the spatial representation of electrophysiological data from one of high dimensionality (number of electrodes or sensors) to one of low dimensionality (number of generators or component clusters). Linear spatial filtering (Bonmassar et al., 1999) is yet another method for computing channel weights based on maximizing the signal-to-noise ratio.

(VII) Joint EEG-fMRI analysis. Calhoun et al. introduced a novel method in which the entire EEG-fMRI dataset is subjected to joint ICA (Calhoun et al., 2006). The same authors extended joint EEG-fMRI ICA to analysis at the group level (Eichele et al., 2008; see also Chapter 3.5 in this volume). Martinez-Montes et al. (2004) have described joint EEG-fMRI analysis based on singular value decomposition rather than maximization of independence. For the present purposes, we classify all joint EEG-fMRI analyses as strategy type VII.

The distinctions between strategies I–VI lie entirely in how the electrophysiological data are analyzed. In all cases, quantities derived from those analyses (e.g., modeled source loci or dipole moment timecourses) are subsequently correlated with functional neuroimaging data. Analysis strategy type VII (*joint* EEG-fMRI analysis) fundamentally differs from strategies I–VI in that the combined dataset is analyzed concurrently rather than sequentially.

A Brief Introduction to Event-Related Potential Paradigms

Much of the combined methodology literature is concerned with specific ERP paradigms that historically have been important in experimental psychology. Below we briefly encapsulate three of these paradigms to make the ensuing discussion more generally accessible.

P300

P300 (also known as "P3") is an ERP phenomenon named after its latency (third positive deflection peaking 300 ms post stimulus presentation). The P3 ERP has a broad, predominantly central scalp distribution and is evoked by low frequency (typically 10%) task-relevant (target) stimuli or unexpected (oddball or distractor) stimuli occurring within a stream mostly containing identical, repeated (standard) items. By far, the greatest part of the P3 literature is exclusively electrophysiological and focused on psychology (for review see Polich, 2007). However, the P3 paradigm is naturally suited to event-related fMRI. Accordingly, the functional anatomy associated with P3-type contrasts (e.g., target vs. standard stimuli) has been determined for both visual and auditory stimulus streams (Kiehl et al., 2001a; Kiehl et al., 2001b).

N400

N400 refers to central-parietal scalp negativity appearing approximately 400 ms after presentation of a semantically incongruent stimulus (Kutas and Hillyard, 1980). The N400 was originally described in relation to anomalous sentence endings (e.g., "I have my tea with cream and *dog*"). It has since become clear that lexicality is not essential and that the same phenomenon can be elicited by semantically incongruous line drawings (Ganis et al., 1996). The N400 is closely related to the P600 (also known as the late positivity), which is more associated with violations of syntax (grammatical errors) than context-inappropriate symbolic content. It is important to remember that surprising, task-irrelevant events (e.g., an unexpected loud buzz) are much more likely to elicit an oddball-P3 than either a N400 or a P600.

Error-Related Negativity (ERN)

ERN refers to midline-frontal scalp negativity that occurs promptly (within 100 ms) after errors of commission, meaning, motor acts committed by the subject that are immediately recognized as mistakes (for reviews see Ullsperger and von Cramon, 2004; Yeung et al., 2004). The ERN is widely believed to reflect discrepancy between intentions and actions. Errors of commission are experimentally studied using tasks with conflicting stimulus-response mappings and instructing subjects to respond as quickly as possible (for a recent review see Roberts and Hall, 2008)). When response speed is emphasized the task is said to be "speeded." In a prototypical ERN paradigm, the Eriksen flanker task, subjects must respond according to the direction of a centrally positioned arrow; the arrow may be surrounded by like arrows (congruent condition) or oppositely pointing arrows (conflict condition). Mistaken responses in the conflict condition reliably elicit the ERN. Inverse dipole localization (Dehaene et al., 1994) as well as event-related fMRI (Carter et al., 1998) suggest that the ERN is generated in or near anterior cingulate cortex. This brain area also is known as the rostral cingulate zone and fronto-median cortex.

Reasons for Combining Electrophysiology and Functional Neuroimaging

We have discussed the physiology relevant to combined electrophysiology-FNI studies, summarized the available data acquisition techniques, categorized the available analysis strategies and have briefly described common ERP protocols. We now are in a position to review what has been achieved by combining electrophysiology with functional neuroimaging. As the relevant literature already is extensive, our review must necessarily be selective. We discuss articles that illustrate particular points or are otherwise noteworthy. This discussion is organized according to scientific objective. We emphasize that these objectives are interrelated and that many of the papers cited below could be discussed under multiple headings.

To Study the Relationship of Electrophysiological Responses to Functional Neuroimaging Signals

It has been understood for over a century that cerebral blood flow and metabolism are coupled to neuronal activity (Raichle, 1987; Malonek et al., 1997). Animal studies have documented tight relations between stimulus intensity, neuronal responses, and optical hemodynamic measures (Devor et al., 2003; Siegel et al., 2003; Sheth et al., 2004). Physiological stimulation causes changes in blood flow, blood volume, and oxygen consumption, although these measures do not all change to the same degree (PT Fox and Raichle, 1986). Indeed, the fact that blood flow changes more than oxygen consumption underlies the physiological basis of BOLD fMRI (Raichle and Mintun, 2006). Optical (NIRS) imaging offers an alternative means of studying the metabolic and hemodynamic responses to physiological stimulation, and moreover, separates signals reflecting oxygenated, deoxygenated, and total hemoglobin (HbO, HbR, HbT, respectively). Thus, it is reasonable to regard optical imaging as a basic tool in the investigation of the relationships between neuronal and vascular responses to behavioral paradigms. Some studies have emphasized non-linear relationships between stimulus intensity and physio-logic (i.e., neuronal and hemodynamic) responses (Devor et al., 2003; Sheth et al., 2004; Franceschini et al., 2008). However, the preponderance of NIRS data indicate that the nonlinearities in question occur in the relations between stimulus intensity and physiologic responses; the induced changes in the various hemoglobin species tend to exhibit a stable proportionality (e.g., $\Delta HbR/\Delta HbO \approx$ const.) (Sheth et al., 2004). Thus, NIRS measurement of the local concentration of deoxyhemogolobin (HbR) may be regarded as a good proxy for the BOLD signal, as has been directly verified (Toyoda et al., 2008).

Human studies have been performed using visual (Obrig et al., 2002; Rovati et al., 2007), somatosensory (Arthurs and Boniface, 2003), auditory (Mulert et al., 2005) and painful (Iannetti et al., 2005) stimuli. Horovitz et al. (Horovitz and Gore, 2004) reported a combined NIRS-ERP experiment using the N400 paradigm. Many experiments have systematically varied stimulus intensity. Other parametric manipulations have included the emotional content of pictures (Herrmann et al., 2008) and the degree to which images are recognizable as cars or faces (Horovitz et al., 2004). Analysis strategy type I (no attempt at inverse dipole localization) generally is sufficient in these experiments, as the scientific question concerns the relation of ERP measures to the hemodynamic response (HDR). The recent report of Arthurs et al. (2007) shows an impressively linear relation (up to a saturation limit) between stimulus intensity and the N20-P25 deflection in the somatosensory evoked potential (SSEP) recorded over the contralateral hemisphere. The BOLD response in contralateral somatosensory cortex also increased linearly with stimulus intensity. Another interesting finding was that the stimulus paradigm (median nerve shocks) elicited negative BOLD responses in ipsilateral somatosensory cortex. These negative responses, unexpected by the authors, were in retrospect consistent with previous reports (Drevets et al., 1995). Critically, the authors did not record SSEPs over ipsilateral somatosensory cortex! Thus, this study provides a very interesting observation worthy of further investigation.

It is commonly assumed that hemodynamic responses are driven by the metabolic requirements of neuronal activity. This view has very recently been challenged (Sirotin and Das, 2009). Thus, awake, behaving monkeys were trained to fixate on a small spot of light briefly presented in an otherwise dark environment. The fixation spot presentation was rhythmic and therefore highly predictable. Anticipatory hemodynamic

(HbT, HbO) responses in visual cortex were clearly observed using optical techniques, but similarly predictive signals were not observed in simultaneously recorded spikes and LFPs. The negative portion of this result seems to undermine the notion that vascular responses are neuronally driven. However several caveats should be mentioned: *(1)* Failure to extract a signal does not prove that it is absent. *(2)* The analysis excluded slow (< 10 Hz) cortical potentials, which in other data have been shown to reflect the local state of cortical excitability (see physiological review above and discussion of resting state EEG/BOLD correspondences below). *(3)* Hemodynamic (BOLD) modulations and single-unit discharge may be dissociable under some circumstances, especially in visual cortex (Maier et al., 2008).

To Study the Correspondence Between "DC" Cortical Potentials and Hemodynamic Responses

Lang et al. conducted the first experiments to link SCPs directly to functional neuroimaging using combined EEG and SPECT (single photon emission tomography) and language tasks (M Lang et al., 1987; W Lang et al., 1987). A more recent example of combined SCP-fMRI experimentation was reported by Lamm et al. (2001). The task was mental rotation of visually displayed 3D objects. fMRI showed activation of visual cortex and specific regions of frontal and parietal cortex that today we recognize as the dorsal attention system (Corbetta and Shulman, 2002). The topography of the task-induced scalp negativity (after sharpening by application of the Laplacian operator) tolerably well matched the BOLD response. Importantly, the SCP began ~600 msec after display onset, incremented over several seconds, and persisted until the end of each trial (trial duration varied between 5 seconds and 2 minutes). Schicke et al. (2006) recently reported a similar experiment with comparable results, in which the task was spatial imagery and the cognitive load was systematically manipulated to obtain a spread of trial durations in the ~1–10 sec range. It is important to keep in mind that here, as in all ERP experiments, the early phase ($< \sim 0.6$ sec) of the evoked response contained transients that probably reflect multiple cognitive processes including stimulus identification and task instantiation. In typical SCP data, a shift toward scalp negativity begins at the termination of the early response phase, but sustained scalp negativity does not fully develop until at least 2–3 s later. Evidence exists that links SCPs to non-neuronal cerebrovascular physiology (Vanhatalo et al., 2003; Voipio et al., 2003; Nita et al., 2004). Hence, it is unclear that task-related SCPs are entirely attributable to synaptic currents. This question most likely can be resolved only by invasive experiments in animals.

To Compare Response Localization by Electrophysiology (Analysis Strategies Types I and II) vs. Functional Neuroimaging

To our knowledge, the first experiment to address this question was conducted in our laboratory using steady-state amplitude modulated vibration (Snyder, 1992). Inverse dipole localization errors (spherical 3-shell head model)

were on the order of 1.5 cm, or about 3 times greater than recently reported somatosensory response localization errors obtained using much more sophisticated methodology (Bai et al., 2007). In most recent experiments on electrophysiological vs. FNI localization, the emphasis has been technical, the principal objective being to demonstrate the feasibility of simultaneous EEG-fMRI acquisition (e.g., Bonmassar et al., 1999; Kruggel et al., 2000; Sammer et al., 2005). Mulert et al. conducted an experiment (2005) primarily to examine the proportionality of ERP vs. BOLD responses to auditory stimuli of graded intensity. However, they used unconstrained inverse generator localization (LORETA) to analyze the ERP results, thereby providing data bearing on the performance of this procedure. To be sure, LORETA found ERP generators in auditory cortex (as did fMRI). Current source densities measured in that region were, to a good approximation, proportional to the BOLD responses. However, even greater current source densities were found in medial frontal cortex (their Figure 2), but there was no corresponding BOLD response (their Figure 3). Considered as a whole, the results reported by Mulert et al. (2005) exemplify a sort of "half empty–half full" situation that characterizes much of the EEG-fMRI literature based on unconstrained inverse generator localization (analysis strategy type II). Much the same conclusion was reached in a systematic comparison of LORETA vs. $[^{15}O]H_2O$ PET in a study pharmacological effects (Gamma et al., 2004).

The experiment of Thees et al. (2003) also illustrates the limitations of unconstrained inverse dipole modeling. The median nerve at the wrist was stimulated using shocks of two easily discriminable intensities. Subjects either simply reported detection of the stimulus (by button press) or discriminated high vs. low intensity (selective button press). The discrimination vs. detection contrast showed expected fMRI activations in contralateral primary and secondary somatosensory cortex (SI and SII) as well as responses in brain regions well known to mediate cognitive control (midline cingulate cortex and bilateral insula). BESA-modeled dipole moment time courses showed discrimination effects primarily in contralateral SII, in good agreement with prior work on spatial attention. These effects were present over two discrete latency windows ($\sim$60 ms and $\sim$200 ms), which is informative regarding the mechanisms underlying sensory discrimination. However, it was not possible to assign dipoles to all significant fMRI foci. Also, foci that were modeled showed localization errors (9 mm distant from fMRI maxima) and the modeled moments did not show discrimination effects at all foci showing BOLD effects. It is probably significant that the same investigators reverted to analysis strategy type I in their most recent study of somatosensory attention (Schubert et al., 2008).

Much of the P3 literature prior to 2005 is framed in terms of comparing localizations obtained by type II analyses vs. fMRI. Again, the results are mixed (for review see Linden, 2005). The inferior parietal lobule and temporo-parietal junction (IPL/TPJ) have been universally identified by all techniques as P3 generators, in accordance with lesion studies (for review of the lesion literature see Knight and Scabini, 1998). Inverse modeling of other P3 generators has been less consistent. Thus, for example, it is now clear that anterior cingulate cortex consistently responds more to targets than standards (Kiehl et al., 2001a; Strobel et al., 2008). Yet this locus was not found by BESA in the study of Bledowski et al. (2004). Within-study comparisons of LORETA and fMRI similarly have revealed both localization correspondences and failures of correspondence (e.g., Mulert et al., 2004). Something approaching ground truth in this area now is better known since Brazdil et al. (2005) reported their systematic comparison of invasive electrophysiological recording vs. fMRI. According to these authors, invasive recording and fMRI generally are in good agreement except in the medial temporal lobe, where P3-like responses have so far been recorded only with invasive techniques (Halgren et al., 1995).

The combined ERP-fMRI N400 literature is very limited. Matsumoto et al. (2005) found correlation across subjects of N400 amplitudes with left superior temporal BOLD response magnitudes. There appears to be substantial disagreement across laboratories regarding even the fMRI correlates of N400-type paradigms (for review see Van Petten and Luka, 2006). One aspect of the phenomenology that has never been explained is that the N400 ERP is essentially symmetric, whereas typical fMRI responses to tasks involving semantic operations generally are lateralized to the left hemisphere (Petersen et al., 1988).

To Study the Correlates of Attentional Response Enhancement

"Attention" is the psychological faculty that controls whether events are noticed or ignored. Well before combined electrophysiology-FNI was first reported, it was known that $[^{15}O]H_2O$ PET as well as ERP responses to stimuli can be enhanced by experimentally manipulating the subject's attention, for example, to the left or the right, or to particular stimulus features (see Heinze et al., 1994, for review). The principal reason for combined experimentation is to determine where in the brain and when (locus and latency) attentional effects occur. Thus, for example, directing attention to the left or right visual field increases the blood flow response in contralateral visual cortex and similarly augments the P1-N1 deflections in the visual evoked response (VEP) recorded from the overlying scalp (Mangun et al., 2001). Combined electrophysiology-FNI studies of spatial attention have used visual (e.g., Noesselt et al., 2002), auditory (Brunetti et al., 2008), and somatosensory (Schubert et al., 2008) stimuli.

To Assign a Correspondence Between Distinct ERP Components and Functional Neuroanatomy

Eichele et al. (2005) conducted a simultaneous BOLD-fMRI study of the P3 type using auditory stimuli (standards and targets only, no distractors). Systematically manipulating the frequency of targets altered the magnitude of specific deflections in the recorded ERP waveform (analysis type I). Trial-to-trial variation in deflection magnitudes was used to construct fMRI regressors. The fMRI analysis based on these regressors showed negative correlations between the P2 (second positive) component of the ERP and the default mode network (Raichle et al., 2001). Similarly, the P3 component was positively correlated with regions that today are identifiable as the parts of the fronto-parietal control system (Vincent et al., 2008). Such results sensibly link electrophysiology and systems neuroscience in a manner that cannot be accomplished except by combined ERP-fMRI experimentation. The authors emphasized the importance of simultaneous acquisition in their study. However, as the ERP waveform variations were induced by manipulating conditions over 25-second duration blocks, it is unclear that comparable results could not have been obtained using separate acquisition. Nevertheless, this is a landmark study demonstrating a novel and potentially useful design.

Calhoun et al. (2006) conducted a similar auditory P3-type experiment (including distractors) and analyzed the data using joint EEG-fMRI ICA (strategy type VII). Joint ICA separated the ERP into components that largely consisted of monophasic deflections at various latencies. The N1 component was associated with activation of auditory cortex, in good agreement with the extant literature and the above-discussed experiment of Eichele et al. (2005). The P3 component was associated with positive BOLD modulation near the temporo-parietal junction (approximately in agreement with most of the P3 fMRI literature) and negative BOLD modulation of the default mode network (DMN). While this latter result is compatible with the extant P3 fMRI literature (which, regrettably, neglects to report negative BOLD responses) it disagrees in detail with Eichele et al. (2005), who assigned default mode network deactivation specifically to the P2 component of the ERP. Thus, we have two experiments based on nearly the same task paradigm but different analysis strategies that are only in partial agreement regarding the correspondence between distinct ERP components and BOLD responses. Additional experimentation will be required to resolve these discrepancies.

To Compare Response Localization by Electrophysiology vs. fMRI and To Determine the Sequence and Timing of Neuronal Activity Using Cortical Surface-Constrained Inverse Generator Modeling (Analysis Strategy Type IV)

The study by Dale et al. (2000) represents one of the more spectacular achievements in the field of combined MEG-fMRI experimentation. Subjects performed a semantic classification task in response to visually presented concrete nouns (judgment of whether or not the named object is more than foot long). All stimuli were presented multiple times. Comparison of responses to novel vs. repeated items isolated the MEG and fMRI correlates of semantic classification. Comparison of the distribution of modeled MEG current sources (in the 185–540 ms latency epoch) showed substantial topographic correspondence with fMRI especially in left hemisphere frontal and inferior temporal regions known to participate in semantic operations. Somewhat less robust MEG-fMRI localization correspondence was observed in parietal and temporal regions shown by fMRI to be activated by the task. The generator time courses (modeled with current flow constrained to the cortical surface normal) suggested that semantic classification mostly occurs in frontal regions at latencies >300 ms. Unfortunately, the dipole moment sign of these time courses could not be reliably determined from the data.

To Determine the Sequence and Timing of the Electrophysiological Correlates of Behavior at Known Loci within the Brain (Analysis Strategy Types III and V)

This objective embodies what arguably is the core purpose of combined electrophysiology-FNI experimentation (Linden, 2007). We know of no experiments in which analysis strategy type V was used in conjunction with cognitive ERP protocols (e.g., P300, N400, ERN). However the basic principle is well illustrated by the study of Vanni et al. (2004), which involved only "passive" viewing of visual stimuli. (This use of "passive" exemplifies conventional but misleading terminology: Neither visual fixation nor perception are truly passive [Yarbus, 1967].) Visual evoked potentials (VEPs) and fMRI data were separately acquired using the identical stimulus paradigm. Responses in multiple visual areas (V1, V2, V3/V3a, LO/V5) were identified by fMRI and the observed focality was combined with structural imaging and cortical surface extraction to implement analysis strategy type V. Thus having defined the geometry of the generators, the authors recovered dipole moment time courses exhibiting a sequence of responses (V1→V3→V5) in the 83 to 113 ms latency range consistent with the hierarchical organization of the visual system. Despite some ambiguities and imperfections (e.g., modeling unexplained variance by including generators of no interest in the linear system), this study is notable for demonstrating that a plausible temporal sequence of signed dipole moment responses may be recovered from scalp potentials even at closely spaced loci. Five years earlier, Ahlfors et al. (1999) performed a similar MEG-fMRI study of visual motion. They seeded dipoles at fMRI response loci but applied no orientation constraints during inverse modeling (analysis strategy type III). The recovered dipole moment waveforms showed early activity (130 ms latency) in area MT+, in accordance with the known role of this region in the perception of motion. However, the generator time courses were, on the whole, less consistent over subjects and less well temporally ordered than those of Vanni et al. (2004). These differences may reflect inherent limitations of MEG (insensitivity to radial current), less efficient use of electrophysiological data (unconstrained dipole orientation), or less precise timing of responses to motion reversals as opposed to flashed stimuli.

Sestieri et al. (2008) reported an MEG-fMRI study of saccadic eye movements to visually presented targets, the objective being to determine which brain structures account for variability of overt response (saccade) latency. Dipole moment time courses were recovered using analysis strategy type III in MT+, frontal, and parietal loci. The shortest latency dipole moment responses (~155 msec) were in MT+, which is consistent with the perceptual role of this structure. Most not all of the variability in saccade latency was attributable to the frontal eye fields.

Bledowski et al. (2006) studied working memory using a delayed match to sample task and meaningless visual stimuli ("BORTS"). The authors explicitly acknowledge response timing as the point of the experiment by including "mental chronometry" in the article title. fMRI results revealed several response foci in areas commonly activated by P3-type paradigms (e.g., temporo-parietal junction, midline frontal cortex), motor cortex (the task involved overt button presses), and higher order visual areas. A total of 14 dipolar generators were "seeded" at these loci and their orientations determined by BESA (strategy type III). Generator time courses evoked by presentation of the test stimulus generally were consistent with prevailing theories of functional localization, e.g., relatively early responses (~174 ms) in areas concerned with stimulus analysis. Response dependence on working memory load (3 items vs. 1 item) was observed mostly in ventro-lateral prefrontal cortex, a structure known to be recruited by recognition memory tasks (Badre and Wagner, 2007; Hampshire et al., 2008). Unfortunately, almost all ERP analyses were confined to the 1 s interval following presentation of the test stimuli: Nothing was said regarding ERPs over the ~7 s delay interval between sample presentation and the test stimuli during which processes corresponding to working memory per se presumably were active. These working memory processes probably contributed to the fMRI responses (Passingham and Sakai, 2004).

The experiment of Debener et al. (2005) exemplifies effective use of combined EEG-fMRI to study the electrophysiological correlates of behavior at known loci. Here, simultaneous acquisition was critical to the experimental design, as the objective was to relate electrophysiology to BOLD modulations on a trial-by-trial basis. Subjects performed the speeded Eriksen flanker task. Trial-by-trial ERN was measured using fixed channel weights that were determined (in each individual) by temporal ICA (analysis strategy VI) informed by prior knowledge of the anatomical locus of the ERN generator. These single-trial ERN measures captured the principal psychological property associated with errors of commission, viz., behavioral adjustment, that is, more deliberate (slower) performance on the next trial. Moreover, fMRI analysis using a regressor constructed from the single-trial ERN measures recovered the BOLD response

in the rostral cingulate zone, which adds to the evidence that the ERN is generated in this structure. Perhaps the most notable feature of this work was the achieved high signal-to-noise ratio of the ERN measure, on which the single-trial analysis depended. The virtues of single-trial designs have been debated (see Bledowski et al., 2007; and for a reply, Debener et al., 2007). This issue is also discussed below.

To Localize Seizure Foci

Simultaneous EEG-fMRI recording is a clinical procedure undertaken to determine the hemodynamic correlates of epileptiform transients in the EEG. In focal epilepsy, seizure foci may be more accurately localized than by EEG alone. Also, characteristic (negative!) BOLD responses can be observed in primary generalized epilepsy. Clinical EEG-fMRI is conceptually identical to conventional event-related fMRI except that the events are electroencephalographic as opposed to behavioral. This topic has been thoroughly reviewed in the recent literature (Laufs and Duncan, 2007; Gotman, 2008; see also Chapter 4.2 in this volume). The critical points to be made here are: *(1)* Simultaneous acquisition is crucial. *(2)* The EEG is used only to identify temporal events. Hence, analysis strategy type I is adequate.

To Study the Hemodynamic Correlates of EEG Rhythms in the Resting State

It has been known since the EEG was first recorded (Berger, 1929) that normal resting humans exhibit spontaneous fluctuations in the amplitude of rhythmic brain activity. Spontaneous fluctuations also are present in the fMRI signal of normal resting humans, although they were not attributed to neuronal activity until 1995 (Biswal et al., 1995). If EEG rhythms and BOLD fMRI both reflect the spontaneously fluctuating state of the brain, then some consistent relation should exist between these two measures. All investigations of this hypothesis are based on simultaneously acquired EEG-fMRI in resting (i.e., not performing any particular task) subjects. The data are analyzed under the reasonable assumption that neuronal activity is reflected in the BOLD signal via convolution with some known (e.g., Boynton et al., 1996) or measureable hemodynamic impulse response function. The preponderance of experimentation in this field has been focused on the BOLD correlates of the occipital alpha rhythm (α; 8–12 Hz). The first paper dealing with this question (Goldman et al., 2002) reported *negative* correlations between occipital alpha power and the BOLD signal in several regions, mostly in posterior parts of the brain. *Positive* correlations were observed principally in the thalamus. These findings have been replicated several times (Feige et al., 2005; de Munck et al., 2007). However, inconsistent results and interindividual differences have emerged as recurrent themes in the resting state EEG-fMRI literature. Thus, Laufs et al. (2003a; Laufs et al., 2003b) performed what is probably the most technically accomplished study in the field and initially reported *negative* α-BOLD correlations in prefrontal and parietal cortex and *positive* beta-2 (17–23 Hz)–BOLD correlations in the default mode network (Raichle et al., 2001). A later reanalysis of these same data (Laufs et al., 2006) omitted all mention of beta-2-BOLD correlations and described the distribution of negative α-BOLD correlations as falling into three different patterns ("occipital-parietal," "fronto-parietal," and "variable"). Intersubject variability per se has been the focus of one report (Goncalves et al., 2006). Some consistency may be present but hidden. For example, if one merges the alpha (8–12 Hz) and beta (24–28 Hz) correlation maps reported by Moosmann et al. (2003, Fig. 5), one obtains a distribution similar to the average α-BOLD result of Laufs et al. (2006, Figure 1). In aggregate, the most consistent EEG α-BOLD correlations in the cerebral cortex have carried a negative sign, that is, decreased BOLD signal in association with increased alpha power. This makes sense, as the presence of the alpha rhythm in the EEG has historically been viewed as a correlate of the awake but relaxed (not cognitively engaged) state. In electrocorticography, high levels of alpha activity indicate local cortical *disengagement* (see above).

In contradistinction, transiently increased EEG theta activity, especially over the frontal midline, has been repeatedly associated with arousal and mental effort (for review see Basar et al., 2001). The metabolic and hemodynamic correlates of theta activity in the resting state were first studied by Pizzagalli et al. (2003) using EEG combined with simultaneously acquired fluoro-deoxyglucose (FDG) PET. Current source density estimates of activity in the 6.5–8.0 Hz band were obtained by LORETA and voxelwise correlated over subjects (N = 29) with the local rate of glucose metabolism. This analysis showed significant correlation primarily in the anterior cingulate cortex, thereby provisionally identifying this region as a major generator of EEG theta activity. More recently, Scheeringa et al. (2008) performed a resting-state EEG-fMRI experiment directed at identifying the BOLD correlates of midline frontal theta (mfθ), which was isolated using a combination of band pass filtering and ICA. Inverse dipole localization of the mfθ component revealed generators in the anterior cingulate cortex, substantially in agreement with prior work and, somewhat more loosely, with the LORETA results of Pizzagalli et al. (2003). The major finding, however, was *negative* mfθ-BOLD correlations within the default mode network (DMN), especially within inferior midline frontal cortex. Similar results were reported by Mizuhara et al. (2004), except that these authors induced mfθ increases and concurrent DMN deactivation by having their subjects perform silent mental arithmetic. Thus, mfθ appears to be correlate of nondefault, that is, goal-directed modes of cognition (Fox et al., 2005). The absence of *positive* mfθ-BOLD correlations in regions that normally are anticorrelated with the DMN remains to be explained.

Mantini et al. (2007) recently described a different but promising approach to examining EEG-BOLD relations. Specifically, instead of first performing a time-frequency analysis of EEG data and then computing activity-BOLD correlations, these investigators first found BOLD resting state networks using spatial ICA (Beckmann et al., 2005) and then determined the spectral characteristics of the EEG corresponding to each component. Several findings were consistent with prior results, including *negative* α-BOLD correlation in occipital cortex and *positive* correlation of beta activity with the DMN (their RSN 1), as initially reported by Laufs et al. (2003a).

Partial least squares (N-PLS; Martinez-Montes et al., 2004) represents yet another method for examining EEG-BOLD relations. This technique is formally related to joint EEG-fMRI ICA (see Chapter 3.5 in this volume) in that the combined data are analyzed simultaneously rather then in sequence. Application of N-PLS to the same dataset acquired by Goldman et al. (2002) produced results that were not visibly different from those obtained using much simpler analyses.

Two recent reports based on invasive human electrophysiology are relevant to the discussion of EEG activity in relation to spontaneous BOLD fluctuations. First, He and colleagues (2008) demonstrated within-subject similarity between the correlation structures of surface potentials recorded by ECoG and resting-state BOLD fluctuations imaged by fMRI. This electrophysiology-BOLD correspondence was found both for the slowest (<4 Hz) components of "raw" ECoG potentials and for spontaneous gamma-band power modulations. Such results add to the accumulating evidence that the large-scale functional organization of the brain, which traditionally has been investigated using task paradigms, can be discerned in the correlation structure of resting activity (for review of the BOLD literature see Fox and Raichle, 2007). The same principle appears to apply as well at the millimeter scale (Kenet et al., 2003). Second, Nir and colleagues (2008) showed that spontaneous electrophysiological signals (single-unit firing rates and gamma-band LFP power) exhibit interhemispheric coherence in homologous regions of auditory cortex. These authors did not acquire resting-state fMRI in their subjects, but it is very likely that BOLD correlations would have been observed in the same homologous regions.

To Study the Hemodynamic Correlates of Sleep

Systematic exploration of sleep stage–dependent regional cerebral blood flow (rCBF) with $[^{15}O]H_2O$ PET began in the 1990s (Madsen, 1993; Braun et al., 1997). In experiments of this type, acquisition is initiated when the EEG indicates that the subject is in a well-defined stage of sleep. There now exists a substantial body of work based on this technique (for review see Maquet et al., 2005). It is well established that rCBF generally is reduced throughout the brain during sleep in comparison to the waking state. However, a more detailed analysis reveals focal effects that depend on sleep stage. Thus, for example, during rapid eye movement (REM) sleep, when vivid dreaming is most prevalent, rCBF is reduced in prefrontal and parietal regions associated with executive control but increased in limbic structures (e.g., hippocampus and amygdala). This intriguing finding is consistent with the heightened emotionality but reduced logicality of dreams.

Directly comparable studies of sleep stage–dependent cerebral activity have not been performed with EEG-fMRI, probably because the signal-to-noise ratio of BOLD imaging is very poor in the appropriate temporal frequency range, which nominally is one cycle per hour, or 0.0003 Hz (see Table 1.3.1). However, it is possible to perform conventional event-related fMRI keyed to specific features of sleep, e.g., the rapid eye movements after which stage REM is named. It has been found that REM events activate visual cortex and related parts of the thalamus (Wehrle et al., 2005), a result that seems eminently reasonable. A similar event-related study of EEG spindles (predominantly a feature of stage II sleep) found activation in paralimbic cortical areas and related parts of the thalamus (Schabus et al., 2007), a result that is novel and informative regarding the functionality of spindles. In a different event-related fMRI study of stage II sleep, Czisch et al. (2004) observed *negative* BOLD responses to auditory stimuli in auditory cortex, i.e., deactivation! This result is opposite to what might be reasonably expected and opposite to what is found in the waking state, and is highly instructive regarding how sleep changes the brain's response to sensory stimuli.

It is also possible to study how sleep affects the second-order statistics of spontaneous BOLD fluctuations in the 0.01–0.1 Hz range. Thus, thalamo-cortical synchrony appears to increase in association with stage REM eye movements (Wehrle et al., 2007). On the other hand, it has been shown (Horovitz et al., 2008; Larson-Prior et al., 2009) that the topography of correlated spontaneous activity within the cortex (resting state networks, or RSNs) appears to be unaffected by degree of arousal as humans transition from wakefulness to light sleep. A combined EEG-fMRI study of monkeys has shown that RSNs are present even during deep anesthesia (Vincent et al., 2007). These RSN observations carry far-reaching implications regarding the physiological significance of spontaneous BOLD fluctuations, which presumably reflect correlated neuronal activity. In particular, the existence of RSNs during sleep and anesthesia implies that resting state activity cannot be attributed solely to uncontrolled cognition. (For additional perspectives on this interesting question see Buckner and Vincent, 2007; Raichle and Snyder, 2007.)

All of the above-discussed studies of sleep employ analysis strategy type I, and often a very limited montage (placement of electrodes on the scalp). This is because the role of EEG in sleep studies is only to report the arousal state of the brain. The question of generator localization is not critical to the science.

Discussion

Combined electrophysiology-FNI experiments fall into two broad classes. First, ERP recording may be combined with fMRI in the context of task performance. This experimental paradigm has been framed as a method for localizing the generators of ERPs (Horwitz and Poeppel, 2002; Babiloni et al., 2004). However, as discussed above, a weakness of this formulation is that fMRI typically discloses more response foci than are needed to explain the ERPs. Hence, a unique answer to the ERP generator question seldom is obtained. The scientific yield of this approach appears to be limited. Curiously, one does not often encounter papers formulated in terms of finding the scalp potential correlates of fMRI responses! On the other hand, if the cortical regions recruited by performance of a particular task are known, it is theoretically possible to use electrophysiology to determine the latency and sequence of the responses with ~10 ms temporal resolution (Dale and Halgren, 2001) provided no attempt is made to distinguish the dipole moment time courses of closely spaced co-linear (pointing along the same axis) generators (Pascual-Marqui, 1999; Bledowski et al., 2006). Optimal implementation of this experimental design (analysis strategy V) requires cortical ribbon extraction together with sophisticated forward modeling of scalp potentials. The associated technical challenges probably account for the fact that analysis strategy V has not been used more often in experimental psychology. Analysis strategy type III is less challenging as it does not involve a priori determination of the orientation of dipolar generators. However, this compromise means that no physiological significance can be attached to the sign of recovered generator time courses.

Second, simultaneously acquired EEG-fMRI may be used to study the BOLD correlates of particular EEG rhythms, or conversely, the EEG correlates of BOLD resting state networks (RSNs). Resting state fMRI studies (not necessarily involving EEG) currently are reported at an exponentially increasing rate: PubMed lists 30, 45, 80, and 117 papers for years 2005–2008, respectively. This development reflects a growing awareness within the neuroscience community that the physiological genesis of behavior cannot be understood only by observing the brain as it responds to (or generates on its own) discrete events (Raichle and Snyder, 2007). It is evident that resting state vs. event-related experiments radically differ in the degree to which the geometrical features of the electrophysiological data are important. Thus, Laufs et al. (2003b, Figure 3) explicitly demonstrate that EEG rhythm–BOLD correlations exhibit little specificity of scalp topography. Contrariwise, if the ERP attributable to a discrete generator is the object of study, than careful attention to scalp topography is essential (e.g., Debener et al., 2005).

Concluding Opinions and Recommendations

Electrophysiology and Functional Neuroimaging Should be Combined in a Manner that Optimally Exploits the Respective Strengths of Each Technique

Scalp potentials and neuromagnetic fields do contain localizing information. However, their principal value is in the temporal domain. Unconstrained inverse generator localization is unreliable. Hence, non-invasive electrophysiology for the primary purpose of response localization is indefensible given that this objective is so much better accomplished by functional neuroimaging. Pursuing this logic leads to the conclusion that *all* geometric aspects of generator models should be determined as far as is possible by prior knowledge, which, in practice amounts to structural + functional imaging (analysis strategy type V). Once this determination is reached, instantaneous generator activity can be computed as a weighted sum over channels. Alternatively, temporal ICA (analysis strategy type VI) may be used to compute channel weights. In all cases, the electrophysiological record is best regarded as a source *only* of temporal information.

EEG/MEG and Functional Neuroimaging are not Symmetrically Complementary When the Objective is Localization of Function

It has been suggested that some neuronal responses may be detected by non-invasive electrophysiologic recording but not by fMRI and vice versa (Nunez and Silberstein, 2000; Herrmann and Debener, 2008), as if the respective weaknesses of these techniques, as regards response detection, were symmetrically arrayed. However, careful thought shows that this proposition is not really true. Certainly, closely spaced but oppositely oriented dipolar generators, e.g., in apposed regions of cortex, may be invisible at the scalp because of mutual cancellation. Also, radially oriented current generally is not well detected by MEG (Hari et al., 1988). However, the best available evidence indicates that neocortical activation and deactivation *always* are accompanied by a corresponding change in the BOLD signal (Logothetis, 2002; Shmuel et al., 2006). One caveat that should be mentioned here is that not all BOLD responses may be detected by fMRI because some parts of the brain are not well imaged by conventional echo-planar sequences (Ojemann et al., 1997). Im et al. (2005) have proposed a strategy for modeling "fMRI invisible" sources; we emphasize that this should be done only at loci clearly affected by compromised imaging. The medial temporal lobe historically has presented problems for both fMRI (Cohen et al., 1999) and scalp recording. Thus, P3-like responses have so far been observed in medial temporal lobe structures *only* by invasive means (Halgren et al., 1995; Brazdil et al., 2005). A similar discrepancy between invasive recording and ERP-fMRI may exist with respect to the hippocampus and memory formation (see Fell et al., 2001; and subsequent discussion, Fernández et al., 2002; Otten and Rugg, 2002). Notwithstanding these exceptions, it is reasonable to regard BOLD fMRI as a much more reliable detector of focal responses than EEG/MEG.

In the Analysis of Task-Related Combined ERP-fMRI Experiments, Response Sign (Positive vs. Negative) is a Crucial Feature of the Data and Should be Retained in the Generator Model

In our early report on a combined ERP–[^{15}O]H$_2$O PET study of verb generation in response to visually presented nouns, we suggested that cortical activation and deactivation correspond, respectively, to surface positivity and negativity (Snyder et al., 1995). The reverse is much more likely to be true: Ample evidence indicates that surface negative transcortical polarization corresponds to the "activated" state (see above). Kotchoubey (2006) suggests that this relation holds very generally, even for stimulus-locked ERP responses in the <300 ms latency range (see also Roland, 2002). A correspondence between surface negativity and "activation" is most clearly supported by observations of sustained responses (e.g., Mackert et al., 2008). However, substantial support for this notion exists also for responses at shorter latencies. For example, Grent-'t-Jong and Woldorff (2007) reported a combined ERP-fMRI study in which subjects directed their attention to either the left or right hemifield in response to a cue. This paradigm generated fMRI responses in the dorsal attention system in good agreement with prevailing theory (Corbetta and Shulman, 2002). The corresponding ERPs showed sustained negativity ("biasing-related negativity") over the contralateral scalp beginning at ~400 ms.

It is physiologically reasonable to hypothesize the existence of a consistent link between superficial layer depolarization and a state of enhanced cortical excitability manifesting as concurrent BOLD signal increases and surface negative transcortical polarization. However, the P3 and memory-related ERP literature present a problem for this theory, as orienting to task-relevant stimuli and item recognition are reliably accompanied by widely distributed scalp *positivity* in the 300 to 800 ms latency range (Miller et al., 2008; Vilberg and Rugg, 2008a). Moreover, systematically increasing the information content of remembered material enhances posterior parietal BOLD responses and increases the magnitude of late (500–800 msec) *positive* ERPs in the overlying scalp (Vilberg and Rugg, 2008b). Kotchoubey argues that the P300 potential reflects the *termination* of stimulus analysis processes ("cognitive closure"), an interpretation endorsed by Polich (2007), who arguably is today the preeminent authority on the P300. One possibility is that a consistent correspondence between cortical surface negativity and fMRI "activation" holds only for sustained processes (nominally, >1000 ms post triggering event). Indeed, strong evidence supporting this view may be seen in Khader et al. (2005): Retrieval of previously memorized human faces or spatial locations was associated with scalp negativity over the plausibly appropriate brain region, but *only* at latencies >1500 ms following presentation of the (lexical) cue. Additional non-invasive investigation of this issue will depend on inverse current source localization procedures that preserve dipole sign, i.e., not LORETA.

Additional Experiments are Needed to Study the Relations Between EEG Rhythms and Spontaneous BOLD Fluctuations

The hypothesis that some consistent relation should exist between the EEG and resting-state BOLD fluctuations is broadly supported by results obtained to date (e.g., Laufs et al., 2006). However, much work remains to be done. Are apparently discrepant findings across laboratories a manifestation of technical factors or true interindividual differences? If the latter, are these differences stable over time within individuals?

As Laufs et al. (2006) note, it may not be appropriate to assume a standard (canonical) hemodynamic impulse response function (HDR) in modeling temporal relations between EEG rhythms and BOLD fluctuations. The observation that the thalamus appears to be (positively) modulated by occipital alpha at unusually short delays (Feige et al., 2005; de Munck et al., 2007) is especially interesting, as there is no good reason to suppose that the thalamic HDR is anomalously prompt. An alternative interpretation (that avoids invoking noncausal models) is that the electrophysiological state of the thalamus is correlated at a lag with cerebral alpha generators, in other words, that the thalamus is causal of alpha. This question should be investigated.

The ICA-based strategy developed by Mantini et al. (2007) appears promising. However, the results obtained so far with this method need to be replicated. Particular attention should be given to RSN 6, which was localized to the fronto-polar regions and associated mostly with EEG activity in the gamma frequency range (30–50 Hz). The recent observations of Yuval-Greenberg et al. (2008) suggest that this activity may be generated by the extraocular muscles.

Additional Experiments are Needed to Study the Relations Between Task-Evoked Rhythmic EEG Activity and BOLD Responses

Although it is well documented that salient events evoke transient increases in midline frontal theta (mfθ; Basar et al., 2001), the BOLD correlates of this phenomenon have not been well studied. Several potentially informative combined EEG-fMRI experiments specifically focused on induced theta (nominally, 3–7 Hz) responses may be

mentioned: Nontarget (i.e., oddball) events appear to be more effective inducers of theta bursting than target events in P3-paradigms (Demiralp et al., 2001). Theta bursting also is characteristically seen as a correlate of the ERN (e.g., Debener et al., 2005). Gruber et al. (2008) have recently reported very interesting observations of induced theta (as well as induced gamma) responses in the context of recognition memory. In the memorization phase of their experiment, subjects viewed images of real objects and performed one of two semantic classification tasks concerning the displayed item. In the test phase they distinguished old from new items (simple recognition) and indicated which classification task had been performed (source or context memory). Correct (but not incorrect) source memory performance was accompanied by induced mfθ activity 600–1200 ms following presentation of the test image. This result links mfθ responses to episodic recall and hence, the limbic system. Given the wealth of fMRI (alone) experiments on source memory (Davachi, 2006), this paradigm presents an attractive possibility for a combined EEG-fMRI study.

It is Unclear that Simultaneous Acquisition is Necessary in all Combined Experimentation

The purpose of all combined electrophysiology-FNI experimentation is to define relations between the two very different types of data by analysis of variation, or, more precisely, covariation, in the combined dataset. Simultaneous EEG-fMRI acquisition is essential when this variation is randomly generated within the subject, e.g., in the resting state (Laufs et al., 2006) or when trial-to-trial response covariation is the chief object of study (e.g., Debener et al., 2005). Thus, simultaneous acquisition is essential also in clinical seizure focus localization and in sleep studies. Simultaneous EEG-fMRI acquisition is not essential when the variation is imposed by the experimentor, i.e., in "parametric" designs (Horovitz et al., 2004). It should be noted that some stochastic variability inevitably is generated within subjects even in parametric design experiments. However, if the parametric dependencies, e.g., on stimulus strength, are separately determined (by averaging) of the electrophysiological and fMRI data, then subject-generated stochastic variability plays no role in the analysis or the science. In some cases, the point of simultaneous acquisition appears to be to demonstrate technical feasibility (e.g., Iannetti et al., 2005). Such demonstrations are important but they should not be confused with neuroscience. It has been argued that it is impossible to exactly duplicate experimental conditions inside and outside the fMRI scanner (Debener et al., 2006). This consideration has merit up to a point. However, it is probably wise to avoid studying phenomena that, by hypothesis, are exquisitely sensitive to environmental conditions of the sort that cannot be made approximately equivalent inside and outside an fMRI scanner. Such sensitivity, if truly present, would compromise the generality of the findings, whatever they were.

A final point regarding simultaneous EEG-fMRI acquisition is that "DC" EEG recording probably is not feasible for technical reasons. Hence, experiments of the type reported by Schicke et al. (2006) can only be performed with separate EEG and fMRI acquisition.

What do Combined ERP-fMRI "Single Trial" Designs Tell us?

Single-trial combined ERP-fMRI designs capture the correlation between electrophysiological and hemodynamic responses in the context of behavioral events (Debener et al., 2006). Operationally, one computes fMRI response maps using a regressor constructed from an ERP. Hence, the computed results reflect two sources of variance: *(1)* a deterministic component linked to the event itself, and *(2)* a stochastic component that reflects trial-to-trial variability within the subject. The BOLD correlates of the deterministic component can be isolated by conventional event-related fMRI (ignoring the electrophysiological data). In principle, the BOLD correlates of the stochastic component can be isolated by analysis of the difference between the "single trial" and the event-related results. It is this stochastic component that can be studied only with simultaneous EEG-fMRI acquisition. Thus, single trial designs and resting state simultaneous EEG-fMRI experiments (e.g., Laufs et al., 2006) both target intrinsic variability within the subject.

Debener et al. (2005) employed temporal ICA to determine the channel weights that were subsequently used to extract the ERN. The objective of ICA in this context is to maximize capture of physiological signal while excluding artifact, e.g., from eye movements. Poolman et al. (2008) described an alternative technique based on forward modeling for maximizing S/N in single trial ERPs. ERPs were recorded from subjects as they performed a target detection task while viewing rapidly presented images. The performance (hit rate) of the single-trial ERP classifier was even better than that of the subjects (87% vs. 27%)! This result is attributable to stochastic variation of the coupling between visual recognition and motor behavior in the context of rapidly presented stimuli. Poolman et al. (2008) did not simultaneously acquire fMRI. However, their paradigm might be highly informative in a combined ERP-fMRI experiment.

ACKNOWLEDGMENTS

The authors' work was supported by NIH NS006833. The authors thank Dr. Richard Leahy for helpful discussion of inverse source localization.

REFERENCES

Ahlfors SP, Simpson GV, Dale AM, Belliveau JW, Liu AK, Korvenoja A, Virtanen J, Huotilainen M, Tootell RB, Aronen HJ, Ilmoniemi RJ (1999) Spatiotemporal activity of a cortical network for processing visual motion revealed by MEG and fMRI. J Neurophysiol 82:2545–2555.

Arthurs OJ, Boniface SJ (2003) What aspect of the fMRI BOLD signal best reflects the underlying electrophysiology in human somatosensory cortex? Clin Neurophysiol 114:1203–1209.

Arthurs OJ, Donovan T, Spiegelhalter DJ, Pickard JD, Boniface SJ (2007) Intracortically distributed neurovascular coupling relationships within and between human somatosensory cortices. Cereb Cortex 17:661–668.

Babiloni F, Mattia D, Babiloni C, Astolfi L, Salinari S, Basilisco A, Rossini PM, Marciani MG, Cincotti F (2004) Multimodal integration of EEG, MEG, and fMRI data for the solution of the neuroimage puzzle. Magn Reson Imaging 22:1471–1476.

Badre D, Wagner AD (2007) Left ventrolateral prefrontal cortex and the cognitive control of memory. Neuropsychologia 45:2883–2901.

Bai X, Towle VL, He EJ, He B (2007) Evaluation of cortical current density imaging methods using intracranial electrocorticograms and functional MRI. Neuroimage 35:598-608.

Basar E, Schurmann M, Sakowitz O (2001) The selectively distributed theta system: functions. Int J Psychophysiol 39:197–212.

Beckmann CF, DeLuca M, Devlin JT, Smith SM (2005) Investigations into resting-state connectivity using independent component analysis. Philos Trans R Soc Lond B Biol Sci 360:1001–1013.

Berger H (1929) On the electroencephalogram of man. Archiv für Psychiatrie und Nervenkrankheiten 87:527–570.

Birbaumer N, Elbert T, Canavan AG, Rockstroh B (1990) Slow potentials of the cerebral cortex and behavior. Physiol Rev 70:1–41.

Biswal B, Yetkin FZ, Haughton VM, Hyde JS (1995) Functional connectivity in the motor cortex of resting human brain using echo-planar MRI. Magn Reson Med 34:537–541.

Bledowski C, Prvulovic D, Hoechstetter K, Scherg M, Wibral M, Goebel R, Linden DE (2004) Localizing P300 generators in visual target and distractor processing: a combined event-related potential and functional magnetic resonance imaging study. J Neurosci 24:9353–9360.

Bledowski C, Cohen Kadosh K, Wibral M, Rahm B, Bittner RA, Hoechstetter K, Scherg M, Maurer K, Goebel R, Linden DE (2006) Mental chronometry of working memory retrieval: a combined functional magnetic resonance imaging and event-related potentials approach. J Neurosci 26:821–829.

Bledowski C, Linden DE, Wibral M (2007) Combining electrophysiology and functional imaging: different methods for different questions. Trends Cogn Sci 11:500–502.

Bonmassar G, Anami K, Ives J, Belliveau JW (1999) Visual evoked potential (VEP) measured by simultaneous 64-channel EEG and 3T fMRI. Neuroreport 10:1893–1897.

Boynton GM, Engel SA, Glover GH, Heeger DJ (1996) Linear systems analysis of functional magnetic resonance imaging in human V1. J Neurosci 16:4207–4221.

Braun AR, Balkin TJ, Wesenten NJ, Carson RE, Varga M, Baldwin P, Selbie S, Belenky G, Herscovitch P (1997) Regional cerebral blood flow throughout the sleep-wake cycle: an H2(15)O PET study. Brain 120 (Pt 7):1173–1197.

Brazdil M, Dobsik M, Mikl M, Hlustik P, Daniel P, Pazourkova M, Krupa P, Rektor I (2005) Combined event-related fMRI and intracerebral ERP study of an auditory oddball task. Neuroimage 26:285–293.

Brunetti M, Della Penna S, Ferretti A, Del Gratta C, Cianflone F, Belardinelli P, Caulo M, Pizzella V, Olivetti Belardinelli M, Romani GL (2008) A frontoparietal network for spatial attention reorienting in the auditory domain: a human fMRI/MEG study of functional and temporal dynamics. Cereb Cortex 18:1139–1147.

Brunia CH, van Boxtel GJ (2001) Wait and see. Int J Psychophysiol 43:59–75.

Buckner RL, Vincent JL (2007) Unrest at rest: default activity and spontaneous network correlations. Neuroimage 37:1091–1096; discussion 1097–1099.

Bullock TH, McClune MC, Achimowicz JZ, Iragui-Madoz VJ, Duckrow RB, Spencer SS (1995) EEG coherence has structure in the millimeter domain: subdural and hippocampal recordings from epileptic patients. Electroencephalogr Clin Neurophysiol 95:161–177.

Buzsaki G, Draguhn A (2004) Neuronal oscillations in cortical networks. Science 304:1926–1929.

Calhoun VD, Adali T, Pearlson GD, Kiehl KA (2006) Neuronal chronometry of target detection: fusion of hemodynamic and event-related potential data. Neuroimage 30:544–553.

Carter CS, Braver TS, Barch DM, Botvinick MM, Noll D, Cohen JD (1998) Anterior cingulate cortex, error detection, and the online monitoring of performance. Science 280:747–749.

Churchland PS, Sejnowski TJ (1988) Perspectives on cognitive neuroscience. Science 242:741–745.

Cohen NJ, Ryan J, Hunt C, Romine L, Wszalek T, Nash C (1999) Hippocampal system and declarative (relational) memory: summarizing the data from functional neuroimaging studies. Hippocampus 9:83–98.

Corbetta M, Shulman GL (2002) Control of goal-directed and stimulus-driven attention in the brain. Nat Rev Neurosci 3:201–215.

Crone NE, Sinai A, Korzeniewska A (2006) High-frequency gamma oscillations and human brain mapping with electrocorticography. Prog Brain Res 159:275–295.

Czisch M, Wehrle R, Kaufmann C, Wetter TC, Holsboer F, Pollmacher T, Auer DP (2004) Functional MRI during sleep: BOLD signal decreases and their electrophysiological correlates. Eur J Neurosci 20:566–574.

Dale AM, Halgren E (2001) Spatiotemporal mapping of brain activity by integration of multiple imaging modalities. Curr Opin Neurobiol 11:202–208.

Dale AM, Sereno MI (1993) Improved localiztion of cortical activity by combining EEG and MEG with MRI cortical surface reconstruction: A linear approach. J Cogn Neurosci 5:162–176.

Dale AM, Fischl B, Sereno MI (1999) Cortical surface-based analysis. I: Segmentation and surface reconstruction. Neuroimage 9:179–194.

Dale AM, Liu AK, Fischl BR, Buckner RL, Belliveau JW, Lewine JD, Halgren E (2000) Dynamic statistical parametric mapping: combining fMRI and MEG for high-resolution imaging of cortical activity. Neuron 26:55–67.

Darvas F, Ermer JJ, Mosher JC, Leahy RM (2006) Generic head models for atlas-based EEG source analysis. Hum Brain Mapp 27:129–143.

Davachi L (2006) Item, context, and relational episodic encoding in humans. Curr Opin Neurobiol 16:693–700.

de Munck JC, Goncalves SI, Huijboom L, Kuijer JP, Pouwels PJ, Heethaar RM, Lopes da Silva FH (2007) The hemodynamic response of the alpha rhythm: an EEG/fMRI study. Neuroimage 35:1142–1151.

Debener S, Ullsperger M, Siegel M, Fiehler K, von Cramon DY, Engel AK (2005) Trial-by-trial coupling of concurrent electroencephalogram and functional magnetic resonance imaging identifies the dynamics of performance monitoring. J Neurosci 25:11730–11737.

Debener S, Ullsperger M, Siegel M, Engel AK (2006) Single-trial EEG-fMRI reveals the dynamics of cognitive function. Trends Cogn Sci 10:558–563.

Debener S, Ullsperger M, Siegel M, Engel AK (2007) Towards single-trial analysis in cognitive brain research. Trends Cogn Sci 11:502–503.

Dehaene S, Posner MI, Tucker DM (1994) Localization of a neural system for error detection and compensation. Psychol Sci 5:303–305.

Demiralp T, Ademoglu A, Comerchero M, Polich J (2001) Wavelet analysis of P3a and P3b. Brain Topogr 13:251–267.

Devor A, Dunn AK, Andermann ML, Ulbert I, Boas DA, Dale AM (2003) Coupling of total hemoglobin concentration, oxygenation, and neural activity in rat somatosensory cortex. Neuron 39:353–359.

Drevets WC, Burton H, Videen TO, Snyder AZ, Simpson JR, Jr., Raichle ME (1995) Blood flow changes in human somatosensory cortex during anticipated stimulation. Nature 373:249–252.

Eichele T, Specht K, Moosmann M, Jongsma ML, Quiroga RQ, Nordby H, Hugdahl K (2005) Assessing the spatiotemporal evolution of neuronal activation with single-trial event-related potentials and functional MRI. Proc Natl Acad Sci U S A 102:17798–17803.

Eichele T, Calhoun VD, Moosmann M, Specht K, Jongsma ML, Quiroga RQ, Nordby H, Hugdahl K (2008) Unmixing concurrent EEG-fMRI with parallel independent component analysis. Int J Psychophysiol 67:222–234.

Engel AK, Singer W (2001) Temporal binding and the neural correlates of sensory awareness. Trends Cogn Sci 5:16–25.

Engel AK, Fries P, Singer W (2001) Dynamic predictions: oscillations and synchrony in top-down processing. Nat Rev Neurosci 2:704–716.

Feige B, Scheffler K, Esposito F, Di Salle F, Hennig J, Seifritz E (2005) Cortical and subcortical correlates of electroencephalographic alpha rhythm modulation. J Neurophysiol 93:2864–2872.

Fell J, Klaver P, Lehnertz K, Grunwald T, Schaller C, Elger CE, Fernandez G (2001) Human memory formation is accompanied by rhinal-hippocampal coupling and decoupling. Nat Neurosci 4:1259–1264.

Fernández G, Fell J, Pascal Fries P (2002) Response: the birth of a memory. Trends Neurosci 25:281–282.

Fox MD, Raichle ME (2007) Spontaneous fluctuations in brain activity observed with functional magnetic resonance imaging. Nat Rev Neurosci 8:700–711.

Fox MD, Snyder AZ, Vincent JL, Corbetta M, Van Essen DC, Raichle ME (2005) The human brain is intrinsically organized into dynamic, anticorrelated functional networks. Proc Natl Acad Sci U S A 102:9673–9678.

Fox PT, Raichle ME (1986) Focal physiological uncoupling of cerebral blood flow and oxidative metabolism during somatosensory stimulation in human subjects. Proc Natl Acad Sci U S A 83:1140–1144.

Fox PT, Miezin FM, Allman JM, Van Essen DC, Raichle ME (1987) Retinotopic organization of human visual cortex mapped with positron-emission tomography. J Neurosci 7:913–922.

Franceschini MA, Nissila I, Wu W, Diamond SG, Bonmassar G, Boas DA (2008) Coupling between somatosensory evoked potentials and hemodynamic response in the rat. Neuroimage 41:189–203.

Fries P (2005) A mechanism for cognitive dynamics: neuronal communication through neuronal coherence. Trends Cogn Sci 9:474–480.

Gamma A, Lehmann D, Frei E, Iwata K, Pascual-Marqui RD, Vollenweider FX (2004) Comparison of simultaneously recorded [H2(15)O]-PET and LORETA during cognitive and pharmacological activation. Hum Brain Mapp 22:83–96.

Ganis G, Kutas M, Sereno MI (1996) The search for "common sense": an electrophysiological study of the comprehension of words and pictures in reading. J Cogn Neurosci 8:89–106.

Goense JB, Logothetis NK (2008) Neurophysiology of the BOLD fMRI signal in awake monkeys. Curr Biol 18:631–640.

Goldman RI, Stern JM, Engel J, Jr., Cohen MS (2002) Simultaneous EEG and fMRI of the alpha rhythm. Neuroreport 13:2487–2492.

Goncalves SI, de Munck JC, Pouwels PJ, Schoonhoven R, Kuijer JP, Maurits NM, Hoogduin JM, Van Someren EJ, Heethaar RM, Lopes da Silva FH (2006) Correlating the alpha rhythm to BOLD using simultaneous EEG/fMRI: inter-subject variability. Neuroimage 30:203–213.

Gotman J (2008) Epileptic networks studied with EEG-fMRI. Epilepsia 49 (Suppl 3):42–51.

Grent-'t-Jong T, Woldorff MG (2007) Timing and sequence of brain activity in top-down control of visual-spatial attention. PLoS Biol 5:e12.

Gross J, Schmitz F, Schnitzler I, Kessler K, Shapiro K, Hommel B, Schnitzler A (2004) Modulation of long-range neural synchrony reflects temporal limitations of visual attention in humans. Proc Natl Acad Sci U S A 101:13050–13055.

Gruber T, Tsivilis D, Giabbiconi CM, Muller MM (2008) Induced electroencephalogram oscillations during source memory: familiarity is reflected in the gamma band, recollection in the theta band. J Cogn Neurosci 20:1043–1053.

Halgren E, Baudena P, Clarke JM, Heit G, Marinkovic K, Devaux B, Vignal JP, Biraben A (1995) Intracerebral potentials to rare target and distractor auditory and visual stimuli. II: Medial, lateral, and posterior temporal lobe. Electroencephalogr Clin Neurophysiol 94:229–250.

Hampshire A, Thompson R, Duncan J, Owen AM (2008) The target selective neural response: similarity, ambiguity, and learning effects. PLoS ONE 3:e2520.

Hari R, Joutsiniemi SL, Sarvas J (1988) Spatial resolution of neuromagnetic records: theoretical calculations in a spherical model. Electroencephalogr Clin Neurophysiol 71:64–72.

He BJ, Snyder AZ, Zempel JM, Smyth MD, Raichle ME (2008) Electrophysiological correlates of the brain's intrinsic large-scale functional architecture. Proc Natl Acad Sci U S A 105:16039–16044.

Heinze HJ, Mangun GR, Burchert W, Hinrichs H, Scholz M, Munte TF, Gos A, Scherg M, Johannes S, Hundeshagen H, et al. (1994) Combined spatial and temporal imaging of brain activity during visual selective attention in humans. Nature 372:543–546.

Herrmann CS, Debener S (2008) Simultaneous recording of EEG and BOLD responses: a historical perspective. Int J Psychophysiol 67:161–168.

Herrmann MJ, Huter T, Plichta MM, Ehlis AC, Alpers GW, Muhlberger A, Fallgatter AJ (2008) Enhancement of activity of the primary visual cortex during processing of emotional stimuli as measured with event-related functional near-infrared spectroscopy and event-related potentials. Hum Brain Mapp 29:28–35.

Horovitz SG, Gore JC (2004) Simultaneous event-related potential and near-infrared spectroscopic studies of semantic processing. Hum Brain Mapp 22:110–115.

Horovitz SG, Rossion B, Skudlarski P, Gore JC (2004) Parametric design and correlational analyses help integrating fMRI and electrophysiological data during face processing. Neuroimage 22:1587–1595.

Horovitz SG, Fukunaga M, de Zwart JA, van Gelderen P, Fulton SC, Balkin TJ, Duyn JH (2008) Low frequency BOLD fluctuations during resting wakefulness and light sleep: a simultaneous EEG-fMRI study. Hum Brain Mapp 29:671–682.

Horwitz B, Poeppel D (2002) How can EEG/MEG and fMRI/PET data be combined? Hum Brain Mapp 17:1–3.

Iannetti GD, Niazy RK, Wise RG, Jezzard P, Brooks JC, Zambreanu L, Vennart W, Matthews PM, Tracey I (2005) Simultaneous recording of laser-evoked brain potentials and continuous, high-field functional magnetic resonance imaging in humans. Neuroimage 28:708–719.

Im CH, Jung HK, Fujimaki N (2005) fMRI-constrained MEG source imaging and consideration of fMRI invisible sources. Hum Brain Mapp 26:110–118.

Juergens E, Guettler A, Eckhorn R (1999) Visual stimulation elicits locked and induced gamma oscillations in monkey intracortical- and EEG-potentials, but not in human EEG. Exp Brain Res 129:247–259.

Kahana MJ (2006) The cognitive correlates of human brain oscillations. J Neurosci 26:1669–1672.

Kenet T, Bibitchkov D, Tsodyks M, Grinvald A, Arieli A (2003) Spontaneously emerging cortical representations of visual attributes. Nature 425:954–956.

Khader P, Heil M, Rosler F (2005) Material-specific long-term memory representations of faces and spatial positions: evidence from slow event-related brain potentials. Neuropsychologia 43:2109–2124.

Kiehl KA, Laurens KR, Duty TL, Forster BB, Liddle PF (2001a) Neural sources involved in auditory target detection and novelty processing: an event-related fMRI study. Psychophysiology 38:133–142.

Kiehl KA, Laurens KR, Duty TL, Forster BB, Liddle PF (2001b) An event-related fMRI study of visual and auditory oddball tasks. J Psychophysiol 15:221–240.

Knight RT (2007) Neuroscience: neural networks debunk phrenology. Science 316:1578–1579.

Knight RT, Scabini D (1998) Anatomic bases of event-related potentials and their relationship to novelty detection in humans. J Clin Neurophysiol 15:3–13.

Kornhuber HH, Deecke L (1965) Changes in the brain potential in voluntary movements and passive movements in man: readiness potential and reafferent potentials. Pflugers Arch Gesamte Physiol Menschen Tiere 284:1–17.

Kotchoubey B (2006) Event-related potentials, cognition, and behavior: a biological approach. Neurosci Biobehav Rev 30:42–65.

Kruggel F, Wiggins CJ, Herrmann CS, von Cramon DY (2000) Recording of the event-related potentials during functional MRI at 3.0 Tesla field strength. Magn Reson Med 44:277–282.

Kutas M, Hillyard SA (1980) Event-related brain potentials to semantically inappropriate and surprisingly large words. Biol Psychol 11:99–116.

Lachaux JP, Fonlupt P, Kahane P, Minotti L, Hoffmann D, Bertrand O, Baciu M (2007) Relationship between task-related gamma oscillations and BOLD signal: new insights from combined fMRI and intracranial EEG. Hum Brain Mapp 28:1368–1375.

Lakatos P, Karmos G, Mehta AD, Ulbert I, Schroeder CE (2008) Entrainment of neuronal oscillations as a mechanism of attentional selection. Science 320:110–113.

Lamm C, Windischberger C, Leodolter U, Moser E, Bauer H (2001) Evidence for premotor cortex activity during dynamic visuospatial imagery from single-trial functional magnetic resonance imaging and event-related slow cortical potentials. Neuroimage 14:268–283.

Lang M, Lang W, Uhl F, Kornhuber A, Deecke L, Kornhuber HH (1987) Slow negative potential shifts indicating verbal cognitive learning in a concept formation task. Hum Neurobiol 6:183–190.Lang W, Lang M, Goldenberg G, Podreka I, Deecke L (1987) EEG and rCBF evidence for left frontocortical activation when memorizing verbal material. Electroencephalogr Clin Neurophysiol Suppl 40:328–334.

Larson-Prior LJ, Zempel JM, Nolan TS, Prior FW, Snyder AZ, Raichle ME (2009) Cortical network functional connectivity in the descent to sleep. Proc Natl Acad Sci U S A 106:4489–4494.

Laufs H, Duncan JS (2007) Electroencephalography/functional MRI in human epilepsy: what it currently can and cannot do. Curr Opin Neurol 20:417–423.

Laufs H, Kleinschmidt A, Beyerle A, Eger E, Salek-Haddadi A, Preibisch C, Krakow K (2003a) EEG-correlated fMRI of human alpha activity. Neuroimage 19:1463–1476.

Laufs H, Krakow K, Sterzer P, Eger E, Beyerle A, Salek-Haddadi A, Kleinschmidt A (2003b) Electroencephalographic signatures of attentional and cognitive default modes in spontaneous brain activity fluctuations at rest. Proc Natl Acad Sci U S A 100:11053–11058.

Laufs H, Holt JL, Elfont R, Krams M, Paul JS, Krakow K, Kleinschmidt A (2006) Where the BOLD signal goes when alpha EEG leaves. Neuroimage 31:1408–1418.

Leistner S, Sander T, Burghoff M, Curio G, Trahms L, Mackert BM (2007) Combined MEG and EEG methodology for non-invasive recording of infraslow activity in the human cortex. Clin Neurophysiol 118:2774–2780.

Leopold DA, Murayama Y, Logothetis NK (2003) Very slow activity fluctuations in monkey visual cortex: implications for functional brain imaging. Cereb Cortex 13:422–433.

Linden DE (2005) The p300: where in the brain is it produced and what does it tell us? Neuroscientist 11:563–576.

Linden DE (2007) What, when, where in the brain? Exploring mental chronometry with brain imaging and electrophysiology. Rev Neurosci 18:159–171.

Linkenkaer-Hansen K, Nikulin VV, Palva S, Ilmoniemi RJ, Palva JM (2004) Prestimulus oscillations enhance psychophysical performance in humans. J Neurosci 24:10186–10190.

Logothetis NK (2002) The neural basis of the blood-oxygen-level-dependent functional magnetic resonance imaging signal. Philos Trans R Soc Lond B Biol Sci 357:1003–1037.

Logothetis NK, Pfeuffer J (2004) On the nature of the BOLD fMRI contrast mechanism. Magn Reson Imaging 22:1517–1531.

Logothetis NK, Pauls J, Augath M, Trinath T, Oeltermann A (2001) Neurophysiological investigation of the basis of the fMRI signal. Nature 412:150–157.

Mackert BM, Leistner S, Sander T, Liebert A, Wabnitz H, Burghoff M, Trahms L, Macdonald R, Curio G (2008) Dynamics of cortical neurovascular coupling analyzed by simultaneous DC-magnetoencephalography and time-resolved near-infrared spectroscopy. Neuroimage 39:979–986.

Madsen PL (1993) Blood flow and oxygen uptake in the human brain during various states of sleep and wakefulness. Acta Neurol Scand Suppl 148:3–27.

Maier A, Wilke M, Aura C, Zhu C, Ye FQ, Leopold DA (2008) Divergence of fMRI and neural signals in V1 during perceptual suppression in the awake monkey. Nat Neurosci 11:1193–1200.

Makeig S, Delorme A, Westerfield M, Jung TP, Townsend J, Courchesne E, Sejnowski TJ (2004) Electroencephalographic brain dynamics following manually responded visual targets. PLoS Biol 2:e176.

Malonek D, Dirnagl U, Lindauer U, Yamada K, Kanno I, Grinvald A (1997) Vascular imprints of neuronal activity: relationships between the dynamics of cortical blood flow, oxygenation, and volume changes following sensory stimulation. Proc Natl Acad Sci U S A 94:14826–14831.

Mangun GR, Hinrichs H, Scholz M, Mueller-Gaertner HW, Herzog H, Krause BJ, Tellman L, Kemna L, Heinze HJ (2001) Integrating electrophysiology and neuroimaging of spatial selective attention to simple isolated visual stimuli. Vision Res 41:1423–1435.

Mantini D, Perrucci MG, Del Gratta C, Romani GL, Corbetta M (2007) Electrophysiological signatures of resting state networks in the human brain. Proc Natl Acad Sci U S A 104:13170–13175.

Maquet P, Ruby P, Maudoux A, Albouy G, Sterpenich V, Dang-Vu T, Desseilles M, Boly M, Perrin F, Peigneux P, Laureys S (2005) Human cognition during REM sleep and the activity profile within frontal and parietal cortices: a reappraisal of functional neuroimaging data. Prog Brain Res 150:219–227.

Martinez-Montes E, Valdes-Sosa PA, Miwakeichi F, Goldman RI, Cohen MS (2004) Concurrent EEG/fMRI analysis by multiway Partial Least Squares. Neuroimage 22:1023–1034.

Matsumoto A, Iidaka T, Haneda K, Okada T, Sadato N (2005) Linking semantic priming effect in functional MRI and event-related potentials. Neuroimage 24:624–634.

Miller BT, Deouell LY, Dam C, Knight RT, D'Esposito M (2008) Spatio-temporal dynamics of neural mechanisms underlying component operations in working memory. Brain Res 1206:61–75.

Miller KJ, Leuthardt EC, Schalk G, Rao RP, Anderson NR, Moran DW, Miller JW, Ojemann JG (2007) Spectral changes in cortical surface potentials during motor movement. J Neurosci 27:2424–2432.

Mitzdorf U (1985) Current source-density method and application in cat cerebral cortex: investigation of evoked potentials and EEG phenomena. Physiol Rev 65:37–100.

Mizuhara H, Wang LQ, Kobayashi K, Yamaguchi Y (2004) A long-range cortical network emerging with theta oscillation in a mental task. Neuroreport 15:1233–1238.

Moon CH, Fukuda M, Park SH, Kim SG (2007) Neural interpretation of blood oxygenation level-dependent fMRI maps at sub-millimeter columnar resolution. J Neurosci 27:6892–6902.

Moosmann M, Ritter P, Krastel I, Brink A, Thees S, Blankenburg F, Taskin B, Obrig H, Villringer A (2003) Correlates of alpha rhythm in functional magnetic resonance imaging and near infrared spectroscopy. Neuroimage 20:145–158.

Mosher JC, Spencer ME, Leahy RM, Lewis PS (1993) Error bounds for EEG and MEG dipole source localization. Electroencephalogr Clin Neurophysiol 86:303–321.

Mulert C, Jager L, Schmitt R, Bussfeld P, Pogarell O, Moller HJ, Juckel G, Hegerl U (2004) Integration of fMRI and simultaneous EEG: towards a comprehensive understanding of localization and time-course of brain activity in target detection. Neuroimage 22:83–94.

Mulert C, Jager L, Propp S, Karch S, Stormann S, Pogarell O, Moller HJ, Juckel G, Hegerl U (2005) Sound level dependence of the primary auditory cortex: simultaneous measurement with 61-channel EEG and fMRI. Neuroimage 28:49–58.

Niessing J, Ebisch B, Schmidt KE, Niessing M, Singer W, Galuske RA (2005) Hemodynamic signals correlate tightly with synchronized gamma oscillations. Science 309:948–951.

Nir Y, Fisch L, Mukamel R, Gelbard-Sagiv H, Arieli A, Fried I, Malach R (2007) Coupling between neuronal firing rate, gamma LFP, and BOLD fMRI is related to interneuronal correlations. Curr Biol 17:1275–1285.

Nir Y, Mukamel R, Dinstein I, Privman E, Harel M, Fisch L, Gelbard-Sagiv H, Kipervasser S, Andelman F, Neufeld MY, Kramer U, Arieli A, Fried I, Malach R (2008) Interhemispheric correlations of slow spontaneous neuronal fluctuations revealed in human sensory cortex. Nat Neurosci 11:1100–1108.

Nita DA, Vanhatalo S, Lafortune FD, Voipio J, Kaila K, Amzica F (2004) Nonneuronal origin of CO_2-related DC EEG shifts: an in vivo study in the cat. J Neurophysiol 92:1011–1022.

Noesselt T, Hillyard SA, Woldorff MG, Schoenfeld A, Hagner T, Jancke L, Tempelmann C, Hinrichs H, Heinze HJ (2002) Delayed striate cortical activation during spatial attention. Neuron 35:575–587.

Nunez PL, Pilgreen KL (1991) The spline-Laplacian in clinical neurophysiology: a method to improve EEG spatial resolution. J Clin Neurophysiol 8:397–413.

Nunez PL, Silberstein RB (2000) On the relationship of synaptic activity to macroscopic measurements: does co-registration of EEG with fMRI make sense? Brain Topogr 13:79–96.

Obrig H, Israel H, Kohl-Bareis M, Uludag K, Wenzel R, Muller B, Arnold G, Villringer A (2002) Habituation of the visually evoked potential and its vascular response: implications for neurovascular coupling in the healthy adult. Neuroimage 17:1–18.

Ohara S, Mima T, Baba K, Ikeda A, Kunieda T, Matsumoto R, Yamamoto J, Matsuhashi M, Nagamine T, Hirasawa K, Hori T, Mihara T, Hashimoto N, Salenius S, Shibasaki H (2001) Increased synchronization of cortical oscillatory activities between human supplementary motor and primary sensorimotor areas during voluntary movements. J Neurosci 21:9377–9386.

Ojemann JG, Akbudak E, Snyder AZ, McKinstry RC, Raichle ME, Conturo TE (1997) Anatomic localization and quantitative analysis of gradient refocused echo-planar fMRI susceptibility artifacts. Neuroimage 6:156–167.

Otten LJ, Rugg MD (2002) The birth of a memory. Trends Neurosci 25:279–281; discussion 281–282.

Pascual-Marqui RD (1999) Review of methods for solving the EEG inverse problem. Int J Bioelectromagn 1:75–86.Pascual-Marqui RD, Michel CM, Lehmann D (1994) Low resolution electromagnetic tomography: a new method for localizing electrical activity in the brain. Int J Psychophysiol 18:49–65.

Passingham D, Sakai K (2004) The prefrontal cortex and working memory: physiology and brain imaging. Curr Opin Neurobiol 14:163–168.

Perrin F, Pernier J, Bertrand O, Giard MH, Echallier JF (1987) Mapping of scalp potentials by surface spline interpolation. Electroencephalogr Clin Neurophysiol 66:75–81.

Petersen SE, Fox PT, Posner MI, Mintun M, Raichle ME (1988) Positron emission tomographic studies of the cortical anatomy of single-word processing. Nature 331:585–589.

Pfurtscheller G (2006) The cortical activation model (CAM). Prog Brain Res 159:19–27.

Pizzagalli DA, Oakes TR, Davidson RJ (2003) Coupling of theta activity and glucose metabolism in the human rostral anterior cingulate cortex: an EEG/PET study of normal and depressed subjects. Psychophysiology 40:939–949.

Pizzella V, Romani GL (1990) Principles of magnetoencephalography. Adv Neurol 54:1–9.

Polich J (2007) Updating P300: an integrative theory of P3a and P3b. Clin Neurophysiol 118:2128–2148.

Poolman P, Frank RM, Luu P, Pederson SM, Tucker DM (2008) A single-trial analytic framework for EEG analysis and its application to target detection and classification. Neuroimage 42:787–798.

Raichle ME (1987) Circulatory and metabolic correlates of brain function in normal humans. In: Handbook of Physiology, Section 1, The Nervous System V. Higher Functions of the Brain, Part 2 (Plum F, ed), pp 643-674. Bethesda: American Physiological Society.

Raichle ME, Mintun MA (2006) Brain work and brain imaging. Annu Rev Neurosci 29:449–476.

Raichle ME, Snyder AZ (2007) A default mode of brain function: a brief history of an evolving idea. Neuroimage 37:1083–1090; discussion 1097–1099.

Raichle ME, MacLeod AM, Snyder AZ, Powers WJ, Gusnard DA, Shulman GL (2001) A default mode of brain function. Proc Natl Acad Sci U S A 98:676–682.

Rektor I, Sochurkova D, Bockova M (2006) Intracerebral ERD/ERS in voluntary movement and in cognitive visuomotor task. Prog Brain Res 159:311–330.

Roberts KL, Hall DA (2008) Examining a supramodal network for conflict processing: a systematic review and novel functional magnetic resonance imaging data for related visual and auditory stroop tasks. J Cogn Neurosci 20:1063–1078.

Roland PE (2002) Dynamic depolarization fields in the cerebral cortex. Trends Neurosci 25:183–190.

Rosler F, Heil M, Roder B (1997) Slow negative brain potentials as reflections of specific modular resources of cognition. Biol Psychol 45:109–141.

Rovati L, Salvatori G, Bulf L, Fonda S (2007) Optical and electrical recording of neural activity evoked by graded contrast visual stimulus. Biomed Eng Online 6:28.

Rush S, Driscoll DA (1968) Current distribution in the brain from surface electrodes. Anesth Analg 47:717–723.

Saalmann YB, Pigarev IN, Vidyasagar TR (2007) Neural mechanisms of visual attention: how top-down feedback highlights relevant locations. Science 316:1612–1615.

Sammer G, Blecker C, Gebhardt H, Kirsch P, Stark R, Vaitl D (2005) Acquisition of typical EEG waveforms during fMRI: SSVEP, LRP, and frontal theta. Neuroimage 24:1012–1024.

Schabus M, Dang-Vu TT, Albouy G, Balteau E, Boly M, Carrier J, Darsaud A, Degueldre C, Desseilles M, Gais S, Phillips C, Rauchs G, Schnakers C, Sterpenich V, Vandewalle G, Luxen A, Maquet P (2007) Hemodynamic cerebral correlates of sleep spindles during human non-rapid eye movement sleep. Proc Natl Acad Sci U S A 104:13164–13169.

Scheeringa R, Bastiaansen MC, Petersson KM, Oostenveld R, Norris DG, Hagoort P (2008) Frontal theta EEG activity correlates negatively with the default mode network in resting state. Int J Psychophysiol 67:242–251.

Scherg M, Picton TW (1991) Separation and identification of event-related potential components by brain electric source analysis. Electroencephalogr Clin Neurophysiol Suppl 42:24–37.

Schicke T, Muckli L, Beer AL, Wibral M, Singer W, Goebel R, Rosler F, Roder B (2006) Tight covariation of BOLD signal changes and slow ERPs in the parietal cortex in a parametric spatial imagery task with haptic acquisition. Eur J Neurosci 23:1910–1918.

Schoffelen JM, Oostenveld R, Fries P (2005) Neuronal coherence as a mechanism of effective corticospinal interaction. Science 308:111–113.

Schubert R, Ritter P, Wustenberg T, Preuschhof C, Curio G, Sommer W, Villringer A (2008) Spatial attention related SEP amplitude modulations covary with BOLD signal in S1-A simultaneous EEG-fMRI study. Cereb Cortex 18:2686–2700.

Sestieri C, Sylvester CM, Jack AI, d'Avossa G, Shulman GL, Corbetta M (2008) Independence of anticipatory signals for spatial attention from number of nontarget stimuli in the visual field. J Neurophysiol 100:829–838.

Sheth SA, Nemoto M, Guiou M, Walker M, Pouratian N, Toga AW (2004) Linear and nonlinear relationships between neuronal activity, oxygen metabolism, and hemodynamic responses. Neuron 42:347–355.

Shmuel A, Augath M, Oeltermann A, Logothetis NK (2006) Negative functional MRI response correlates with decreases in neuronal activity in monkey visual area V1. Nat Neurosci 9:569–577.

Siegel AM, Culver JP, Mandeville JB, Boas DA (2003) Temporal comparison of functional brain imaging with diffuse optical tomography and fMRI during rat forepaw stimulation. Phys Med Biol 48:1391–1403.

Siegel M, Donner TH, Oostenveld R, Fries P, Engel AK (2007) High-frequency activity in human visual cortex is modulated by visual motion strength. Cereb Cortex 17:732–741.

Sirotin YB, Das A (2009) Anticipatory haemodynamic signals in sensory cortex not predicted by local neuronal activity. Nature 457:475–479.

Snyder AZ (1991) Dipole source localization in the study of EP generators: a critique. Electroencephalogr Clin Neurophysiol 80:321–325.

Snyder AZ (1992) Steady-state vibration evoked potentials: descriptions of technique and characterization of responses. Electroencephalogr Clin Neurophysiol 84:257–268.

Snyder AZ, Abdullaev YG, Posner MI, Raichle ME (1995) Scalp electrical potentials reflect regional cerebral blood flow responses during processing of written words. Proc Natl Acad Sci U S A 92:1689–1693.

Strobel A, Debener S, Sorger B, Peters JC, Kranczioch C, Hoechstetter K, Engel AK, Brocke B, Goebel R (2008) Novelty and target processing during an auditory novelty oddball: a simultaneous event-related potential and functional magnetic resonance imaging study. Neuroimage 40:869–883.

Thees S, Blankenburg F, Taskin B, Curio G, Villringer A (2003) Dipole source localization and fMRI of simultaneously recorded data applied to somatosensory categorization. Neuroimage 18:707–719.

Towle VL, Yoon HA, Castelle M, Edgar JC, Biassou NM, Frim DM, Spire JP, Kohrman MH (2008) ECoG gamma activity during a language task: differentiating expressive and receptive speech areas. Brain 131:2013–2027.

Toyoda H, Kashikura K, Okada T, Nakashita S, Honda M, Yonekura Y, Kawaguchi H, Maki A, Sadato N (2008) Source of nonlinearity of the BOLD response revealed by simultaneous fMRI and NIRS. Neuroimage 39:997–1013.

Ullsperger M, von Cramon DY (2004) Neuroimaging of performance monitoring: error detection and beyond. Cortex 40:593–604.

Van Petten C, Luka BJ (2006) Neural localization of semantic context effects in electromagnetic and hemodynamic studies. Brain Lang 97:279–293.

Vanhatalo S, Tallgren P, Becker C, Holmes MD, Miller JW, Kaila K, Voipio J (2003) Scalp-recorded slow EEG responses generated in response to hemodynamic changes in the human brain. Clin Neurophysiol 114:1744–1754.

Vanni S, Warnking J, Dojat M, Delon-Martin C, Bullier J, Segebarth C (2004) Sequence of pattern onset responses in the human visual areas: an fMRI constrained VEP source analysis. Neuroimage 21:801–817.

Varela F, Lachaux JP, Rodriguez E, Martinerie J (2001) The brainweb: phase synchronization and large-scale integration. Nat Rev Neurosci 2:229–239.

Vilberg KL, Rugg MD (2008a) Memory retrieval and the parietal cortex: a review of evidence from a dual-process perspective. Neuropsychologia 46:1787–1799.

Vilberg KL, Rugg MD (2008b) Functional significance of retrieval-related activity in lateral parietal cortex: evidence from fMRI and ERPs. Hum Brain Mapp 30:1490–1501.

Vincent JL, Kahn I, Snyder AZ, Raichle ME, Buckner RL (2008) Evidence for a frontoparietal control system revealed by intrinsic functional connectivity. J Neurophysiol 100:3328–3342.

Vincent JL, Patel GH, Fox MD, Snyder AZ, Baker JT, Van Essen DC, Zempel JM, Snyder LH, Corbetta M, Raichle ME (2007) Intrinsic functional architecture in the anaesthetized monkey brain. Nature 447:83–86.

Voipio J, Tallgren P, Heinonen E, Vanhatalo S, Kaila K (2003) Millivolt-scale DC shifts in the human scalp EEG: evidence for a nonneuronal generator. J Neurophysiol 89:2208–2214.

Wehrle R, Czisch M, Kaufmann C, Wetter TC, Holsboer F, Auer DP, Pollmacher T (2005) Rapid eye movement-related brain activation in human sleep: a functional magnetic resonance imaging study. Neuroreport 16:853–857.

Wehrle R, Kaufmann C, Wetter TC, Holsboer F, Auer DP, Pollmacher T, Czisch M (2007) Functional microstates within human REM sleep: first evidence from fMRI of a thalamocortical network specific for phasic REM periods. Eur J Neurosci 25:863–871.

Yarbus AL (1967) Eye movements and vision. New York: Plenum Press.

Yeung N, Botvinick MM, Cohen JD (2004) The neural basis of error detection: conflict monitoring and the error-related negativity. Psychol Rev 111:931–959.

Yodh AG, Boas DA (2003) Functional imaging with diffusing light. In: Biomedical photonics handbook (Vo-Dinh T, ed), pp 21–45. Boca Raton, FL: CRC Press.

Yuval-Greenberg S, Tomer O, Keren AS, Nelken I, Deouell LY (2008) Transient induced gamma-band response in EEG as a manifestation of miniature saccades. Neuron 58:429–441.

Part 2

Technical Basics of Recording Simultaneous EEG-fMRI

2.1 ⊞ Ingmar Gutberlet

Recording EEG Signals Inside the MRI

Introduction

The wish to perform parallel (but not necessarily concurrent) recordings of EEG and fMRI signals largely stems from the differences in the characteristics of the signals measured. While both the EEG and fMRI are capable of quantifying aspects of the changes occurring in the brain's activity in response to exogenous and endogenous stimuli, they differ vastly in their temporal and spatial resolution (Ives et al., 1993). They can thus be seen as disparate, or as we shall see in later chapters, also as complementary if properly used in so-called combined or simultaneous measurements (Horwitz and Poeppel, 2002; Debener et al., 2005; Debener et al., 2006).

The EEG measures the changes in electrical discharge of cortical neuronal populations and can (at least theoretically) characterize these signal variations at arbitrary speeds, thus allowing full characterization of the evolution of the electrical processes as they occur. However, its spatial resolution has to be seen as poor, even with EEG recordings of 256 or more channels. This poor resolution is attributable to the dispersion of the electrical signals along their projected path from the neuronal sources through the layers of CSF, skull, and scalp to the superficially attached EEG electrodes, and to the decay of the signals with distance. These influences limit the spatial in-plane resolution achievable as well as the spatial depth of measurements possible with EEG recordings (see Chapter 1.1 in this volume).

Functional magnetic resonance imaging, on the other hand, is vastly superior to EEG in its spatial depth and resolution, spanning the entire brain based on voxels of only a few millimeters. But at the same time fMRI has a rather slow acquisition rate, typically on the order of 60–100 ms per slice acquired, which leads to acquisition times for fMRI volumes of the entire brain volume that are on the order of seconds, an eternity in EEG terms. Furthermore, the signal measured by fMRI is not a rapidly time-varying signal

as in the case of the EEG, but instead consists of the rather slow and somewhat slurred evolution of the hemodynamic response to the exogenous or endogenous stimulation, and thus only gives indirect information on the processes involved (see Chapter 1.2 in this volume).

While these differences in domain, signal content, and spatial and temporal resolution certainly contain many challenges, the benefit from performing parallel and concurrent EEG and fMRI measurements is vast, and since the late 1990s much attention has focused on the development of equipment suitable for the integration of these two signal domains (Salek-Haddadi et al., 2003; Menon and Crottaz-Herbette, 2005; Ritter and Villringer, 2006; Herrmann and Debener, 2008; Laufs et al., 2008).

Parallel Versus Concurrent Acquisition

In many cases, a parallel acquisition, where the same subject is measured with the same experimental paradigm in the EEG laboratory and in the MR scanner on separate occasions may suffice (cf. Chapter 3.7 in this book). This holds true particularly for situations where conducting the same experiment in succession does not lead to memory or learning effects and where no habituation or sensitization has to be expected to occur. Several groups have successfully applied parametric approaches to integrating the data from separately recorded EEG and fMRI session (Horovitz et al., 2002; Schicke et al., 2006).

However, the validity of data acquired for the EEG and fMRI domains in separate sessions is not only dependent on aspects related to the experimental paradigm, but also depends profoundly on differences in the measurement environment. One important factor contributing to this is the restricted space available in the scanner bore in conjunction with the explicit requirement to avoid any movement, which makes this a situation with substantial claustrophobic potential for many subjects. The position of the subject in the scanner typically is supine rather than sitting upright, as in the EEG lab situation, which can have a profound effect on behavioral and bodily processes (Caldwell et al., 2003; Debener et al., 2006). And last but not least, the loud noise caused by the mechanical resonances related to magnetic gradient switching in the MR environment not only makes experiments with auditory stimulation more challenging, but also physically acts as a distractor for experimental stimuli of other modalities and reduces the available attentional capacity.

Taken together, all of these factors very likely alter the time course and pattern of processing for the nominally same experimental stimuli sufficiently to cast serious doubt on the assumption that EEG and fMRI data acquired in subsequent experimental runs will show similar or even the same experimental effects (Sammer et al., 2005; Debener et al., 2006).

While the concurrent acquisition of EEG and MR/fMRI will certainly not alleviate the environmental effects that hamper the performance of experimental paradigms in the scanner bore, it clearly would help to keep these factors constant for the EEG data as well as for the fMRI data. In other words, while a certain paradigm with well-known effects may not elicit the expected effects in as pure a form as can be expected for measurements outside the scanner, the combined EEG and fMRI measurement will nonetheless allow researchers to explore the commonalities of the processes elicited by the experimental stimulation in the fast EEG domain and concurrently in the highly resolved fMRI domain. Moreover, within-subject analyses of brain dynamics, e.g., ongoing and trial-by-trial changes of hemodynamic and electrical activity, can only be performed using simultaneously acquired EEG and fMRI data (Debener et al., 2005; Debener et al., 2006).

Challenges in Recording EEG in the MR

Performing EEG measurements in the scanner environment has many technical and safety related challenges. This section deals primarily with technical challenges of recording EEG in the MR environment. For a discussion of safety related issues see below.

Technically, the MR bore has to be seen as a "hostile" environment for the recording of EEG. There are several reasons for this, mostly related to the homogeneous and gradient-switching magnetic environment of the MR bore.

While the EEG systems available for combined EEG/MR recordings differ in their technical setup and thus also in the exposure of the equipment to the MR environment (and vice versa), one thing that is common to all systems is that the measurements have to be made using electrode caps with greatly differing electrode counts that are fitted on the subject's head while the subject is lying supine in the magnet.

This exposes the cap, electrodes, and electrode leads to the strong homogeneous static magnetic field of the scanner and also, more importantly, to the rapidly changing variable magnetic fields generated by gradient switching. Finally, the cap, electrodes, and electrode leads are also exposed to the profound radio frequency (RF) energy emitted during the scan sequence (Grandolfo et al., 1992; Schenck, 2000; Den Boer et al., 2002; Nitz et al., 2005).

Because of the electrical nature of the EEG signals to be measured, the electrodes and electrode leads used in EEG systems have to be made of electrically conducting materials (typically, Ag/AgCl for the electrodes and stranded copper or carbon fibers for the leads). In accord with Faraday's law, any changes in the magnetic field, including those induced by the switching of the magnetic gradients but also any movement of the subject's head or individual cables, induce currents in the electrodes and leads (Hill et al., 1995; Lemieux et al., 1997). The voltage potentials resulting from this current flow are measured along with the EEG signals as artifacts with amplitudes of up to two orders of magnitude above the spontaneous EEG and at equally enormous rates of change that are often three orders of magnitude faster than those of the EEG acquired (Allen et al., 2000; Ritter et al., 2007). The amplitude and frequency characteristics of these gradient artifacts superimposed on the EEG signals largely depend on the strength and slew rate of the gradients being switched as well as on the input stage and filter characteristics of the EEG amplifier. They will also vary with the length of the electrode leads, since longer electrode leads tend to have a more antenna-like characteristic and are often routed through more inhomogeneous portions of the scanner's magnetic field, resulting in stronger magnetic induction (Laufs et al., 2008; also see the section on patient safety, below, regarding cable length).

The RF energy emitted during slice acquisition is coupled onto the electrode leads and dissipated at the points of highest thermal resistance, which typically is the contact point between the electrode terminal and the scalp across the conductive EEG gel, associated with the risk of heating and potentially also of burning (Angelone et al., 2004; Angelone et al., 2006; Laufs et al., 2008). However the RF energy will also dissipate on the input stages of the amplifier, and sophisticated engineering efforts are required to guard the input stages against this energy dissipation and at the same time retain the sensitivity and frequency response desired from a modern EEG amplifier.

The EEG signals afflicted with these artifacts are typically contaminated to the point where no EEG is discernible in the ongoing EEG traces at standard vertical resolutions. Chapter 2.3 in this volume shows examples of this and gives an account of the various methods used for the reduction/removal of these gradient artifacts from the EEG traces.

Types of MR Compatible Equipment

Despite the strong interest in this field, documented by the steadily increasing number of publications and the strong focus on the topic at large international conferences, there are few commercially available EEG systems for simultaneous EEG/fMRI acquisition.

The reasons for this apparent discrepancy surely lie in the technical challenges inherent to the design of EEG equipment capable of withstanding the technical hostility of the MR environment. All elements of the EEG hardware that are exposed to the strong homogeneous magnetic field, to the time-varying gradient fields, and to the RF pulses emitted have to be designed with the various MR scanner effects considered. Add to this the need to complement the MR-compatible hardware with online/offline software capable of removing the artifacts caused by combined EEG/MR recordings, and it becomes clear that not many EEG equipment manufacturers would have the developmental prowess, manpower, and market exposure to make such a complete new system development manageable and feasible.

Currently, the market for EEG/MR equipment is dominated by two companies whose equipment differs vastly in the technical approach taken to the EEG/MR problem. Beyond those, a few smaller companies have positioned their equipment mostly in niches, such as an adjunct to clinical applications or in animal research. However, several further additions to this group are currently making their entrance into the EEG/fMRI market; and while it is clearly too early to judge the EEG/MR data quality achievable with these upcoming systems, the technical approaches taken seem well founded and in part even technically innovative, and these systems therefore deserve mention. It would also be unfair to neglect the early pioneering efforts of individual research groups to engineer their own "home grown" EEG/MR amplifiers, many of which resulted in working and quite effective EEG/MR machines (e.g., Ives et al., 1993, Allen et al., 2000; Goldman et al., 2000). However, since the focus of this chapter is on the application of EEG/MR for the larger scientific community, we shall limit our discussion to commercially and thereby readily available EEG/MR equipment.

The manufacturers of currently available and upcoming EEG/MR equipment take different approaches both to the "hostility" of the MR recording environment and to the reduction of the gradient artifacts. And generally speaking, the currently available MR-compatible EEG systems fall into two categories: EEG systems that reside in the scanner control room during recording, and EEG systems that reside in the scanner enclosure or even in the scanner bore during combined recordings.

EEG Systems Positioned Outside of Scanner Room (EEG/MR Cap Systems)

Positioning the EEG system used for a combined EEG/MR recordings in the scanner control room has its definite advantages, but it also has drawbacks. One major advantage for the manufacturer of such equipment is that the amplifier system is not exposed to the strong magnetic field of the MR system and therefore does not have to be designed specifically for MR compatibility and MR safety. In fact, such EEG systems can be technically equivalent to their non-MR counterparts, which means that there is almost none of the cost that would otherwise be incurred by the design, manufacturing, testing, and marketing of an amplifier specifically intended for use *inside* the scanner chamber. Another potential advantage, closely related to the first, is that there can be no direct electromagnetic influence either on the amplification circuitry or on the electronics that control the amplifier itself. The operation of the amplifier thus can not be compromised by the MR environment; this condition is otherwise quite challenging to achieve.

However, there are drawbacks: The most notable of these is that the distance between the amplifier deriving the EEG signals and the electrodes on the subjects head is very long, typically on the order of 8–10 meters, since the orientation of most MR scanners is with the subject's head pointing away from the scanner control room. This means that the electrode leads have to extend through the entire MR enclosure and through the filter panel into the MR control room to connect to the amplifier. This is technically challenging for several reasons: The induction of gradient artifacts in the electrode leads varies with the length of the cables used, and longer cables will also cause EEG signal decay and instability. It can also be more difficult to keep long leads from moving or being moved, e.g., by gradient-switching induced resonances, which in turn would induce artifacts into the EEG data recorded. However, the most critical aspect is that the entire electrode cable matrix needs to be passed through the MR filter panel into the scanner control room, which requires a conduit with a diameter large enough to pass through the cable matrix including its multi-channel connector. Furthermore, this setup creates an electrical connection between the scanner enclosure and the scanner control room, which can lead to severe leakage of RF energy into the sealed MR chamber. This can only be counteracted with the help of special RF filter devices installed on the MR filter panel, which makes such EEG/MR setups rather bulky and a more or less a permanent installation. There is, however, no reason to assume that this setup, if implemented well, will lead to reduced data quality. The challenges are not fundamental, but instead technical.

One currently available commercial system that is designed in this fashion is the MagLink™ EEG/MR system (Compumedics Limited, Abbotsford, Australia). It is specified for up to 128 channels of concurrent EEG and MRI/fMRI and for field strengths of up to 4T.

To deal with the aforementioned problem of electromagnetic and RF cross conductance onto the very long lead assembly passing through the entire MR chamber and into the scanner control room, an impedance matching buffer amplifier is available, which boosts the EEG signal and thus increases the signal-to-noise ratio (SNR) of the signal along its transmission path.

EEG Systems Positioned in the Scanner Room (EEG/MR Amplifier Systems)

Irrespective of the data quality achievable with setups where the EEG amplifier is located outside of the scanner enclosure, it is the specific technical challenges and effort involved that make it seem more desirable to place the amplifier inside the scanner enclosure instead.

The major advantage with these setups is that the mass of cables coming off the electrode cap does not have to be routed over a long distance, thus reducing the chance for significant MR gradient and RF signal induction and cable movement artifacts. And finally and most importantly, the connection that forwards the signals from the amplifier to the recording computer after analog/digital (AD) conversion can be constructed with fiber optical leads, which are immune against magnetic or RF coupling and consequently also do not hold the risk of creating an RF leak between the scanner control room and MR chamber (Allen et al., 2000).

Most systems that fall into this category essentially are nonetheless shielded versions of non–MR compatible amplifiers, where a standard amplifier is enclosed in an MR shielding box equipped with RF filters, fiber optical transmission links, and a rechargeable battery. An EEG system enclosed in such an MR shielding case can then safely be placed inside the MR scanner chamber, albeit not inside the scanner bore. This solution shares the advantage of lower development cost, with the systems located completely outside of the MR chamber, since the amplifier system itself does not have to be redesigned.

However, this solution nonetheless means some additional technical effort and cost, not only for the design and production of the MR-compatible casing, RF filters, and battery pack, but also because these essentially non-MR amplifiers typically have further inputs—for example, event or trigger inputs—located on the amplifier itself that would normally receive information from devices that are located in the scanner control room. To avoid passing these signals to the amplifier via electrical connections through the MR chamber filter panel, which would again potentially cause RF leakage, these electrical signals are then integrated by an interface device residing in the scanner control room and are then forwarded to the amplifier via fiber optical connections. Figure 2.1.1 shows a schematic illustration of the arrangement of such a system in the scanner chamber and the scanner control room.

There have recently been some additions to the commercially available EEG/MR systems in this category and one good example of this is the "fMRI Upgrade Package" available from Electrical Geodesics Inc. (EGI, Eugene, USA) for their Net Amps 300™ amplifier. This system uses a "Field Isolation Containment System" (FICS), essentially a magnetically shielded box, to achieve MR compatibility. This FICS box also contains the additionally required components mentioned above such as RF filters, optical-electrical converters for signal transmission, and a rechargeable battery. The amplifier itself is modified only slightly, compared to the standard amplifier version, to enhance its compatibility with the MR environment (personal communication, Phan Luu, EGI). The system uses an MR compatible version of EGI's HydroCel Geodesic Sensor Net 120 and is specified to work with up to 256 channels of EEG. Figure 2.1.2 shows the "Field Isolation Containment System" with the NetAmps 300™ amplifier halfway inserted.

Currently, there is only one commercially available EEG/MR system explicitly designed to work directly inside the scanner bore with the idea being to minimize the length of all electrical connections and to thereby minimize the influence of the gradient switching on the data acquired. The BrainAmp MR system by Brain Products (Brain Products GmbH, Gilching, Germany) is a modular amplifier consisting of units of 32 unipolar channels each. It is specified for up to 128 channels and for field strengths of up to 4T, but due to its explicit MR design has been shown to work without fault in field strengths of up to 7T. A special bipolar amplifier is available for the derivation of bipolar (e.g., EMG, EKG) or sensor-based signals (e.g., galvanic skin response, temperature, respiration) and can be combined with the EEG amplifiers. The BrainAmp MR amplifier system is battery powered and communicates with the recording software via a two-channel fiber optics connection made through an intelligent USB interface located in the scanner control room. This interface contains most of the more sensitive electronics circuitry needed to operate the amplifiers, such as the acquisition clock electronics and the circuit for the synchronization with an external clock signal, and also contains the logic for integrating external events. In this way, all electronically critical components of the EEG system can be kept in the scanner control room, while the amplifier itself can be made robust enough to reside in the scanner bore and directly behind the head coil for virtually any field strength. Also, having been designed explicitly for use inside the scanner, this EEG system does not require any shielding enclosure or external RF filters for its operation, thus giving it a small footprint. Furthermore, since the only connection between the amplifier and the scanner control room is a two channel fiber optics cable of approximately 4 mm diameter, this system not only has a small footprint, but also is highly mobile and can be set up and removed in a few minutes. Figure 2.1.3 shows the placement of such an amplifier in the scanner bore. Please note the sandbags used to weigh down the electrode leads in order to avoid scanner gradient,

GES 300 MR Package within the MR Environment

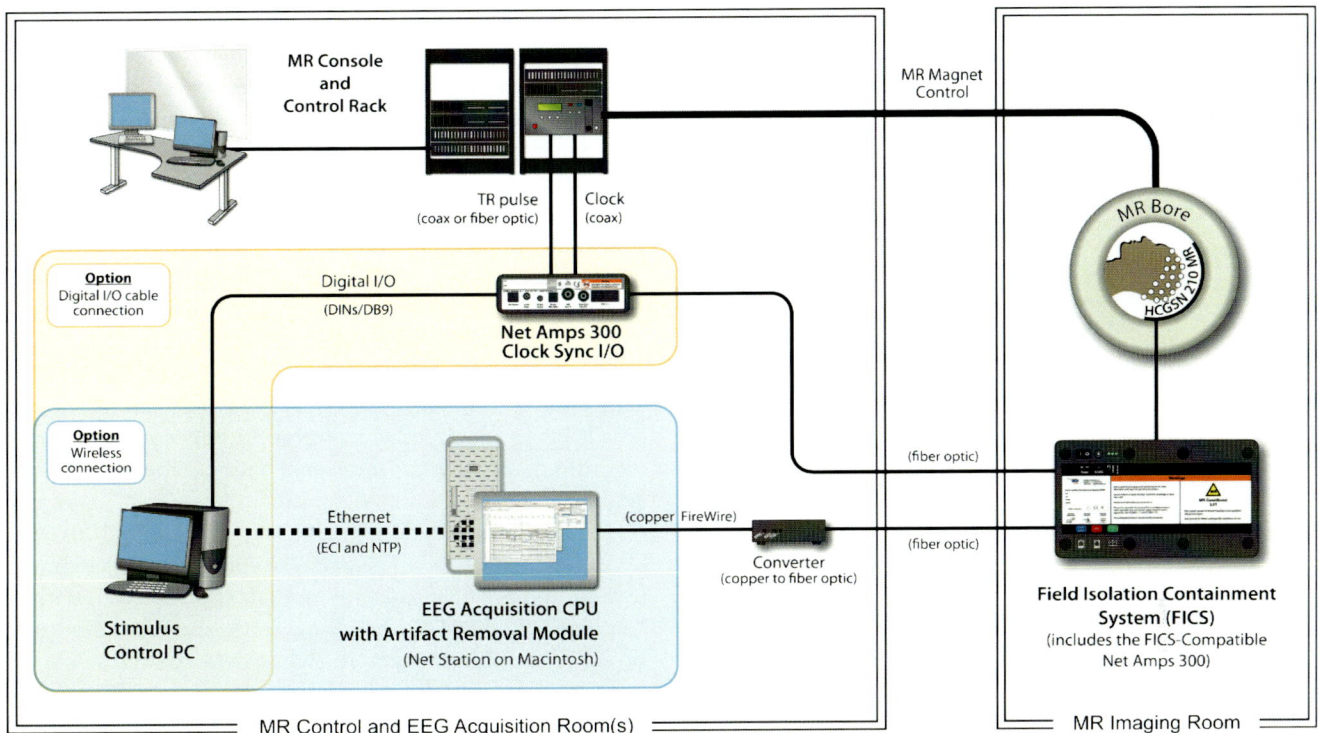

Figure 2.1.1. A schematic diagram of the arrangement of a shielded amplifier used in the scanner environment. The amplifier resides in the MR chamber and communicates with the recording equipment in the MR control room via fiber optical connections. Volume onset pulses, clock signals, and some stimulus related events are received in the scanner control room, converted to optical pulses and forwarded to the amplifier in the MR chamber, where the event codes are reintegrated with the EEG/MR data acquired and are sent back to the scanner control room for storage. (Figure reprinted with kind permission of Electrical Geodesics Incorporated, Eugene, USA.)

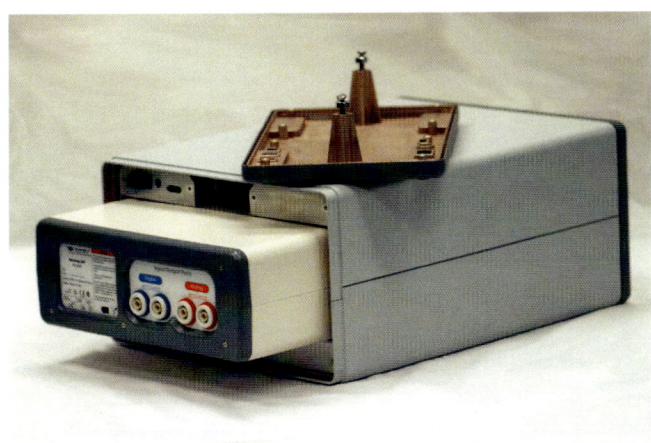

Figure 2.1.2. Example of a shielding box used to encapsulate EEG amplifiers that are either not MR compatible, or as in this case (EGI NetAmps 300) essentially are MR compatible, but need some additional hardware for the operation in the MR environment. This typically means RF filters, electrical-to-optical converters for the EEG signals derived as well as an MR compatible rechargeable battery. (Figure reprinted with kind permission of Electrical Geodesics Incorporated, Eugene, USA.)

Helium pump, and subject head movement induced artifacts (Benar et al., 2003; Hill et al., 1995).

In summary it can be said that there are now a few mature commercially available EEG systems on the market for combined EEG/MR recordings, with new competitors finally emerging. However, all of the above machines share the same common approach to the measurement of EEG in the MR, which is to record the EEG signal plus the superimposed MR artifacts as they appear at the amplifier inputs.

Only recently, though, another contender has entered the EEG/MR market with a technically innovative EEG cap system (Kappametrics Inc., Chantilly, USA). This system aims to reduce or even remove the gradient artifacts from the EEG signal directly on the electrode cap and thus *before* the data is even routed to the amplifier inputs. Their technology, termed **fEEG**™ uses a special cap consisting of several layers, one of which is connected to the scalp (measurement layer), while another is not (reference layer). A third layer creates an ionic-conductive reference loop between the electrodes that matches the loop at the scalp for the same

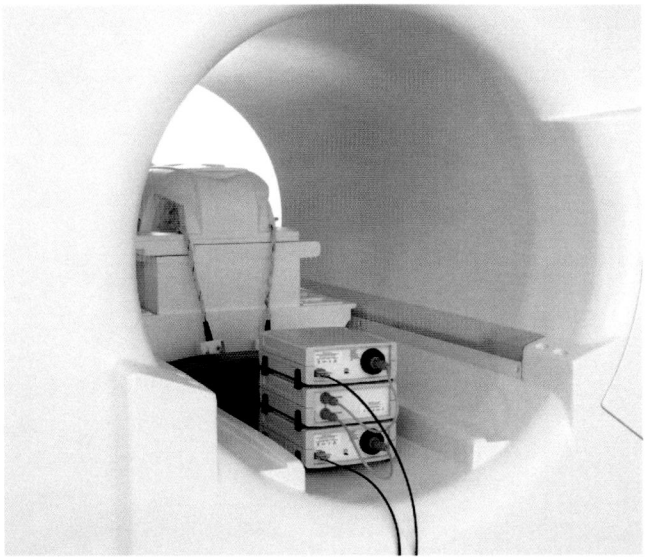

Figure 2.1.3. Example of the typical placement of a fully MR compatible and MR safe EEG amplifier directly in the scanner bore and typically behind the head coil. The arrangement shown consists of two EEG amplifiers at the top and bottom with a rechargeable power pack positioned in the middle. Cap connections are made with standard flat ribbon cables at the front of the amplifiers. Please note the sandbags used to fix the electrode cables in place to avoid cable movement induced by mechanical resonances caused by gradient switching and by the action of the Helium pump. (Figure reprinted with kind permission of Brain Products GmbH, Gilching, Germany.)

recording time, clearly is worthwhile, and Kappametrics should be applauded for attempting this with their fEEG™ system.

Some further developments should be noted here, that have not (yet) made it onto the market of commercially available equipment, but that nonetheless have great technical potential.

In 2006, Hanson et al. presented a multi-channel bio-signal amplifier that resides directly in the scanner bore and transmits the measured biosignals modulated onto discrete parts of the unused MR recording bandwidth. This means that the biosignals are automatically stored along with the MR image data and in absolute synchrony with the MR signals themselves. Unfortunately, this also means that acquisition of the biosignal data is only possible when MR data is being acquired, which requires fully continuous MR recordings for ongoing biosignal measurements (Hanson et al., 2006).

Another notable development is that of printed *InkCaps* by Vasios et al. (2006). The primary aim of this development was to address the issue of mutual SNR deterioration of combined EEG/fMRI recordings and also the important problem of subject safety at higher field strengths. This is done by replacing the metallic materials normally used in EEG/fMRI caps with printed structures based on conductive ink; preliminary results regarding SNR and the safety features of the *InkCap* are very encouraging (Vasios et al., 2006).

electrodes. Since the reference loop is not in contact with the scalp, but is co-located with (on) its scalp electrode counterpart, it will theoretically measure the same amount of gradient and RF artifact, but no EEG. The electronically derived difference signal between the local reference electrode and its scalp counterpart is thus, at least in theory, the artifact-free EEG. For lack of openly available data, publications or even experience with this system, one can only speculate on the true promise of this technology. For this to work, the impedance at the reference electrode must indeed be perfectly matched to that at the scalp electrode. If this were not the case, then more or less pronounced residuals would remain in the data. Another implicit assumption of this approach is that changes in impedance at the scalp electrode will be followed by corresponding changes in the conductivity at the reference electrode. If not, then not only will there be the more or less pronounced residuals mentioned above, but these will actually appear in a time varying fashion, which would more or less void the technical nature of the artifact and necessitate more involved secondary correction methods (e.g., adaptive filtering) than for the currently used EEG systems, where simple artifact template subtraction alone often yields very good results.

However this may turn out, the idea of taking the hardware one step further in order to reduce or even remove the gradient artifacts completely, at the recording site and at

Equipment Safety During Combined Recordings

With regard to equipment safety we can differentiate between aspects of the safety of the MR hardware and its operation and those related to EEG hardware safety.

All manufacturers of EEG equipment used in combined recordings are well aware of the special safety aspects that need to be heeded in the MR environment. Thus, no direct danger from the EEG equipment to the MR system or its electronics has to be feared. There may be issues of minimum distances to keep for some of the externally MR shielded, but inherently non–MR compatible amplifiers, but these requirements will be communicated by the manufacturer as binding and thus should be common knowledge where such systems are used.

Possible dangers to the MR hardware and electronics are thus only conceivable in cases where additional equipment is introduced into the scanner bore or is attached to the scanner electronics. On the part of additional equipment this could mean stimulation devices such as headphones, goggles, or response devices as well as non–MR compatible biosignal sensors or electrodes. The prime risk is of course that such equipment can contain or be made of ferromagnetic materials, which could cause attraction to and damage of the interior of the scanner bore (Schenck, 2000), but admittedly, patient safety would be much more at risk than scanner hardware in these situations.

Another possible danger to the scanner hardware are electrical connections made between the EEG system and the scanner electronics. Such connections would typically be needed to obtain a master clock signal from the MR device that can be used to drive the EEG amplifier clock and to achieve clock synchrony between the two devices. Attaching such devices can harm the scanner electronics, e.g., by drawing too much current from the clock output terminal or by detuning the MR system clock due to influences of the synchronization hardware attached. It is therefore of the utmost importance that any devices attached to the MR scanner electronics are built to the highest technical standards, with optical decoupling of all signal connections between the scanner and the device (if possible) and with all necessary power for operation being sourced from the synchronization device (see section on clock synchronization for more details).

Patient Safety During Combined Recordings

Patient safety during combined EEG/MR recordings is and has to be of the highest concern. The MR scanner is an environment where physical forces are either present at all times, such as with the static magnetic field (Schenck, 2000), or are induced during the MR acquisition with the switched gradient magnetic fields (Den Boer et al., 2002) and with the RF excitation of the tissue to be scanned (Grandolfo et al., 1992; Nitz et al., 2005), all of which pose particular dangers to the subject undergoing a combined EEG/MR measurement.

The most profound risk for the subject or patient is the heating of bodily tissue due to the RF energy being deposited onto the electrodes during slice excitation. Placing EEG electrode caps with multiple electrodes on the scalp and establishing contact to the scalp with the help of conductive gel creates surfaces of high conductivity and with high thermal resistance. The RF energy causes large surface current densities in these materials, effectively shielding the inside of the skull from the RF energy emitted (Angelone et al., 2004; Angelone et al., 2006; Laufs et al., 2008). This typically means that higher RF transmit energies are necessary to achieve the desired flip angle and to avoid image deterioration. At the same time, the energy deposited at the electrode terminal will dissipate as warming or even heating at the scalp/gel border (Achenbach et al., 1997; Nitz et al., 2001). Figure 2.1.4, taken from a masters thesis on this topic, shows this effect for three commonly used MR sequences, EPI, SPGR, and FSE (Meriläinen, 2003).

It is easy to see from Figure 2.1.4a that there is a profound difference between the three sequence types in the amount of heating observed. While the *Echo Planar Imaging* (EPI) sequence showed virtually no warming at all and the *Spoiled Gradient* (SPGR) sequence only showed marginal warming, the picture is quite dramatic for the *Fast Spin Echo* (FSE) sequence, and it becomes clear that the temperature development observed would lead to heating/burning if allowed to develop over more time. As can be seen in Figure 2.1.4b, this effect could be modeled nearly perfectly using a simple physical model based on the RF energy emitted over time and on the heating and cooling constants from physics. This effect is thus entirely RF energy dependent and can simplistically be said to be reflected by the number of RF excitation and inversion pulses during any MR sequence. Clearly, Figure 2.1.4a shows that it would be a bad idea to perform combined EEG/MR recordings with an FSE sequence or any sequence with equivalent RF emission parameters.

Another safety relevant issue is RF energy coupling onto cable loops, which would again dissipate the energy through heat emitted, e.g., to the tissue or to the material of the loop itself (Lemieux et al., 1997). If an electrode cable assembly is looped, the RF induction effect can be severe enough to cause the cable sheath to melt at the points where the cables crosses its own path to form the loop. It is therefore important that loops be avoided at all cost (Dempsey and Condon, 2001; Dempsey et al., 2001).

However, this effect is not limited to cable loops. Any cable, straight or looped, can act as an RF antenna and cause severe burning, especially at its ends, if its length and shape is such that it becomes resonant at the particular MR scanner's Larmor frequency (42.58 Mhz/T) or at any harmonic of that frequency. This effect is affected by the scanner's field strength and thus its frequency as well as the cable length, but is also dependent on a number of other parameters such as cable shape and orientation (Konings et al., 2000; Nitz et al., 2001; Pictet et al., 2002; Armenean et al., 2004). Since these are a complex set of parameters, it is immensely important to verify—before any measurements are made—that the particular setup to be used does not induce any heating. This can either be done empirically, by having a "confederate" test subject pay particular attention to sensations of warming at the electrode or cable positions, or—if this is not feasible or possible—by using an MR compatible/safe thermometer to measure the ongoing temperature during scanning. MR thermometers with one to many channels are readily available from a number of commercial vendors (e.g. Neoptix, Quebec, Canada; Luxtron, Santa Clara, USA; FISO, Quebec, Canada). Additionally, some EEG manufacturers will provide their customers with MR compatible thermometers for testing if need arises, thus also testifying to their own particular awareness of the need for rigid patient-safety testing.

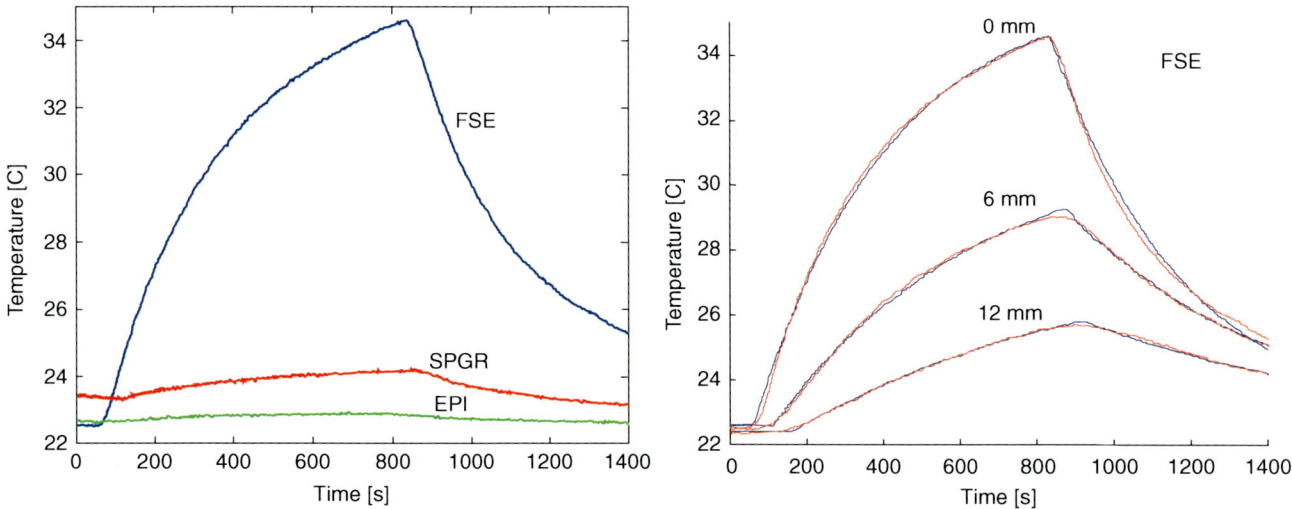

Figure 2.1.4. Figure (a) on the left shows temperature changes induced by three different MR sequences in a frontopolar EEG electrode on a sheep's head. MR scanning was performed for 900 seconds with each sequence. Temperature changes differ dramatically between the sequences, with a standard Echo Planar Imaging (EPI) sequence showing only a very slight amount of warming of approximately 0.3°C and with the Spoiled Gradient Recalled Acquisition (Nomenclature: GE: SPGR, Siemens: FLASH, Philips: T1 FFE) showing a warming of approximately 0.6°C over the 900-second measurement. The Fast Spin Echo (GE: FSE, Siemens, Philips: TSE) sequence shows a dramatic increase in surface temperature of 12°C and with the temperature asymptote not nearly having been reached. Figure (b) on the right shows the result of modeling of the FSE heating effect with a simple script using only the RF induction and the heating and cooling constants as model parameters. Figure (b) very clearly shows that the heating effect is owed entirely to the RF induction over time. (Reprinted with kind permission of the author, Veera Meriläinen, Helsinki, Finland.)

To further reduce the risk of RF-induced cable heating, a number of measures can be and typically are taken by the manufacturers of EEG/MR equipment.

- Only non-ferromagnetic leads and electrode plates must be used. Leads are typically made from carbon fibers or stranded copper, and electrode plates are mostly made from high quality sintered Ag/AgCl materials or from gold.
- All scalp electrodes must have RF shielding resistors conductively attached (e.g., conductively glued) to the electrode surface. The RF shielding resistors typically vary in resistivity between 5 and 15 kOhms, depending on the field strength of the scanner and on the length of the cable assembly (Lemieux et al., 1997).
- The scalp electrode leads should be routed as straight as possible toward a bundled exit from the cap and on to a common connector or common input.
- The scalp electrode leads must be routed on top of the textile cap fabric to avoid direct lead contact with the skin.
- All electrode leads must be fixed to the textile fabric to avoid lead movement and inadvertent loop formation.
- Peripheral leads such as those for EKG acquisition, which have to be routed along the subject's back, must be sheathed in heat resistant tubing.

Figure 2.1.5 shows a typical EEG/MR electrode cap assembly highlighting the safety features described above, and Figure 2.1.6 shows a typical EKG electrode used in

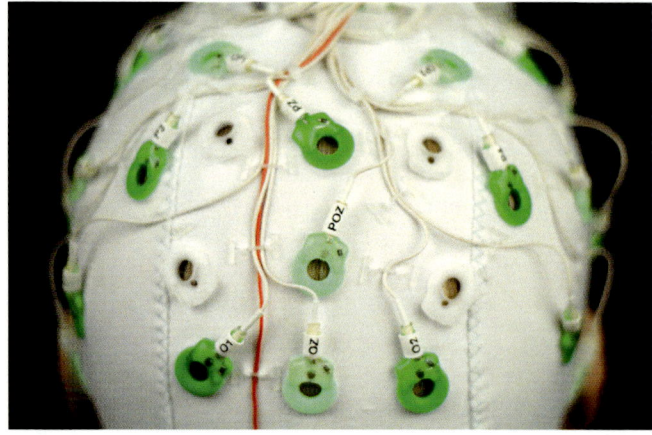

Figure 2.1.5. Back view of a commonly used MR-compatible EEG cap system (BrainCap MR, Brain Products GmbH, Gilching, Germany). Safety features on this cap are: *(1)* plastic electrode holders to avoid direct contact of Ag/AgCl element with the scalp, *(2)* RF shielding resistor on electrode (e.g., black "dot" on electrode POz), *(3)* fixation of electrode cables with nylon "Ts," and *(4)* routing of electrode cables together in bundles of increasing numbers of electrodes. Note the empty electrode shells left and right of POz and at P1 and P2 used to distribute the head's pressure more evenly across a larger number of points in the posterior plane. (Figure reprinted with kind permission of Brain Products GmbH, Gilching, Germany.)

EEG/MR measurements. Please note the heat resistant tubing used. The electrode itself is embedded in the red plastic holder and does not make contact with the subject's

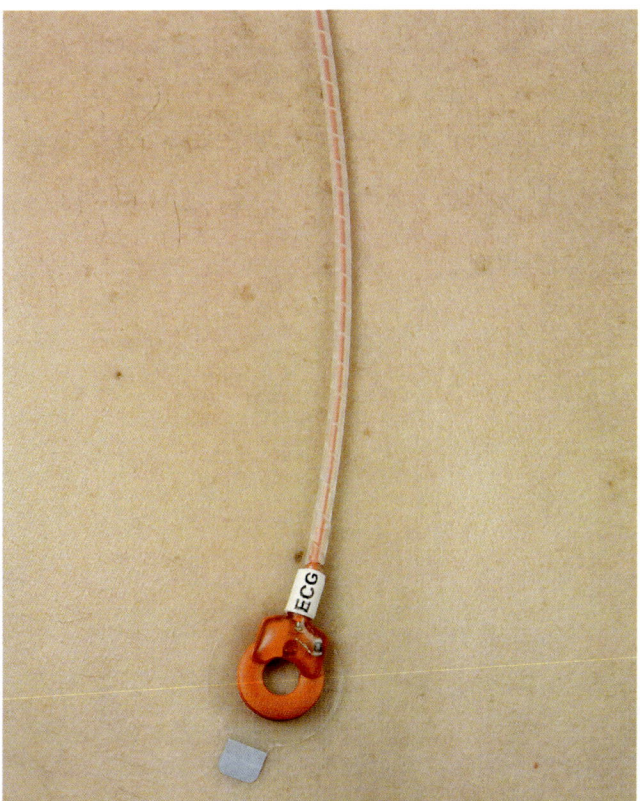

Figure 2.1.6. Example of an ECG electrode used in combined EEG/MR recordings and typically placed slightly laterally on the lower back. Please note the plastic electrode body and the use of an adhesive pad for electrode application in order to avoid direct contact with the skin. The RF shielding resistor on this electrode is 15 kOhm to suppress the increased MR gradient and RF energy induction caused by the long lead and location outside the homogeneous part of the magnetic field. Please note the heat resistant sheathing required to avoid any potential heating of the lateral electrode lead causing heating/burns on the skin on the back. This is particularly important for this electrode, since the heat discrimination ability on the back is by far inferior to that on the scalp. (Figure reprinted with kind permission of Brain Products GmbH, Gilching, Germany.)

skin. Also note the SMD RF shielding resistor bonded to the electrode holder surface (BrainCap MR, Brain Products GmbH, Gilching, Germany).

Some manufacturers give specific and binding information on the intended use of their EEG/MR equipment, last but not least for liability reasons. However, the topic of patient/subject safety in the MR is so important that any researcher should be aware of the issues involved. If, on the other hand, the manufacturer of a particular set of equipment does not give rules and guidelines, it would be wise to proactively query these to avoid any potential harm being done due to negligence on the part of the researcher or—in fact—of the manufacturer.

However, if the critical points raised here are taken into consideration, then performing combined EEG/MR recordings will not pose any additional risk to the subjects or patients when compared to normal MR-only measurements.

Data Acquisition Considerations

Performing recordings of EEG in the MR scanner during ongoing MRI/fMRI requires the use of acquisition parameters that take into account the characteristics of the gradient switching effects on the amplifier input stages. Parameters of particular importance are the low pass filter (band limiter) of the amplifier input stage, the sample rate, the amplifier gain and the amplifier high pass setting, as well as—more indirectly related—EEG and MR system clock synchronization methods and settings.

Low Pass Filter (Band Limitation)

The gradient systems of modern scanners are immensely powerful, and the energy emitted by the switching of the directional moving gradients is extremely large in comparison to the EEG signal power. The gradient artifact signal also covers a broad spectrum extending from very low frequencies well within the typically used EEG spectrum all the way to several thousand Hertz (Allen et al., 2000). This can make it difficult to contain the gradient energy within the effective bandwidth of the EEG amplifier and to avoid the appearance of aliasing artifacts in the resulting EEG data.

At the sample rate of 5000 Hz used by some of the most commonly used equipment for EEG/MR derivations, the highest frequency represented in the recorded data is of course 2500 Hz (Nyquist frequency), which would seem like a broad recording bandwidth. However, the bandwidth of the gradient artifact signal often extends well beyond 2500 Hz and, since it consists of discrete frequency peaks and their harmonics at a great range of frequencies, it does not typically show the 1/f power decrease seen in EEG recordings, and even frequencies that are very close to Nyquist can contain very large energy. It is therefore immensely important to employ a high quality analog band limiting filter in the signal path of the EEG system that is capable of reducing the signal energy in such a way that none or virtually no energy at or beyond the Nyquist frequency of 2500 Hz is recorded, since this would otherwise lead to aliasing artifacts being introduced into the signal. Figure 2.1.7 shows the slightly smoothed raw spectrum of an EEG channel recorded at 5000 Hz and with a band limiter of 1000 Hz @ 30 dB/Octave in a Siemens 1.5T Magnetom scanner running a standard EPI BOLD sequence.

It is easy to see from Figure 2.1.7 that the band limiter set at 1000 Hz did not fully succeed in containing the gradient energy to the frequency band available. While the continuation of the spectral power contribution of the scanner beyond Nyquist can of course only be inferred from the spectral content immediately below Nyquist, and although the average energy below Nyquist is not very high, it nonetheless stands to reason that this band limiter would not have been a

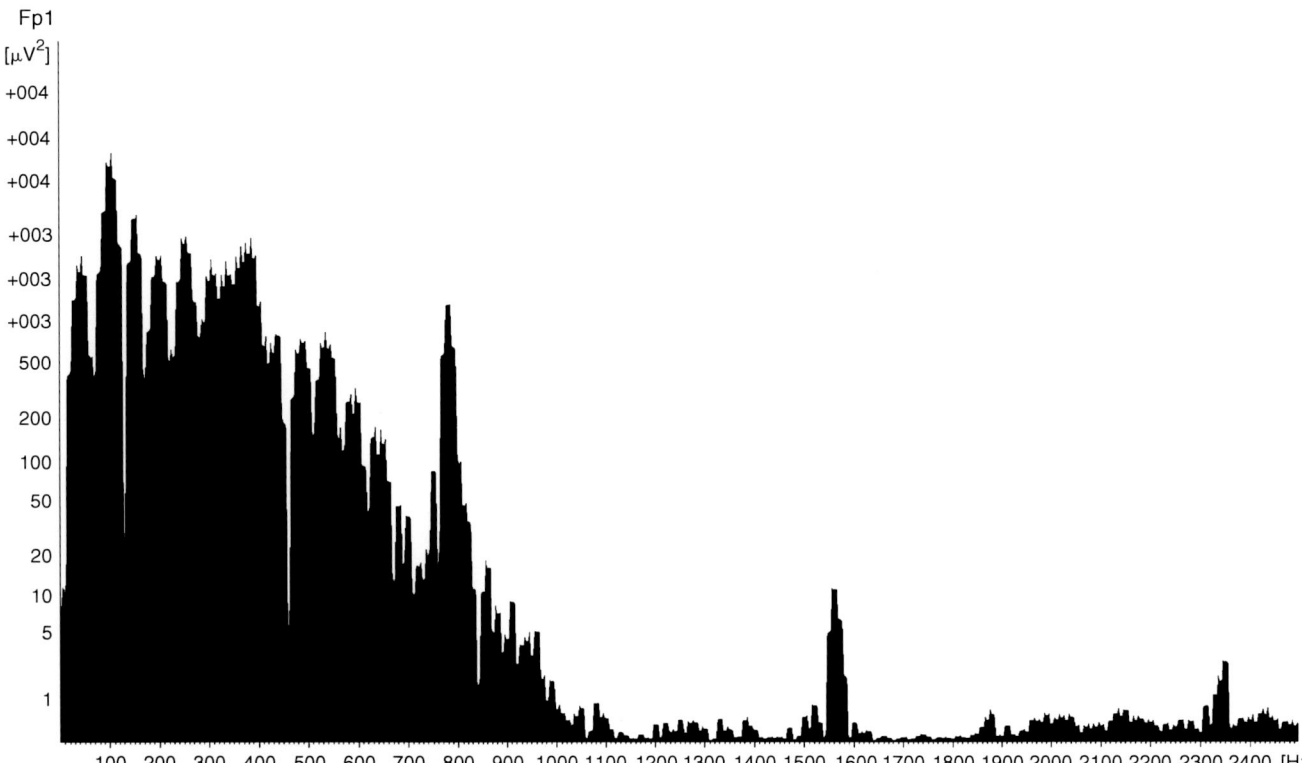

Figure 2.1.7. Slightly smoothed (10 Hz moving window) raw spectrum of an EEG/MR acquisition in a 1.5T MR machine and using a hardware band limiter with 1000 Hz at 30 dB/Octave. Note that while the main spectral power is located within the first 800 Hz of the spectrum, there are spectral lines with substantial power all the way up to the Nyquist frequency of 2500 Hz, making aliasing artifacts very likely for this recording. Modern scanners with their very fast and strong gradient systems therefore demand band limiter (low pass) settings that are as low as 10% of Nyquist to properly contain the gradient energy and avoid aliasing artifacts.

wise choice to completely avoid aliasing artifacts in the data recorded. In fact, for recordings done in most newer scanner models, with their immensely strong and fast gradient systems, the analog band limiter oftentimes has to have its edge frequency set as low as 10% of Nyquist (e.g. 250 Hz @ 30 dB/Octave) in order to fully avoid the induction of aliasing artifacts. As a logical consequence the effective bandwidth of the EEG amplifier would then also be limited to those 250 Hz.

Sample Rate Considerations

As we will see in Chapter 2.3 in this volume, correcting the MR gradient–induced artifacts in the EEG requires that the true onset of each volume's gradient activity can be detected and marked in the EEG data. For this, almost all modern MR scanners have a configurable TTL or fiber optical output readily available at the scanner console, which gives a short signal pulse at the exact time point of every slice or volume acquisition onset.

However, if the EEG system were acquiring its data at a typical data rate of 500 Hz, then the EEG system would only "see" this onset pulse with its next data acquisition point,

which means that the worst case would be a detection of the volume/slice onset just under 2 ms after it actually occurred: An eternity in MR timing.

Worse yet, since the EEG system is oblivious to the fact that it is missing the true onset by some small fraction of time, it will record whatever gradient amplitude is present at the time of its next scheduled EEG data point acquisition, and the resulting EEG signal will show this lack of timing exactness as inflated standard deviation at the supposed gradient onset time point and also throughout the entire gradient correction template.

In these cases it is therefore important to sample the EEG data with a high enough sample rate, since higher EEG data rates will sample the fast rising gradient signal at shorter time intervals and the resulting smaller amplitude steps between successive EEG sample points will help to reduce the standard deviation and thus the correction uncertainty in the gradient correction template.

In theory this would mean that the EEG sample rate should be at least twice as high as the true highest frequency in the gradient switching spectrum. However, it can be shown empirically that an EEG sample rate of 5000 Hz is perfectly adequate for EEG/ERP recordings. The reason for this is that the data would typically be down sampled (e.g., to

250 or 500 Hz) and subsequently low pass filtered during the artifact correction process, the combination of which effectively eliminates all potentially existing (high frequency) gradient correction residuals. Using higher sample rates therefore typically does not improve the data quality, unless down sampling and low pass filtering are not possible for whatever reasons.

In fact, higher sample rates simply translate into better approximation of the true onset of volume acquisition and thus into better *synchronization* between the EEG and MR system clocks. However, raising the sample rate clearly is a poor choice when the aim is clock synchronization, since this can be achieved much more economically, e.g., by directly coupling the EEG and MR clocks to have the MR system clock drive the EEG acquisition clock.

Clock Synchronization

There are several ways in which the EEG data obtained can be synchronized with the clock of the MR system. These methods can generally be separated into online and offline methods and since this section is concerned with recording considerations, we will only deal with online methods here. Please see Chapter 2.3 in this volume for an account of performing template optimization with offline synchronization.

Hardware Clock Synchronization

Hardware methods for EEG-MR clock synchronization require a physical (electrical) connection to the MR scanner electronics hardware and must tap into a clock signal that is phase synchronous with the scanner's gradient system. This clock signal is then used to generate the new and synchronized EEG acquisition clock (Mandelkow et al., 2006; Gebhardt et al., 2008).

All major commercially available MR scanners provide clock signals that lend themselves to this purpose and all signals in question are readily available on commonly used connectors such as 50 Ohm BNC or QLA types. These clock outputs are typically unused by the MR system itself during normal operation, which makes them freely available for clock synchronization without having to worry about the electrical side effects of branching off an already used output. The frequency of these clock signals may vary, but all major scanner brands (also) have a 10 MHz clock that can be used for this purpose.

As was described above, the synchronization hardware has to optically decouple this signal from the MR scanner for technical safety reasons, but also to avoid drawing power from the MR system circuit. Since the MR system electronics cabinets are typically located behind the scanner enclosure and thus on the opposite side from the scanner control room, the clock signal furthermore has to be stabilized in a way that

allows transport of the signal over a distance of typically 20 to 30 meters without decay or slurring of the signal edges, since these are needed for high frequency phase alignment. This signal is then fed into a clock divider circuit, which down samples the 10 MHz signal into a clock signal that can be used directly by the EEG amplifier. Figure 2.1.8 shows a schematic example of a typical clock synchronization setup.

The synchronization of the EEG system with the external clock is dependent on the temporal accuracy of the external clock signal, which can typically be assumed to be excellent with an MR derived clock signal. However, there are many factors such as the length of the cable, the amount of noise present in the environment of the cable, etc., that can at least potentially influence the quality of the clock signal. The synchronization device should therefore also be able to evaluate the signal quality and frequency stability and to generate information on the synchronization status. This information should then be stored together with the EEG data to allow later reconstruction of the synchronization status, should this be necessary.

Recently, a different approach to achieving a similar effect for combined EEG/MR datasets has been published (Cohen, 2007; U.S. Patent No. 7,286,871) and found its first implementation in the EGI "FICS" system described above. This method uses the volume onset pulses from the MR device to trigger the (resting) acquisition of a number of EEG data points corresponding to one MR volume's length (time of repetition, TR), upon completion of which the EEG system goes into a resting state again in order to await the next trigger. The actual EEG acquisition is thus based on the original EEG system clock, and while this method indeed achieves an effect similar to clock synchronization with regard to artifact timing homogenization, it is not based on clock synchronization as defined here, but instead is based on the well-established method of *triggered burst mode acquisition*.

A logical consequence of the volume-length based acquisition is that this method relies on an absolute invariance of the volume TR used and secondly, also requires that the TR be evenly divisible by the EEG data acquisition rate to achieve a continuous EEG recording. If either of these prerequisites is not met, partial data points or even multiple data points will be missing at the end of the acquisition burst, thus leading to noncontinuous data.

As a final note, it must be said that the attachment of any electrical device to the scanner electronics hardware can void the MR manufacturer's warranty. Permission must therefore be obtained from the manufacturer prior to making such connections to the MR device electronics in order to avoid technical or potentially even legal issues.

MR Sequence–Based Clock Synchronization

Another interesting method for achieving clock synchrony between the MR scanner and the EEG system is the so called "Stepping Stone Sequence" method (Anami et al., 2003). This

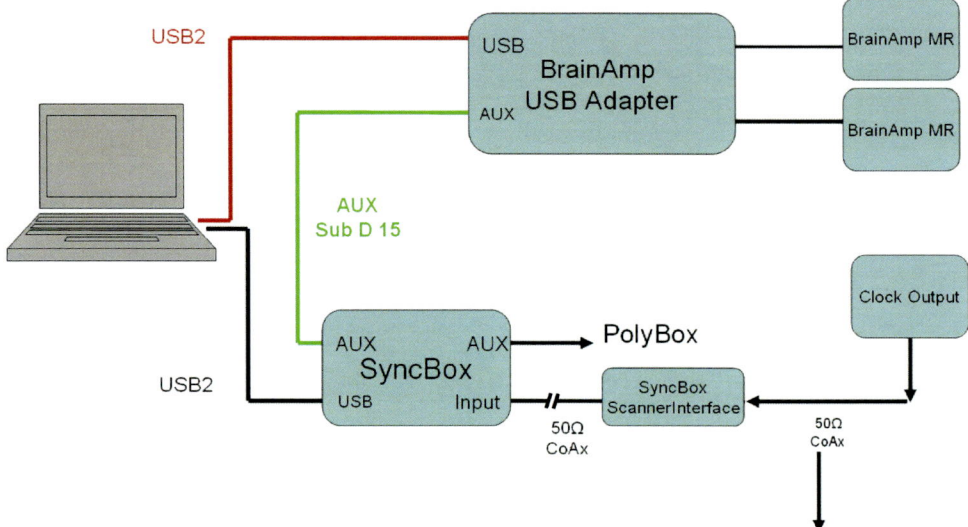

Figure 2.1.8. A schematic diagram of an EEG/MR setup utilizing hardware clock synchronization. The MR clock on the lower right is fed into the "SyncBox Scanner Interface" installed locally in/at the scanner electronics cabinet. The signal is stabilized and transported 20–30 meters to the "SyncBox Main Unit" located in the scanner control room. The SyncBox down samples the MR clock into a clock signal usable by the MR amplifier and feeds it into the clock circuit on the USB2 interface hosting the amplifier clock logic. The SyncBox is under control of the EEG recording software and evaluates and feeds back information on clock signal quality and synchronization status to the recording system. This information is stored together with the EEG data and event markers recorded. (Figure reprinted with kind permission of Brain Products GmbH, Gilching, Germany.)

synchronization method works on the basis of special MR sequences that are custom built for a given scanner. The idea behind the stepping stone technique is to separate perfectly the time points at which gradient switching is taking place from those time points at which an EEG data point is being acquired. In order to further assure that these discrete time points are correctly met during EEG acquisition, this method employs hardware based clock synchronization as given above.

This assures minimal influence of the gradient activity on the EEG data acquired at the price of having to individually program custom sequences for a given scanner and measurement paradigm. This method has not been widely adopted due to the high effort involved in developing a stepping stone sequence, but it is nonetheless a noteworthy method since it significantly improves the acquired EEG signal's SNR and allows for a much easier subsequent artifact correction. As such, using this method would be beneficial beyond using hardware clock synchronization alone (Anami et al., 2003; Ritter et al., 2006).

Amplifier Gain Considerations

When selecting the amplifier gain for a combined EEG-fMRI study one has to keep in mind that the gradient artifact peaks can reach amplitudes that are more than 100 times larger than those of the ongoing spontaneous EEG and that these gradient artifacts rise at speeds that often exceed the rate of change of ongoing EEG by factors of 1000 and more. The maximal amplifier gain that can be employed in the presence

of such massive artifacts is of course largely dependent on the amplifier's AD bit count and its dynamic range, but of course the strength of the gradients being switched play an important role in this as well. And it may well turn out that certain MR paradigms can not safely be run without risking amplifier saturation.

However, there is another aspect that should be taken into consideration: If a high amplifier gain is used, then much larger artifact amplitudes will result. At any given frequency and band limitation, the phase jitter inherent at least to nonsynchronized measurements will then lead to a large inflation of the standard deviations in the correction template, which will in fact degrade and not improve the correction quality. Higher amplifier gains should therefore always be accompanied either by sampling at proportionally higher frequencies or with hardware clock synchronization employed. Since it was shown above that increasing the sample rate is by far the more ineffective method for achieving enhanced signal synchrony, hardware clock synchronization would be strongly advised for measurements at higher amplifier gains.

High Pass Filter Settings

From a theoretical standpoint it would be advisable to record EEG/MR data with a DC-capable amplifier, since an AC-coupled amplifier could show ringing of the signal in response to the very fast and very powerful gradient switching signals. And in fact, this may just be the case.

However, as can be shown empirically, this potentially present ringing is technical in nature, meaning that it occurs in a virtually invariant fashion across subsequent gradient switching episodes. With that being so, this part of the MR artifact is equally well characterized by the commonly used gradient artifact correction procedures as the gradient artifacts themselves are and is removed along with them. There is therefore no direct need to acquire EEG/MR data in DC mode. As a matter of fact, data acquisition in DC mode typically increases the risk of spontaneous or gradual amplifier saturation especially in amplifiers with limited dynamic range, which can often make AC-coupled recordings the better choice.

Subject Considerations

Generally speaking, any subject that qualifies for MR measurements can also participate in a combined EEG/MR measurement, if properly instructed and possibly, trained. However, there are some subject-related aspects of combined measurements that need to be considered:

- The available space in the head coil is further reduced due to the cap and electrodes. This can enhance any existing tendencies toward claustrophobia.
- The subject is connected to the amplifier and can not exit the scanner on their own. This is not desired anyhow, but the inability to do so, e.g., in case of a panic attack, becomes obvious to the subject and can serve to promote such anxiety.
- The subject is lying supine on the posterior portion of the electrode cap and the weight of the head is typically placed on a rather sparse number of electrodes present at posterior sites. This can cause discomfort in itself, but taken together with the explicit instruction not to move the head, can lead to subjectively increasing pressure and even painful sensations at the pressure points over the course of the EEG/MR measurement.
- The addition of more equipment to be tended to in preparation of and during the combined EEG/MR measurements can and in most cases will lead to longer measurements and oftentimes also to longer "quiet spells" in between measurement phases, which can again serve to promote a feeling of having been left alone and can thereby promote feelings of apprehension or anxiety.

The above points clearly show which subjects should not be considered for combined EEG/MR measurements. This would primarily be subjects with a known history of claustrophobia or other tendencies toward anxious or panic related reactions, but also subjects who are particularly sensitive to feelings of pain or discomfort in general.

However, some of the potentially problematic characteristics of combined measurements can also actively be avoided or at least reduced. The effect of the subject lying on only a few electrodes can be remedied with a number of measures: It is possible to insert a few additional electrode holders or dummy electrodes in the posterior plane of the cap to distribute the pressure more evenly over a larger number of electrodes (for an example, see Figure 2.1.5). This effect can be reduced further with the use of a memory foam cushion, which assumes and then retains a shape impressed into it, thereby effectively helping to distribute the pressure more evenly across the entire posterior plane. The potentially enhanced claustrophobic effect of combined measurements can be reduced by communicating all aspects of the experiment in more detail than one would normally do for simple MR or EEG recordings. Explicitly informing the subject about the equipment used, its location, and its function and reassuring the subject that he/she is in control and can be heard at all times typically helps not only avoid anxiety, but also has proven to be very helpful in reducing head and body movement in the scanner. In experimental paradigms where subjects with anxiety disorders are the target population it has proven very helpful to train the subjects in a mock scanner. This can help to reduce the general anxiety and arousal induced by the experimental environment and procedure per se, which could otherwise obscure any specific anxiety/arousal effects of the experimental stimulation itself.

Conclusion

In recent years, the hardware and software used for combined recordings of EEG and MR/fMRI have matured to the point that such recordings are no longer technically challenging or out of the ordinary. Several different EEG/MR systems are now commercially available along with powerful commercial as well as free software for the correction of the gradient and ballistocardiogram artifacts, with resulting EEG readings generally being of excellent quality (see Chapter 2.3 in this volume for details).

However, safety aspects must remain at the top of the list of priorities to tend to during every single measurement, since the subject's safety is the responsibility both of the EEG researcher and of the MR personnel. Since even simple parameter or sequence changes that would be entirely noncritical in purely MR measurements can prove potentially dangerous in combined EEG/MR measurements, there is a great need for both the MR and EEG personnel to receive proper training with regard to the operation and safety procedures and limits of combined EEG/MR measurements.

REFERENCES

Achenbach S, Moshage W, Diem B, Bieberle T, Schibgilla V, Bachmann K (1997) Effects of magnetic resonance imaging on cardiac pacemakers and electrodes. Am Heart J 134:467–473.

Allen PJ, Josephs O, Turner R (2000) A method for removing imaging artifact from continuous EEG recorded during functional MRI. Neuroimage 12:230–239.

Anami K, Mori T, Tanaka F, Kawagoe Y, Okamoto J, Yarita M, Ohnishi T, Yumoto M, Matsuda H, Saitoh O (2003) Stepping stone sampling for retrieving artifact-free electroencephalogram during functional magnetic resonance imaging. Neuroimage 19:281–295.

Angelone LM, Potthast A, Segonne F, Iwaki S, Belliveau JW, Bonmassar G (2004) Metallic electrodes and leads in simultaneous EEG-MRI: specific absorption rate (SAR) simulation studies. Bioelectromagnetics 25:285–295.

Angelone LM, Vasios CE, Wiggins G, Purdon PL, Bonmassar G (2006) On the effect of resistive EEG electrodes and leads during 7 T MRI: simulation and temperature measurement studies. Magn Reson Imaging 24:801–812.

Armenean C, Perrin E, Armenean M, Beuf O, Pilleul F, Saint-Jalmes H (2004) RF-induced temperature elevation along metallic wires in clinical magnetic resonance imaging: influence of diameter and length. Magn Reson Med 52:1200–1206.

Benar C, Aghakhani Y, Wang Y, Izenberg A, Al-Asmi A, Dubeau F, Gotman J (2003) Quality of EEG in simultaneous EEG-fMRI for epilepsy. Clin Neurophysiol 114:569–580.

Caldwell JA, Prazinko B, Caldwell JL (2003) Body posture affects electroencephalographic activity and psychomotor vigilance task performance in sleep-deprived subjects. Clin Neurophysiol 114:23–31.

Cohen MS (2007) Method and apparatus for reducing contamination of an electrical signal In: (Office USP, #7,286,871), p 37. Oakland, CA: Regents of the University of California.

Debener S, Ullsperger M, Siegel M, Fiehler K, von Cramon DY, Engel AK (2005) Trial-by-trial coupling of concurrent electroencephalogram and functional magnetic resonance imaging identifies the dynamics of performance monitoring. J Neurosci 25: 11730–11737.

Debener S, Ullsperger M, Siegel M, Engel AK (2006) Single-trial EEG-fMRI reveals the dynamics of cognitive function. Trends Cogn Sci 10:558–563.

Dempsey MF, Condon B (2001) Thermal injuries associated with MRI. Clin Radiol 56:457–465.

Dempsey MF, Condon B, Hadley DM (2001) Investigation of the factors responsible for burns during MRI. J Magn Reson Imaging 13:627–631.

Den Boer JA, Bourland JD, Nyenhuis JA, Ham CL, Engels JM, Hebrank FX, Frese G, Schaefer DJ (2002) Comparison of the threshold for peripheral nerve stimulation during gradient switching in whole body MR systems. J Magn Reson Imaging 15:520–525.

Gebhardt H, Blecker CR, Bischoff M, Morgen K, Oschmann P, Vaitl D, Sammer G (2008) Synchronized measurement of simultaneous EEG-fMRI: a simulation study. Clin Neurophysiol 119:2703–2711.

Goldman RI, Stern JM, Engel J, Jr., Cohen MS (2000) Acquiring simultaneous EEG and functional MRI. Clin Neurophysiol 111:1974–1980.

Grandolfo M, Polichetti A, Vecchia P, Gandhi OP (1992) Spatial distribution of RF power in critical organs during magnetic resonance imaging. Ann N Y Acad Sci 649: 176–187.

Hanson LG, Skimminge A, Lund TE, Hanson CG (2006) Encoding of EEG in MR images. Neuroimage 31:S131.

Herrmann CS, Debener S (2008) Simultaneous recording of EEG and BOLD responses: a historical perspective. Int J Psychophysiol 67:161–168.

Hill RA, Chiappa KH, Huang-Hellinger F, Jenkins BG (1995) EEG during MR imaging: differentiation of movement artifact from paroxysmal cortical activity. Neurology 45:1942–1943.

Horovitz SG, Skudlarski P, Gore JC (2002) Correlations and dissociations between BOLD signal and P300 amplitude in an auditory oddball task: a parametric approach to combining fMRI and ERP. Magn Reson Imaging 20:319–325.

Horwitz B, Poeppel D (2002) How can EEG/MEG and fMRI/PET data be combined? Hum Brain Mapp 17:1–3.

Ives JR, Warach S, Schmitt F, Edelman RR, Schomer DL (1993) Monitoring the patient's EEG during echo planar MRI. Electroencephalogr Clin Neurophysiol 87:417–420.

Konings MK, Bartels LW, Smits HF, Bakker CJ (2000) Heating around intravascular guidewires by resonating RF waves. J Magn Reson Imaging 12:79–85.

Laufs H, Daunizeau J, Carmichael DW, Kleinschmidt A (2008) Recent advances in recording electrophysiological data simultaneously with magnetic resonance imaging. Neuroimage 40:515–528.

Lemieux L, Allen PJ, Franconi F, Symms MR, Fish DR (1997) Recording of EEG during fMRI experiments: patient safety. Magn Reson Med 38:943–952.

Mandelkow H, Halder P, Boesiger P, Brandeis D (2006) Synchronization facilitates removal of MRI artefacts from concurrent EEG recordings and increases usable bandwidth. Neuroimage 32:1120–1126.

Menon V, Crottaz-Herbette S (2005) Combined EEG and fMRI studies of human brain function. Int Rev Neurobiol 66:291–321.

Meriläinen V (2003) Magnetic resonance imaging with simultaneous electroencephalography recording: safety issues. In: Department of electrical and communications engineering, p 84. Helsinki: Helsinki University of Technology (Master Thesis).

Nitz WR, Oppelt A, Renz W, Manke C, Lenhart M, Link J (2001) On the heating of linear conductive structures as guide wires and catheters in interventional MRI. J Magn Reson Imaging 13:105–114.

Nitz WR, Brinker G, Diehl D, Frese G (2005) Specific absorption rate as a poor indicator of magnetic resonance-related implant heating. Invest Radiol 40:773–776.

Pictet J, Meuli R, Wicky S, van der Klink JJ (2002) Radiofrequency heating effects around resonant lengths of wire in MRI. Phys Med Biol 47:2973–2985.

Ritter P, Villringer A (2006) Simultaneous EEG-fMRI. Neurosci Biobehav Rev 30:823–838.

Ritter P, Freyer F, Becker R, Anami K, Curio G, Villringer A (2006) Recording of ultrafast (600-Hz) EEG oscillations with amplitudes in the nanovolt range during fMRI- acquisition periods. In: 14th scientific meeting ISMRM. Seattle: ISMRM.

Ritter P, Becker R, Graefe C, Villringer A (2007) Evaluating gradient artifact correction of EEG data acquired simultaneously with fMRI. Magn Reson Imaging 25:923–932.

Salek-Haddadi A, Friston KJ, Lemieux L, Fish DR (2003) Studying spontaneous EEG activity with fMRI. Brain Res Brain Res Rev 43:110–133.

Sammer G, Blecker C, Gebhardt H, Kirsch P, Stark R, Vaitl D (2005) Acquisition of typical EEG waveforms during fMRI: SSVEP, LRP, and frontal theta. Neuroimage 24:1012–1024.

Schenck JF (2000) Safety of strong, static magnetic fields. JMRI-J Magn Reson Im 12:2–19.

Schicke T, Muckli L, Beer AL, Wibral M, Singer W, Goebel R, Rosler F, Roder B (2006) Tight covariation of BOLD signal changes and slow ERPs in the parietal cortex in a parametric spatial imagery task with haptic acquisition. Eur J Neurosci 23:1910–1918.

Vasios CE, Angelone LM, Purdon PL, Ahveninen J, Belliveau JW, Bonmassar G (2006) EEG/(f)MRI measurements at 7 Tesla using a new EEG cap ("InkCap"). Neuroimage 33:1082–1092.

2.2 Andrew P. Bagshaw and Christian-G. Bénar

Scanning Strategies for Simultaneous EEG-fMRI Recordings

Introduction

The simultaneous recording of EEG and fMRI has opened several new perspectives within the field of functional MRI. It allows the detailed temporal and spectral information contained in EEG to be incorporated into the analysis of fMRI signals. In addition, it permits the study of spontaneous brain activity that can only be observed with EEG, such as epileptic spikes, sleep spindles, or alpha waves. Finally, it is a first step in the construction of a meta-modality with both high temporal and high spatial resolution.

However, the price to pay for this technical advance is the deterioration of the quality of both signals, and in particular of EEG. EEG is highly affected by the presence of the magnetic fields, both constant and time-varying, used in the fMRI procedure. In particular, significant artifacts that can obscure the physiological EEG appear as a result of movements of electrodes and leads associated with cardiac pulsation (the ballistocardiogram or 'pulse' artifact, which is present whenever the subject is within the static magnetic field), and as a result of switching gradient fields during scanning (the gradient artifact). As a result of this, many early studies avoided the reduction of EEG quality associated with recording in the MRI scanner by conducting separate sessions of EEG and fMRI, with the same task performed in both sessions. Comparisons were then made between the responses observed with the two modalities. As a step toward a more integrated use of EEG and fMRI, while avoiding contamination by gradient artifacts, simultaneous EEG-fMRI studies have also been performed with a sparse fMRI procedure, which alternates scanning with nonscanning sections. This leads to periods with an EEG of better quality, which is used for further analysis. However, progress in artifact removal procedures and in synchronization of the EEG and MRI clocks have improved the quality of continuous recordings made during fMRI scanning, and the question remains of which strategy to use, sparse or continuous acquisition.

The first two sections of this chapter review the pros and cons of sparse and continuous EEG-fMRI. The third section introduces advanced recording strategies that aim at improving the quality of EEG within a continuous sampling scheme.

Sparse fMRI Acquisition

Attempts to record EEG in the MRI scanner started soon after the development of fMRI, with the clear motivation of allowing the two techniques to be combined to provide a more accurate representation of the spatiotemporal dynamics of brain activity. The first report of the acquisition of EEG data in the MRI scanner came from Ives and colleagues in 1993 (Ives et al., 1993), and at that time the focus was on the technological challenges associated with safely recording EEG, rather than the optimal strategy for doing so. Once this technical obstacle had been overcome, several groups proceeded to apply EEG-fMRI in different ways.

The approaches adopted in the first few years of EEG-fMRI were based on the assumption that the gradient artifact precludes the acquisition of usable EEG data during fMRI scanning. The main distinction between the different approaches related to the type of EEG activity that was of interest. The clinical application of EEG-fMRI was a driving force from the beginning, and so interictal epileptiform discharges (IEDs, often called "epileptic spikes") formed one common event type, which was characterized by random occurrence. On the other hand, many groups were interested in evoked potentials, which incidentally provided more scope for experimental control of the relationship between EEG and fMRI acquisition.

Spike-Triggered EEG-fMRI

IEDs are transient events characteristic of patients with epilepsy, lasting from around 100 ms in focal epilepsies to several seconds for spike and wave discharges in patients with generalized epilepsy. They are distinct from seizures, having no clinical manifestation, but provide information about the regions of the brain involved in the patient's epilepsy (Gavaret et al., 2006; see Badier and Chauvel 1995, Bartolomei et al 2008, Rosenow and Lüders, 2001, for an introduction to the link between cortical regions and epileptogenicity). IEDs are apparent upon visual inspection of the EEG by a trained neurophysiologist, facilitating the EEG-fMRI acquisition strategy that was quite widely used in early studies: spike-triggered EEG-fMRI (Krakow et al., 1999a, 1999b; Patel et al., 1999; Seeck et al., 1998; Symms, 1999; Warach et al., 1996).

In spike-triggered EEG-fMRI a short sequence of fMRI scanning, ranging from one to a few image volumes, is initiated each time the neurophysiologist observes an IED on the continuously monitored EEG. Ideally, the image acquisition will begin a few seconds after the observation of the IED to allow time for the BOLD response to reach its maximum amplitude. Spike-triggered EEG-fMRI allowed the hemodynamic correlates of IEDs to be investigated for the first time, but as a methodology it has a number of disadvantages. Perhaps chief among these is the requirement for a trained neurophysiologist to observe the EEG for the duration of the scanning session, which could last for over an hour, and make an immediate decision about the occurrence or otherwise of an IED. Especially given the distortions of the EEG that were present in the early EEG-fMRI recordings, this procedure is not straightforward.

As well as the practical difficulty of spike-triggered EEG-fMRI, there is another important problem related to the sampling of the hemodynamic response (HR) to the IED. The issue of HR sampling relates not only to those situations where explicit characterization of the HR is required, but more fundamentally to the statistical power of the experiment. In spike-triggered EEG-fMRI there is no guarantee that the image volumes will be acquired near the peak of the HR. Since statistical maps are created by comparison of the signal in the IED volumes with that in separately acquired baseline volumes, acquisition of the IED volumes at anything other than the peak of the HR will result in a reduced ability to detect true activations. Sparse acquisition also does not allow the large baseline fluctuations present in fMRI signals to be accounted for. Furthermore, spike-triggered EEG-fMRI is only applicable to situations in which the EEG event of interest occurs sparsely and is clearly visible on the raw EEG, which in practice has limited its use to IEDs in patients with epilepsy. There is some evidence that HR to IEDs are more variable than those to normal brain function (Bagshaw et al., 2004; Gotman et al., 2004; Hawco et al., 2007; Lu et al., 2006; but see Lemieux et al., 2008), again making it difficult to ensure that the imaging volumes are acquired at the appropriate time.

Alternative Sparse Sampling Approaches

While spike-triggered EEG-fMRI was being applied to the study of IEDs, a different approach was taken in studies that involved external stimulation. Although IEDs have the advantage that they are large enough to be visible on the raw EEG, the fact that their timing is entirely random and independent of any control by the experimenter limits the scanning strategies that can be applied. When the subject is stimulated by the experimenter, for example in a sensory or cognitive paradigm, the timing of the events of interest is known and controlled. This means that the acquisition of fMRI data can be linked to the stimulation such that the EEG response of interest, such as an evoked potential, is acquired in the absence of gradient artifacts. The sluggishness of the HR means that there are several seconds between the completion of an event-related EEG response and the peak of the HR. As with spike-triggered EEG-fMRI, fMRI acquisition starts 2–3 seconds after the event. However, it is not triggered by a neurophysiologist observing the EEG but is instead controlled by the known timing of the experimental paradigm. There are several variants of this strategy, which differ in the details of the fMRI acquisition in relation to the stimulation.

Bonmassar et al. (2001) recorded EEG in the MRI scanner, but performed the stimulation twice, effectively having separate sessions for the recording of the EEG and fMRI signals. FMRI was recorded in relatively long blocks (~30s, with stimuli intermixed with fixation), and the paradigm was then repeated during an EEG window without fMRI. Portas et al. (2000) took a similar approach, but in this case the EEG during the fMRI silent periods was used to classify sleep stages.

Recording EEG and fMRI in separate blocks is an extension of previous studies that had completely separate sessions, with the EEG session occurring outside of the scanner. It has an advantage over separate sessions in that the EEG and fMRI recordings are interleaved, reducing the overall experimental time and the effects of habituation and fatigue that can complicate separate session recordings. However, EEG and fMRI responses to the same stimuli are not recorded, limiting the experimental questions that can be asked and the data integration strategies that can be applied.

The next step toward continuous and simultaneous EEG-fMRI involves sparse acquisition of the fMRI data. This has the advantage that the EEG and fMRI responses are generated in response to exactly the same stimuli. There are at least two ways of acquiring the fMRI data, both of which require a relatively long TR and few slices, but which differ in terms of the temporal acquisition. On the one hand, all slices can be acquired at the beginning of each TR, leaving a gap at the end of each TR free from gradient artifact. Alternatively, slices can be evenly spaced throughout the TR, with long gaps between each slice acquisition during which artifact-free EEG can be observed. Both of these strategies have been successfully applied (Bonmassar et al., 1999; Christmann et al., 2007; Feige et al., 2005; Goldman et al., 2000, 2002; Kruggel et al., 2000, 2001; Scarff et al., 2004), with the former being more common. For example, Laufs et al. (2003a; Laufs et al., 2003b) were interested in examining the relationship between spontaneous fluctuations in EEG spectral power and the BOLD signal. They used an fMRI protocol that acquired 19 slices in 2.8 s but had 4 s between the acquisition of successive volumes. Just over one second in each TR was thus free from gradient artifact, and it was from this period that the spectral power was quantified for use in the fMRI analysis.

Sparse acquisition suffers from some of the same limitations as spike-triggering, particularly that the hemodynamic response is not necessarily sampled efficiently. This can be a problem if there is an unusual delay in the HRF, or if accurate characterization of the HRF is desired (see Figure 2.2.1, below).

In summary, several variations of sparse sampling data acquisition strategies have been applied successfully over the past few years. The use of sparse sampling acquisition is based on the assumption that the gradient artifact is the

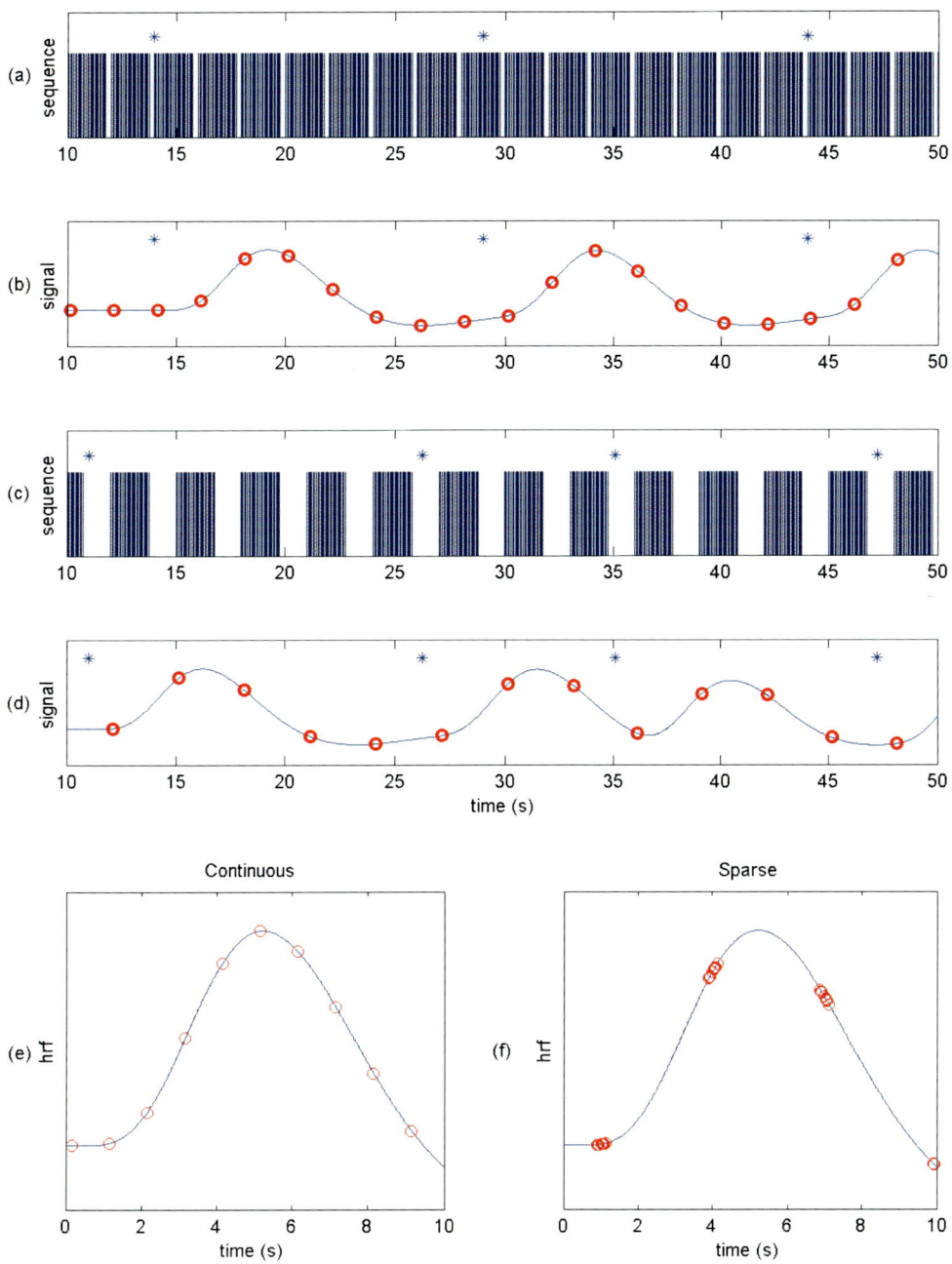

Figure 2.2.1. The effect of fMRI acquisition strategy on sampling of the HRF. In a) and b) we see continuous scanning, while c) and d) illustrate a sparse acquisition. Asterisks (*) represent events, while open circles (O) represent the timing of image acquisition. In e) and f) the effect of the acquisition strategy on the sampling of the HRF is shown. Much more complete characterization of the HRF is achieved with continuous scanning.

biggest hurdle to recording good quality EEG data. In fact, several studies have now shown that the data quality obtained with continuous scanning is generally as good as that obtained with sparse sampling (see below), at least in the low frequency range (<15 Hz) and that the ballistocardiogram artifact is potentially more problematic. With this in mind, and given the extra constraints on the fMRI acquisition when sampling is sparse, continuous scanning is now more widely used.

Continuous fMRI Acquisition

As mentioned in the introduction, the main EEG artifacts that affect simultaneous EEG fMRI are *(1)* the pulse artifact or "ballistocardiogram" (BCG) following each heartbeat, and *(2)* the induced currents due to the switching of the gradients ("gradient artifact"). Another source of artifact is the helium pump, which can be switched off during acquisition.

The pulse artifact is independent of the scanning strategy, and only depends on the MR static field (B0). With continuous fMRI acquisition, contrary to sparse sampling, the gradient artifact completely obscures the EEG traces: it is at least one order of magnitude higher than the background EEG signal (Bénar et al., 2003; Salek-Haddadi et al., 2003a). As a consequence, it needs to be removed in order to reveal the EEG activity of interest that is hidden behind it. The residuals of this filtering may impact on the retrieval of the activity of interest, especially at high frequency, as discussed below.

Despite the technical constraint of artifact filtering, continuous acquisition has several advantages, which we present in the first section below. In the second section, we discuss the impact of scanning on the EEG signal. In the third section, we review some of the studies that have demonstrated that it is possible to retrieve EEG signals of interest despite continuous scanning.

Advantages of Continuous fMRI Scanning

The first advantage of continuous scanning over sparse acquisition is that it permits a better sampling of the hemodynamic response (see Figure 2.2.1). Signals are sampled more frequently and consistently and, in a stimulation paradigm as done in event-related fMRI, the timing of the fMRI slices can be more easily decorrelated with the stimulation time. Continuous scanning also puts less constraint on the protocol, as the timing of the stimuli can be decided independently of the fMRI sequence. Finally, it is likely that the steady fMRI noise is less distractive than alternating noise with silent periods, which can be an advantage for resting state or sleep studies. In a cognitive paradigm, it gives a stable auditory environment, with no gaps to act as "cues" that a stimulus will be presented.

Therefore, generally speaking, a continuous paradigm is advantageous as it gives both more information on the hemodynamic response, which can improve the detection power, and more degrees of freedom for the protocol design. However, the impact on the EEG traces has to be carefully assessed in relation to the activity of interest.

Impact of Scanning on the EEG Traces

A typical fMRI sequence involves the acquisition of around 30 closely spaced slices (see Figure 2.2.2). The first important parameter is the frequency of acquisition of the slices, which is typically of the order of 15 per second. As a consequence, this produces the gradient artifact with a fundamental frequency at the slice acquisition frequency (in this example, 15 Hz). This fundamental frequency is followed by harmonics, which would in this case be at 30 Hz, 45 Hz, and so on (see Figure 2.2.3).

The second important frequency is that of gradient switching during the spatial encoding within a slice. For example, with 64 lines per image, this would produce a peak frequency at $64 \times 15 = 960$ Hz. This second frequency is much higher than the band of interest. However, as the signal is of very high energy this puts a constraint on the anti-aliasing filter that needs to remove this activity. If this is not the case, this activity could be aliased into and contaminate the low frequency band during the EEG sampling.

The most common method to remove the gradient artifact is the subtraction of a template constructed by averaging several realizations of the artifact (Allen et al., 2000). Despite this subtraction, there are some remnant artifacts due to the variability of the gradient-related waveform from one frame to the next. Several methods have been proposed to remove the residual artifacts, for example adaptive filtering based on the timing of the slices.

The variability in the gradient artifact has two sources. The first is the different timing between the EEG sampling and the fMRI acquisition, resulting in a sampling of the artifact waveform at slightly different times from one frame to the other. The synchronization of EEG and fMRI acquisition drastically reduces the remnant signals after subtraction, as discussed in more detail in the next section. The second source is the slight variation of the position of the EEG cables in the scanner that can happen during a session because of movements of the head. This can be reduced by placing the head in a vacuum cushion, but rapid variations of the head position are problematic. Of course, a large movement will produce a large artifact on the EEG traces, and the underlying EEG signals of interest will most likely have to be discarded from further analysis. Still, one has to be careful to avoid incorporating frames with large movements in the construction of the artifact template as they would contaminate the average artifact.

It can be seen directly from the spectrum (Figure 2.2.3) that frequencies below the slice acquisition frequency are well preserved. This implies that, with an acquisition frequency of the order of 15 Hz, signals such as evoked potentials, spikes, or alpha waves can be reasonably well recovered. This has indeed been demonstrated by several studies (see below). For signals

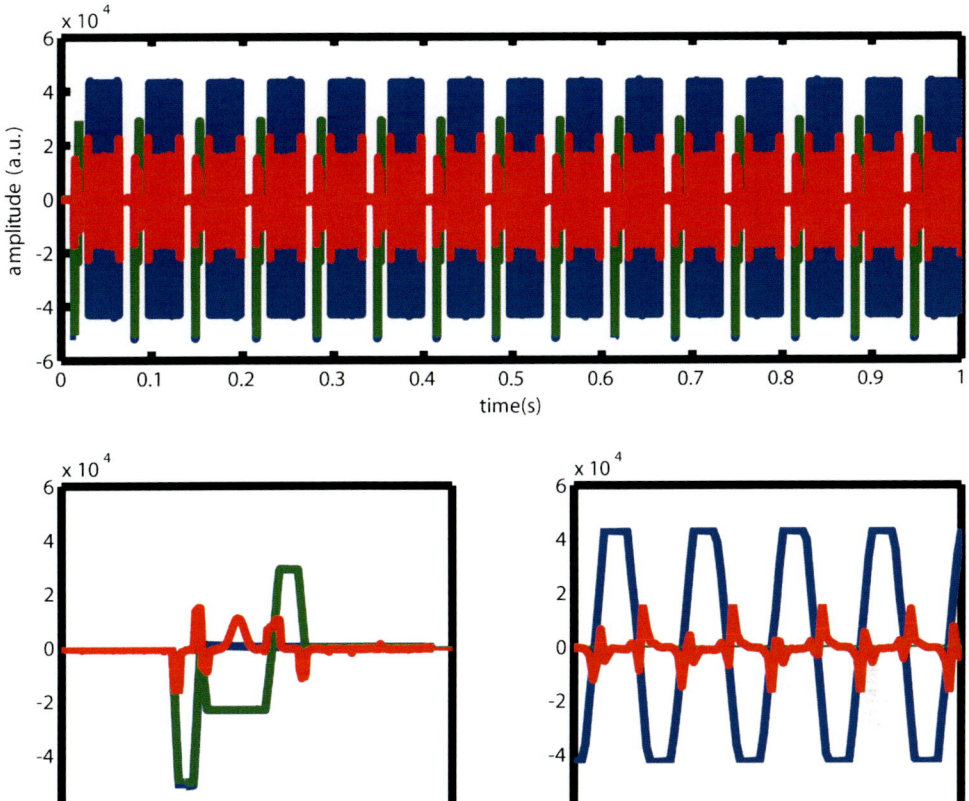

Figure 2.2.2. Comparison of the gradient artifact waveform and the fMRI sequence timing, with a 20 kHz sampling. Data were recorded on a phantom. The color code is: red for the gradient artifact, blue for the x_direction gradient (line encoding), green for the z-gradient (slice selection). Upper graph: one second of data (15 slices with the TR). Lower left: zoom on the slice encoding part. Lower right: zoom on the line encoding part.

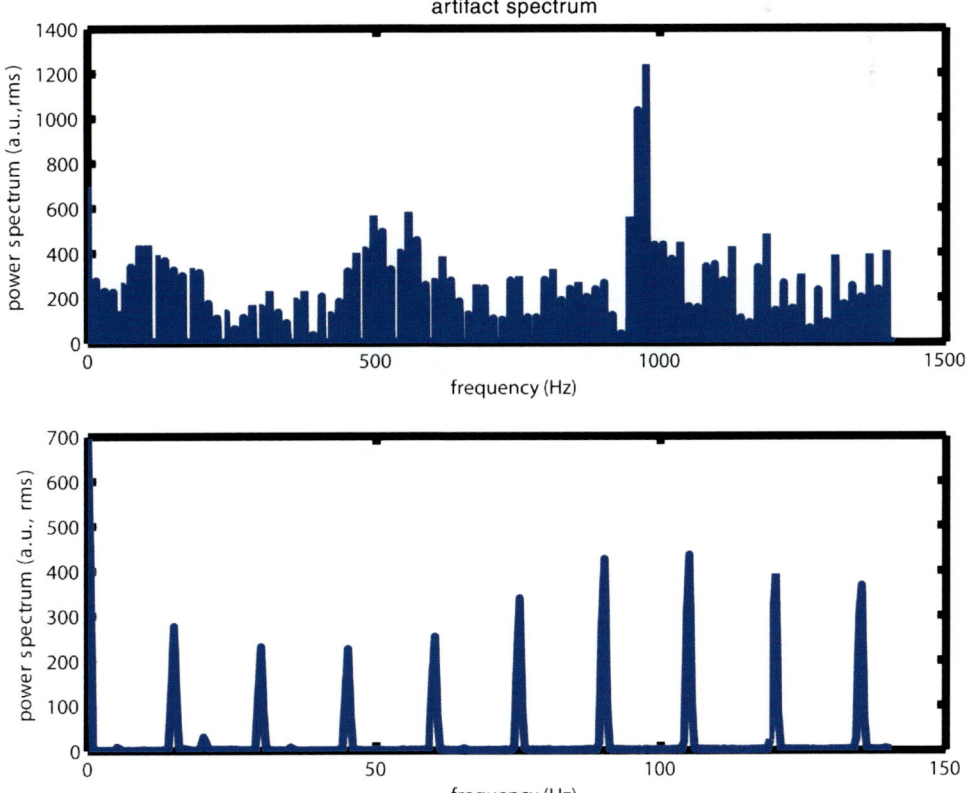

Figure 2.2.3. (top) Spectrum of the gradient artifact on the phantom. There is a large peak at 960 Hz corresponding to line encoding gradient switching (15 slices per second × 64 lines per slice). There is a peak at 15 Hz (slice acquisition frequency), followed by large harmonics. (bottom) Zoom on the 0–150 Hz band.

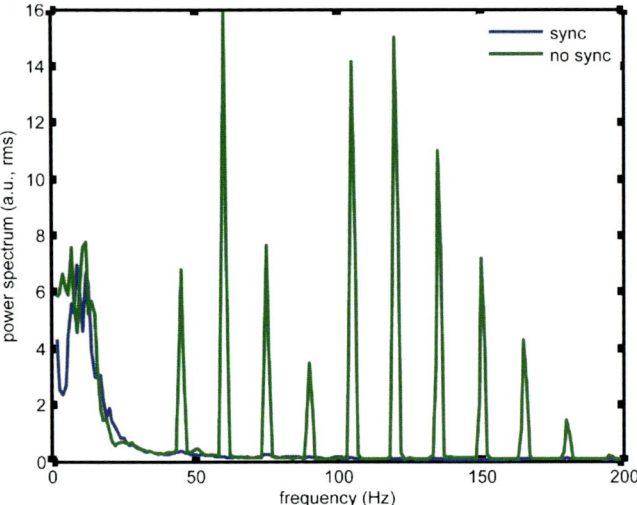

Figure 2.2.4. Comparison of EEG spectra from two subjects, after gradient artifact subtraction, with and without synchronization, from electrode O1. The synchronization has removed the gradient artifact almost completely.

with higher frequencies, such as oscillations in the beta band, or the gamma band (above 40 Hz), considerable care has to be taken with respect to the reduction of the artifact at the source, for example by synchronization (see the "Advanced Recording Strategies" section below), and at the post-processing level, by using advanced filtering methods.

An interesting development is that of real-time artifact filtering, which permits the quality of EEG signals to be monitored during the fMRI recording session (Garreffa et al., 2003; Masterton et al., 2007), but obviously places considerable constraints on the speed and accuracy of the artifact removal algorithms. The extent to which such monitoring will affect the progress of an experimental session remains to be seen, but it could prove useful for example to assess the level of fatigue or movement of the subject.

Advanced Recording Strategies

Continuous recording is the most common strategy for data acquisition, because of the advantages that have been discussed. However, with the standard implementation of continuous recording, the EEG and MRI hardware are entirely separate and the data are acquired independently. By moving in the direction of more explicit integration of the EEG acquisition system and MRI scanner, a number of improvements can be made to the data quality, particularly at high frequency ($f > 30$ Hz).

Perhaps the most straightforward of these advanced acquisition strategies is to synchronize the EEG and MRI clocks (Mandelkow et al., 2006; Mullinger et al., 2008). The purpose of synchronization is to maximize the accuracy with which the gradient artifact is recorded on the EEG, reducing residual variance caused by inconsistencies in the sampling of the EEG relative to the MRI. Improved characterization of the gradient artifact means that standard artifact removal methods are more successful. This is particularly important when the EEG signal of interest is at relatively high frequency, for example in the gamma band ($\sim$40–100Hz). Without synchronization, residual harmonics of the gradient artifact corrupt the EEG power spectrum (see Figures 2.2.3 and 2.2.4), making quantification of changes due to task performance difficult. In practice, synchronization is relatively straightforward and involves the use of an additional piece of hardware containing a frequency divider and phase-locking device.

Anami et al. (2003) adopted a different strategy to achieve the same goal of more accurate gradient artifact removal. They accurately characterized the temporal properties of the gradient artifact by digitizing at a sampling rate of 20 kHz, determining which parts of the fMRI sequence were responsible for the largest artifacts. Using this information, the fMRI sequence was then modified to reduce the artifacts generated by gradient pulses, rather than RF pulses. By driving the EEG acquisition by the MRI scanner clock to ensure accurate relative timing between the EEG and modified fMRI sequence, similarly to Mandelkow et al. (2006), they were able to reduce the gradient artifact at source by approximately a factor of ten. The disadvantage of this "stepping stone sampling" is that it requires considerable modification of the MRI sequence. However, the procedure whereby the major contributions to the gradient artifact are identified and reduced is clearly an interesting approach.

In terms of the BCG artifact, it is most common to use the ECG lead from the EEG system to provide the information necessary for artifact removal (R-peak detection). This makes the recording of a good ECG signal of paramount importance, since if R-peak detection fails artifact removal is not possible. One of the main problems associated with the recording of the ECG signal is saturation of the amplifier, since larger gradient artifacts tend to be measured relative to the ECG leads because of the longer lead length between the ECG electrode and reference (Mullinger et al., 2008). Mullinger et al. (2008) developed an alternative method that made use of the physiological monitoring apparatus attached to the scanner, specifically the vectorcardiogram (VCG). The VCG is more commonly used for cardiac gating of MRI scans, and requires the application of four ECG electrodes arranged in a cross on the thorax (Chia et al., 2000). These multiple ECG signals are converted into planar VCG signals, leading to much more robust identification of the QRS complex, which can then be used to perform a standard BCG artifact subtraction protocol. In addition, the VCG signals are inherently less sensitive to gradient artifacts because of the short lead length and the low pass filtering that is applied at the hardware stage. The disadvantage of this approach is that four additional electrodes need to be applied to the participant's chest and, since the EEG and VCG are recorded by separate systems, they must be explicitly temporally synchronized.

As a final example of the integration of EEG and fMRI data acquisition, some efforts have been made in the direction of integrated hardware, either by incorporating EEG electrodes directly in the RF antenna (van Auderkerke et al., 2000) or using surplus bandwidth in the MRI scanner to encode EEG or other physiological signals (Hanson et al., 2007). The former approach would allow more fixed and reproducible positioning of the EEG leads, potentially with a connection to the scanner similar to that for the head coil. The level of hardware integration proposed by Hanson et al. (2007) should make it more straightforward to apply modifications of the MRI sequence of the type proposed by Anami et al. (2003), hence reducing artifacts at source and the reliance on artifact correction algorithms. Clearly, wide use would require a considerable commitment by the MRI scanner manufacturers, which suggests that a clear clinical use of EEG-fMRI must first be demonstrated.

Applications of Continuous Scanning

Since well-validated and efficient methods are available for gradient and BCG artifact removal, and it is clear that good quality EEG data can be extracted from scanning periods, continuous EEG-fMRI has been applied to a wide range of neuroscientific questions. As will be discussed in more detail in later chapters, most algorithms for gradient artifact removal are variations on the template subtraction method proposed by Allen et al. (2000), while template subtraction and more complex methods such as independent component analysis (ICA) have been used for BCG artifact removal (Allen et al., 1998; Bénar et al., 2003; Mantini et al., 2007a; Niazy et al., 2005). Several studies have shown that it is feasible to obtain average evoked potentials of good quality during simultaneous scanning (Becker et al., 2005; Comi et al., 2005; Niazy et al., 2005; Sammer et al., 2005; Warbrick and Bagshaw., 2008). In particular, comparison between average ERPs during or outside scanning have shown little or no difference between the signals (Becker et al., 2005; Bregadze and Lavic., 2006).

The first example of the use of continuous EEG-fMRI was for the study of epileptic spikes (Lemieux et al., 2001a; 2001b). This remains the primary clinical application of the technique, and work is continuing to effect the transition from the research to the clinical environment (Zijlmans et al., 2007). Application to epilepsy was followed by simultaneous EEG-fMRI recordings of several spontaneous events: alpha rhythm (Goldman et al., 2000; Goldman et al., 2002; Laufs et al., 2003b; Moosmann et al., 2003), sleep spindles, and generalized spike-and-wave bursts (see Salek-Haddadi et al., 2003b, for a review).

The primary interest in simultaneous recording of evoked potentials is to obtain EEG and fMRI signals in exactly the same conditions. However, another motivation is the possibility of performing trial-to-trial coupling of the signals. In this method, the amplitude of the EEG signal is estimated for each trial, and fMRI voxels are tested for a correlation with the EEG-derived parameters. This application puts a high demand on the quality of the EEG signal. Simple filtering methods have been used (Bénar et al., 2007) and there is also a growing interest in ICA to extract the signals for the single-trial estimation (Debener et al., 2005; Eichele et al., 2005). Recently, several studies have successfully used single-trial coupling of EEG and fMRI, demonstrating the quality of the evoked potentials at the single-trial level (Bénar et al., 2007; Debener et al., 2005; Eichele et al., 2005; Mulert et al., 2008). Such single-trial analysis is of great interest in the wider field of MEG and EEG, especially with the surge of brain-computer interfaces, and it is likely that future developments will arise in this field (for example, Bénar et al., 2009; Quian Quiroga and Garcia 2003; Ranta-aho et al., 2003).

There have been fewer studies of higher frequency activity, which is generally the most difficult portion of the EEG signal to study reliably. In terms of spontaneous activity, Laufs et al. (2003a) demonstrated the feasibility of tracking the spontaneous fluctuations in the beta band. More recently, Mantini et al. (2007b) performed a similar resting-state study up to the gamma band, using ICA of the fMRI signal to identify resting-state networks, which were subsequently correlated with fluctuations in the EEG power spectrum. It is likely that the use of EEG-fMRI to study higher frequencies in the EEG spectrum will become increasingly widespread as new methods are developed to improve artifact rejection and consequently the EEG quality. Some of these methods were discussed in the last section.

Conclusions

Until recently, simultaneous recording of EEG and fMRI was not a widely used technique, but one restricted to a handful of centers with the motivation and technical expertise required to obtain good quality signals. It is now clear that to a large extent the technical obstacles have been overcome, although as discussed in the "Advanced Recording Strategies" section above, improvements can be expected. With this in mind, and with the availability of several commercial EEG systems, it is now possible to record good quality EEG-fMRI data relatively straightforwardly, meaning that many imaging centers now include EEG-fMRI as an available technique.

Perhaps the most important question that remains is how the data can most appropriately be fused to gain the high spatiotemporal resolution that is promised. To date, the most advanced data fusion strategies are probably single-trial coupling and probabilistically constrained source localization. Both of these, and indeed any other existing or future strategies, contain assumptions about the underlying link between the EEG and fMRI signals. As an example, single-trial coupling implicitly assumes that the variation in evoked potential amplitude on a trial-by-trial basis is reflected in the

BOLD signal. While this seems to be valid from the empirical success of studies that have applied the technique, little is known about the factors that affect the link between EEG and fMRI at this level of detail. It will only be via this basic work that simultaneous EEG-fMRI will achieve its full potential. Improved understanding of neurovascular coupling as accessed via the macroscopic, non-invasive techniques of EEG and fMRI will lead to better methods of data integration, and consequently more detailed spatiotemporal information about the brain's function. This is the goal of EEG-fMRI, and the challenge for the future.

REFERENCES

Allen PJ, Polizzi G, Krakow K, Fish DR, Lemieux L (1998) Identification of EEG events in the MR scanner: the problem of pulse artifact and a method for its subtraction. Neuroimage 8:229–239.

Allen PJ, Josephs O, Turner R (2000) A method for removing imaging artifact from continuous EEG recorded during functional MRI. Neuroimage 12:230–239.

Anami K, Mori T, Tanaka F, Kawagoe Y, Okamoto J, Yarita M, Ohnishi T, Yumoto M, Matsuda H, Saitoh O (2003) Stepping stone sampling for retrieving artifact-free electroencephalogram during functional magnetic resonance imaging. Neuroimage 19:281–295.

Badier JM, Chauvel P. Spatio-temporal characteristics of paroxysmal interictal events in human temporal lobe epilepsy. J Physiol Paris. 1995;89(4–6):255–64.

Bagshaw AP, Aghakhani Y, Bénar C-G, Kobayashi E, Hawco C, Dubeau F, Pike GB, Gotman J (2004) EEG-fMRI of focal epileptic spikes: analysis with multiple haemodynamic functions and comparison with gadolinium-enhanced MR angiograms. Hum Brain Mapp 22:174–192.

Bartolomei F, Chauvel P, Wendling F. (2008) Epileptogenicity of brain structures in human temporal lobe epilepsy: a quantified study from intracerebral EEG. Brain. 2008 Jul;131(Pt 7):1818–30.

Becker R, Ritter P, Moosmann M, Villringer A (2005) Visual evoked potentials recovered from fMRI scan periods. Hum Brain Mapp 26:221–230.

Bénar C-G, Aghakhani Y, Wang Y, Izenberg A, Al-Asmi A, Dubeau F, Gotman J (2003) Quality of EEG in simultaneous EEG-fMRI for epilepsy. Clin Neurophysiol 114:569–580.

Bénar C-G, Schön D, Grimault S, Nazarian B, Burle B, Roth M, Badier J-M, Marquis P, Liegeois-Chauvel C, Anton J-L (2007) Single-trial analysis of oddball event-related potentials in simultaneous EEG-fMRI. Hum Brain Mapp 28:602–613.

Bénar CG, Papadopoulo T, Torrésani B, Clerc M. 2009 Consensus Matching Pursuit for multi-trial EEG signals. J Neurosci Methods. 2009 May 30;180(1):161–70.

Bonmassar G, Anami K, Ives J, Belliveau JW (1999) Visual evoked potential (VEP) measured by simultaneous 64-channel EEG and 3T fMRI. Neuroreport 10:1893–1897.

Bonmassar G, Schwartz DP, Liu AK, Kwong KK, Dale AM, Belliveau JW (2001) Spatiotemporal brain imaging of visual-evoked activity using interleaved EEG and fMRI recordings. Neuroimage 13:1035–1043.

Bregadze N, Lavic A (2006) ERP differences with vs without concurrent fMRI. Int J Psychophysiol 62:54–59.

Christmann C, Koeppe C, Braus DF, Ruf M, Flor H (2007) A simultaneous EEG-fMRI study of painful electric stimulation. Neuroimage 34:1428–1437.

Chia JM, Fischer SE, Wickline SA, Lorenz CH (2000) Performance of QRS detection for cardiac magnetic resonance imaging with a novel vectorcardiographic triggering method. J Magn Reson Imag 12:678–688.

Comi E, Annovazzi P, Martins Silva A, Cursi M, Blasi V, Cadioli M, Inuggi A, Falini A, Comi G, Leocani L (2005) Visual evoked potentials may be recorded simultaneously with fMRI scanning: a validation study. Hum Brain Mapp 24:291–298.

Debener S, Ullsperger M, Siegel M, Fiehler K, von Cramon DY, Engel AK (2005) Trial-by-trial coupling of concurrent electroencephalogram and functional magnetic resonance imaging identifies the dynamics of performance monitoring. J Neurosci 25:11750–11737.

Eichele T, Specht K, Moosmann M, Jongsma MLA, Quian Quiroga R, Nordby H, Hugdahl K (2005) Assessing the spatiotemporal evolution of neuronal activation with single-trial event-related potentials and functional MRI. Proc Natl Acad Sci U S A 102:17798–17803.

Feige B, Scheffler K, Esposito F, Di Salle F, Hennig J, Seifritz E (2005) Cortical and subcortical correlates of electroenceph alographic alpha rhythm modulation. J Neurophysiol 93:2864–2872.

Garreffa G, Carni M, Gualniera G, Ricci CB, De Carli D, Morasso P, Pantano P, Colonnese C, Roma V, Maraviglia B (2003) Real-time MR artifacts filtering during continuous EEG/fMRI acquisition. Magn Reson Imag 21:1175–1189.

Gavaret M, Badier J-M, Marquis P, McGonigal A, Bartolomei F, Regis J, Chauvel P (2006) Electric source imaging in frontal lobe epilepsy. J Clin Neurophysiol 23:358–370.

Goldman RI, Stern JM, Engel J, Jr., Cohen MS (2000) Acquiring simultaneous EEG and functional MRI. Clin Neurophysiol 111:1974–1980.

Goldman RI, Stern JM, Engel J, Jr., Cohen MS (2002) Simultaneous EEG and fMRI of the alpha rhythm. Neuroreport 13:2487–2492.

Gotman J, Bénar C-G, Dubeau F (2004) Combining EEG and fMRI in epilepsy: methodological challenges and clinical results. J Clin Neurophysiol 21:229–240.

Hanson LG, Lund TE, Hanson CG (2007) Encoding of electrophysiology and other signals in MR images. J Magn Reson Imag 25:1059–1066.

Hawco CS, Bagshaw AP, Lu Y, Dubeau F, Gotman J (2007) BOLD changes occur prior to epileptic spikes seen on scalp EEG. Neuroimage 35:1450–1458.

Ives JR, Warach S, Schmitt F, Edelman RR, Schomer DL (1993) Monitoring the patient's EEG during echo planar MRI. Electroenceph Clin Neurophysiol 87:417–420.

Krakow K, Allen PJ, Symms MR, Fish DR, Lemieux L (1999a) Imaging of interictal epileptiform discharges using spike-triggered fMRI. Int J Bioelectromag 1:96–101.

Krakow K, Woermann FG, Symms MR, Allen PJ, Lemieux L, Barker GJ, Duncan JS, Fish DR (1999b) EEG-triggered functional MRI of interictal epileptiform activity in patients with partial seizures. Brain 122:1679–1688.

Kruggel F, Wiggins CJ, Herrman CS, von Cramon DY (2000) Recording of the event-related potentials during functional MRI at 3.0 Tesla field strength. Magn Reson Med 44:277–282.

Kruggel F, Herrmann CS, Wiggins CJ, von Cramon DY (2001) Hemodynamic and electroencephalographic responses to illusory figures: recording of the evoked potentials during functional MRI. Neuroimage 14:1327–1336.

Laufs H, Krakow K, Sterzer P, Eger E, Beyerle A, Salek-Haddadi A, Kleinschmidt A (2003a) Electroencephalographic signatures of attentional and cognitive default modes in spontaneous brain activity fluctuations at rest. Proc Natl Acad Sci U S A 100:11053–11058.

Laufs H, Kleinschmidt A, Beyerle A, Eger E, Salek-Haddadi A, Preibisch C, Krakow K (2003b) EEG-correlated fMRI of human alpha activity. Neuroimage 19:1463–1476.

Lemieux L, Salek-Haddadi A, Josephs O, Allen P, Toms C, Krakow K, Turner R, Fish DR (2001a) Event-related fMRI with simultaneous and continuous EEG: description of the method and initial case report. Neuroimage 14:780–787.

Lemieux L, Krakow K, Fish DR (2001b) Comparison of spike-triggered functional MRI BOLD activation and EEG dipole model localization. Neuroimage 14:1097–1104.

Lemieux L, Laufs H, Carmichael D, Paul JS, Walker MC, Duncan JS (2008) Non-canonical spike-related BOLD responses in focal epilepsy. Hum Brain Mapp 29:329–345.

Lu Y, Bagshaw AP, Grova C, Kobayashi E, Dubeau F, Gotman J (2006) Using voxel-specific hemodynamic response function in EEG-fMRI data analysis. Neuroimage 32:238–247.

Mandelkow H, Halder P, Boesiger P, Brandeis D (2006) Synchronization facilitates removal of MRI artefacts from concurrent EEG recordings and increases usable bandwidth. Neuroimage 32:1120–1126.

Mantini D, Perrucci MG, Cugini S, Ferretti A, Romani GL, Del Gratta C (2007a) Complete artifact removal for EEG recorded during continuous fMRI using independent component analysis. Neuroimage 34:598–607.

Mantini D, Perrucci MG, Del Gratta C, Romani GL, Corbetta M (2007b) Electrophysiological signatures of resting state networks in the human brain. Proc Natl Acad Sci U S A 104:13170–13175.

Masterton RA, Abbott DF, Fleming SW, Jackson GD (2007) Measurement and reduction of motion and ballistocardiogram artefacts from simultaneous EEG and fMRI recordings. Neuroimage 37:202–211.

Moosmann M, Ritter P, Krastel I, Brink A, Thees S, Blankenburg F, Taskin B, Obrig H, Villringer A (2003) Correlates of alpha rhythm in functional magnetic resonance imaging and near infrared spectroscopy. Neuroimage 20:145–158.

Mulert C, Seifert C, Leicht G, Kirsch V, Ertl M, Karch S, Moosmann M, Lutz J, Möller HJ, Hegerl U, Pogarell O, Jäger L (2008) Single-trial coupling of EEG and fMRI reveals the involvement of early anterior cingulate cortex activation in effortful decision making. Neuroimage 42:158–168.

Mullinger KJ, Morgan PS, Bowtell RW (2008) Improved artifact correction for combined electroencephalography/functional MRI by means of synchronisation and use of vectorcardiogram recordings. J Magn Reson Imag 27:607–616.

Niazy RK, Beckmann CF, Iannetti GD, Brady JM, Smith SM (2005) Removal of fMRI environment artifacts from EEG data using optimal basis sets. Neuroimage 28:720–737.

Patel MR, Blum A, Pearlman JD, Yousuf N, Ives JR, Saeteng S, Schomer DL, Edelman RR (1999) Echo-planar functional MR imaging of epilepsy with concurrent EEG monitoring. Am J Neuroradiol 20:1916–1919.

Portas CM, Krakow K, Allen O, Josephs O, Armony JL, Frith CD (2000) Auditory processing across the sleep-wake cycle: simultaneous EEG and fMRI monitoring in humans. Neuron 28:991–999.

Quian Quiroga R, Garcia H (2003) Single-trial event-related potentials with wavelet denoising. Clin Neurophysiol 114:376–390.

Ranta-aho P, Koistinen A, Ollikainen J, Kaipio J, Partanen J, Karjalainen P (2003) Single-trial estimation of multichannel evoked-potential measurements. IEEE Trans Biomed Eng 50:189–196.

Rosenow F, Lüders H (2001) Presurgical evaluation in epilepsy. Brain 124:1683–1700.

Salek-Haddadi A, Lemieux L, Merschhemke M, Diehl B, Allen PJ, Fish DR (2003a) EEG quality during simultaneous functional MRI of interictal epileptiform discharges. Magn Reson Imag 21:1159–1166.

Salek-Haddadi A, Friston KJ, Lemieux L, Fish DR (2003b) Studying spontaneous EEG activity with fMRI. Brain Res Rev 43:110–133.

Sammer G, Blecker C, Gebhardt H, Kirsch P, Stark R, Vaitl D (2005) Acquisition of typical EEG waveforms during fMRI: SSVEP, LRP and frontal theta. Neuroimage 24:1012–1024.

Scarff CJ, Reynolds A, Goodyear BG, Ponton CW, Dort JC, Eggermont JJ (2004) Simultaneous 3-T fMRI and high density recording of human auditory evoked potentials. Neuroimage 23:1129–1142.

Seeck M, Lazeyras F, Michel CM, Blanke O, Gericke CA, Ives J, Delavelle J, Golay X, Haenggeli CA, de Tribolet N, Landis T (1998) Non-onvasive epileptic focus localization using EEG-triggered functional MRI and electromagnetic tomography. Electroenceph Clin Neurophysiol 106:508–512.

Symms MR, Allen PJ, Woermann FG, Polizzi G, Krakow K, Barker GJ, Fish DR, Duncan JS (1999) Reproducible localization of interictal epileptiform discharges using EEG-triggered fMRI. Phys Med Biol 44:N161-N168.

van Auderkerke J, Peeters R, Verhove M, Sijbers J, Van der Linden A (2000) Special designed RF-antenna with integrated non-invasive carbon electrodes for simultaneous magnetic resonance imaging and electroencephalography acquisition at 7T. Magn Reson Imag 18:887–891.

Warach S, Ives JR, Schlaug G, Patel MR, Darby DG, Thangaraj V, Edelman RR, Schomer DL (1996) EEG-triggered echo-planar functional MRI in epilepsy. Neurology 47:89–93.

Warbrick T, Bagshaw AP (2008) Scanning strategies for simultaneous EEG-fMRI evoked potential studies at 3T. Int J Psychophysiol 67:169–177.

Zijlmans M, Huiskamp G, Hersevoort M, Seppenwoolde J-H, van Huffelen AC, Leijten FSS (2007) EEG-fMRI in the preoperative work-up for epilepsy surgery. Brain 130:2343–2353.

2.3

Tom Eichele, Matthias Moosmann, Lei Wu, Ingmar Gutberlet, and Stefan Debener

Removal of MRI Artifacts from EEG Recordings

Introduction

The simultaneous recording of electroencephalogram (EEG) and functional magnetic resonance imaging (fMRI) provides several advantages over multimodal integration based on separate EEG and fMRI recording protocols (Debener et al., 2006). However, the recording and analysis of simultaneous EEG-fMRI is not without pitfalls. The potential benefits of simultaneous recordings come at the expense of a massive, inevitable presence of artifacts, which corrupt the EEG signals recorded in the MR environment. It therefore comes as no surprise that many researchers find it difficult to obtain a reasonable EEG data quality in simultaneous EEG-fMRI recordings, or prefer separate protocols (Bledowski et al., 2007). However, the past few years have seen significant progress. With the advent of reliable hardware solutions, and increasing experience in artifact processing, multimodal integration has become feasible. The present chapter surveys the major types of artifacts evident in inside-scanner EEG recordings. With a focus on the most prominent artifacts, it presents different methods of EEG artifact correction; it also discusses the limitations of currently available approaches as well as possible future directions. For a discussion of MRI image quality, see Chapter 2.4.

Prominent MRI Artifacts in EEG Recordings

Depending on the MRI scanner field strength (B_0), the MR protocol applied, the subject's behavior in the scanner, and the recording equipment used, EEG data recorded inside the MRI appear massively obscured to totally indiscernible. A typical example of continuous EEG recorded inside the scanner is illustrated in Figure 2.3.1, showing a few channels of an EEG recording taken during an fMRI echo planar imaging (EPI) recording in a 3 Tesla MRI scanner. As can be seen, visual inspection of the raw EEG traces appears impossible and necessitates further processing of the data. In fact, the application of offline artifact removal techniques is mandatory to enable a meaningful interpretation of the EEG signal. The principle assumption of such artifact removal is that the original EEG is linearly mixed with the artifact, the latter dominating the recording and thus rendering the visual inspection of typical EEG features such as occipital alpha oscillations impossible. Indeed, one particular type of artifact, which is related to MR image acquisition, contributes signals that can easily be several orders of magnitude larger than neural contributions to the EEG recording. Moreover, it is not just one artifact, but rather a number of qualitatively different artifact types that obscure the signal and contaminate the data over a broad frequency range overlapping with the frequency range of interest (0–100 Hz) of the physiological EEG. Following Allen et al. (2000), three groups of artifact can be distinguished:

Motion Related Artifacts

The movement of conductive materials, such as EEG electrodes and cables, in the static magnetic field induce an electromotive force. The strength of the induced current varies with a number of factors, such as the area of the conductive loop, the velocity, and the amount of motion and the strength of the static magnetic field (Huang-Hellinger et al., 1995). Accordingly, all kinds of motion listed below should be reduced to a minimum in simultaneous EEG-fMRI. This holds true in particular for transient, gross head motion, which can distort the EEG signal beyond recovery. Since head motion also deteriorates fMRI image quality, both modalities profit from the application of procedures preventing transient head motions (e.g., vacuum pillows, cushions) as well as more slowly occurring changes in head position. It is important to recognize that, compared

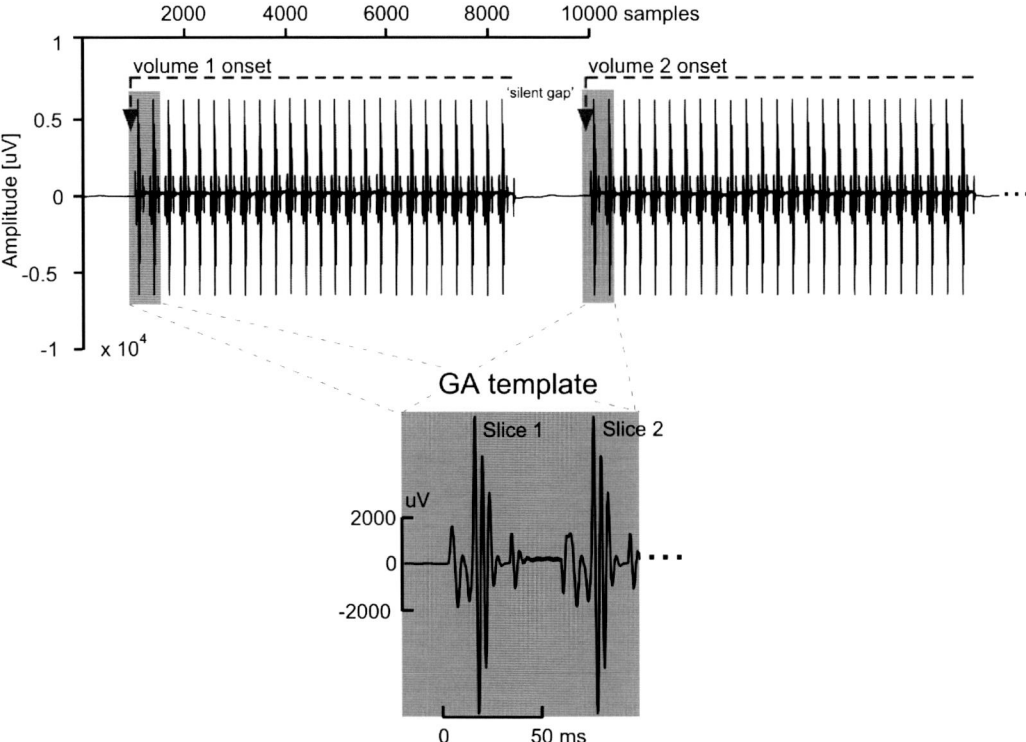

Figure 2.3.1. Example of EEG recordings during EPI image acquisition of two consecutive volumes.

to mere fMRI recordings, the problem of head motion can be significantly amplified in simultaneous EEG-fMRI recordings, simply because of the discomfort caused by the posterior EEG electrodes, which the subject is lying on. In addition, at least two types of vibration-induced motion can contaminate the EEG signal. Vibration-induced motion can be related to the MRI scanner cryogen pump, a problem that could be bypassed by transiently switching off the cooling system. Vibration can also be caused by the gradient switching itself, which, of course, cannot be fully avoided. It is important to note that both types of vibration can induce motion of the subject and/or of EEG recording equipment (i. e., cables and amplifier). Therefore, beyond head fixation, the fixation of EEG cables and amplifiers may be beneficial (this and related recording procedures are covered in Chapter 2.1). And finally, *endogenous* and inevitable artifacts are induced by subtle head movement related to respiration and the cardiac cycle. The latter in particular forms another group of artifacts that will be discussed in more depth below.

MR Imaging–Related Artifacts

The switching of magnetic gradients is necessary for MRI image acquisition; and the related EEG signal distortions cannot be avoided by any shielding. Interleaved designs, where EEG recordings are analysed during the "silent" interval between MR scanning, have been used, but they do not solve the principle problem and restrict the efficiency of

the experiment. The two types of imaging artifact that can be distinguished are the gradient artifact (GA), which causes a massive distortion of the EEG, and radio frequency (RF) artifact. Because the latter has a much higher frequency than the EEG signal, it can be effectively suppressed by analog low pass filtering. Analog low pass filtering is mandatory anyway to avoid EEG amplifier saturation and aliasing problems. Accordingly, the GA represents the major source of MR imaging artifact. The GA is a technical or exogenous artifact that reflects the imaging slice acquisition. Its major contribution is a very steep rising, transient signal with gradients that can be in the order of millivolts per millisecond. Most of the signal distortion visible in Figure 2.3.1 represents the GA. The GA completely dominates the EEG recording during MR image acquisition periods. Unlike the RF, the GA distorts the EEG spectrum over a broad frequency, including the frequency range of interest (< 100 Hz), and therefore cannot be fully accounted for by filtering (Allen et al., 2000). In fact, for many purposes, the GA is one of the two major artifacts that need to be dealt with statistically. Different ways of GA correction, and the challenges involved in it, will be discussed below.

Cardiac-Related Artifacts

Unlike the GA, which occurs only during slice acquisition periods, the ballistocardiogram (BCG) is always present in the scanner's magnetic field. The BCG contributes to the low

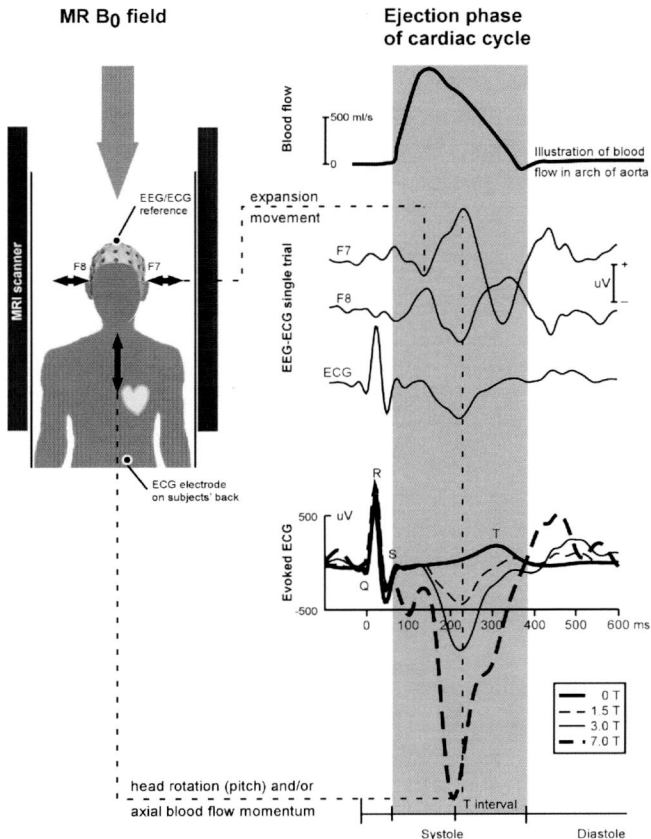

Figure 2.3.2. A schematic diagram illustrating possible factors causing the BCG. Two different types of movement are indicated, axial nodding rotation of the head and expansion movement at lateral and temporal scalp sites. The left part of the figure illustrates a subject in supine position inside an MRI scanner. The locations of EEG electrodes, EEG/ECG reference site, and ECG recording site at the lower back are indicated. Lower right part of the figure shows the evoked ECG from one individual, recorded outside the MRI (0 T) and inside three different MRI scanners (1.5, 3.0, 7.0 T). Above the evoked ECG traces, a typical single trial of ECG and EEG activity is shown, and on top, the blood-flow time course in the arch of aorta, as it can be adapted from cardiac physiology textbooks. As highlighted by the grey background, the BCG mostly occurs during the ejection phase of the cardiac cycle. (This figure is reprinted from Debener et al. 2007, with kind permission from Elsevier Publishers.)

frequency portion of the EEG signal (< 15 Hz). A concurrent recording of the EEG with the electrocardiogram (ECG) reveals that the periodic distortion present in most EEG channels is related to the cardiac cycle. While the exact origin of the BCG is not known yet, it is likely that the pulsatile flow of blood associated with the cardiac cycle induces a rocking, nodding head motion (Anami et al., 2002). Figure 2.3.2 provides a schematic. Another source of influence could be that EEG electrodes (or cables) over, or adjacent to, pulsatile blood vessels are in steady motion. And finally, according to the Hall effect, the acceleration of blood, which is electrically conductive, could be a source of current induction that is registered in the EEG.

Consequently, it is important to recognize that the BCG is of mesogenous rather than purely exogenous or endogenous origin. It is a major problem for EEG recordings acquired in the MRI environment and approximately scales with the static magnetic (B_0) field (Debener et al., 2008). However, its temporal variability reflects changes in heart rate and blood-flow parameters, which are under autonomous nervous system control. Accordingly, the BCG is subject to substantial temporal fluctuations, making its removal challenging.

Removal of the GA

The GA is generated by the magnetic field inside the scanner changing due to rapidly switching varying gradient fields and by the RF pulse, both of which are necessary to produce MR images. They represent a technical type of artifact that shows little fluctuation over time (see Figure 2.3.1). Accordingly, consecutive occurrences of MR volume (or slice) acquisitions can be expected to lead to similar EEG signal distortions. Another important characteristic of the GA is that it generates fast transients with large amplitudes on the order of 25000 μV/ms. Fortunately, MR-compatible EEG hardware solutions provide effective analog low pass filters that prevent the amplifier from drifting into saturation. Thus, the recorded signal, though carrying very large artifact amplitudes, contains the normal EEG signal "riding on top" of the GA. This linear mixing renders the statistical removal of the GA possible.

Under the assumption of similarity of repetitive GAs, a GA template can be created by using the onset of each GA (per slice or per volume, respectively) as the time-locking event and then averaging over repeated GAs. Given enough trials, this effectively averages out the non–volume locked EEG signal and leaves a GA template that can be used subsequently to subtract out the GA from every single trial. This general procedure is known as average artifact subtraction (AAS) and was originally proposed by Allen et al. (2000). Previous attempts to deal with the GA included, among others, adaptive filtering (Sijbers et al., 1999) and frequency domain methods (Hoffmann et al., 2000), but proved less practical. Note that the morphologies and amplitudes of the GA (template) systematically differ between EEG channels, due to the different positions and orientations of the electrodes and cables with respect to the gradients, and other factors (see Hoffmann et al., 2000, for details). Hence, the GA template calculation and the corresponding GA correction is done for each channel separately.

A second important aspect concerns the temporal precision assumption, that is, the accuracy by which the GA is recorded and digitized. Given the enormous slope of the GA, an EEG sampling rate of, e.g., 250 Hz would mean that the GA amplitude could easily jump in steps of 100 μV (or more) from sample to sample. Accordingly, sampling rates are generally high in simultaneous EEG-fMRI experiments, in order to capture the steep GA slopes. Any temporal jitter that could for instance be introduced by asynchronous MR scanner and EEG recording computer clocks would then result in systematic errors, that is, residual artifact amplitudes that could still be larger than the EEG signal of interest.

In fact, both assumptions mentioned above are in reality not perfectly met: the GA amplitude and morphology fluctuates a little over time, and the precision by which the GA is recorded can suffer from temporal jitter, causing even more problems. Taking these two problems into account is the challenge for all GA correction procedures, and this has inspired a number of researchers to develop more sophisticated procedures, which generally include a number of processing steps, not just template subtraction. Allen et al. (2000) already combined the template subtraction approach with an upsampling procedure and adaptive noise cancellation, and these two procedures are still included in several currently used GA reduction implementations, albeit in different ways.

Challenges in GA Removal

As already noted, one complicating factor is that the GA can change over time, for instance due to different types of head movement (slow, involuntary movement; fast voluntary, temporally restricted movements). Because these types of head movement result in a different position and orientation of the EEG electrodes in the gradient field, the GA can be substantially different. Thus, a mean template based on the average across all recorded volumes may not be representative for single GA events. To compensate for the potential problem that single artifact instances could compromise the quality of the GA template (because they could be overlayed by other artifacts, say, gross head movement), Allen et al. proposed to include only those GA events that correlate with an initial GA template (based on the mean of the first five volumes) above r = 0.975, thus effectively removing outlier events.

Now consider the scenario that an individual's head position shifts a little, but continuously, over the EEG-fMRI recording duration. In this case, one would expect nearby GA events to be highly similar, whereas those being more distant in time would correlate to a much lesser amount. Following this line of reasoning, several AAS removal implementations now offer to calculate the GA template based on a moving average of adjacent volumes. Combined with an outlier identification procedure such as the one used by Allen, this would then account for involuntary head movements over time. To account for possible drifts in the GA over time, Becker et al. (2005) introduced a weighted average based on an exponential decay function, thereby ensuring that adjacent artifact volumes have a stronger influence on the local template than artifact volumes that are more distant and thus might have a different morphology.

In addition to slow head movements, participants also move their head abruptly during data acquisition. It was shown that abrupt head movements larger than 1 mm head deflection do happen in about 30% of fMRI studies (Moosmann et al., 2009). This ratio is likely to be higher in simultaneous EEG-fMRI studies, in which discomfort may be caused by the EEG electrodes on which the subjects are lying. Abrupt head movements alter the geometry of electrodes and cables in the magnetic field and consequently the induced GA properties change. This leads to an increased heterogeneity of the GA and thus impairs EEG signal quality after GA correction (Laufs et al., 2008). The correction techniques mentioned above are adequate for homogeneous data or slow drifts of the artifact properties but cannot optimally represent transitions, i.e., when abrupt changes of the artifact properties occur. Whereas head movements in fMRI data are commonly corrected by the realignment preprocessing procedure (Friston et al., 1996), this issue has not been addressed for MR gradient–contaminated EEG data. Therefore modifications of the moving average algorithm have been proposed recently (Moosmann et al., 2009; Sun and Hinrichs, 2009) that take the head movement parameters from the fMRI preprocessing into account to estimate improved artifact templates that serve as local filters to correct the distorted EEG. More precisely, the subject's movement information is used to calculate a correction matrix that codes the position of the window of GA volumes being part of a specific template. Movements above a certain threshold act as a barrier in order to avoid averaging over discontinuities of artifact properties. Templates for GA volumes before/after a head movement are generated from GA volumes before/after the movement only (See Figure 2.3.3 for an illustration of the method). The application of this method (Moosmann et al., 2009) will result in a better signal-to-noise ratio and a smaller residual variance around events of head movements compared to standard template correction methods. The realignment parameter–informed algorithm has now been realized as a Matlab plug-in for the open-source EEGLAB environment (Delorme and Makeig, 2004).

As mentioned above, the GA amplitude and morphology fluctuates over time due to a lack of temporal precision, the so-called jitter-problem. Because of an inaccuracy of the internal clocks of the EEG and MR system, the temporal properties of the gradient switching process (GHz) and limits in the sampling rate of the EEG (kHz), the GA is not always digitized at the same location in time, introducing a variation in the shape of the GA from volume to volume. An upsampling up to 100 kHz was proposed to adequately sample the slope of the gradient followed by a phase correction via a temporal alignment using a cross-correlation function (Allen et al., 2000; Becker et al., 2005; Niazy et al., 2005). Goncalves et al. (2007) proposed a selective average subtraction on slice and on volume level to meet jitter-related GA variations. Niazy et al. (2005) further introduced the fMRI artifact template removal (FASTR) procedure, which is implemented as part of the FMRIB toolbox, a plug-in for EEGLAB. FASTR reduces jitter-related temporal variations of the GA by generating a unique artifact template for each

volume. It combines a local moving average as a template with a linear combination of basis functions, which are derived from a temporal principal component analysis (PCA) on the residual artifacts.

However, jitter-related issues can be avoided by synchronizing scanner clock and the EEG recording computer clock (Anami et al., 2003; Mandelkow et al., 2006; Mullinger et al., 2008). The synchronization of the systems results in more homogeneous GA volumes, which better meet the assumptions of the template-based correction methods and thus result in cleaner EEG signals after GA correction.

Anami and colleagues went one step further and modified the fMRI imaging sequence timing parameters. They programmed MR gradients to be switched during the times when no EEG data point was sampled, theoretically resulting in minimal GA (Anami et al., 2003).

As discussed above, template-based GA correction methods have been proven to be very successful to correct GA. However, since the assumptions for applying any of the proposed algorithms are not always met, the corrected EEG data might still be contaminated by residual artifacts. To correct residual artifacts a second processing step was proposed. Niazy and colleages (2005) employed optimal basis sets of orthogonal components to filter residual imaging artifacts. This method is discussed in more detail in the paragraph on the removal of ballistocardiographic artifacts below. Brookes et al. (2008) suggested a spatial beamformer technique, which uses spatial filters that extract the components of a signal with

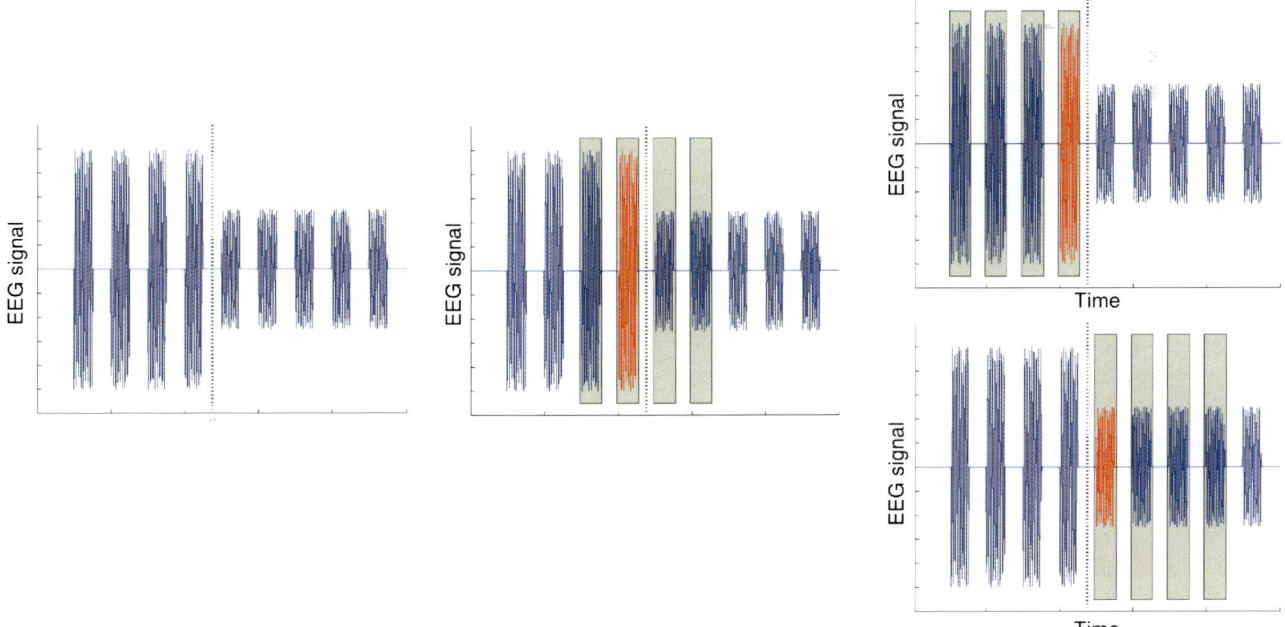

Figure 2.3.3. Illustration of the RP-informed algorithm. In the event of a head movement (vertical dashed line) the artifact properties may change abruptly as schematically indicated on the left. The conventional moving average algorithm corrects by averaging over the discontinuity caused by the head movement (middle) while the realignment parameter–informed algorithm (RP-informed) respects the discontinuity (right). The grey blocks indicate which artifacts are taken into account to calculate the template to correct the red artifact.

a specific spatial characteristic. It is able to localize electrical activity as well as to remove residual artifacts that may not be eliminated by the AAS technique. Mathematically, the filter is based on a weighted sum of measurements made at each of the EEG electrodes. This weighted sum gives an estimate of local electrical source strength at some predetermined location in the brain. Sequential application of the spatial filter to a number of locations (voxels) in the brain will then yield a volumetric image of source power. To correct residual artifacts related to head movements Masterton et al. proposed a method using wire loops that were attached to the electrode cap to measure subject movements (Masterton et al., 2007). Linear adaptive filtering based on recursive least squares was used to reduce the artifact power online while preserving the physiological EEG signal.

Properties and Removal of the BCG

In most recording conditions the BCG is clearly visible after gradient artifact removal. In the absence of scanning it contributes signals to the frequency range that are close to the range of the EEG. Although it exists in EEG recordings outside the scanner, the large amplitude BCG in the scanner arises due to the interaction between the active cardiovascular system (endogenous contribution) and the main static (B_0) field inside the MRI scanner (exogenous contribution), rendering it a mixed, or mesogenous artifact. This characterization already outlines some potential problems associated with the variability inherent in the BCG, i.e., the MRI environment (e.g., the scanner field strength) and the cardiovascular characteristics (e.g., heart rate variability) influence the resulting BCG.

The BCG is usually present in all recorded EEG channels, albeit to a different extent; as a rule of thumb, EEG electrodes far from the EEG reference electrode express larger amplitudes, and a high field MRI scanner causes larger amplitudes than a scanner with lower field strength (Debener et al., 2008), as the BCG amplitude is proportional to the MRI scanner B_0 field strength (Tenforde et al., 1983). Note the general temporal pattern inherent in the BCG is synchronized to the cardiac cycle. This becomes apparent when comparing the EEG traces with the simultaneously recorded electrocardiogram (ECG) signal. Importantly, this comparison reveals a delay of approximately 200 ms between the ECG R peak and the peak amplitude of the BCG in the EEG traces (Allen et al., 1998). Due to its close relationship to the cardiac cycle, however, fluctuations in the subject's heart rate (and likely in other cardiovascular parameters) result in fluctuations in the BCG. Also, BCG peak latencies and BCG morphologies can be different across channels, suggesting a complex spatiotemporal activity pattern that the BCG contributes to the EEG.

The BCG represents a rather complicated, dynamic contribution to the EEG and therefore requires attention when BCG removal procedures are developed, applied, and compared. The spatial complexity of the BCG has only recently

(Nakamura, et al., 2006) been investigated in more detail. A spatial analysis may help to characterize important properties of the BCG with possible implications for its reduction or removal (Debener et al., 2008). Figure 2.3.4 illustrates the main spatial features of the BCG, showing the time-domain averaged signal. The upper traces in the figure show the evoked BCG activity at all EEG electrodes together with the mean global field power (GFP). It can be seen that the BCG starts approximately 150 ms after the ECG Q peak and is characterized by two main power maxima at approximately 230 and 330 ms. Also, the BCG lasts at least until approximately 500 ms after the ECG Q peak. Corresponding voltage maps at selected GFP peak latencies reveal several interesting features: First, in most cases the BCG topography can be characterized by a low spatial frequency, meaning that most electrodes contribute to generally smooth topographies. Therefore, the BCG can best be studied based on adequate spatial coverage of the head sphere. Second, as noted above, these topographies change substantially over time. At first glance, it appears that several topographies recur at later latencies (for example, compare maps at 176 and 464 ms in Figure 2.3.2). However, closer inspection reveals that these maps appear slightly rotated to each other. This rotational aspect demonstrates that the BCG does not simply contribute a single topography. Rather, it appears that the BCG represents very dynamic (moving, rotating, and polarity-inverting) activity.

The lower part of Figure 2.3.4 shows all single ECG trials, along with the averaged ECG. Note that the ECG morphology is also compromised by the magnetic field influence. Bear in mind that this illustrates a single subject, based on 30-channel EEG recordings obtained in a 1.5 Tesla MRI scanner. The illustrated BCG features appear to be similar across subjects and MRI scanners. However, some important differences can be expected as well. First of all, because the BCG scales approximately in proportion to the MRI B_0 field (Tenforde et al., 1983), the BCG is much smaller in amplitude at 1.5 Tesla compared to 3 or 7 Tesla recordings, which has consequences for the choice of the BCG removal technique (Debener et al., 2008). Second, individuals differ in fluctuations of cardiac activity, such as heart rate changes. Therefore, for those individuals with a higher heart rate, the BCG activities between adjacent cardiac cycles may overlap to some extent, which could further complicate BCG removal issues (Vincent et al., 2007). The peak latencies (and the exact morphologies) shown in Figure 2.3.2 will differ between subjects (Allen et al., 1998). The features discussed above seem to be fairly consistent across subjects and scanner sites. Among them is the ~200 ms delay as well as the general topography, with its dynamic, rotational, and polarity-inverting aspects. In fact, it was consistently found that the moving topographical BCG pattern is irrespective of the number of EEG channels (30 to 62), the MRI scanner manufacturer (Siemens, Philips), the MRI scanner type (head scanner, whole body scanner), or the MRI B_0 field strength (1.5, 3, and 7 Tesla).

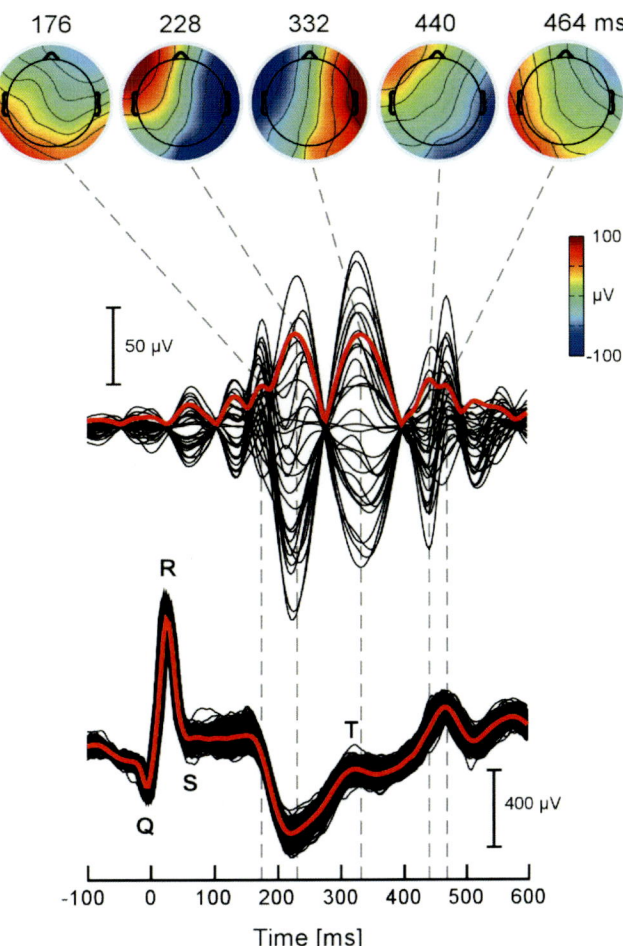

Figure 2.3.4. Temporal characteristics of the BCG, based on a typical 30-channel EEG recording in a 1.5 Tesla MRI scanner. The upper traces show the evoked BCG at all EEG channels. Overlayed in red is the mean global field power (GFP), which corresponds to the spatial standard deviation. Voltage maps are shown for selected GFP peak latencies. Note that while some maps (176 and 464 ms; 228 and 440 ms) look similar, they are differently rotated, illustrating the temporal dynamics and spatial nonstationarity of the BCG. The BCG also compromises the ECG, which is shown in the bottom part of the figure (see legend of Figure 2.3.1 for ECG recording details). Here, black traces refer to all recorded single cardiac cycles, with the Q peak used as the time-locking event and the red trace representing the average ECG. Waveform T of the cardiac cycle can be identified at about 300 ms, on top of the approximately 150 to 450 ms BCG-caused deflection. The polarity of the BCG-deflection in the ECG trace depends on the orientation of the MRI B_0 field, thus can be different at different MRI scanner sites.

Challenges in BCG Removal

Allen and colleagues introduced the average artifact subtraction (AAS) approach (Allen et al., 1998), which has been among the most influential and frequently used methods for BCG removal. While different implementations and developments of the AAS exist (Laufs et al., 2008), the basic principle of the AAS is common to all variants.

Figure 2.3.5 illustrates and highlights several features of the AAS. First, the AAS approach requires estimates of the onset of each cardiac-cycle from the concurrently recorded ECG. The next step is then to define an artifact template; this is done with a moving average procedure for each EEG channel separately through averaging the EEG time-locked to each cardiac cycle onset. The resulting average represents the evoked BCG, and this template can then be subtracted from each EEG epoch, thus removing the major fraction of the BCG. This procedure often yields satisfactory EEG data quality (e.g., Sammer et al., 2005; Hamandi et al., 2008). Another strength of the AAS is the straightforward possibility for a real-time implementation that then affords an online evaluation of the EEG.

However, experience with the AAS has led to the identification of several potential pitfalls, and has motivated the further development of the original approach. For example, the ECG channel itself is also contaminated with gradient and BCG artifact contributions, making it sometimes hard to identify the onset of each heartbeat cycle in the ECG. As a result, automatic R-peak detection algorithms that work on

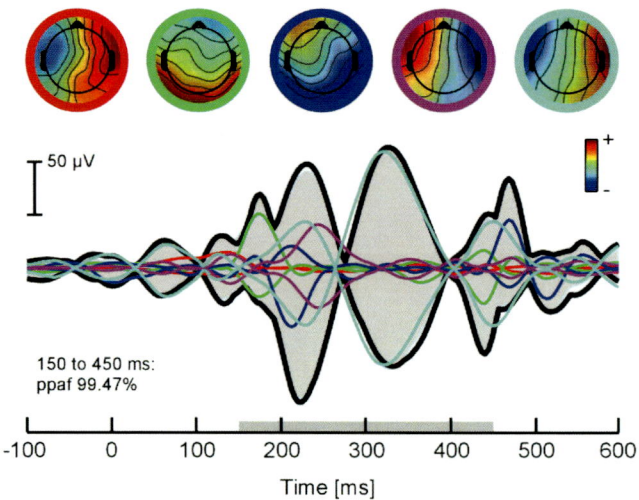

Figure 2.3.5. Typical example of the use of ICA for removing the BCG. Using the EEGLAB function *envtopo*, those independent components explaining most of the variance of an evoked signal in a specified time range (here 150 to 450 ms) can be identified. In this case, five components were selected and accounted for > 99% of the variance of the evoked signal. Shown is the envelope of the sensor data (black), which reflects the minima and maxima across all channels, and the envelope of the joint back-projection of the five independent components shown above (grey shaded area). For each component, the map (i.e., inverse weights) and the envelope of the back-projection (colored traces) is shown. ppaf = percentage of power accounted for.

artifact-free ECG recordings sometimes fail on inside scanner recordings and result in an inaccurate positioning of the event markers (Debener et al., 2008). Some software packages such as BrainVision Analyzer (Brain Products GmbH, Munich, Germany) already take jitter information into account, and automatically align markers statistically such that the overall jitter is minimized before the AAS correction is performed. A second main problem of this approach is the assumption of similarity between adjacent BCG occurrences. That is, within the chosen moving average window size, it is assumed that the BCG contribution to the EEG channel artifact is very similar at adjacent cardiac cycles and changes only slowly over time. This assumption may not always be correct. Shortening the moving average window size can not fully address this problem (as a smaller moving average window would leave more residual EEG activity in the template). Several groups have suggested alternative template constructions that are based on weighted averages (Goldman et al., 2000) or median instead of mean values (Sijbers et al., 2000). Also, some implementations allow for the selection of trials contributing to the template generation to depend on whether they correlate sufficiently with other trials or not. This option helps to ensure that trials containing other EEG artifacts are excluded, thus improving the quality of the final template being used. While all these features may improve the BCG correction quality, they do not fully address the basic problem, as they still rest on the assumption of local BCG similarity, and assume that one template is sufficient for each BCG epoch.

These latter problems have been addressed by Niazy and colleagues (Niazy et al., 2005), and similarly by Negishi et al.

(2004), who proposed a new way of constructing a BCG template. These authors suggested generating BCG templates based on a channel-wise temporal principal components analysis (PCA), thereby not assuming any local BCG similarity. Niazy and colleagues named this approach the optimal basis set (OBS) method, which refers to the view that the first few principal components represent several distinct BCG templates and at the same time explain most of the BCG variance in any given EEG channel. These templates are jointly used to regress out the BCG from the EEG data. The OBS approach does not assume that adjacent BCGs are more similar than more distant ones, and accounts for the possibility of different artifact shapes. It has received considerable attention, and indeed several groups have used it successfully. This tool is a freely available Matlab plug-in that interacts with the open-source EEGLAB environment (Delorme and Makeig, 2004). However, the number of principal components used as BCG templates in the OBS approach has to be chosen by the user, such that bias and over- and under-fitting become relevant issues.

A further problem that is common to all channel-by-channel template subtraction approaches is the choice of template length. With a constantly changing interbeat (R-R) interval, the length of the template may also need some adjustment over time. A template covering an inappropriately short or long interval may either leave residual activity in, or add spurious activity to, the EEG traces. Indeed, because the interbeat interval changes over time (e.g., due to respiratory arrhythmia), an AAS template that may be of appropriate length for some cardiac cycles may not be adequate for other cycles. This has led to the introduction of alternative template generation schemes that either scale the BCG template with a percentage of the mean R-R period in the moving average window (Ellingson et al., 2004) or that build a template that incorporates the BCG data for all R-R period lengths present in the current moving average window (BrainVision Analyzer software). In the latter case, this template is then adaptively applied to each heartbeat based on its R-R period, thus ensuring that no portion of the BCG artifact remains uncorrected due to a suboptimal template length.

Other channel-by-channel correction approaches exist that account for the template duration problem. Bonmassar and colleagues for instance utilized an adaptive Kalman filter approach (Bonmassar et al., 2002), but this requires an extra motion sensor signal to be recorded as a reference signal and, while producing good corrections, appears to be computationally demanding. Other methods such as the wavelet-based non-linear reduction of the BCG (Wan et al., 2006) are also computationally demanding and therefore unlikely to replace the AAS in the near future. Recently, Vincent and colleagues (2007) proposed a moving general linear model approach (mGLM). These authors point to a potentially important problem of the AAS and related BCG temporal template correction approaches: they fail to account for BCG artifacts that last longer than a cardiac cycle. It remains to be determined whether this is indeed a significant problem, and whether the mGLM approach provides a substantial improvement over the AAS.

Removing the BCG Using Spatial Pattern Removal Approaches

The BCG can also be characterized by a number of prototypical topographies. The potential virtue of spatial approaches, aiming at removing those topographies, is that exact knowledge about the onset of each cardiac cycle is not necessarily required. In principle, a spatial approach can avoid problems that are inherent in AAS and OBS as discussed above.

Motivated by the success of spatial approaches for the removal of ocular artifacts, two spatial BCG correction approaches have been proposed (Bénar et al., 2003): principal components analysis (PCA) and independent component analysis (ICA). The assumption behind these is that the BCG contribution is statistically independent of, or in the case of PCA uncorrelated to, ongoing EEG activity. Therefore, BCG activity can be expected to be identified by few components, whereas all other EEG activity should be represented by other components. In the original work by Bénar and colleagues, BCG components were visually identified by exploring the similarity of all component time courses to the simultaneously recorded ECG signal (Bénar et al., 2003). Back-projection of all but the identified components then reduced the BCG in the EEG recordings. Bénar and colleagues found both ICA and PCA well suited for this

task, as they eliminated BCG activity while preserving the relative amplitude of epileptic spikes.

However, an obvious problem of this approach is selection of components based of subjective criteria. Indeed, it can be rather difficult to visually identify and select the components representing BCG activity beyond the first few strongest and most obvious. Therefore, other methods of BCG component identification have been proposed. Srivastava and colleagues (2005), for instance, proposed the identification-by-correlation approach, by which all ICA time courses are correlated with the simultaneously recorded ECG channel and those components expressing the highest correlations with the ECG are identified as BCG-components. Alternatively, BCG-related components can be identified by the amount of variance they contributed to the evoked BCG. When compared to the identification-by-correlation criterion, this latter approach gives better results (Debener et al., 2008).

Several groups have reported success in using ICA for BCG removal (Bénar et al., 2003; Eichele et al., 2005; Briselli et al., 2006; Nakamura et al., 2006; Mantini et al., 2007) in 1.5 T MRI scanners, while the experiences in a 3 Tesla MRI scanner were much less positive (Debener et al., 2007). Note that a model assumption of temporal ICA is that the sources contributing to the linearly mixed signals are spatially *stationary*. In a recent study, the properties of the BCG artifact and the performance of ICA at 1.5, 3 and 7 Tesla were compared. Compared to ICA decompositions based on outside MRI scanner data, it was found that the ICA results obtained from 1.5 Tesla recordings were only moderately affected in their quality. At 3 and 7 Tesla, however, the typical topographies could hardly be recovered anymore. While it appears that ICA is robust to violation of the stationarity assumption at lower field strength, it is more sensitive and requires more components to model the convolutive (moving, rotating) properties of the BCG artifact at higher field strengths.

Currently, the available evidence suggests that the spatial filtering approaches such as ICA and PCA are not as efficient as template methods and in particular at fields of 3 Tesla and higher. Nevertheless, as will be pointed out in the next section, the application of ICA *in combination* with other approaches such as AAS or OBS seems very attractive, as it provides several advantages that may otherwise be impossible to achieve, and does so even at higher field strengths (Debener et al., 2006).

Combining and Comparing Different BCG Removal Approaches

It appears that no single method exists that performs optimally under all circumstances, and many authors consider the combination of different BCG removal algorithms a very attractive option. Kim and colleagues, for instance, combined a wavelet-based denoising approach with recursive adaptive filtering as post-processing only in the case that AAS gave not satisfactory results (Kim et al., 2004). Likewise, the FMRIB plug-in developed by Niazy et al. (2005) offers application of adaptive noise cancellation following OBS to increase performance. Also, BrainVision Analyzer provides flexibility in combining different methods, such as optimized AAS and subsequent ICA with automatic determination of the BCG components to remove.

In the study mentioned above (Debener et al., 2007), three different BCG removal approaches were compared, namely ICA with the identification-by-correlation approach (Srivastava et al., 2005), OBS (Niazy et al., 2005), and a combination of both, where ICA was applied *after* BCG removal with OBS (Debener et al., 2005b). It was found that ICA, when used on its own, while reducing the BCG substantially, also reduced the SNR of ERPs, suggesting that artifact and signal could not be well disentangled by ICA. However, when used after OBS, which, as expected, reduced the BCG and improved the ERP SNR, infomax ICA could further improve the ERP SNR and the ERP topography. This pattern of finding suggests that ICA, *after* most of the BCG is removed with a channel-wise procedure such as AAS of OBS, is able to deal with residual artifact, which is well in line with the earlier argument. Moreover, in this combination, the other advantages of ICA can be utilized, that is, the removal of further EEG artifacts such as eye blinks, and the separation of brain-related signals from each other (Debener et al., 2005a; Debener et al., 2005b; Debener et al., 2006). It is important to note that not only the amount of BCG artifact removed should be considered. Analyzing whether the BCG is reduced or not does not make it possible to determine whether the separation from ongoing (or event-related) EEG activity was successful. It is therefore a better strategy to always analyze the data with regard to the amount of BCG correction *and* with regard to one or more measures of the quality of the EEG variable of interest. When the focus is on event-related potentials (ERPs) consider the signal-to-noise ratio (SNR) of the ERP component of interest. The topographical quality of the resulting ERPs could be quantified if a reference topography is available, or if information about the source configuration of the ERP component of interest exists (Debener et al., 2007). Also, measures of the recovery of the EEG spectrum can be included, in particular if the EEG variable of interest is in the frequency or time-frequency domain (Allen et al., 1998).

Conclusion

This chapter describes the different types of artifacts caused by the static and changing magnetic fields of the MR and the possibilities of their removal. The GA, due to its large amplitudes, is quite dominant on first sight but it has been shown to be more easily controllable than the the cardiac-related artifacts. This is mainly due to the fact that the GA is caused by an external source that is reliable in its temporal properties. Template-based correction methods have been shown to be most successful and convenient as a first step of GA

removal. Modifications for dealing with motion-induced alteration of the geometry of the electrodes and cables were discussed. We believe that future work should focus on how to avoid or attenuate MR-related imaging artifacts altogether, or at least reduce the heterogeneity of the GA in order to further increase signal quality. Dedicated fMRI sequences should be designed that are tuned for EEG-fMRI recordings as it was pioneered by Anami and colleagues (2003). Recently developed "silent" fMRI sequences (Schmitter et al., 2008) could be advantageous because acoustic resonance peaks of the MR system during the gradient switching process are avoided. Consequently this would result in less vibration-induced motion of the EEG electrodes and cables.

Removal of cardiac-related artifacts remains challenging since their origins are partly physiologically caused. As the fMRI community moves on to larger field strengths to increase sensitivity, and the pulse artifacts scale with it, the issues of removing cardiac-related artifacts become even more challenging. It was shown that different methods and especially their combination have to be adapted to the given situation.

Improved artifact correction techniques may result from a better understanding of the mechanisms that give rise to the MR induced artifacts (Yan et al., 2009). In other words, a better knowledge about the different mechanisms causing GA and BCG should help to optimize recording conditions as well as offline data correction approaches, and thus contribute to a better EEG signal quality. Given the promises of simultaneous EEG-fMRI (e.g., Debener et al., 2006), this seems a worthwhile goal.

REFERENCES

Allen PJ, Polizzi G, Krakow K, Fish DR, Lemieux L (1998) Identification of EEG events in the MR scanner: the problem of pulse artifact and a method for its subtraction. Neuroimage 8:229–239.

Allen PJ, Josephs O, Turner R (2000) A method for removing imaging artifact from continuous EEG recorded during functional MRI. Neuroimage 12:230–239.

Anami K, Saitoh O, Yumoto M (2002) Reduction of ballistocardiogramwith a vacuum head-fixating system during simultaneous fMRI and multi-channel monopolar EEG recording. Recent Adv Hum Brain Mapp 1232:427–431.

Anami K, Mori T, Tanaka F, Kawagoe Y, Okamoto J, Yarita M, Ohnishi T, Yumoto M, Matsuda H, Saitoh O (2003) Stepping stone sampling for retrieving artifact-free electroencephalogram during functional magnetic resonance imaging. Neuroimage 19:281–295.

Becker R, Ritter P, Moosmann M, Villringer A (2005) Visual evoked potentials recovered from fMRI scan periods. Hum Brain Mapp 26:221–230.

Bénar C, Aghakhani Y, Wang Y, Izenberg A, Al-Asmi A, Dubeau F, Gotman J (2003) Quality of EEG in simultaneous EEG-fMRI for epilepsy. Clin Neurophysiol 114:569–580.

Bledowski C, Linden DE, Wibral M (2007) Combining electrophysiology and functional imaging: different methods for different questions. Trends Cogn Sci 11:500–502.

Bonmassar G, Purdon PL, Jaaskelainen IP, Chiappa K, Solo V, Brown EN, Belliveau JW (2002) Motion and ballistocardio-gram artifact removal for interleaved recording of EEG and EPs during MRI. Neuroimage 16:1127–1141.

Briselli E, Garreffa G, Bianchi L, Bianciardi M, Macaluso E, Abbafati M, Grazia Marciani M, Maraviglia B (2006) An independent component analysis-based approach on ballistocardiogram artifact removing. Magn Reson Imaging 24:393–400.

Brookes MJ, Mullinger KJ, Stevenson CM, Morris PG, Bowtell R (2008) Simultaneous EEG source localisation and artifact rejection during concurrent fMRI by means of spatial filtering. Neuroimage 40:1090–1104.

Debener S, Makeig S, Delorme A, Engel AK (2005a) What is novel in the novelty oddball paradigm? Functional significance of the novelty P3 event-related potential as revealed by independent component analysis. Brain Res Cogn Brain Res 22:309–321.

Debener S, Ullsperger M, Siegel M, Fiehler K, von Cramon DY, Engel AK (2005b) Trial-by-trial coupling of concurrent electroencephalogram and functional magnetic resonance imaging identifies the dynamics of performance monitoring. J Neurosci 25:11730–11737.

Debener S, Ullsperger M, Siegel M, Engel AK (2006) Single-trial EEG-fMRI reveals the dynamics of cognitive function. Trends Cogn Sci 10:558–563.

Debener S, Strobel A, Sorger B, Peters J, Kranczioch C, Engel AK, Goebel R (2007) Improved quality of auditory event-related potentials recorded simultaneously with 3-T fMRI: removal of the ballistocardiogram artefact. Neuroimage 34:587–597.

Debener S, Mullinger KJ, Niazy RK, Bowtell RW (2008) Properties of the ballistocardiogram artefact as revealed by EEG recordings at 1.5, 3 and 7 T static magnetic field strength. Int J Psychophysiol 67:189–199.

Delorme A, Makeig S (2004) EEGLAB: an open source toolbox for analysis of single-trial EEG dynamics including independent component analysis. J Neurosci Methods 134:9–21.

Eichele T, Specht K, Moosmann M, Jongsma ML, Quiroga RQ, Nordby H, Hugdahl K (2005) Assessing the spatiotemporal evolution of neuronal activation with single-trial event-related potentials and functional MRI. Proc Natl Acad Sci U S A 102:17798–17803.

Ellingson ML, Liebenthal E, Spanaki MV, Prieto TE, Binder JR, Ropella KM (2004) Ballistocardiogram artifact reduction in the simultaneous acquisition of auditory ERPS and fMRI. Neuroimage 22:1534–1542.

Friston KJ, Williams S, Howard R, Frackowiak RS, Turner R (1996) Movement-related effects in fMRI time-series. Magn Reson Med 35:346–355.

Goldman RI, Stern JM, Engel J, Jr., Cohen MS (2000) Acquiring simultaneous EEG and functional MRI. Clin Neurophysiol 111:1974–1980.

Goncalves SI, Pouwels PJ, Kuijer JP, Heethaar RM, de Munck JC (2007) Artifact removal in co-registered EEG/fMRI by selective average subtraction. Clin Neurophysiol 118:2437–2450.

Hamandi K, Laufs H, Noth U, Carmichael DW, Duncan JS, Lemieux L (2008) BOLD and perfusion changes during epileptic generalised spike wave activity. Neuroimage 39:608–618.

Hoffmann A, Jager L, Werhahn KJ, Jaschke M, Noachtar S, Reiser M (2000) Electroencephalography during functional echo-planar imaging: detection of epileptic spikes using post-processing methods. Magn Reson Med 44:791–798.

Huang-Hellinger FR, Breiter HC, McCormack GM, Cohen MS, Kwong KK, Savoy RL, Weisskoff RM, Davis TL, Baker JR, Belliveau JW, Rosen BR (1995) Simultaneous functional magnetic resonance imaging and electrophysiological recording. Hum Brain Mapp 3:13–23.

Kim KH, Yoon HW, Park HW (2004) Improved ballistocardiac artifact removal from the electroencephalogram recorded in fMRI. J Neurosci Methods 135:193–203.

Laufs H, Daunizeau J, Carmichael DW, Kleinschmidt A (2008) Recent advances in recording electrophysiological data simultaneously with magnetic resonance imaging. Neuroimage 40:515–528.

Mandelkow H, Halder P, Boesiger P, Brandeis D (2006) Synchronization facilitates removal of MRI artefacts from concurrent EEG recordings and increases usable bandwidth. Neuroimage 32:1120–1126.

Mantini D, Perrucci MG, Cugini S, Ferretti A, Romani GL, Del Gratta C (2007) Complete artifact removal for EEG recorded during continuous fMRI using independent component analysis. Neuroimage 34:598–607.

Masterton RA, Abbott DF, Fleming SW, Jackson GD (2007) Measurement and reduction of motion and ballistocardiogram artefacts from simultaneous EEG and fMRI recordings. Neuroimage 37:202–211.

Moosmann M, Schonfelder VH, Specht K, Scheeringa R, Nordby H, Hugdahl K (2009) Realignment parameter-informed artefact correction for simultaneous EEG-fMRI recordings. Neuroimage 45:1144–1150.

Mullinger KJ, Morgan PS, Bowtell RW (2008) Improved artifact correction for combined electroencephalography/functional MRI by means of synchronization and use of vectorcardiogram recordings. J Magn Reson Imaging 27:607–616.

Nakamura W, Anami K, Mori T, Saitoh O, Cichocki A, Amari S (2006) Removal of ballistocardiogram artifacts from simultaneously recorded EEG and fMRI data using independent component analysis. IEEE Trans Biomed Eng 53:1294–1308.

Negishi M, Abildgaard M, Nixon T, Constable RT (2004) Removal of time-varying gradient artifacts from EEG data acquired during continuous fMRI. Clin Neurophysiol 115:2181–2192.

Niazy RK, Beckmann CF, Iannetti GD, Brady JM, Smith SM (2005) Removal of FMRI environment artifacts from EEG data using optimal basis sets. Neuroimage 28:720–737.

Sammer G, Blecker C, Gebhardt H, Kirsch P, Stark R, Vaitl D (2005) Acquisition of typical EEG waveforms during fMRI: SSVEP, LRP, and frontal theta. Neuroimage 24:1012–1024.

Schmitter S, Diesch E, Amann M, Kroll A, Moayer M, Schad LR (2008) Silent echo-planar imaging for auditory FMRI. Magma 21:317–325.

Sijbers J, Michiels I, Verhoye M, Van Audekerke J, Van der LA, Van Dyck D (1999) Restoration of MR-induced artifacts in simultaneously recorded MR/EEG data. Magn Reson Imaging 17:1383–1391.

Sijbers J, Van Audekerke J, Verhoye M, Van der Linden A, Van Dyck D (2000) Reduction of ECG and gradient related artifacts in simultaneously recorded human EEG/MRI data. Magn Reson Imaging 18:881–886.

Srivastava G, Crottaz-Herbette S, Lau KM, Glover GH, Menon V (2005) ICA-based procedures for removing ballistocardiogram artifacts from EEG data acquired in the MRI scanner. Neuroimage 24:50–60.

Sun L, Hinrichs H (2009) Simultaneously recorded EEG-fMRI: Removal of gradient artifacts by subtraction of head movement related average artifact waveforms. Hum Brain Mapp Apr 13 [Epub ahead of print].

Tenforde TS, Gaffey CT, Moyer BR, Budinger TF (1983) Cardiovascular alterations in Macaca monkeys exposed to stationary magnetic fields: experimental observations and theoretical analysis. Bioelectromagnetics 4:1–9.

Vincent JL, Larson-Prior LJ, Zempel JM, Snyder AZ (2007) Moving GLM ballistocardiogram artifact reduction for EEG acquired simultaneously with fMRI. Clin Neurophysiol 118:981–998.

Wan X, Iwata K, Riera J, Ozaki T, Kitamura M, Kawashima R (2006) Artifact reduction for EEG/fMRI recording: nonlinear reduction of ballistocardiogram artifacts. Clin Neurophysiol 117:668–680.

Yan WX, Mullinger KJ, Brookes MJ, Bowtell R (2009) Understanding gradient artefacts in simultaneous EEG/fMRI. Neuroimage 46:459–471.

2.4 Karen Mullinger and Richard Bowtell

Influence of EEG Equipment on MR Image Quality

Introduction

The effects of concurrent MRI on the quality of EEG recordings, which have been discussed in previous chapters, are immediately apparent in the raw EEG data and extremely detrimental to the data quality if not corrected. However, the effects of the EEG equipment on the MRI data quality are more subtle and it has thus proved possible to acquire fMRI data in the presence of EEG equipment without making significant modifications to MRI techniques or hardware. The subtleness of these effects has meant that only a limited number of groups have investigated the extent of MR image degradation due to the presence of EEG equipment. However, as simultaneous EEG and fMRI is applied across more areas of research and at higher field strengths, it is becoming ever more important to understand fully the effect that the combined approach has on the quality of the data acquired using both modalities.

To understand the effects of the EEG cap on data collected in fMRI experiments it is necessary to explore the physical mechanisms underlying the collection of MR data and how these are affected by the presence of EEG equipment. Although there are a number of sources of image degradation, the most important ones to consider are: *(1)* magnetic susceptibility effects, and *(2)* the perturbation of the RF fields involved in excitation and detection of the MR signal.

In this chapter, we first focus on the detrimental effect of main magnetic field inhomogeneity in MRI, focusing on the particular effects of the differences in magnetic susceptibility between the materials used in EEG recording (electrodes and leads) and the human head. We then continue by considering the importance of a uniform RF field in MRI and analyzing how the presence of an EEG cap may affect the homogeneity of this field, thus reducing image quality. The ways in which these phenomena affect the signal-to-noise ratio (SNR) and cause local signal loss in EPI data collected

for fMRI experiments are then discussed. The safety aspect of simultaneous EEG-fMRI, which is an extremely important consideration, is then explored. Guidance is given relating to how to test the safety of an experimental set-up and the importance of testing each new EEG recording arrangement in the scanner is emphasized. Finally we suggest some methods that may be used to overcome the problems of reduced MR image quality, which can be encountered when performing simultaneous EEG and fMRI.

Magnetic Susceptibility Effects (B_0-Inhomogeneity)

Introduction to B_0-Inhomogeneity

The process of MR imaging relies on the presence of a homogeneous static magnetic field, B_0. Hydrogen nuclei align with this magnetic field, producing a net nuclear magnetization, which precesses about the axis of the B_0-field when perturbed from alignment with this field. Differences in the magnitude of the static magnetic field cause the frequency of precession, ω, (known as the Larmor frequency) to vary. Varying the magnitude of the static magnetic field in a controlled manner using magnetic field gradients enables spatial encoding of the MR signals, which forms the basis of magnetic resonance imaging (for further details of the principles of MRI please refer to Morris, 1990; Hashemi et al., 2004).

All materials have a magnetic susceptibility, χ. This is a measure of how readily a material develops a magnetic moment when exposed to an external magnetic field (Levitt, 2005). The value of χ can be either positive or negative. Materials with $\chi > 0$ are said to be paramagnetic, while those with $\chi < 0$ are known as diamagnetic materials. In most paramagnetic and diamagnetic materials the magnetic moment induced in an applied field is relatively small, so that the magnetic field perturbation produced by the material is much smaller than the applied field. Ferromagnetic materials on the other hand can have a very large magnetic moment, which may persist in the absence of an applied field. The strong forces that such materials experience in spatially varying magnetic fields mean that ferromagnetic objects must be excluded from the environment of an MR scanner: if brought into proximity with the magnet such objects are dragged into the bore of the magnet, usually becoming a dangerous projectile in the process (Shellock, 2004). Paramagnetic and diamagnetic materials can be brought inside the bore of an MR scanner, but differences in the magnetic susceptibility of these materials generate spatially varying magnetic fields, which can cause image degradation, as we shall now explore.

The EEG cap causes unwanted magnetic field inhomogeneity if the wires, electrodes, or conductive gel have a significantly different magnetic susceptibility from the tissues of the head. Although the differences in magnetic susceptibility are likely to be small ($\chi \approx 0$ for air, $\chi = -9 \times 10^{-6}$ for water, and $\chi = -9.2 \times 10^{-6}$ for copper), the resulting field deviation can cause a significant variation in the NMR resonance frequency, ω. This is because

$$B = (1 + \chi)\mu_0 H \qquad (1)$$

(where H is the magnetic field intensity, produced by the large electric current flowing in the main magnet, and B is the magnetic flux density), and:

$$\omega = \gamma B \qquad (2)$$

where γ is the magnetogyric ratio, which is equal to 42.58 MHz/T for ^{1}H nuclei. The large value of γ means that a small change in the local magnetic field due to a change in magnetic susceptibility can lead to a significant variation in ω. Consequently the presence of the EEG electrodes and leads can introduce artifacts in MR images due to the magnetic field inhomogeneity (Schomer et al., 2000; Bonmassar et al., 2001; Iannetti et al., 2005; Stevens et al., 2007a; Mullinger et al., 2008a). These artifacts take two main forms. First, field inhomogeneities may cause image distortion. If we take the average field offset due to the changes in χ to be ΔB_0, and the range of fields produced across the slice that is being imaged to be δB_0, then

$$\Delta\omega_0 = \gamma\Delta B_0 \qquad (3a)$$

$$\delta\omega_0 = \gamma\delta B_0 \qquad (3b)$$

where $\Delta\omega_0$ is the average frequency offset and $\delta\omega_0$ is the frequency range across the slice. If $\Delta\omega_0/2\pi$ is similar in magnitude or greater than the frequency separation of pixels (typically 10–50 Hz in echo planar images), distortion of the image will occur. This is a consequence of the fact that in the process of image reconstruction all frequency variation is assumed to result from the effect of the applied magnetic field gradients, which impose a linear variation of field with spatial coordinate. Any additional field offset, due for example to magnetic susceptibility effects,

therefore translates into a spatial misregistration of signal contributions.

The other effect that may occur as a result of field inhomogeneity is local signal loss, often known in this context as signal drop-out. If the variation in frequency across the imaging slice is large, the signal in gradient echo images is reduced as the spins at different locations across the slice precess at different rates and consequently get out of phase with one another during the echo time, TE. Significant dephasing and consequent signal loss occurs in gradient echo images if the product of $\delta\omega_0$ and TE approaches 2π in magnitude. The extent of signal drop-out and image distortion resulting from magnetic susceptibility effects depends on how greatly the magnetic susceptibilities of the materials used differ, and on the spatial arrangements of electrodes and leads with respect to the subject's head and applied field, since these factors control the strength and spatial form of the magnetic field inhomogeneity that is produced.

Signal Loss due to Magnetic Susceptibility Effects of EEG Caps

Signal loss has been observed by a number of groups when imaging phantoms in the presence of EEG electrodes and leads (Krakow et al., 2000; Bonmassar et al., 2001; Iannetti et al., 2005; Stevens et al., 2007a; Mullinger et al., 2008a; Negishi et al., 2008). These reductions in signal are generally localized to the sites of electrodes and only penetrate on average distances of the order of 10 mm into the phantom. Therefore given the average scalp-brain distance is 13.8 mm (Krakow et al., 2000) the signal loss is not often observed within the brain. However, investigations by Krakow et al. (2000) demonstrate that if injudiciously chosen components are used in the cap then the depth to which significant signal loss occurs can be much greater than this (19 mm for a carbon composition resistor).

Mapping B_0 Inhomogeneity

Signal loss observed in gradient echo EPI data or in other T_2^*-weighted images may be a consequence of the susceptibility effects discussed above or due to interactions of the EEG cap with the RF field, which will be explored later in this chapter. Directly mapping the perturbation of the B_0-field (Ericsson et al., 1995) due to the EEG recording system is therefore valuable since it allows differentiation of the effects of B_0 and RF inhomogeneity and consequently provides a greater awareness of the exact interactions between the EEG and MRI hardware. A clearer understanding of the source of any artifacts also means that the correct methods can be used to overcome the image distortion and signal loss encountered when performing simultaneous EEG-fMRI. B_0-mapping conducted by Stevens et al. (2007a) demonstrated that the composition of the EEG electrodes has a strong effect on the magnitude

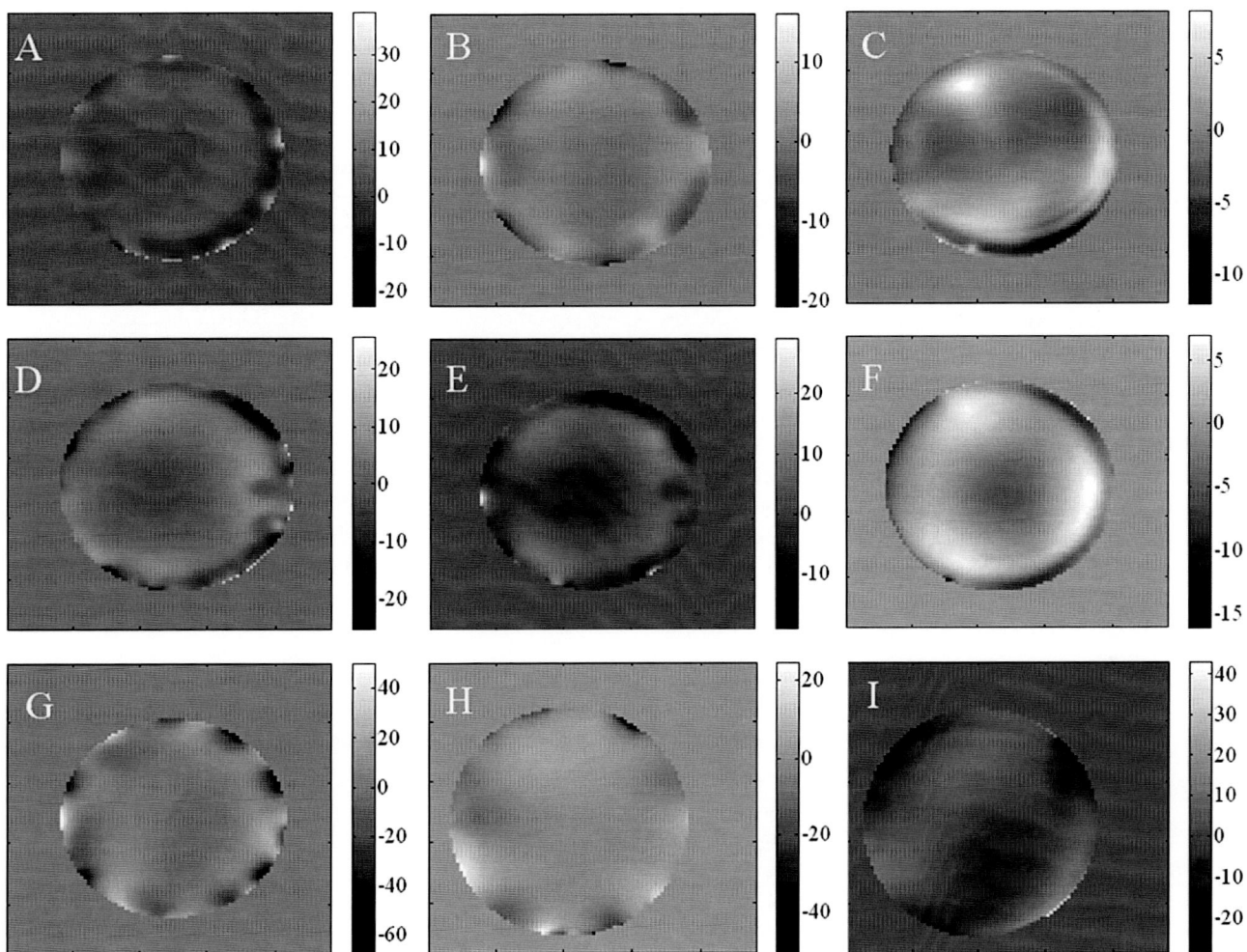

Figure 2.4.1. B_0 field maps (in Hz) acquired from the phantom, shown after removal of large-scale field variations at 1.5 T (A–C), 3 T (D–F) and 7 T (G–I) with the 64-electrode cap (left), 32-electrode cap (center), and no cap (right) on. From Mullinger et al. (2008a).

of the B_0-inhomogeneity. An electrode with a thin layer of ferromagnetic nickel plating was found to perturb the B_0-field 10 times more than electrodes made up entirely of diamagnetic materials. B_0-mapping in the presence of commercially available EEG caps carried out by Mullinger et al. (2008a) showed that caps carrying 32 and 64 electrodes cause similar perturbations of B_0. However, the greater number of electrodes in the 64-electrode cap meant that a greater proportion of the periphery is affected by this cap (Figure 2.4.1). This work also showed that the leads of the EEG system did not cause significant B_0 perturbations. These leads were composed of braided copper wire (3 mm in diameter). The extent of the perturbations from the electrodes became more pronounced with field strength as would be expected from Equations 1 and 2.

The presence of the cap was also shown to increase the width of the distribution of field values measured inside the phantom. At 3 T, 95 % of the measured field values lay within a range of 30 Hz in the presence of a 64 electrode cap, but this range was reduced to 16 Hz with no cap present. These values were however, recorded on a phantom and when similar measurements were performed on data acquired on a human head there was no discernable change in the distribution of field values between data collected in the presence of the cap and that collected with no cap. This is because in the head the magnetic field inhomogeneity resulting from the difference in magnetic susceptibility of brain tissue, bone, and air has the dominant effect on the field distribution. From Equations 1 and 3 one would expect the range of field offsets to scale in direct proportionality with B_0. However, it was found that width of the field distribution grew less rapidly with field than expected. This is probably due to the better field shimming systems that were available at 3 and 7 T compared to 1.5 T, which allowed improved correction of the B_0 inhomogeneities. With advances in shimming methodology (Koch et al., 2006) it may be possible to reduce further the B_0-inhomogeneity resulting from the presence of an EEG cap, thus improving MR image quality during simultaneous EEG-fMRI experiments.

Effect on EPI Data

The B_0 distortions observed in Figure 2.4.1 can be seen to manifest themselves as signal loss and distortion in the corresponding EPI data (Figure 2.4.2).

However such signal loss and distortion was not observed in echo planar images of the brain due to the limited extent of the field perturbations, which means that the effect of an electrode positioned on the scalp does not extend across the ~1 cm distance between scalp and brain. Work carried out by Mirsattari et al. (2004) clearly demonstrates the reason for the differences in signal loss in EPI data sets acquired on the phantom compared with those acquired on the head. Figure 2.4.3 shows how the susceptibility effects of the cap may influence the image quality of different types of MR image. The greatest signal loss is observed in the T_2^*-weighted image, with a negligible loss observed in the T_2- or diffusion-weighted images. This shows that the signal-loss is caused by dephasing of spins across the slice, since such dephasing does not occur when a spin-echo acquisition is used (as in the T_2- and diffusion-weighted data). However, the signal losses seen in the T_2^*-weighted image do not extend into the brain tissue. This shows why signal losses observed in phantoms are not normally seen in the brain in EPI data sets.

Conclusion: B_0-Inhomogeneity Effects

Given the experimental findings that have been summarized here, it is clear that B_0-inhomogeneities due to the EEG recording system do not cause significant distortions or signal loss in fMRI data sets. This is because manufacturers have carefully chosen the type and amount of materials used in electrodes and leads so as to produce minimal magnetic field inhomogneity. The residual effects that are observed are generally less than those caused by natural susceptibility variations in the human head: the most significant such effect is due to the tissue-air boundaries of the sinuses (Jezzard and Balaban, 1995). Therefore B_0-effects should not significantly compromise magnetic resonance image quality when simultaneous EEG-fMRI is performed.

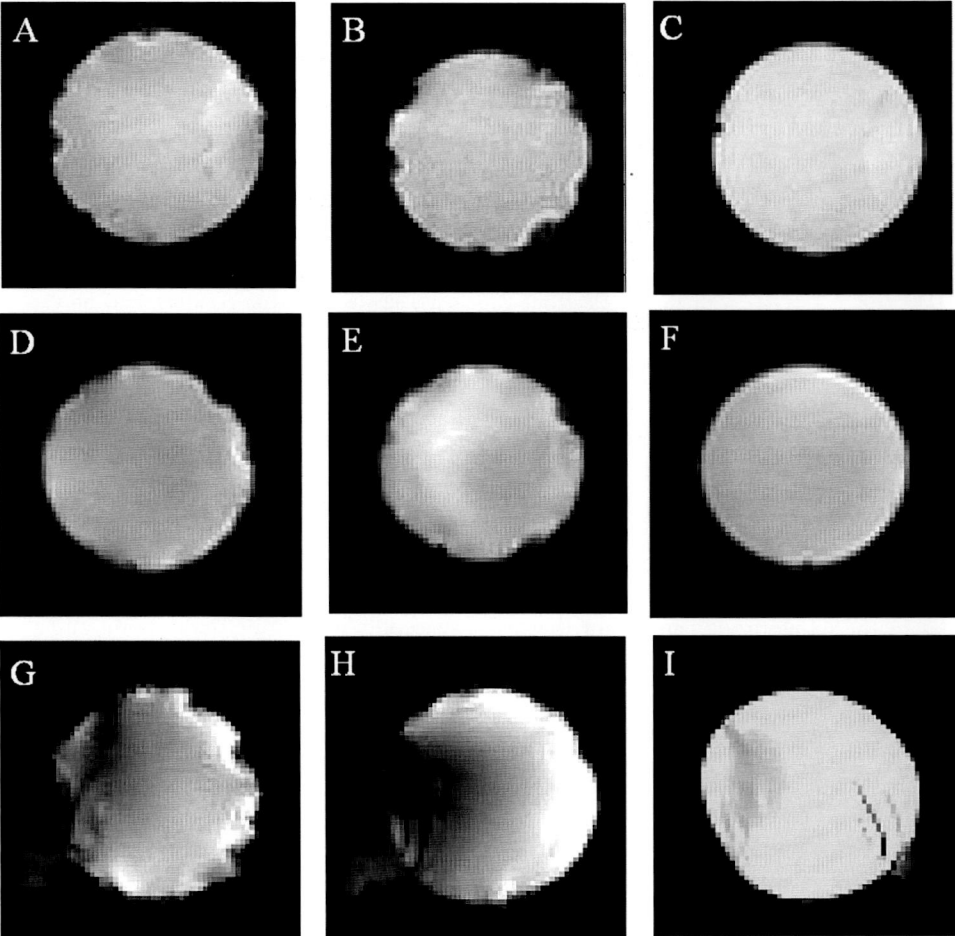

Figure 2.4.2. EPI data of a similar slice of the phantom at 1.5 T (A–C), 3 T (D–F) and 7 T (G–I) with 64-electrode cap (left), 32-electrode cap (center), and no cap on (right). From Mullinger et al. (2008a).

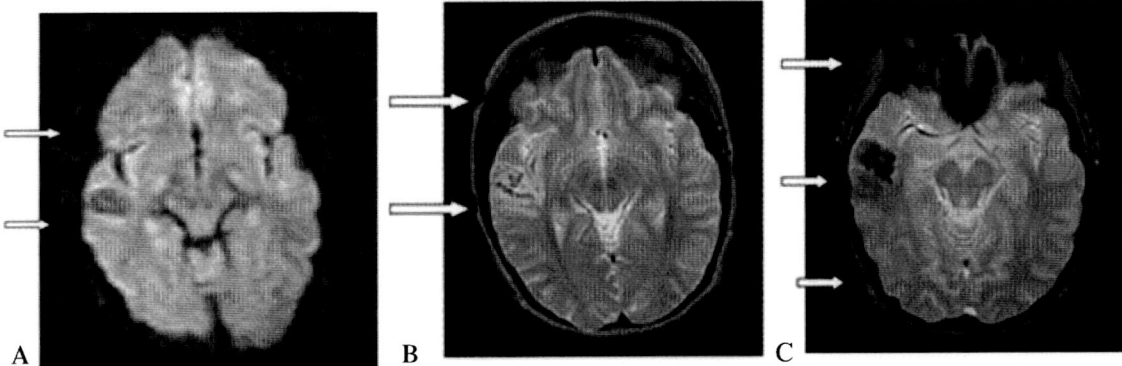

Figure 2.4.3. Cranial MRI with EEG electrodes on the scalp during various sequences: (A) Diffusion-weighted image (Trace image). (B) T2-weighted image (TR/TE 2200/80 ms, 5 mm slice thickness). (C) T2* gradient echo image (TR/TE 600/20 ms, flip angle 20 degrees, 5 mm slice). All images were acquired at 1.5 T. Arrows point to areas of signal loss on skin surface secondary to electrode contact. Adapted from Figure 4 of Mirsattari et al. (2004).

B_1-inhomogeneity

Introduction to RF Field Homogeneity

A magnetic field varying in time at the Larmor frequency, which lies in the radio-frequency (RF) region of the electromagnetic spectrum, is required in addition to the static B_0-field for the generation of MR images. This RF magnetic field (B_1-field) is used to excite the nuclear magnetization into precession. The precessing nuclear magnetization produces an RF signal, which is detected using a tuned radio frequency coil (for further details on MR image formation refer to Morris 1990; Hashemi et al., 2004).

Degradation of MR images due to RF interference caused by the presence of EEG hardware (Huang-Hellinger et al., 1995; Krakow et al., 2000) was reported in some of the first EEG-fMRI experiments. Corruption of MRI data sets occurs when interfering RF signals at, or close to, the Larmor frequency reach the RF coil. Sources of interference can include radio stations, electrical motors, electrical lighting, and computers. Interference from such external radio frequency sources is normally prevented from reaching the RF coil by siting the scanner inside an RF screened room. This is essentially a box formed from electrically conducting material which greatly attenuates high frequency electromagnetic fields. It is generally necessary to provide apertures in the screened room to allow access for services, such as medical gases. Provided these apertures are formed from appropriately sized conducting tubes, known as wave-guides, they do not compromise the efficacy of screening. If, however, an electrically conducting wire is passed through the waveguide, RF interference can easily be conducted into the scanner room, where it is picked up by the RF coil. Electrical devices such as EEG amplifiers that must be sited close to the subject inside the room can also generate RF interference themselves.

The effect that RF interference has on MR images depends on its frequency content and also on the imaging sequence that is employed. If the bandwidth is narrow then an alternating black and white pattern, known as a zipper artifact (Bushberg et al., 2002), is often produced across images acquired using gradient echo sequences involving multiple excitations. In images acquired using echo planar imaging the artifact is likely to appear as a small number of bright spots. If the noise has a wide bandwidth then the contrast of images produced using a range of sequences will be reduced and a "herringbone" artifact may be produced (Bushberg et al., 2002). Clearly such artifacts are detrimental to image quality and should be avoided by careful design of any equipment that must be introduced into the magnet hall.

The majority of EEG systems that are now in use employ fiber-optic cables to transfer data from the EEG amplifier inside the shielded room to a recording system placed outside. This prevents transmission of externally generated RF interference into the shielded room and also has the advantage of electrically isolating the subject from the recording system. In addition, a high degree of RF screening of the EEG amplifier, along with the incorporation of RF filters, is used to prevent any interference generated by the amplifier electronics from reaching the RF coil. Provision of an optically isolated EEG system, which allows high quality recording of EEG data relies on high-quality construction of the EEG amplifiers. If the system is not constructed to a high standard then either RF interference will be introduced into the MR scanner or the EEG signals will not be amplified sufficiently, resulting in poor EEG data quality.

Perturbation of the RF magnetic field can be a major cause of unwanted spatial variation in signal intensity in magnetic resonance images and of global variation in SNR. In all MRI sequences, pulsed RF is used to rotate the nuclear magnetization from alignment with the main field, producing a net component of the magnetization that is perpendicular to the strong static magnetic field and that precesses around it. The local amount of this precessing transverse magnetization determines the image intensity and depends on the angle, α, through which the RF pulse initially rotates the magnetization. The flip-angle, α, produced by an RF pulse with magnetic field amplitude, B_1, and duration, τ, is given by

$$\alpha = \gamma B_1 \tau \qquad (4)$$

so that variation of the time that the RF pulse is applied for, or its magnitude, B_1, changes the angle through which the magnetization is tipped, thus changing the strength of the signal that is subsequently produced. Consequently, if the magnitude of the applied B_1-field varies spatially over the region that is being imaged, unwanted spatial variation of the signal intensity will be produced. In addition to the effect of B_1-inhomogeneity on the process of signal excitation, the strength of the signal received from a given region is also dependent on the local value of B_1, and this effect can give rise to further intensity variation in images acquired in the presence of any RF inhomogeneity.

When materials of high electrical conductivity are exposed to RF, large surface current densities that act to screen the RF field from the interior of the material are generated. These currents also disturb the B_1-field in regions that are in close proximity to the conductor. Consequently it can be expected that electrically conducting material in EEG caps will cause some perturbation of the B_1-field, leading to artifactual intensity variation in MR images. In addition, the interaction between the RF field and conducting material increases the effective resistance of the RF coil. Since any resistance acts as a source of noise, this effect can lead to a reduction in the SNR of images obtained in combined EEG-fMRI studies (Scarff et al., 2004; Mullinger et al., 2008a).

A particularly significant disturbance of the RF field can occur if the wires of the EEG cap have a length that is close to an integer multiple of half the RF wavelength, since a standing wave may then be set up in the wire. This resonance can produce a large perturbation of B_1 around the lead. To excite the spins, the frequency of the applied RF pulse must be chosen to match the Larmor frequency. From Equation 2 it is clear that the required frequency and therefore the wavelength of the RF pulse depends on the applied B_0-field and therefore the resonant effect will occur for leads of different length as the field strength changes. The consequences of this type of interaction for MR images and the relationship to lead-lengths are discussed in detail later in this chapter (refer to "Mapping B_1-inhomogeneity," below).

There is also the possibility that the gradient switching during MRI can cause eddy currents to be set up in the conductive materials of the EEG cap thus producing magnetic fields, which might distort the image (Lemieux et al., 1997). However, these effects are minimized by using small electrodes and preventing large, highly conducting loops being formed in the cap design.

Mapping B_1-Inhomogeneity

Although a number papers have discussed the potential problem of increased B_1-field inhomogeneity in combined EEG-fMRI studies (Krakow et al., 2000; Schomer et al., 2000; Iannetti et al., 2005; Stevens et al., 2007a; Mullinger et al., 2008a), until recently few investigators have tried to quantify the effect that the EEG cap has on the RF field. Stevens et al. (2007a) considered the RF shielding due to EEG electrodes made from three different materials. In this study a single electrode was placed on a hemispherical oil phantom and a T_2-weighted multi-slice spin echo sequence was then used to measure the signal reduction close to the electrode; imaging took place at 4 T. Stevens et al. (2007a) reported that the shielding caused by brass, silver, and conductive plastic electrodes was similar, being manifested as a signal loss of greater than 5% of the signal amplitude at distances up to 11.2 mm along projections normal to the center of the electrodes. This distance was measured for an electrode made of Ag/AgCl, although the other two electrode compositions produced the 5% signal losses at similar distances (less than 1.2 mm difference between electrodes). This study did not however consider the interactions between the EEG leads and the RF field.

The same group have also evaluated the effect of EEG lead length on MR image artifacts and the use of RF chokes to prevent lead-related artifacts (Stevens et al., 2007b). They tested whether standing waves were set up in wires of specific lengths and also evaluated the effect such waves had on image quality. They studied wires of two different lengths (35 and 70 cm) with and without RF chokes in place. The experiments were conducted on a cylindrical agar phantom in a 4 T MR scanner. They found with the 35 cm wire a large region of signal loss was produced as a result of a resonance being set up in the wire. When an RF choke was placed half way along the wire no image artifact was produced, indicating that the added inductance eliminated the standing wave. With the longer wire no artifact was observed when there was no RF choke in place, but in the presence of the choke two 35 cm wires were effectively created causing a large artifact in the MR image. This study demonstrates the strong effects that standing waves can have on image quality and the importance of avoiding resonance effects.

Mullinger et al. (2008a) considered the effect of entire EEG caps on B_1-homogeneity. In this study the effects of commercially available EEG caps (EasyCap, Herrsching, Germany) carrying (1) 32 and (2) 64 electrodes were considered at field strengths of 1.5, 3, and 7 T. Each cap employed an equidistant montage of electrodes and was connected to a BrainAmp EEG amplifier (BrainProducts, Munich, Germany). Flip angle maps were generated by using a double-delayed, spoiled gradient echo sequence (Yarnykh and Yuan, 2004) applied to a spherical, 17 cm inner diameter saline filled phantom that was doped with Gd-DTPA to yield a T_1 of ~700 ms at 3T, similar to that of white matter. Maps were generated at the three field strengths with the two different caps fitted around the

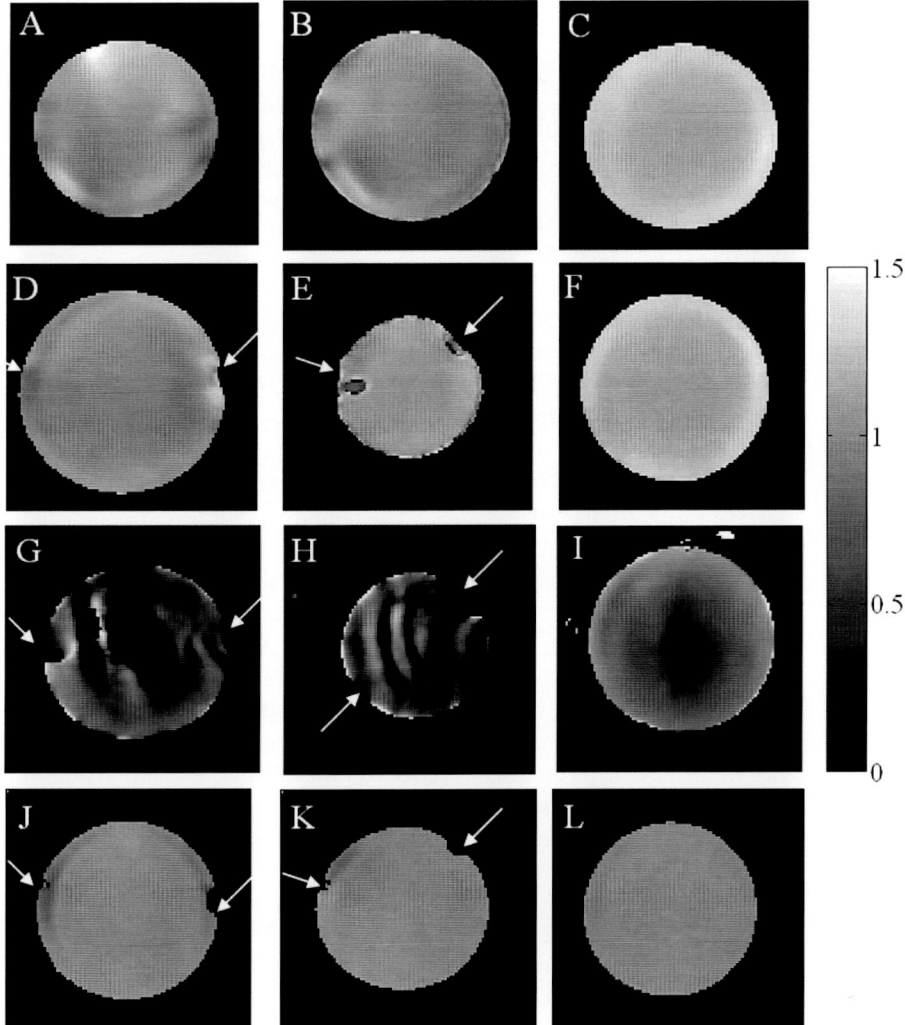

Figure 2.4.4. Flip angle maps of the phantom (normalized to average flip angle) with the 64-electrode cap (left), the 32-electrode cap (center), and no cap (right). A–C show maps acquired at 3 T from similar slices to that shown in Figure 2.2.2. The maps shown in the rest of figure are taken from more inferior slices and show the effect of B_1 perturbations occurring in proximity to the ECG and EOG wires (highlighted with arrows) at 3 T (D–F), 7 T (G–I) and 1.5 T (J–L). A more inferior slice is shown for the 64-electrode cap compared with the 32-electrode cap as the path of the EOG and ECG wires was different on these caps. The thresholding process led to the generation of significantly sized areas in the 7 T maps (G–I), where the flip angle could not be characterized. From Mullinger et al. (2008a).

phantom and with no cap in place. Flip angle maps of the human head were also created at 1.5 and 3 T with and without the 32-electrode cap. The flip angle maps acquired from this study on the phantom are shown in Figure 2.4.4. This figure shows that the electrodes did not cause significant B_1 distortions (Figure 2.2.4, A–C).

However, it was apparent from analysis of the standard deviation of the flip angle across the phantom that the presence of either EEG cap caused a significant increase in the spatial variation of the flip angle across the phantom. Examination of the flip angle maps obtained from more inferior axial slices (Figure 2.2.4, D–L) revealed that this was mainly due to the significant flip angle variation that was produced in regions of the phantom that lay close to the

path of the ECG and EOG leads. Similar effects were also observed in flip angle maps acquired on the human subject, where the inhomogeneity occurred in occipital and frontal regions that lay under the ECG and EOG leads. These leads are much longer (20 and 58 cm respectively) than all the other leads present in the cap design and it is likely that it is this difference in length that causes the interaction with the RF field although the precise form of the interaction is still not fully understood. However, since the artifact is present at all field strengths it is unlikely to be a resonant, standing wave effect. To test if the increased length of these leads is the cause of the image degradation RF chokes could be placed in line with them, thus reducing the length of wire "seen" by the RF field while still maintaining the leads' physical length (Stevens et al., 2007b).

Conclusion: B_1-Homogeneity

The problem of RF interference can be eliminated by appropriate screening of the EEG amplifier electronics and by eliminating electrical connections between the amplifier, sited inside the scanner's shielded room, and the recording system, located outside. This is most commonly done via use of a fiber-optic link, but interestingly it is also possible to encode the EEG data as an RF signal that is recorded by the scanner itself in spectral regions that do not contain any useful information about the MR signal (Hanson et al., 2007). Analysis of the effect of EEG recording apparatus on the B_1-homogeneity has shown that the electrodes generally have very little effect, but the longer copper leads used to connect to the ECG and EOG electrodes on one commercially available EEG cap were shown to cause significant B_1-inhomogeneity-related signal loss in the areas of the brain directly beneath the wires. Further investigation is needed to elucidate the origin of this effect.

Signal-to-noise Ratio

As mentioned earlier, the presence of an EEG cap can also cause increased loading of the RF coil(s) used for signal reception and thus a reduction in the global signal-to-noise ratio (SNR) of MRI data.

Measurements of the changes in SNR due to the presence of EEG caps have been carried out by Scarff et al. (2004). In their study, the SNR was calculated by considering the average pixel intensity in a region of interest (ROI), placed in the white matter of brain images recorded using echo-planar imaging (EPI), and then dividing by the standard deviation of the pixel intensity in a region of the same size located in an image region lying outside the head. They carried out this measurement using caps containing 64, 128, and 256 electrodes on a 3 T MR system. The results showed that there was a significant reduction in SNR with increasing electrode density, and although data quality was still acceptable when 64 or 128 electrodes were employed, their 256 electrode cap reduced the SNR by such an extent that data was unusable (Scarff et al., 2004).

Vasios et al. (2006) used a similar method for testing SNR when investigating the effect that their specially designed "InkCap" had on the SNR of EPI data acquired at 7 T. This cap was designed using conductive ink technology with the aim of improving both the EEG and fMRI data quality when performing simultaneous imaging. These authors reported that there was a 12% decrease in SNR in the presence of the InkCap, but this did not significantly effect the quality of fMRI results obtained when the InkCap was present compared with those acquired with no cap in place.

Iannetti et al. (2005) also considered the intrinsic SNR variation due to the presence of a 30-channel EEG cap placed on an agar gel phantom in a 3 T MR scanner. Here comparisons were made between data acquired with no cap, with a cap in place, but disconnected from the rest of the EEG system, and finally with the cap in place and connected to the EEG system. They found that the intrinsic SNR did not significantly change when the cap was present and connected to the amplifier. This group of authors also considered the temporal variation of the signal intensity in image time series acquired using EPI. This temporal variation provides a more relevant measure of SNR for fMRI experiments. To measure the temporal stability a large ROI was taken and the mean signal from the ROI for each acquisition was calculated. The ratio of the average to the standard deviation of the resulting time course was then found. This measure of SNR also showed that the presence of the EEG cap and associated hardware had no significant effect on the temporal stability of the MR images.

The temporal SNR was also considered by Mullinger et al. (2008a) across 1.5, 3, and 7 T MR field strengths. In this work measurements were made with no cap and with 32- and 64-electrode caps applied to a human subject. The measure of SNR was taken to be the temporal standard deviation of the pixel signal intensity averaged over an ROI positioned in white matter, divided by the mean signal in the same region. This study showed that neither cap had a strong effect on the SNR at 3 T and also that at 1.5 T the number of electrodes did not have significant effect on the reduction in SNR, which was measured to be approximately 27%. At 7 T, increasing the number of electrodes had a greater effect, with the SNR reduction due to the cap's presence being 18% and 28% with 32- and 64-electrode caps, respectively. The finding that the SNR reduction was smallest at 3 T is likely to be due to a combination of factors. Assuming that the NMR signal strength is unaffected by the presence of the cap, the change in SNR depends largely on the ratio of the magnitude of the extra noise due to the cap's loading of the RF coil to the magnitude of other noise sources. Although both would be expected to increase with field strength it appears that between 1.5 and 3 T the latter increases more rapidly, while between 3 and 7 T the increase in cap-induced noise is greater.

In this study, the SNR was also shown to increase with field strength both with and without the cap present, and it was noted that the SNR measured in the EPI data acquired at 7 T with the cap present was still greater than that measured at 3 T with no cap present. This indicates that the effort required to implement simultaneous EEG-fMRI at higher field strengths is worthwhile (Vasios et al., 2006; Mullinger et al., 2008b).

Effect on fMRI Data

Along with the studies of the underlying effects of the EEG cap on MR image quality several groups have also carried out comparisons of the results of fMRI experiments based on simple sensory paradigms, where data was collected with and without an EEG cap present. Iannetti et al. (2005) showed that during a laser stimulation task the blood oxygenation level dependent (BOLD) responses obtained with a 30-electrode EEG cap present were similar to previously published results showing nociceptive-related brain activity (Peyron et al., 2000; Tracey et al., 2002). Vasios et al. (2006) carried out a direct measurement of the effect that their 64-channel InkCap had on fMRI data collected at 7 T. Using an auditory paradigm they found that there were no significant differences between the BOLD responses obtained with or without the InkCap present. Bonmassar et al. (2001) drew similar conclusions from their work on retinotopic mapping in the presence of a nonmagnetic, custom-made 64-channel cap (Bonmassar et al., 1999) at 3 T. Both these groups therefore concluded that the presence of the EEG cap did not affect the quality of the BOLD responses obtained.

In contrast however, Kruggel et al. (2001) noted signal losses in the uppermost slices of their EPI data set, but did not comment directly on the effect that this had on the BOLD responses observed. Mullinger et al. (2008a) also discuss how the signal loss due to cap-induced B_1-inhomogeneity will lead to spatial variation in the sensitivity of detection of activation in fMRI data analysis. In areas of greater signal loss, a larger fractional BOLD signal change will be necessary to enable statistically significant activation to be detected.

Safety of Simultaneous EEG-fMRI

The interactions between the EEG hardware and the MR image quality that have been discussed in this chapter indicate that the EEG cap has a detectable effect on the magnetic fields used in MR imaging. The interactions of the cap with the RF-field and gradients used for image acquisition are of particular concern when considering subject safety while conducting simultaneous EEG-fMRI experiments.

Both the magnetic and electric field associated with the time-varying B_1-field can cause a number of interactions that may compromise patient safety and therefore should be considered carefully. These interactions are discussed in detail by Lemieux et al. (1997). The main cause for concern is heating due to induced currents in current-limiting resistors, leads, electrodes, and gel resulting from the applied RF-field. Interactions with the time-varying fields used in MRI may cause a number of health risks to the subject including heating or burning (due to high frequency current flow), ulcers (due to electrolysis caused by the flow of current), and electric shock (due to currents flowing at frequencies below 100 Hz) (Lemieux et al., 1997).

Standard modifications of EEG systems to make them MR compatible include the introduction of 5 kΩ resistors between each lead and electrode. This reduces the magnitude of the induced currents and therefore reduces the level of RF heating (Lemieux et al., 1997). Fiber optic cables are also employed to transmit the EEG signals out of the scanner room, thus optically isolating the subject from as many sources of danger as possible. After careful study of safety issues, Lemieux et al. (1997) concluded that with the correct precautions it was safe to conduct combined EEG-fMRI at 1.5 T, and commercial EEG systems have now been certified safe up to 3 T (BrainProducts, 2004).

Given the potential interactions between the EEG recording apparatus and MR scanner, it is important to define the exact experimental set-up, including the wire paths, used in simultaneous EEG-fMRI acquisitions. It is necessary to consider the positions of the EEG cable-bundles as well as those of individual leads relative to the RF coil used for transmission, as the interactions of the RF with the leads are strongly position dependent.

It is also important to reconsider the safety issues when moving between scanners operating at different field strengths: the associated change in the frequency of the B_1-field changes the interactions with the EEG cap, as discussed in the section "B_1-inhomogeneity," above. A number of groups have carried out safety testing on a variety of EEG caps at a range of magnetic field strengths. Along with Lemieux et al. (1997), Lazeyras et al. (2001) conducted some experimental work at 1.5 T, finding that heating effects occurred when sequences with high specific absorption rates (SAR) were used in the presence of an EEG cap. They found the extent of the heating increased almost linearly with SAR, showing it is important to test an EEG system with the actual pulse sequence that it is intended to use or to use a pulse sequence with a higher SAR value for testing purposes. A maximum increase in temperature of 6.1 °C was measured over a three-minute period when using a sequence with a SAR value of 2.6 Wkg^{-1}. Although significant, these heating effects were still within safety guidelines.

A number of groups have also investigated safety concerns relating to the implementation of simultaneous EEG-fMRI at higher field strengths, where the RF wavelength may approach that of the length of the wires used in the EEG system. Angelone et al. (2004) carried out simulations with the aim of evaluating the change in SAR with field strength and number of electrodes applied to the scalp. Their simulations used a model of the EEG system with electrodes and leads represented as perfect electric conductors. They found that the introduction of the conducting components of the EEG system at 7 T caused a significant increase in the calculated value of the peak local SAR. This effect became stronger as the number of electrodes/leads was increased (a maximum of 124 leads/electrodes were considered) and was larger at 7 T than at 3 T. In further work, the same group have made experimental measurements of RF heating at 7 T on a conducting, head-shaped phantom, with a variety of EEG electrode and lead arrangements using a TEM RF coil with an end-cap (Angelone et al., 2004; Vasios et al., 2006). Despite the long, 33-minute, experimental duration and the very high maximum local SAR of 15.5 Wkg^{-1} that was employed, the largest temperature rise that was measured in these experiments was only about 10° C, occurring in the conducting paste of electrode Cz. These authors suggested that the RF power input to the system should be scaled relative to their findings, so that SAR limits for tissue are not exceeded when EEG systems are present.

In related work carried out at 7 T by Vasios et al. (2006), temperature changes in the presence of their "InkCap" (described earlier in this chapter), a standard EEG cap, and a QuickCap (CompumedicsUSA, Ltd.; this cap is MRI-compatible up to 4 T) were recorded. In this study, significant temperature rises (up to 6.6° C) were measured at a number of electrode sites on the standard EEG cap and the Quickcap when a high-powered TSE sequence (SAR = 15.5 Wkg^{-1}) was applied. However, temperature increases measured using the InkCap were not significantly different from those measured on the phantom alone. The InkCap was subsequently used successfully in the first combined EEG-fMRI experiment carried out at 7 T (Vasios et al., 2006).

Experimental investigations were also carried out by Mullinger et al. (2008b) at 7 T. Here the heating effects on the commercially available Brain Products 32-channel MR compatible EEG cap were measured. A relatively high-SAR, TSE sequence (SAR $\approx$ 2 Wkg^{-1}) was run for 20 minutes using a head, transmit-receive RF coil. A maximum temperature rise of just 0.5°C was measured over the 8 electrode and wire positions that were monitored, and these investigators therefore concluded that it was safe to record on humans at 7 T using this set-up. However, the maximum SAR levels of this scanner are limited by the manufacturers to a conservative value, and therefore caution should be exercised when using this EEG system on other ultra-high field MR systems or with different RF transmit coils, as higher SAR values may be produced.

Limiting the Reduction of MRI Data Quality During Simultaneous EEG-fMRI

The increasing availability of scanners operating at magnetic fields in excess of 3 T, which provide improved sensitivity for fMRI, along with the general increase in the interaction between EEG recording apparatus and the magnetic fields applied in MRI, mean that the degradation of MR data quality in combined EEG-fMRI experiments has become an important consideration. Fortunately there are several approaches that should in the future help to ameliorate the effects that have been highlighted in this chapter. The use of higher resistance material for lead fabrication (e.g., carbon rather than copper), as in the system designed by Vasios et al. (2006), has been shown to improve the SNR of MRI data relative to a standard cap, as a result of a reduction in RF interactions. Recent measurements by Negishi et al. (2008) supported this finding, showing that carbon wires and

electrodes improved the MR data quality compared with conventional Ag/AgCl electrodes that are often used in EEG caps. However, care must be taken when using high resistance materials not to compromise the EEG data quality and there may also be issues of physical robustness when nonmetallic leads are used.

A second method for ameliorating the effects of the EEG-cap-induced B_1-inhomogeneity at high field may be the use of parallel transmit technology, which forms an area of active research (Adriany et al., 2005; Katscher and Bornert, 2006) and is already being used at high field.

By careful choice of electrode and resistor materials it is likely that even at very high magnetic field unwanted effects of magnetic susceptibility differences between EEG cap materials and the human head, such as image distortion and signal loss, can be limited to acceptable levels in the brain. Stronger shim systems and improved shimming approaches, such as dynamic shim updating, in which shim values are varied on a slice-by-slice basis in multislice echo planar imaging may also help in this regard (Koch et al., 2006).

REFERENCES

Adriany G, Van de Moortele PF, Wiesinger F, Moeller S, Strupp JP, Andersen P, Snyder C, Zhang XL, Chen W, Pruessmann KP, Boesiger P, Vaughan T, Ugurbil K (2005) Transmit and receive transmission line arrays for 7 Tesla parallel imaging. Magn Reson Med 53:434–445.

Angelone LM, Potthast A, Segonne F, Iwaki S, Belliveau JW, Bonmassar G (2004) Metallic electrodes and leads in simultaneous EEG-MRI: specific absorption rate (SAR) simulation studies. Bioelectromagnetics 25:285–295.

Bonmassar G, Anami K, Ives J, Belliveau J (1999) Visual evoked potential (VEP) measured by simultaneous 64-channel EEG adn 3T fMRI. Neuroreport 10:1893–1897.

Bonmassar G, Hadjikhani N, Ives JR, Hinton D, Belliveau JW (2001) Influence of EEG electrodes on the BOLD fMRI signal. Hum Brain Mapp 14:108–115.

BrainProducts (2004) BrainAmp operating instructions.

Bushberg JT, Seibert JA, Leidholdt EM, Boone JM (2002) The essential physics of medical imaging: Chapter 15. Philadelphia: Lippincott Williams and Wilkins.

Ericsson A, Weis J, Hemmingsson A, Wikstrom M, and Sperber GO (1995) Measurements of magnetic field variations in the human brain using a 3D-FT multiple gradient echo technique. Magn Reson Med 33:171–177.

Hanson LG, Lund TE, Hanson CG (2007) Encoding of electrophysiolofy and other signals in MR images. J Magn Reson Im 25:1059–1066.

Hashemi RH, Bradley WG, Jr., Lisanti CJ (2004) MRI the basics. Philadelphia: Lippincott Williams and Wilkins.

Huang-Hellinger FR, Breiter HC, McCormack G, Cohen MS, Kwong K, Sutton JP, Savoy RL, Weisskoff RM, Davis TL, Baker J, Belliveau J, Rosen BR (1995) Simultaneous functional magnetic resonance imaging and electrophysiological recording. Hum Brain Mapp 3:13–23.

Iannetti GD, Niazy RK, Wise RG, Jezzard P, Brooks JCW, Zambreanu L, Vennart W, Matthews PM, Tracey I (2005) Simultaneous recording of laser-evoked brain potentials and continuous, high-field functional magnetic resonance imaging in humans. Neuroimage 28:708–719.

Jezzard P, Balaban RS (1995) Correction for geometric distortion in echo planar images from B0 field variations. Magn Reson Med 34:65–73.

Katscher U, Bornert P (2006) Parallel RF transmission in MRI. NMR Biomed 19:393–400.

Koch KM, McIntyre S, Nixon TW, Rthman DL, De Graaf RA (2006) Dynamic shim updating on the human brain. J Magn Reson 180:286–296.

Krakow K, Allen PJ, Symms MR, Lemieux L, Josephs O, Fish DR (2000) EEG recording during fMRI experiments: image quality. Hum Brain Mapp 10:10–15.

Kruggel F, Herrmann CS, Wiggins CJ, Cramon DY von (2001) Hemodynamic and electroencephalographic responses to illusory figures: recording of the evoked potentialduring functional MRI. Neuroimage 14:1327–1336.

Lazeyras, F, Zimine I, Blanke O, Perrig SH, Seeck M (2001) Functional MRI with simultaneous EEG recording: feasibility and application to motor and visual activation. J Magn Reson Im 13:943–948.

Lemieux L, Allen PJ, Franconi F, Symms MR, Fish DR (1997) Recording of EEG during fMRI experiments: patient safety. Magn Reson Med 38:943–952.

Levitt, MH (2005) Spin dynamics: basics of nuclear magnetic resonance: Chapter 2. Chichester, UK: John Wiley & Sons.

Mirsattari SM, Lee DH, Jones D, Bihari F, Ives JR (2004) MRI compatible EEG electrode system for routine use on the epilepsy monitoring unit and intensive care unit. Clin Neurophysiol 115:2175–2180.

Morris PG (1990) Nuclear magnetic resonance imaging in medicine and biology. Oxford: Oxford University Press.

Mullinger KJ, Debener S, Coxon R, Bowtell RW (2008a) Effects of simultaneous EEG recording on MRI data quality at 1.5, 3 and 7 tesla. Int J Psychophysiol 67:178–188.

Mullinger KJ, Brookes MJ, Stevenson CM, Morgan PS, Bowtell RW (2008b) Exploring the feasibility of simultaneous EEG-fMRI at 7 T. Magn Reson Imaging: 26:607–616.

Negishi M, Laufer I, Abildgaard M, Nixon T, Constable RT (2008) Abstract #1059: an EEG system with carbon wire electrodes and an anti-polarization circuit for simultaneous EEG-fMRI. ISMRM.

Peyron R, Laurent B, Garcia-Larrea L (2000) Functional imaging of brain reponses to pain: A review and meta-analysis. Clin Neurophysiol 30:263–288.

Scarff CJ, Reynolds A, Goodyear BG, Ponton CW, Dort JC, Eggermont JJ (2004) Simultaneous 3-T fMRI and high-density recording of human auditory evoked potentials. Neuroimage 23:1129–1142.

Schomer DL, Bonmassar G, Lazeyras F, Seeck M, Blum A, Amani K, Schwartz D, Bellivau JW, Ives J (2000) EEG-linked functional magnetic resonace imaging in epilepsy cognitive neurophysiology. J Clin Neurophysiol 17:43–58.

Shellock FG (2004) Reference manual for magnetic resonance safety, implants and devices. Los Angeles: Biomedical Research Publishing Group.

Stevens TK, Ives JR, Klassen LM, Bartha R (2007a) MR compatibility of EEG scalp electrodes at 4 tesla. J Magn Reson Im 25:872–877.

Stevens TK, Ives J, Bartha R (2007b) Abstract #1078: avoiding resonant lengths of wire with RF chokes at 4 tesla. Berlin: ISMRM.

Tracey I, Ploghaus A, Gati JS, Clare S, Smith S, Menon RS, Matthews PM (2002) Imaging attentional modulation of pain in the periaqueductal gray in humans. J Neurosci 22:2748–2752.

Vasios CE, Angelone LM, Purdon PL, Ahveninen J, Belliveau J, Bonmassar G (2006) EEG/(f)MRI measurements at 7 Tesla using a new EEG cap ("InkCap"). Neuroimage 33:1082–1092.

Yarnykh VL, Yuan C (2004) Actual flip angle imaging in the pulsed steady state. In: Proceedings of ISMRM. Kyoto, Japan.

Part 3 ⊞

Multimodal Data Integration

3.1 Stefan Debener, Jeremy Thorne, Till R. Schneider, and Filipa Campos Viola

Using ICA for the Analysis of Multi-Channel EEG Data

Introduction

It has been known for several decades that electric potential recordings provide a wealth of information about brain function. Electroencephalogram (EEG) signals inform about various types of processes, from basic brain function via sensory processing to higher order cognition such as language, memory or awareness, to name a few. Accordingly, the EEG technique provides a "window of the mind" (Nunez and Srinivasan, 2006). However, what types of information the EEG signal might contain that can help us to advance our understanding of the relationship between mind, brain, and behavior is not well understood (Sauseng and Klimesch, 2008). Here we take the view that the statistical decomposition of multi-channel EEG signals provides an important means to gain a better recognition and understanding of the various types of processes that are reflected in the EEG signal. Specifically, this chapter is concerned with the application of independent component analysis (ICA) to EEG data. ICA is a linear decomposition technique that aims to reveal the underlying statistical sources of mixed signals. That the EEG signal consists of a mixture of various brain and nonbrain contributions can hardly be questioned. Accordingly, a valid and powerful unmixing tool promises a better, more accessible representation of the statistical sources contributing to the mixed recorded signal. ICA, being potentially such a tool, may therefore help in the detection of signal sources that cannot be identified on the raw data level alone using other, more conventional techniques. An example illustrating this claim is shown in Figure 3.1.1. Here, the electrical signal of an unborn baby's heartbeat was recovered from multi-channel electric potential recordings taken from a pregnant woman's abdomen. Note that the infant's heartbeat was not evident from the raw data, which was dominated by the mother's heartbeat. Neither was it recoverable using other techniques such as filtering or averaging. So, under favorable circumstances, ICA can identify even small signal sources that otherwise would be missed.

Excellent books covering the mathematical details and different implementations of ICA have been published (Hyvärinen et al., 2001; Stone, 2004); the application of ICA to multi-channel EEG recordings has been reviewed (Onton et al., 2006); and a conceptual framework for using ICA for the study of event-related brain dynamics exists (Makeig et al., 2004a). Indeed, the application of ICA to EEG signals has become popular, as it provides two key features: it is a powerful way to remove artifacts from EEG data (Jung et al., 2000a; Jung et al., 2000b), and it helps to disentangle otherwise mixed brain signals (Makeig et al., 2002). In some fields of EEG research, such as EEG-fMRI integration, these two key characteristics have clearly fostered progress in the field (Debener et al., 2006). Not surprisingly, this book contains several chapters on ICA for EEG-fMRI integration, so the topic will not be considered further here. Instead, the present chapter is concerned with a more basic issue, namely, evaluating and optimizing EEG decompositions by means of ICA. We will first show typical ICA results and discuss these with reference to artifact- and brain-related components. After this we will discuss different EEG preprocessing steps, considered in light of the statistical assumptions underlying ICA. Accordingly, we will present examples showing that the quality of ICA decompositions depends at least partly on the adequate preprocessing of the EEG data and discuss examples that help to evaluate decomposition quality. As such, the motivation for this chapter is to provide some practical guidelines for those researchers who wish to successfully decompose multi-channel EEG recordings.

A   Recorded data (mixed)

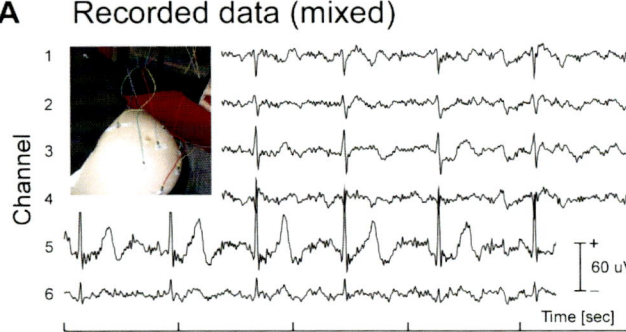

B   Component activations (unmixed)

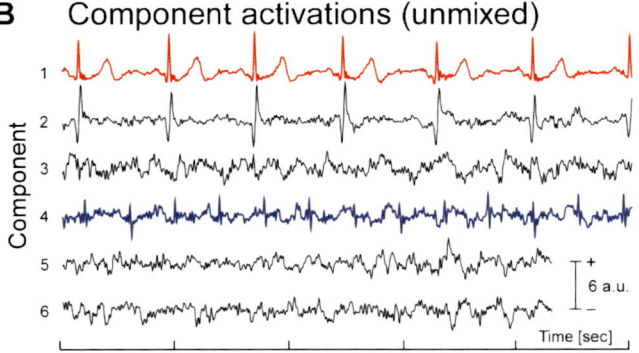

Figure 3.1.1. Example illustrating the blind decomposition of mixed multi-channel biopotential recordings into statistical sources. A: Data were recorded from six electrodes attached to a pregnant woman's abdomen. Shown is a 5-second section, dominated by the mother's electrical heartbeat activity. B: Same section of data after decomposition with ICA. Shown are maximally temporally independent time courses, with component 1, in red, reflecting the mother's electrical heartbeat activity, and component 4 reflecting the unborn baby's heartbeat that was not visible from the mixed channel recordings shown in A.

Basic ICA Model

ICA decomposes multi-channel recordings into a weighted (linear) mixture of different processes or signal sources. Let us call the recorded EEG data a 2-D matrix X consisting of a number of channels (rows) and time points (columns). The outcome of a complete form of ICA is a square matrix W of the size of the number of channels. W enables the modeling, or recovery, of the independent component activity time courses, A, such that

$$A = WX \qquad (1)$$

A is revealed by matrix multiplication of W with the raw data X and has the same size as X. However, A now refers to independent components (ICs), not channels, and the columns represent the activity profiles from ICs that are maximally temporally independent from each other. The recorded data X can be fully reconstructed by

multiplication of the inverse of W with A. Thus, W^{-1} is known as the mixing matrix:

$$X = W^{-1}A \qquad (2)$$

The left-hand part of Equation 2 is usually referred to as the channel or signal space, meaning that the values stored in X have a proper physical unit (μV for EEG recordings). The right-hand part of Equation 2 can be considered the source space. For practical reasons outlined below, it is important to keep in mind that the data in the source space are arbitrarily scaled. However, arbitrary scaling does not mean that sign and magnitude information are lost, just that the sign and magnitude information for each IC are distributed between W^{-1} and A. For this and several further reasons, it is generally helpful to consider both the inverse weights and the activations for the functional interpretation of each IC: just as EEG data in the raw signal space usually require the consideration of temporal and topographical information for interpretation, ICA results similarly require an interpretation.

For each IC, the rows of matrix W^{-1} contain the weights at each recording channel and may be best considered a spatial filter. This provides the topographical information for an IC of interest, that is, the contribution of each channel to the respective IC time course stored in A, and could be plotted as a map. So, while A reflects the activity profile that changes over time, W^{-1} stores the spatial weights that apply equally to all time points. This is illustrated in Figure 3.1.2, providing a more comprehensive illustration of Equation 2.

In order to obtain the actual contribution of one or several ICs to the raw signal, it is possible to back-project single ICs of interest. Similarly, ICs that are identified as artifacts can be removed by back-projection of all but those ICs. This can be done by making use of Equation 2 and zeroing out the columns (in W^{-1}) or the rows (in A) of those ICs that are not to be considered further. Figure 3.1.3 shows an example. The segment of raw EEG data shown, matrix X, contains two eye blinks plus ongoing oscillations in the EEG alpha frequency range. Unmixing of these data by means of ICA reveals IC time courses (A) and maps (W^{-1}). It can be seen that the first component, IC 1, captures the eye blinks, whereas IC 3 and IC 4 seem to represent oscillations in the alpha frequency range. Note the similarity between the eye blink topography shown in the raw data and the map of IC 1, as well as the time course of this component with the time course of the eye blinks. Back-projection of all but the first two components returns corrected EEG data (X_c), as shown in the upper right part of Figure 3.1.3. A comparison of the eye blink topographies before and after artifact correction enables a quality check. In the present example, the map after eye blink correction does not suggest residual eye blink activity, indicating very good correction

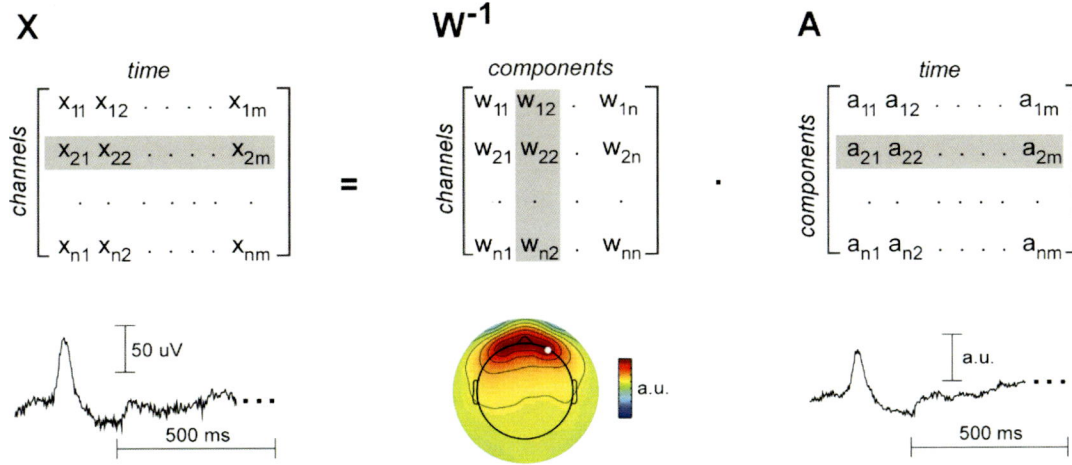

Figure 3.1.2. Linear decomposition of multi-channel EEG data (X). Inverse weights (W^{-1}) represent the spatial pattern of each source time course. Matrix-multiplication of W^{-1} with the maximally temporally independent time courses (in A) gives the mixed channel data, a process called back-projection. For illustration purposes, one component/channel vector is highlighted in grey and shown below the corresponding matrices.

quality. Note also that occipital alpha oscillations can now be observed during the eye blink interval. This interpretation would not have been possible without accurate eye blink correction.

More generally, a comparison between the original data X and the back-projected data X_c provides several opportunities. For instance, it enables the quantification of the amount of variance accounted for by one IC, or a group of ICs, in the raw data. This procedure has been used to identify the contribution of ICs to event-related potential (ERP) components of interest (e.g., Debener et al., 2005a). Moreover, further quality checks can also be done by comparing measures derived from X and X_c. For instance, the signal-to-noise ratio (SNR) improvement for an ERP component of interest could be determined by comparing the SNR of the ERP based on trial averages of X versus the SNR of the ERP based on trial averages of X_c (e.g., Debener et al., 2007). An additional advantage of back-projected data is that they are scaled in physical units, thus solving the sign and magnitude ambiguity that needs to be considered at the source level. Therefore, for practical reasons, it can be convenient to perform further processing on back-projected data instead of source data, even if only one IC per decomposition is of interest (e.g., Debener et al., 2005a).

While more advanced ICA algorithms—that often promise solutions to some of the problems outlined in the next section—are under development and have been published, they have not yet been tested on EEG data rigorously enough to justify their consideration here. Infomax ICA on the other hand has been extensively applied to EEG data and seems to be among the most powerful ICA algorithms (e.g., Delorme et al., 2007a). Therefore, all further statements and illustrations refer to the well-established and freely available infomax ICA algorithm.

ICA Assumptions

Like other statistical procedures, the application of ICA rests on several statistical assumptions. Are these assumptions reasonably fulfilled for EEG data? It is our experience that a consideration of these assumptions can improve the outcome of the ICA decomposition. Indeed, many failures and disappointments with ICA may arise from suboptimal EEG recording or preprocessing. Accordingly, the argument put forward here is that EEG preprocessing steps can be adjusted to ensure as good as possible compliance of the EEG data with ICA assumptions. The possible relationship between EEG preprocessing and ICA model assumptions will be discussed and illustrated below, after a brief summary of the most relevant ICA assumptions.

Imagine the situation where several groups of people are in a room and talk to each other, all in the presence of background noise. Background noise might be the humming of an air conditioning unit, some jazz music, and the sound of a cocktail-shaker—hence the name cocktail party problem. Let us also assume that we are recording this mixture of sounds by placing a number of microphones positioned at different places in the room. It would certainly be very hard, if not impossible, to follow any single conversation by listening to the sounds recorded by the different microphones. This is because each microphone will have picked up sounds from all sources, albeit with a different level.[1] So, which assumptions must be fulfilled, such that ICA can correctly identify these different sound sources from the cocktail party recordings, and how similar is the cocktail party scenario to EEG?

More Sensors than Sources

To solve the cocktail party problem, there must be at least as many microphones in the room as there are sound sources.

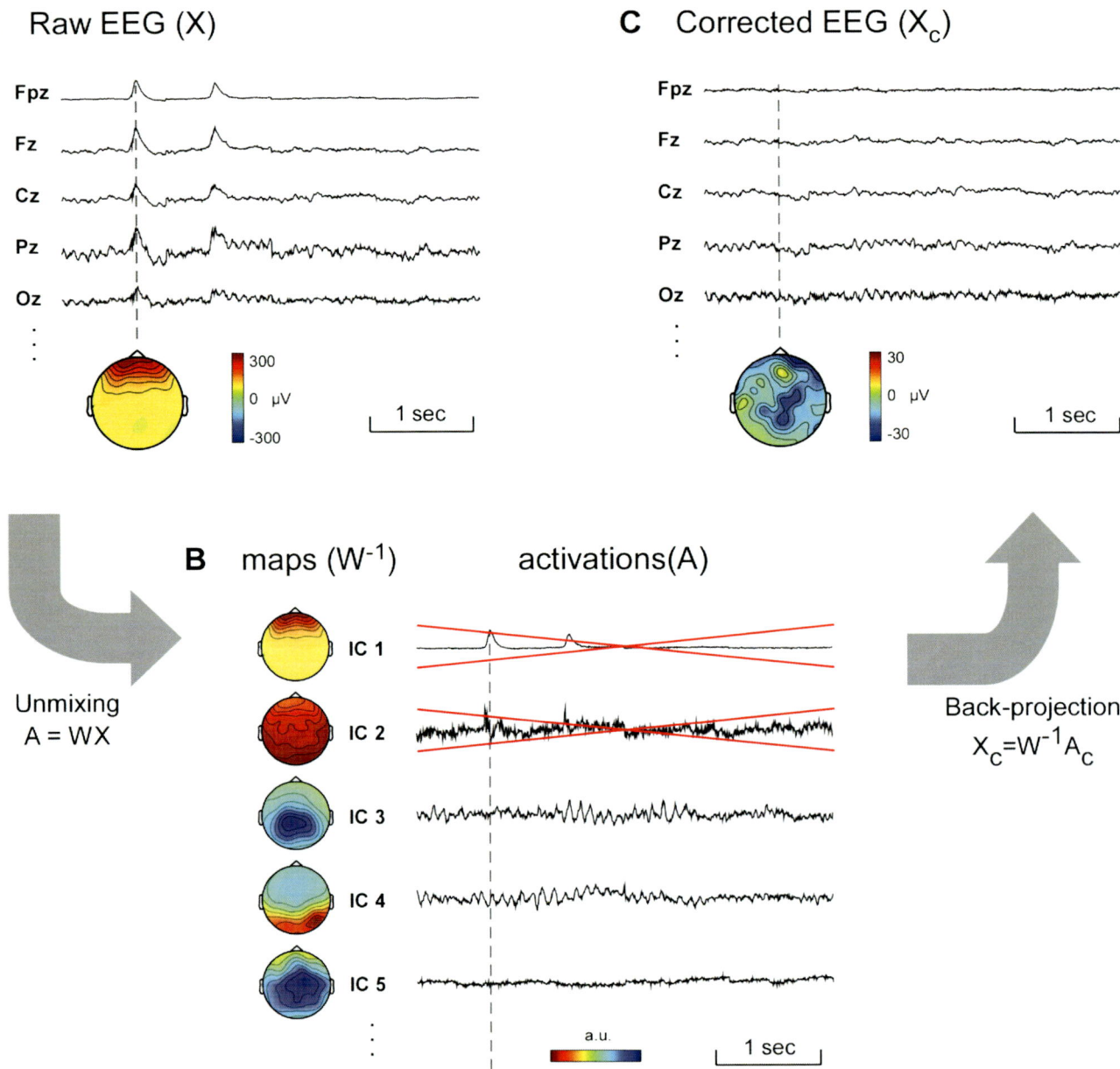

Figure 3.1.3. Illustration of artifact removal by means of ICA. A: Section of selected channels from a multi-channel EEG recording is shown, with ongoing EEG oscillations in the alpha range evident at occipital electrodes and two eye blinks at fronto-polar channels. B: Unmixing of the EEG data into a set of independent components. Each component can be described on the basis of a spatial pattern (map) and a time course (activation). C: Back-projection of all but components 1 and 2 reveals artifact-corrected EEG data.

Ideally, the number of microphones should be equal to the number of sound sources. The problem of course is that for real recordings of biological signals, we don't know how many sources there are that contribute to the recordings. This is particularly the case for the decomposition of EEG signals. How many EEG electrodes are needed for ICA? What types of problems can arise from either undercomplete (i.e., there are more sensors than sources), or overcomplete scenarios (i.e., there are more sources than sensors)? We will show ICA examples from 30, 68, and 128 channel recordings and

illustrate some practical aspects of the assumption that there are at least as many sensors as sources in each case.

Spatial Stationarity (Fixed Sources-Sensor Configuration)

Another assumption is that the location of the sources does not change relative to the location of the microphones. Different scenarios that could potentially violate this assumption should be considered, such as the relocation of microphones during the recording, or the movement of signal sources (such as guests at the cocktail party). If either of this happens, ICA is not very effective and a decomposition would likely return unsatisfactory results. Does this problem apply to EEG or magnetoencephalography (MEG)? In the case of multi-channel EEG recordings, individuals may touch the electrode cap during the recording. The cap can also be dislocated as a result of gross head movement, facial expressions, pulling on the electrode cables, or bad fit. It is our experience that some electrode cap systems and configurations are more susceptible to various forms of dislocation than others. Fortunately, for MEG, the sensors are fixed in a helmet, making it impossible for the relative position between the sensors to change. Here, the source of the problem is rather that the position of the head relative to the helmet can change as a result of head movement. Clearly, this scenario would also violate the spatial stationarity assumption. The second scenario is the movement of signal sources and seems to be a problem for EEG/MEG recordings in only a very few, limited recording situations. Some sleep patterns and certain epileptic sources have been reported to contribute moving projections to the EEG signal, and those data can pose a problem for ICA. However, most neural signals picked up by EEG and MEG are generated by pyramidal neurons, which do not move. Thus, this latter issue seems much less of a problem. However, sensor dislocation (EEG) and head movement (MEG) should be avoided or kept at a minimum to facilitate good ICA decompositions. Finally, single channel drifts, as sometimes occur in EEG recording, can be seen as violating the spatial stationarity (and the more signals than sources) assumption, as they would result in stationarity distortions of the "true" underlying signals and can add complexity to the whole dataset.

Linear Mixing

The signals received by each microphone are considered as an instantaneous linear mixture of a number of source signals. The assumption of instantaneous mixing is indeed a problem for acoustic signals, because it takes some time for a sound to travel a distance, meaning that microphones placed further away pick up a signal from a sound source later than those nearby. However, for EEG/MEG, this issue seems negligible. Based on the laws of conductance, the assumption of instantaneous superposition is usually considered to be fulfilled for EEG/MEG.

Independence of Sources

Now let us assume that the host of the cocktail party uses two cocktail shakers perfectly simultaneously and synchronously. Would ICA be able to separate these two sounds? Indeed, the independence assumption is often criticized as being not very plausible for EEG/MEG data, as some form of organized

temporal structure is probably present in large-scale, inter-regional brain activity. It seems unlikely that large-scale brain areas contributing to the EEG have "nothing to do with each other." A more plausible view would be to assume some form of functional coupling or connectivity between distant cortical regions, and this seems to be in contrast to the independence assumption. However, as long as two sources are not perfectly coupled during the recording, they may express some degree of temporal independence, and this amount of partial independence (or partial connectivity) may be sufficient for ICA to achieve a good degree of unmixing. Several publications report that ICA can deal with even those artifacts that appear to be perfectly phase-locked to event-related potentials (ERPs) of interest (Debener et al., 2008). Moreover, the success of ICA in recovering dipolar patterns of brain activity, as shown below, suggests that large-scale brain regions may not be perfectly coupled (with the possible exception of some homologous brain areas), but rather express some dynamics in their coupling.

Non-Gaussian Distribution

Another assumption is that (at least some) sources must not contribute a perfectly Gaussian distribution. Mixed signals such as EEG data are often characterized by Gaussian distributions. This can be explained by the central limit theorem, which states that the sum of a number of independent random variables is characterized by a more Gaussian distribution than that of the independent variables. The opposite interpretation is however not justified: Just because we are recording a signal with a Gaussian distribution we cannot infer that this signal consists of a mixture of non-Gaussian sources. Therefore, as with the independence assumption, it seems impossible to tell whether this assumption is reasonable. However, given the practical value of ICA and the quality of many ICA decompositions, we conclude that the assumptions of independence and non-Gaussian distribution seem to be reasonably plausible for EEG data.

ICA Outcome

In this section, we will first illustrate some typical artifact and brain ICs that can often be identified across laboratories, recording set-ups, subjects, and experiments. Subsequently, we will discuss potential problems that can arise when the reliability of ICA solutions is low.

ICs Representing Artifacts

According to the model outlined above, ICA should separate EEG artifacts from brain activity patterns. Some of the most common artifacts typically identified by ICA are shown in Figure 3.1.4. Eye blinks, for instance, can often be easily identified by their characteristic topography (W^{-1}) and time

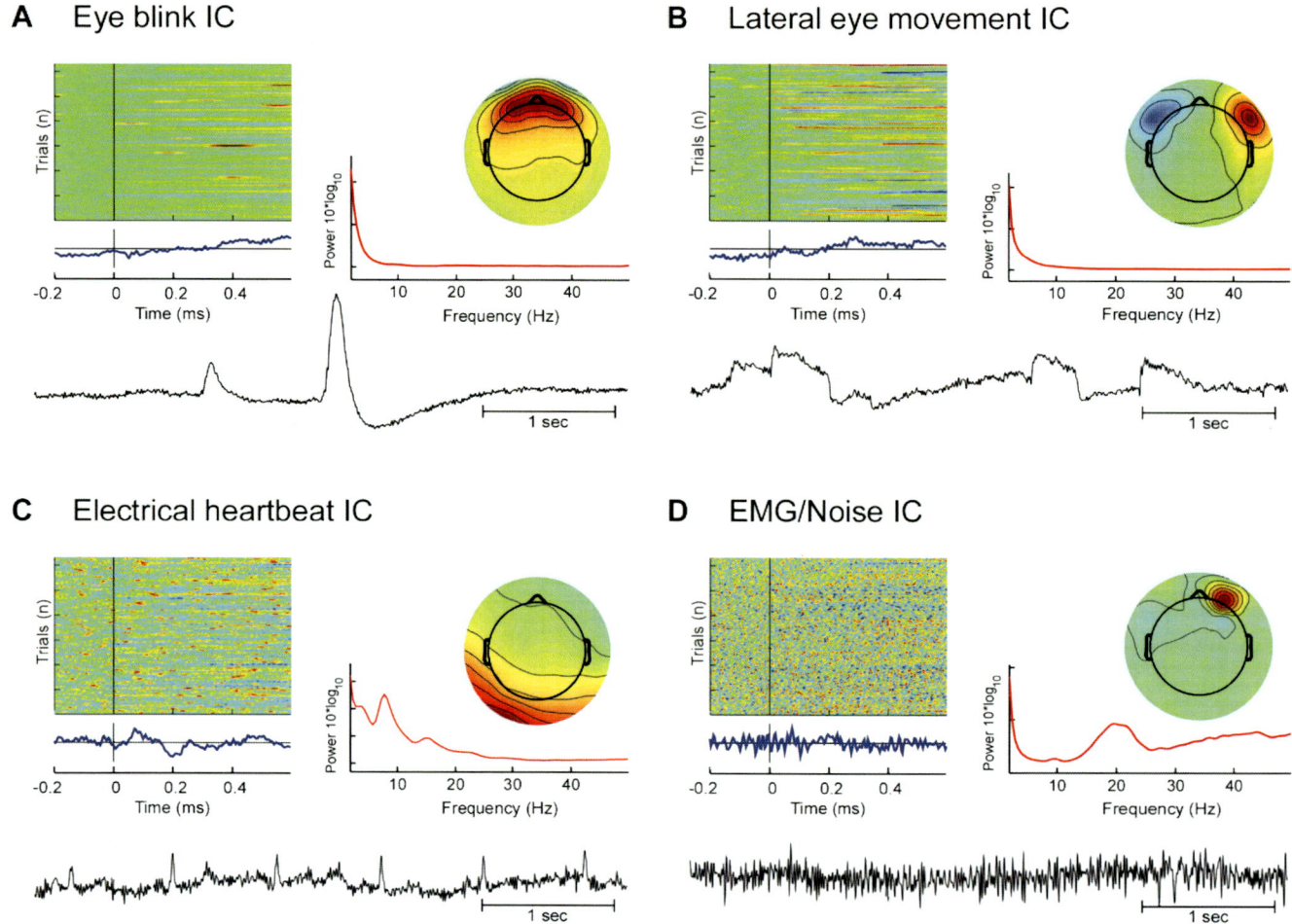

Figure 3.1.4. Typical EEG artifacts as identified by ICA. A: Eye blink artifact components. Shown are the IC map, the single-trial activity as an image, the time-domain average, i.e., the ERP (blue) and the spectrum (red), along with a representative section of ongoing activity (below). B: Same for lateral eye movements. C: Same for electrical heartbeat artifact. D: Same for muscle/noise activity.

course (A), but provide limited spectral information (Viola et al., 2009). Whether these and other artifact ICs show event-related activity such as an evoked response usually depends on the task. The presentation of visual stimuli for instance often induces event-related eye blinks, which could then be characterized by an eye-blink IC ERP. The examples shown in Figure 3.1.4 are taken from an auditory experiment while the participant watched a silent movie. Accordingly, lateral eye movements and eye blinks were rather common, as illustrated in the single-trial visualization, the ERP image, but did not evoke much event-related activity. Note that even with the occurrence of artifacts that seem perfectly phase-locked to ERPs, ICA has been demonstrated to be of significant help (e.g., Debener et al., 2008).

Technically, ICA allows all artifacts that can be safely identified to be removed by back-projection. This requires, of course, the correct identification of artifact ICs. However, the decomposition of high-density EEG recordings often results in more than one IC representing the same type of artifact. This general problem might indicate overfitting, or

an undercomplete decomposition, that is, the separation of the identical source process on different ICs (see Gómez-Herrero et al., 2005; Särelä and Vigário, 2004, for in depth discussion and examples). Alternatively, it might suggest that different types of eye blinks (e.g., voluntary and spontaneous) were identified due to their slightly different time courses. Another common artifact that is usually represented by a single IC results from lateral eye movements. The lateral eye movement IC is easy to identify by the characteristic time course and topography, and is often found to be highly correlated with bipolar horizontal electrooculogram (HEOG) recordings.

Also very common in EEG recordings are ICs reflecting electromyogram (EMG) or muscle activity, which are sometimes hard to distinguish from channel noise or overfitting problems. ICA from high-density EEG recordings typically reveals a number of these ICs, sometimes clearly representing different muscle groups and/or different EEG channels. The distinction between EMG and channel noise seems not easy, since both contribute high frequency activity to the EEG signal. In our experience, EMG ICs tend to express a more tangential dipolar pattern, whereas channel-noise IC maps specifically point (radially) to a single channel.

One artifact type that receives less attention in EEG/ERP research is related to electrical heartbeat activity. ICA often represents this activity in one IC (or sometimes two), as shown in Figure 3.1.4C. It is plausible to expect that the location and orientation of the heartbeat dipole is reflected in an asymmetry of the IC map. The characteristic R peaks represented by the IC time course often go undetected in the mixed channel signal, probably due to their relatively small contributions to the ongoing EEG signal. However, while electrical heartbeats may not show substantial event-related activity patterns in typical ERP experiments, they may nevertheless represent a serious source of artifact, in particular for a topographical analysis in the frequency domain: The highly characteristic, asymmetric topography of this component, together with its broad-band spectral contribution, suggests that measures such as posterior EEG alpha asymmetry, which have been used to study individual differences, could be substantially biased by this artifact and thus profit from its removal.

If the focus is on artifact removal, a good strategy seems to be to remove those ICs that can be classified as representing artifacts. The necessary classification of these components could be done by visual inspection of various component properties, such as those shown in Figure 3.1.4. More objective and efficient component identification approaches have been developed (e.g., Viola et al., 2009), but we nevertheless recommend a careful visual inspection of the ICA outcome, since the separation of artifacts from brain-related activity is not always satisfactory. However, the use of ICA for artifact removal often achieves good data quality in ERP research, which enables, for instance, the dipole source localization of single subject data (e.g., Hine, 2008), the recovery of ERPs that otherwise would be completely buried in artifact (e.g., Debener et al., 2008) or the study of trial-by-trial event-related brain activity (e.g., Makeig et al., 2002). The following section will present a few examples of ICs reflecting brain activity.

ICs Representing Brain Activity

Various examples have been published demonstrating the potential of ICA for the identification of event-related brain activity patterns (e.g., Debener, et al., 2005a; Debener et al., 2005b; Delorme et al., 2007b; Makeig et al., 2002; Onton et al., 2005). These studies have combined ICA with single-trial EEG analysis, thereby exploring brain dynamics beyond the evoked fraction of the signal that is preserved in the ERP. Summarizing this growing body of work is clearly beyond the scope of this chapter. Instead, we will illustrate the basic view that some ICs represent brain-activity as clearly as others represent artifact. Based on this assumption, ICA should disentangle not only different artifacts, but also different brain processes from each other.

To briefly illustrate the capability of ICA for achieving this, data from an audiovisual speech discrimination experiment recorded in our lab are shown in Figure 3.1.5. This experiment included multisensory audiovisual (AV) as well as unisensory auditory (A) and visual (V) trials. ICA decomposition was performed for concatenated single-trial data that included the trials from all three experimental conditions A, V, and AV, with the main purpose of removing artifacts. However, inspection of the other, nonartifact ICs clearly suggested that some were specifically related to auditory or visual processing. Two representative ICs are shown in Figure 3.1.5. The top row of this figure shows the channel data and scalp maps at the peak latency of the P1 VEP (left) and the peak latency of the AEP N1 (right). Panel B shows IC 6, which explained about one third of the VEP in the P1 latency range 70 to 126 ms, but did not contribute to the AEP in the N1 range 88 to 166 ms. This suggests that IC 6 represented mainly visual event-related activity. The bottom panel shows the same analysis for another component, IC 1, which contributed little to the VEP variance in the P1 latency range, but more than 50% of the AEP in the N1 range.

Note the substantial similarity between the channel-based evoked potentials at the ERP peak latencies and the respective IC 1 and IC 6 maps. Again, these ICs were defined across all experimental conditions, but explained condition-specific variance, which can be taken as important information for the functional interpretation of ICs reflecting event-related brain activity. Of further importance is the notion that these ICs can be studied on the single-trial level, thereby allowing the assessment of event-related activity beyond the phase-locked portion (not illustrated here). And finally, inspection of further ICs indicates that several ICs commonly contribute to the scalp-ERP, although it often seems the case that few ICs explain a large amount of variance, whereas many others contribute little each. Accordingly, a number of ICs usually represent event-related activities, among which some may be condition-specific, as shown in Figure 3.1.5, whereas others may contribute similarly to different conditions.

ICA Reliability

A very important practical consideration is that the stability or reliability of any ICA decomposition cannot be taken for granted. Unlike principal components analysis (PCA), which always returns identical decompositions when applied repeatedly, ICA can produce different results from repeated application to identical data. This is because the unmixing weights (W) are learned over repeated iterations, which use randomly chosen samples from the training data submitted (X). As a result, the outcome may differ to some extent. It is therefore important to consider the factors that contribute to the reliability of ICA decompositions.

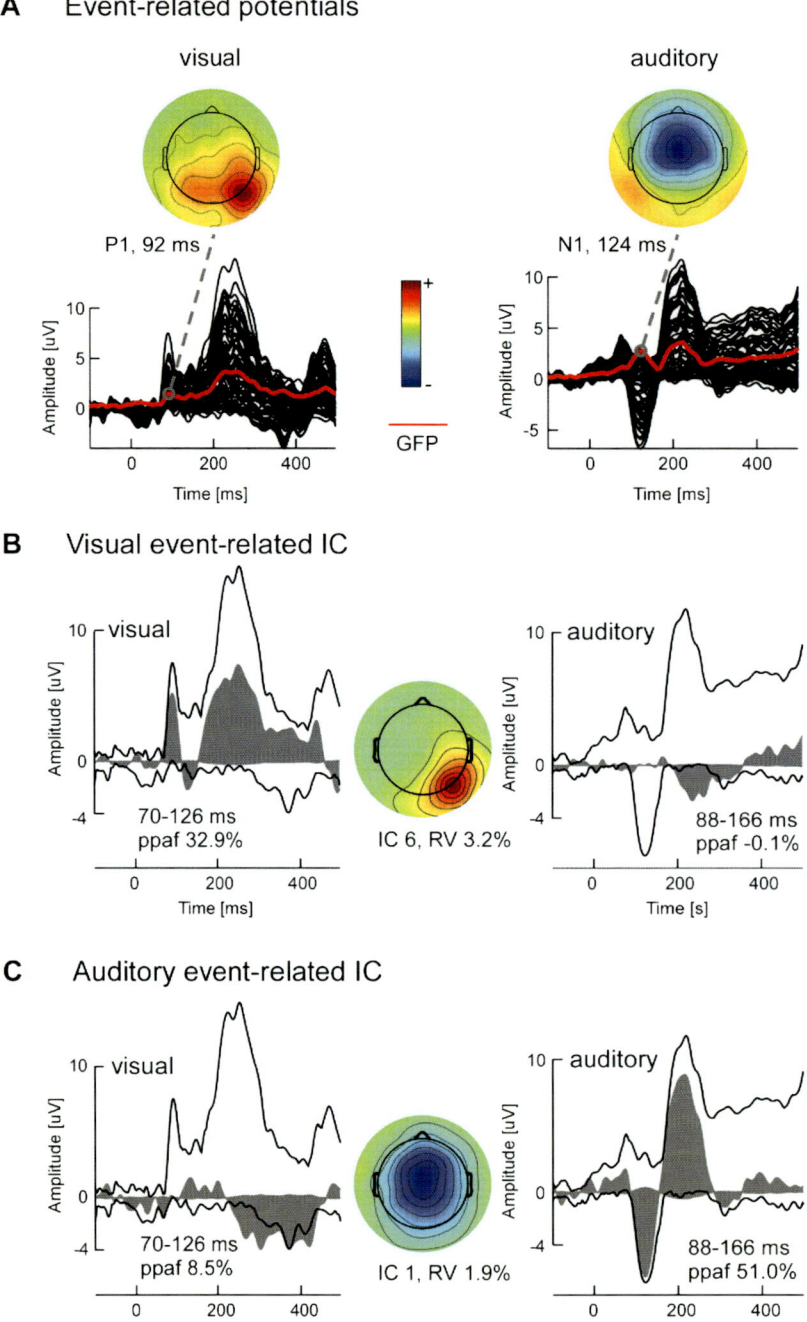

Figure 3.1.5. Two example ICs representing event-related brain activity. A: ERPs from a single subject in response to acoustic and visual stimulation. Shown are VEPs and AEPs, respectively, for all recorded channels (black traces) and the topography for the indicated VEP at the P1 peak latency (92 ms) and for the AEP at the N1 peak latency (124 ms). B: Contribution of IC 6 to the VEP (left) and AEP (right), indicated by showing the channel ERP envelope (the minima-maxima across all recording channels, black traces) and, in grey, the envelope of the back-projection of this component, explaining approximately 32% of the total variance of the VEP in the 70-126 ms interval. The same IC does not contribute to the AEP N1 interval (88-166 ms). C: Contribution of IC 1 to the VEP (left) and AEP (right). This component explained 51% of the variance in the N1 latency range (88–166 ms), but did not contribute substantially to the VEP in the 70–126 ms interval. PPAF = percentage of power accounted for; GFP = global field power; RV = residual variance.

First, reliability depends on the amount of data submitted to the algorithm. ICA requires a sufficient number of training data to produce near identical solutions for the repeated decomposition of the identical data. It is difficult to estimate how much data are needed but high density data require more training data than low density data, because n^2 weights need to be trained (where n refers to the number of channels). An illustration of the effect of the number of training

A   Subject #1   **B**   Subject #2

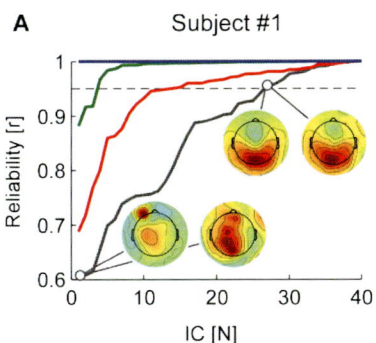
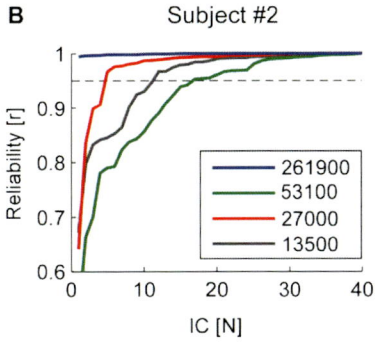

Figure 3.1.6. Effect of the number of training data on ICA reliability for two representative subjects (A, B). Time courses reflect the degree of correlation between the ICA maps of a first and second decomposition of the identical data, sorted in ascending order. Blue line reflects decomposition of all epochs (after rejection of those containing nonstereotype artifacts, see below), other lines a subsample of approx. 20% (green), 10% (red) and 5% (grey) of all data. For the 5% condition from subject #1, two pairs of IC maps are shown, illustrating maps with very high and very low reliability. Note that only the decomposition of all epochs (blue line) revealed near-perfect reliability for both subjects and all ICs.

data on the reliability of ICA is given in Figure 3.1.6. A rule of thumb has suggested at least $20^\star n^2$ data as a minimum number of training data (Onton et al., 2006).

According to the rule of thumb mentioned above, for a 68-channel dataset at least 92480 data points (training data) would be necessary to achieve a reliable decomposition. To test this we applied ICA twice to identical data, and correlated the weights from the first and second applications to identify maximum correlations for each component. This was done for 40 dimensions and the concatenated epochs that remained after rejection of epochs containing atypical activity (Delorme et al., 2007a). The correlation procedure was repeated for all data (261900), which exceeded the $20^\star n^2$ criterion, and sub-samples of the data epochs, representing about 20, 10, and 5% of the available data points, thus not passing this criterion. This enabled us to study the effect of the length of the training data on the reliability of ICA. Shown are the reliability values for each IC, sorted in ascending order. As can be seen for subject 1 (Figure 3.1.6A), all ICs trained on the total data were retest reliable, as evidenced by correlation values of r >.99. The 20% subsample of these data (green line) also indicated good retest reliability, with 37 out of 40 ICs showing correlations of r >.95. However, the results for the 10% (red) and 5% (gray) subsamples show that retest-reliability was further reduced to an unacceptable level. In the 5% dataset, only 17 ICs could be considered retest reliable, if one applies the r >.95 criterion, strongly indicating an insufficient amount of data.

The results shown in Figure 3.1.6A clearly support the common statement that ICA needs "a lot" of training data to achieve a stable decomposition. However, the conclusion that "more is always better" may be a bit premature. To illustrate this, data from another representative subject are shown in Figure 3.1.6B. As for subject 1, the decomposition of the total data from subject 2 revealed near perfect retest reliability. However, a comparison of the 20% dataset (green line) with the 10% and 5% subsamples shows that retest reliability was higher for the smaller compared to the larger number of training data (Figure 3.1.6B). In the 10% dataset (red line), 36

ICs correlated with r >.95, whereas in the 20% dataset, only 24 ICs met this criterion. Accordingly, it can be speculated that, in addition to the quantity of the data, the quality of the data plays an important role as well. It is likely that the data from subject 2 contained sections that were not in accord with the ICA assumptions. For the 100% dataset, which also included these sections and was of the size of approximately $56^\star n^2$, this did not affect retest reliability. In other words, for very large numbers of training data, temporally constrained violations of ICA assumptions seem to be tolerable. However, the 20% dataset, which was of the size of approximately $11^\star n^2$, was apparently substantially affected by these data sections. This illustrates that in cases where large numbers of training data are not available, a better retest reliability may be achieved by using fewer but more consistent data for ICA decomposition. Similarly, ICA decompositions of ERPs tend to return disappointing results, probably because not enough training data is provided. It can also be argued that most of the information that could be used to define independence might be lost in the average (Makeig et al., 2004a). Finally, the rule of thumb mentioned above should in our opinion be considered in light of the low-pass filter used, not the sampling rate. Using a low low-pass filter in combination with a high sampling rate may not help in achieving good reliability, because this does not add information to the existing data. Instead, the frequency of the recording low-pass filter may be considered to estimate the required number of samples for a reproducible decomposition. In any case, it is recommended that the reliability of data of interest be assessed (Groppe et al., 2009). This could be done by simple correlation statistics as outlined here, or by using more advanced tools such as ICASSO (http://www.cis.hut.fi/projects/ica/icasso/).

Good Components, Bad Components

Keeping the reliability problem in mind, it is important to note that most ICA solutions of EEG data are rarely fully considered and analyzed. That is, in most practical cases,

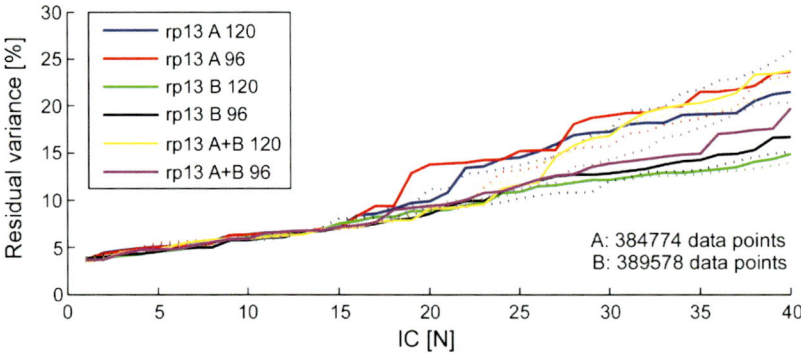

Figure 3.1.7. Relationship between the reliability and dipolarity of independent components, illustrated for a single subject 128 channel EEG recording. Plotted is the residual variance (RV) of 40 independent components, in ascending order, for several different ICA models. Solid lines refer to the first, dotted lines to the repeated decomposition of the identical model/data, with color indicating different models. A = data of the first half of a 128 channel EEG recordings, B = data of the second half of the recording, A+B = all data. 120, 96 = number of components decomposed. Note that for the dipolar ICs (those with residual variance <10%), lines overlap each other near perfectly.

researchers tend to choose some ICs, but do not usually consider all available components. This raises the important question as to whether those ICs of scientific interest are retest reliable or not. In the former case, the issue of training data quantity becomes less significant practically, but in the latter case, it would raise substantial concerns about the usage of ICA. Figure 3.1.6A shows two pairs of ICs from the 5% training dataset, one pair expressing high retest reliability (here r =.96) and one with low retest reliability (r =.61). As can be seen, the reliable pair expressed a dipolar-like topography, that is, a map that could be reasonably well modeled by a single dipole or by two symmetric dipoles. Dipolarity has been used as a criterion for the selection of ICs representing brain activity (e.g., Makeig et al., 2004a; Makeig et al., 2004b; see also Figure 3.1.5), and it is therefore of interest to consider the relationship between the dipolarity and reliability of ICs. Are dipolar ICs more reliable than non-dipolar ones? In order to explore this issue, we repeatedly decomposed a 128 channel EEG recording in several different ways, the results of which are summarized in Figure 3.1.7. Each model was repeated once (dotted lines), and six different models are shown (in different colors). Here, either all data (A + B; 777352 data points) or the first (A; 384774 data points) or second (B; 389578 data points) half of the recording were used. Additionally, different numbers of dimensions were considered by employing PCA reduction to either 120 or 96 components. Shown are the sorted dipolarity values for each model, as revealed by single equivalent current dipole modeling using the DIPFIT EEGLAB plug-in and a spherical head model (www.sccn.eeglab.edu).

As can be seen, the lines substantially overlap each other for those ICs expressing a high dipolarity (i.e., low residual variance, RV). This holds for the different models as well as for the replication of the identical model (solid versus dotted lines). We repeatedly observed this pattern in several subjects, and interpret this as evidence for the view that dipolar ICs tend

to be more reliable than non-dipolar ICs. Accordingly, the focus on dipolar ICs seems a reasonable strategy. High dipolarity of ICs representing brain activity seems to indicate a successful and reliable unmixing process.

EEG Preprocessing and ICA Outcome

According to the model outlined above, ICA should separate EEG artifacts from brain activity patterns. Moreover, ICA should also separate different brain activity patterns originating from different areas of the brain from each other (see Onton et al., 2006, for discussion). Accordingly, ICs reflecting brain activity can be assumed to express an equivalent current dipolar pattern to the EEG signal, representing the contribution from one cortical area (or in some cases two homologous areas), and a maximally temporally independent activity profile. IC 6 in Figure 3.1.5 shows one example of a dipolar IC probably representing brain activity from right occipital cortex and contributing predominantly to the visual evoked potential. In addition to the issue of training data quantity discussed in section 3.2.5, what other factors might favorably affect ICA quality?

Rejection of Nonstereotype Artifacts

One strategy recommended by several labs employing ICA regularly is the rejection of nonstereotyped artifacts, such as those due to gross head movement, cable movement, or swallowing. All these contributions usually occur only for small sections of EEG recordings, but may unfavorably change the "More signals than sources" ratio of ICA. Accordingly, the data should be "pruned" from those nonstereotype sections before they are submitted to ICA. In contrast, more common and frequent EEG artifacts such as eye blinks or eye movements seem repeatedly to express the same source signal to the EEG, and it can therefore be considered a good investment to spend a few ICs on modeling (and thereby potentially removing) their activity patterns. Note that nonstereotyped artifacts are not specifically identified by a simple amplitude criterion, as this would find eye blinks for instance as well. Also, some nonstereotyped artifacts may not necessarily contribute high-amplitude signals to the EEG. It is therefore recommended to use more advanced artifact identification algorithms, such as those operating on the probability of amplitude distributions (Delorme et al., 2007a).

Removal of Channel Drifts

Given the enormous dynamic range of modern EEG amplifiers, many researchers tend to record EEG data now with the filters wide open. In the low frequency range, this usually comes at the expense of recording high amplitude drifts in the <1 Hz frequency range, which may be largely caused by electrode potentials or sweating artifacts, among other things. We find that these low-frequency contributions, which are often spatially unstable and fluctuate substantially over time, have an adverse effect on ICA quality. This may be because these low-frequency contributions add spatially nonstationary signals to the EEG, and compromise the "More sensors than sources" assumption. It is therefore recommended that those portions are removed by application of a suitable high-pass filter or by de-trending of the data. In our experience, this tends to return more reliable, and more dipolar ICs. At first glance, this recommendation may prevent using ICA for DC-recorded EEGs and the study of slow potentials (e.g., Schicke et al., 2006). However, a solution to this problem would be to train the ICA weights on high pass filtered data and apply the results to the unfiltered data. This approach would allow, for instance, the use of ICA for eye blink removal in DC EEG recordings.

Decomposition of Continuous Data Versus Concatenated Single Trials

Much less clear is the issue of whether continuous EEG recordings or concatenated single trials should be submitted to ICA. In light of the reliability issue, one might argue for the decomposition of continuous recordings, as this would, for most experimental paradigms, result in more data points and thus the likelihood of improved ICA reliability. However, following the assumptions of the additive ERP model, neural sources that cause ERP deflections may be regarded as contributing activity to the EEG recording specifically for rather small intervals that are phase-locked to some events of interest. Accordingly, if the aim is to identify ICs that refer to classical ERP components, it might be advisable to constrain ICA training to these intervals of interest, which could be done by concatenating the corresponding single trials or epochs. However, doubts have been expressed over the adequacy of the additive ERP model, and it is not yet known whether the additive model is more valid than alternative accounts (e.g., Sauseng and Klimesch, 2008). One of these alternative accounts would state, in contrast, that there is no clear distinction between sources contributing to the ongoing EEG and those contributing to the event-related EEG (e.g., Makeig et al., 2004a). According to this view, EEG alpha oscillations for instance should be modeled as carefully as possible to study how they might contribute to visual evoked potentials (Makeig et al., 2002). Accordingly, concatenated long epochs or even the continuous recordings should be submitted to ICA, as this increases the likelihood of returning a better identification and separation of ICs representing ongoing alpha activity. In short, no clear recommendation can be given for the decomposition of epoched versus continuous data, as this depends on the research question asked and is linked to the view a researcher may have about event-related brain function.

Low-Pass Filtering and Down Sampling

One of the commonly mentioned disadvantages of ICA is that it can take considerable time for the algorithm to converge to a solution. Among other issues, the size of the training data is an important determinant of computation time, and therefore, reducing the number of training data— within the limits of reliable solutions—is a practical consideration. One way to achieve a substantial speed-up would be to down-sample the recorded data, which are usually recorded over-sampled, in order to prevent aliasing problems. Thus, if the focus is on ERPs and/or other low frequency EEG activity, it may be advisable to down-sample EEG data recorded at 1000 Hz (with a 200 Hz analog low-pass filter) to a sampling rate of 250 Hz, after further low-pass filtering (e.g., 80 Hz). As a result, a substantial reduction in computation time can be expected. However, it should be noted that the degree of low-pass filtering can have a negative effect. While low-pass filtering yields an important noise reduction, very substantial low-pass filtering has also been reported to increase the likelihood of over-fitting the input data (Gómez-Herrero et al., 2005). Care should be taken to not remove too much information from the EEG data by using a too narrow passband before ICA decomposition.

Removal of Bad Channels

Another practical consideration is the management of bad channels, that is, electrodes that have lost good contact to the scalp or show other forms of malfunctioning during the recording. It seems to be the case that some EEG cap and electrode systems are more prone to creating bad channels than others, and it would of course be best to use systems and procedures that avoid the occurrence of bad channels. However, unforeseen circumstances may counteract this standard, raising the question of how ICA outcome could be affected by inclusion of bad channels. The signal contributed by bad channels can be seen as further inflating the dimensionality of EEG data and also increasing the risk of nonstationarity. Thus, activity from bad channels should be removed before ICA decomposition, as it can massively deteriorate otherwise good decomposition results. If bad channel replacement is implemented by means of spatial interpolation, it should be kept in mind that the dimensionality of the data set is reduced by the number of the interpolated bad channels. The resulting rank-deficiency can cause problems for ICA algorithms to converge, and the procedure of bad channel interpolation may therefore be combined with a subsequent dimensionality reduction step to prevent this.

Conclusion

Over the past decade, ICA has become increasingly popular in EEG/MEG research. Besides the significant achievements that have been made by using ICA, the increased experience with this technique requires us to draw some practical conclusions, simply because the success of ICA should not overshadow the potential limitations inherent in it. First, using ICA does not necessarily guarantee an unmixing into physiologically plausible components. Although it is sometimes forgotten that this argument does not selectively apply to ICA, the plausibility of independent components is a matter of interpretation and not given inherently by the data. Second, unmixing multi-channel EEG/MEG data with ICA does not necessarily return a reliable decomposition. We have discussed some of the main factors that seem to contribute to the reliability of ICA decompositions. In particular, we argue that different preprocessing steps should be selected and adjusted keeping the ICA model assumptions in mind. This allows one to appreciate that, when adequately chosen, preprocessing can help to produce more reliable solutions. Third, there is at least preliminary evidence that these two issues, interpretability and reliability, are closely related. In terms of physiological plausibility, it makes sense to assume dipolar or near dipolar independent components (see Makeig et al., 2004a, for discussion), and independent components contributing with a dipolar spatial pattern to the EEG tend to be more reliable than non-dipolar ones. Dipolar components are also more robustly observed across subjects than non-dipolar ones. However, it is not yet fully understood how dipolarity and reliability of independent components relate to each other, and this issue clearly requires further research. And finally, more recent ICA algorithm developments may also help to further optimize the amount of information that can be identified in, and used from, EEG/MEG recordings. Careful comparison and validation studies are needed to advance our knowledge on which algorithm performs best for a given type of data or problem. It is unlikely that any single algorithm is superior to all others for all practical questions that can be addressed with ICA-based EEG/MEG analysis. However, future developments will bring better algorithms and better validation criteria and it is evident that, while not perfect, ICA can be expected to continue providing a significant contribution to cognitive brain research.

NOTE

1. Here, for the sake of simplicity, we ignore the problem of sound travel time delays which greatly complicates the unmixing process. A similar problem does not however exist for EEG recordings.

REFERENCES

Debener S, Makeig S, Delorme A, Engel AK (2005a) What is novel in the novelty oddball paradigm? Functional significance of the novelty P3 event-related potential as revealed by independent component analysis. Cognitive Brain Res 22:309–321.

Debener S, Ullsperger M, Siegel M, Fiehler K, von Cramon DY, Engel AK (2005b) Trial-by-trial coupling of concurrent electroencephalogram and functional magnetic resonance imaging identifies the dynamics of performance monitoring. J Neurosci 25:11730–11737.

Debener S, Ullsperger M, Siegel M, Engel AK (2006) Single-trial EEG/fMRI reveals the dynamics of cognitive function. Trends Cogn Sci 10:558–563.

Debener S, Mullinger KJ, Niazy RK, Bowtell RW (2007) Properties of the ballistocardiogram artefact as revealed by EEG recordings at 1.5, 3 and 7 T static magnetic field strength. Int J Psychophysiol 67:189–199.

Debener S, Hine J, Bleeck S, Eyles J (2008) Source localization of auditory evoked potentials after cochlear implantation. Psychophysiology 45:20–24.

Delorme A, Sejnowski T, Makeig S (2007a) Enhanced detection of artifacts in EEG data using higher-order statistics and independent component analysis. Neuroimage 34:1443–1449.

Delorme A, Westerfield M, Makeig S (2007b) Medial prefrontal theta bursts precede rapid motor responses during visual selective attention. J Neurosci 27:11949–11959.

Gómez-Herrero G, Huupponen E, Värri A, Egiazarian K, Vanrumste B, Vergult A, De Clercq W, Van Huffel S, Van Paesschen W (2005) Independent component analysis of single trial evoked brain responses: is it reliable? In: Proceedings of IEEE/IEE International Conference on Computational Intelligence in Medicine and Healthcare (CIMED'2005), pp 69–76. Costa da Caparica, Portugal.

Groppe DM, Makeig S, Kutas M (2009) Identifying reliable independent components via split-half comparisons. Neuroimage 45:1199–211.

Hine J, Davis A, Debener S (2008) Does unilateral deafness change auditory evoked potential asymmetries? Clin Neurophysiol 119:576–586.

Hyvärinen A, Karhunen J, Oja E (2001) Independent component analysis. New York: John Wiley & Sons.

Jung TP, Makeig S, Humphries C, Lee TW, McKeown MJ, Iragui V, Sejnowski TJ (2000a) Removing electroencephalographic artifacts by blind source separation. Psychophysiology 37:163–178.

Jung TP, Makeig S, Westerfield M, Townsend J, Courchesne E, Sejnowski TJ (2000b) Removal of eye activity artifacts from visual event-related potentials in normal and clinical subjects. Clin Neurophysiol 111:1745–1758.

Makeig S, Westerfield M, Jung TP, Enghoff S, Townsend J, Courchesne E, Sejnowski TJ (2002) Dynamic brain sources of visual evoked responses. Science 295:690–694.

Makeig S, Debener S, Onton J, Delorme A. (2004a) Mining event-related brain dynamics. Trends Cogn Sci 8:204–210.

Makeig S, Delorme A, Westerfield M, Jung TP, Townsend J, Courchesne E, Sejnowski TJ (2004b) Electroencephalographic brain dynamics following manually responded visual targets. Plos Biology 2:747–762.

Nunez PL, Srinivasan R (2006) Electric fields of the brain: The neurophysics of EEG. Oxford: Oxford University Press.

Viola FC, Thorne J, Edmonds B, Schneider T, Eichele T, Debener S (2009) Semi-automatic identification of independent components representing EEG artifact. Clin Neurophysiol. 120: 868–77.

Onton J, Delorme A, Makeig S (2005) Frontal midline EEG dynamics during working memory. Neuroimage 27:341–356.

Onton J, Westerfield M, Townsend J, Makeig S (2006) Imaging human EEG dynamics using independent component analysis. Neurosci Biobehav R 30:808–822.

Särelä J, Vigário R (2004) Overlearning in marginal distribution-based ICA: analysis and solutions. J Mach Learn Res 4:1447–1469.

Sauseng P, Klimesch W (2008) What does phase information of oscillatory brain activity tell us about cognitive processes? Neurosci Biobehav R 32:1001–1013.

Schicke T, Muckli L, Beer AL, Wibral M, Singer W, Goebel R, Rösler F, Röder B (2006) Tight covariation of BOLD signal changes and slow ERPs in the parietal cortex in a parametric spatial imagery task with haptic acquisition. Eur J Neurosci 23:1920–1918.

Stone JV (2004) Independent component analysis: a tutorial introduction. Cambridge, MA: MIT Press.

3.2

Giancarlo Valente, Fabrizio Esposito, Federico de Martino, Rainer Goebel, and Elia Formisano

Using ICA for the Analysis of fMRI Data

Introduction

Noninferential or data-driven multivariate methods are being increasingly used in functional magnetic resonance imaging (fMRI) data analysis. The rationale of their application is substantially different from the most commonly used inferential or hypothesis-driven approach, in which one or few predefined activation contrasts are tested voxel-by-voxel using univariate statistics (e.g., general linear model [GLM]).

Exploratory methods provide a characterization of the fMRI time series in terms of spatiotemporal modes. Importantly, this characterization does not require detailed knowledge and modeling of the signals of interest and noise. Whereas a statistical analysis based on the GLM is blind to all those brain activations and artifacts that are not modeled within the design matrix, a data-driven approach may pinpoint interesting effects or identify and correct for confounding factors whose spatiotemporal profile could not be anticipated.

The most used exploratory approaches in fMRI are principal component analysis (PCA) (Friston et al., 1993), independent component analysis (ICA) (McKeown et al., 1998b; McKeown et al., 1998a; McKeown and Sejnowski, 1998), and statistical clustering (Baumgartner et al., 1997; Baumgartner et al., 2000). Both PCA and ICA are based on a *linear mixture model*, i.e., the observed data are interpreted as a linear mixture of a set of spatiotemporal modes that can be retrieved by means of suitable criteria. While PCA is based on the maximization of the explained variance within an orthogonal basis, ICA accounts for spatial (or temporal) independence of patterns of brain activity (see below).

It has been noted that the interpretation of the principal components of an fMRI data set may be troublesome (Petersson et al., 1999). In fact, fMRI principal components are constrained to be orthogonal both in the spatial and the temporal dimension. Considering that the temporal profile

of various effects of interests and artifacts may be correlated (e.g., activation in gray matter and in large vessels), it is likely that a principal component includes a mixture of these effects. ICA overcomes the limitations inherent to PCA by seeking statistical independence in one dimension (normally in the spatial dimension) while leaving the other dimension unconstrained.

An illustrative example of the principles underlying the use of ICA is the *cocktail party problem* (Hyvarinen et al., 2001). Assume that n conversations are being held in a room, and that n microphones are placed in different positions. Each microphone records all the conversations with different weights (according to the position, and assuming negligible delays in signal propagation). The aim of blind source separation (BSS) techniques—such as ICA—is to "recover" the original conversations (*sources*) from the different mixtures (*observations*). This problem is generally ill-posed, as both the sources and the weights of the sources in each observation have to be estimated. However, if the sources are *statistically independent*, then the solution is unique (under some very general assumptions, Comon, 1994).

In fMRI, in analogy to the cocktail effect, each functional scan can be regarded as a microphone, and spatial patterns of activations represent the conversations; each volume is thus modeled as a mixture of different sources, which are statistically independent.

This chapter examines the most relevant aspects concerning the use of ICA for the analysis of fMRI data. In particular, after illustrating the fMRI-ICA model ("Problem formulation and application to fMRI"), the chapter compares the most commonly used ICA algorithms in the context of fMRI data analysis ("Algorithms and performance"). The problems of choosing the dimensionality of the ICA decomposition and of selecting the "meaningful" components are considered in "Selection and interpretation of fMRI independent components." Optimizations of the ICA algorithms for

135

dealing with the specific spatiotemporal properties of the fMRI data and extensions of the ICA to multisubject fMRI studies are described in "Tailoring ICA to fMRI" and "ICA in multisubject fMRI studies." For each of these aspects, different approaches from various groups are briefly reviewed; greater emphasis, however, is posed on the recent methodological contributions from our group.

Problem Formulation and Application to fMRI

The multivariate statistical nature of ICA allows decomposing a four-dimensional fMRI data set into a set of activity patterns based on spatial or temporal independence.

The linear model considered in ICA is:

$$\mathbf{X} = \mathbf{AS} \qquad (1)$$

where X represents the fMRI data set and it is expressed as a linear combination of independent *sources* S by means of *mixing matrix* A. This model does not specifically account for noise in its formulation (*noiseless ICA*), as the noise is embedded among the sources.

Two different versions of ICA for fMRI can be considered, according to the dimension on which statistical independence is considered (Calhoun et al., 2001b). In spatial ICA (sICA) a dataset X is decomposed into a set of spatially independent activity patterns, with associated *unconstrained* time courses, while in temporal ICA (tICA) the dataset is decomposed into a set of temporally independent time courses with associated *unconstrained* spatial maps.

In sICA, a $t \times v$ matrix X (t = number of volumes, v = number of voxels) is decomposed into an $n \times v$ source matrix S, that has up to t rows and whose rows are (maximally) statistically independent, and a $t \times n$ mixing matrix A, whose columns are the time courses associated with the independent components. Conversely, in tICA data are decomposed such that the columns of A are maximally statistically independent. Given the typical dimensions of fMRI datasets, the spatial ICA model is usually preferred both for the plausibility of the underlying neurophysiological model (see below) and for computational requirements. In fact, as the number of voxels is much larger than the number of scans, temporal ICA may be computationally very demanding and therefore it is seldom applied to fMRI (Biswal and Ulmer, 1999; Calhoun et al., 2001b; Seifritz et al., 2002). Note that in sICA no orthogonality constraint is considered for the time-courses associated with the independent maps, and thus sICA proves more flexible than PCA in dealing with multiple spatiotemporal patterns with correlated time courses (Formisano and Goebel, 2003).

The sICA model for fMRI data was first proposed by McKeown et al. (1998b; McKeown et al., 1998a; McKeown

and Sejnowski, 1998; see Figure 3.2.1). Each of the n independent maps (left) contributes with different weights to the generation of the fMRI measurements (right side). The weights of this mixing process can be seen as shared time courses of the *whole* map, and all the maps with their associated time courses sum up linearly to give the measured signal.

McKeown and colleagues (McKeown and Sejnowski, 1998) also pointed out the assumptions underlying the use of ICA in fMRI data analysis and the requirements on the mixing model:

- Maps associated with independent activation in the brain are *sparse* and mostly *non-overlapping*, although some overlap may occur.
- The mixing coefficients are *constant* throughout the brain.
- The components *mix up linearly* to form the fMRI measurements.
- The number of components contained in data is limited to the number of time points in the measurements.

Subsequently, many brain imaging studies employing ICA have been published. In (Quigley et al., 2002) a comparison of classical hypothesis-driven methods and ICA was made on clinical functional MR images, showing that both techniques are able to identify spatiotemporal patterns of activity, with ICA being more robust in case of data sets corrupted by motion or by incorrect task performance. In Lange et al. (1999) the ICA analysis (based on INFOMAX algorithm) was compared to several other data methods on simulated

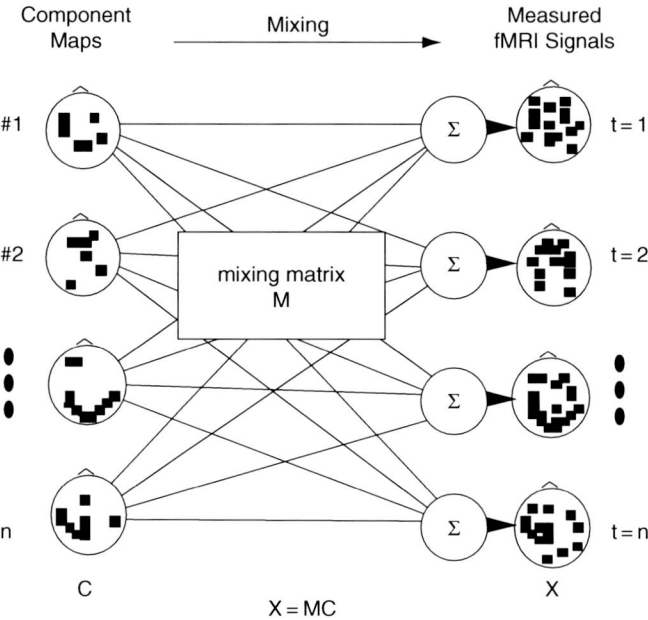

Figure 3.2.1. Spatial ICA model proposed in (McKeown et al., 1998a; McKeown and Sejnowski, 1998). Volumes are decomposed as sums of independent spatial maps with associated mixing coefficients. (Figure from McKeown et al. (1998a)).

and real fMRI data, proving that ICA was able to identify locations of activity not accessible by simple correlation, t-test, or GLM-based methods.

ICA has also been employed in challenging neuroscientific problems, e.g., involving visual ambiguous stimulations and bi-stable perception (Castelo-Branco et al., 2002), scanner-generated auditory stimulation (Seifritz et al., 2002), and spontaneous hallucinatory events (van de Ven et al., 2005). Considering the generality of its model, ICA is well suited for the analysis of data collected either with very complex sensory and cognitive stimulation (such as during simulated driving, Calhoun et al., 2002; or the natural vision of a movie, Bartels and Zeki, 2005) or with no stimulation at all, as in the study of resting state (van de Ven et al., 2004; De Luca et al., 2006) and default mode function (Greicius et al., 2004). Moreover, ICA has been employed effectively in fMRI preprocessing (Thomas et al., 2002; Liao et al., 2005), as the independent components corresponding to artifacts and noise can be removed from the data.

Algorithms and Performance

Solving an ICA problem consists of finding an unmixing matrix $W = A^{-1}$ such that an estimate of the components $S' = WX$ are maximally statistically independent.

As it proves difficult to estimate the joint probability density function of the components directly, several methods have been proposed for estimating their independence. In general, to find an ICA decomposition of the observed mixture, an *objective function* denoting independence is defined, and an optimization procedure is chosen for maximizing it. Both the objective function and the optimization procedure affect the overall performances of the ICA. The objective function influences the statistical properties, like consistency, asymptotic variance, and robustness, while the optimization procedure influences the algorithmic properties, like convergence speed, memory requirement and numerical stability (Hyvarinen et al., 2001).

For what concerns the objective functions, they can be grouped into those that estimate all the components together, and those that estimate one component at a time. Even if the first class seems to be more "related" to the problem of estimating independence (as independence is defined *among* all the components), the one-unit objective functions have some appealing properties from both computational and algorithmic stability point of view.

Many of the objective functions proposed stem from information theoretic criteria, or from non-linear decorrelation principles. For comprehensive reviews, refer to Hyvarinen et al. (2001) and Chicocki and Amari (2002). In the next part of this section, two of the most employed algorithms for ICA of fMRI data analysis are briefly described. Both INFOMAX (Bell and Sejnowski, 1995) and FastICA (Hyvarinen and Oja, 1997; Hyvarinen, 1999) have been extensively used in fMRI data analysis, and their performances have been compared using simulated and real fMRI data (Esposito et al., 2002).

Infomax

Minimization of mutual information is a "natural" way of looking for independence. In fact, if n random variables are statistically independent, their mutual information is zero.

A neural network approach has been proposed in Bell and Sejnowski (1995), where, by maximizing the differential entropy of the output it is possible to minimize its mutual information.

The maximization of output entropy of the network, whose transfer function is $g(x)$, is obtained when the high density parts of probability density function of x are aligned with the high sloping parts of nonlinearity $g(x)$. For instance, a logistic transfer function can be chosen for this purpose:

$$g(x) = \frac{1}{1 + e^{-u}}, \quad u = wx + w_0 \tag{2}$$

Output entropy maximization is performed by means a stochastic gradient optimization, which leads to the learning rules for the two parameters of the transfer function w and w_0:

$$\Delta w \propto \frac{1}{w} + x(1 - 2y) \tag{3}$$

$$\Delta w_0 \propto x(1 - 2y) \tag{4}$$

There are some cases, however, where the Infomax algorithm, as presented in (Bell and Sejnowski, 1995), fails to recover the sources. This happens in the presence of *sub-Gaussian* sources (i.e., with negative kurtosis, see Hyvarinen et al., 2001). To overcome this drawback, an extension of the algorithm has been proposed, based on maximum likelihood estimation, and it is commonly referred to as "Extendend Infomax" (Lee et al., 1999).

FastICA

The algorithm known as FastICA (Hyvarinen and Oja, 1997; Hyvarinen, 1999) is one of the most popular ICA algorithms, and both its speed and accuracy make it one of the most used in various applications including fMRI. The principle of FastICA is the maximization of non-Gaussianity, which is estimated by means of a negentropy approximation.

Non-Gaussianity maximization is closely related to independence by means of the central limit theorem (Papoulis, 1991; Ross, 1997). Loosely speaking, this theorem states that the (standardized) sum of n random variables tends to be distributed with a Gaussian probability density function (PDF), in the limit of n going to infinity. However, if the variables have the same distribution, around 30 signals will be enough such that the distribution of the sum is Gaussian. Moreover, in the case of smooth densities, a value of n as low as 5 can be used (Papoulis, 1991).

Source S is estimated as the linear combination of observed data X that has maximally independent components. This problem can be reformulated in terms of non-Gaussianity maximization. Since the original sources have a non-Gaussian distribution (at most there can be only one with such PDF (Comon, 1994)), the Central Limit Theorem indicates that a linear combination of them has a pdf that is closer to a Gaussian or at most equal to one of the sources. Therefore, the linear combinations that maximize non-Gaussianity are an estimate of independent sources.

A suitable function for non-Gaussianity is *kurtosis*, which is defined as the fourth-order cumulant, and has the property of being always zero for Gaussian distributions and nonzero for (almost) all non-Gaussian distributions. Kurtosis, however, lacks robustness to outliers, and usually more robust

measures, like *negentropy* (Hyvarinen, 1999) are employed. Negentropy is defined as:

$$J(y) = H(y_{Gauss}) - H(y) \qquad (5)$$

where H denotes the (differential) entropy and y_{Gauss} denotes a variable with the same mean and standard deviation as y, but with a Gaussian distribution. Negentropy is always nonnegative and is zero only if y has a Gaussian distribution (a Gaussian variable has the *largest* entropy among *all* the random variables having the same mean and variance, Cover and Thomas, 1991). Moreover, it is scale-invariant, making it a suitable contrast function for ICA.

In (Hyvarinen, 1999) a robust approximation of Negentropy by means of a non-linearity G has been proposed:

$$J(y) \propto \left[E\{G(y)\} - E\{G(v)\} \right]^2 \qquad (6)$$

where v is a normally distributed variable with the same mean and variance as y. The quality of the approximation depends on the choice of function G, whereas a smoothly growing G helps having a robust estimation. In

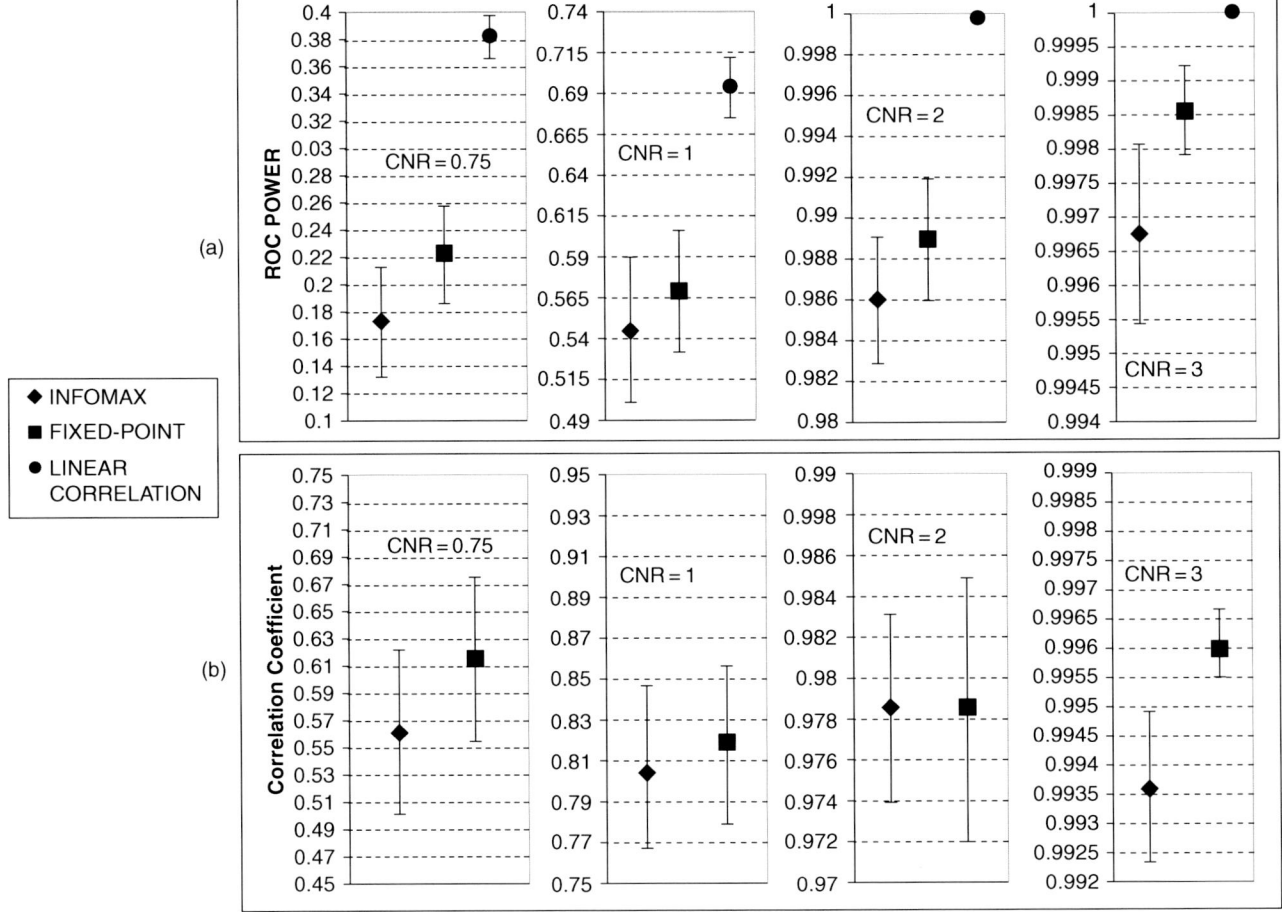

Figure 3.2.2. Results of the comparison between the Infomax and the Fixed-Point ICA algorithms on simulated activation data (Esposito et al., 2002). a): Spatial accuracy (as assessed by ROC analysis) of ICA maps and linear correlation maps. b): Temporal accuracy (as assessed by correlation analysis) of the time courses of the task-related ICA components.

(Hyvarinen, 1999) several functions have been proposed and tested.

FastICA is a fixed point algorithm optimizing the negentropy approximation in Equation 6 (Hyvarinen, 1999); each iteration of the algorithm consists of three steps: weight update, decorrelation, and normalization steps. These steps can be performed by extracting either one component at a time (*deflation* approach) or all the components together (*symmetric* approach).

Comparison on Simulated and Real fMRI Data

Esposito et al. (2002) compared the performances of Infomax and FastICA for spatial ICA of fMRI data using simulated motor, and real motor and visual activation fMRI time-series and an ensemble of performance measures.

The authors performed a *Likelihood analysis*, characterizing the extracted components by means of *Minus Log–Likelihood* of the data, computed for each voxel included in the analysis and averaged across all voxels (or regions of interest) (McKeown et al., 1998a). This analysis was performed on real activation data and showed that the increase of the number of the principal components selected by the preliminary PCA and used in the ICA decomposition produced a progressive decline of the averaged Minus-Log-Likelihood estimate (corresponding to an improved likelihood of the decomposition). This reduction is normally greater for the Infomax algorithm compared to the FastICA algorithm.

The effectiveness of the two algorithms in estimating the temporal dynamics of the task-related effects was evaluated in terms of the cross-correlation coefficients between the time course of activity of the most consistently task-related components (Baumgartner et al., 2000; Esposito et al., 2002) and the reference time courses of the experiment. Spatial accuracy was evaluated using receiver operating characteristics (ROC) methodology (Sorenson and Wang, 1996; Skudlarski et al., 1999; Esposito et al., 2002) for either simulated (where it is possible to separate with infinite precision false and true activation areas) and real activation data. In this latter case, standard linear correlation maps were used as benchmarks.

Figure 3.2.2 shows the comparison results of the performances of the two algorithms on the artificial data at four different contrast-to-noise ratios (CNRs) of the simulated activation signal (CNR = 0.75, 1, 2, and 3). The measures of spatial and temporal accuracy indicate that the FastICA ensures slightly superior performances in terms of ROC power and correlation coefficient; however, the difference between the performances becomes significant only in the case of the highest CNR, suggesting that only strong activation phenomena, less corrupted by noise, tend to be better detected by the FastICA.

In conclusion, both algorithms produced comparable and highly accurate results; the FastICA slightly outperformed Infomax in terms of spatial and temporal accuracy as long as inferential statistics were employed as benchmarks. Conversely,

the Infomax sICA was superior in terms of global estimation of the ICA model and noise reduction capabilities.

Selection and Interpretation of fMRI Independent Components

When analyzing an fMRI dataset with ICA, the experimenter is usually confronted with the problems of: *(1)* choosing the number of independent components to be estimated (*dimension reduction*) and, after the estimation has been performed, *(2)* selecting and interpreting a subset of "interesting" and "meaningful" components (*component selection*).

Dimensionality and Reliability: How Many Components?

Dimension reduction is usually performed by means of PCA, selecting the subspace associated with the highest eigenvalues of the covariance matrix. Several methods have been proposed for guiding the choice of a PCA cut-off and separating between signal and noise variance/covariance subspaces (Calhoun et al., 2001c; Beckmann and Smith, 2005; Cordes and Nandy, 2006). Nonetheless, the number of ICs is often chosen using empirical approaches (van de Ven et al., 2008) or simple rules of thumb (Greicius et al., 2007) instead of being estimated from the data (Calhoun et al., 2009).

One criticism to PCA-based methods for dimension estimation is that they only examine the variance contribution of orthogonal components, which seems to contradict the fact that properties other than variance drive the actual ICA decomposition. The simulation below shows that *(1)* reliable independent components can still be recovered below a cut-off dimension determined using PCA-based methods, and *(2)* a range of dimensions can be indentified where reliable components remain stable, despite the reliability of some components decreases with increasing dimensions.

In this simulation five spatial sources were added to real resting-state fMRI data (180 whole-brain echoplanar volumes at TR of 2*s*) by injecting artificial activation signals in five non-overlapping regions whose volumes ranged between 0.01% and 0.1% of a whole-brain fMRI slab; the CNR of 5 sources was graded from 5.0 down to 0.5. At these CNR values it was found that all five injected sources were successfully recovered and selected with 30 dimensions kept at the preliminary PCA stage, whereas a PCA-based dimensionality reduction (using, e.g., PPCA [Beckmann and Smith, 2004]) suggested a cut-off of 20 and 21 dimensions respectively for the resting-state (*RS*) and resting-state + 5 simulated sources (*RS+5S*) data sets. We also noted that only three out of five true sources were recovered by ICA with 21 dimensions kept for the *RS+5S* data set. This example illustrates the potential limitations of PCA-based approaches in recovering weak sources.

An alternative useful concept for understanding the effect of data dimensionality on the ICA output is the reliability or stability of the ICA decomposition. Given the stochastic nature of ICA algorithms, two ICA runs performed on the same data set from different initial conditions will produce different sets of components; nonetheless, some of the components of the second ICA run will be very "similar" to some of the components of the first ICA run. Thereby, a given ICA component is said to be reliable or stable when its characteristic pattern (spatial layout and time-course of activity) remains stable across many ICA runs, (re)started from different (random) initial conditions (*randomization approach*). Since data dimensionality controls the amount of residual noise in the data, it seems natural to investigate the stability of ICA runs with respect to the dimensionality and, thus, the number of components extracted.

In order to asses the reliability of an entire set of components, such as a full ICA decomposition, similarity and clustering are used in a method called ICASSO (Himberg et al., 2004). In this framework, ICA is repeated many, e.g., 50, times, with randomized initial conditions and all components from all runs are submitted to a hierarchical clustering algorithm that explores the similarity between all components and produces partitions of them with the desired number of components per cluster. In a given partition and for each cluster, the similarity between the "average" component, cluster centroid, and all other components of the cluster (within-cluster similarity) provides an estimate of "compactness" of that cluster and, therefore, of the reliability of the member components. As is the case for the dimensionality, the optimal number of components per clusters (i.e., the optimal partition) is not known in advance. Nonetheless, it is possible to explore the tendency of components toward forming more or less compact clusters when changing the desired partition for discriminating between more and less reliable components. In fact, starting from the trivial case that only one component per cluster is allowed and increasing this number, those clusters with most reliable components tend to "preserve" themselves as highly compact clusters across new and more stringent partitions, whereas less reliable components tend to be joined together in less compact clusters.

To illustrate visually the issue of reliability of the independent components and its qualitative relation to dimensionality, image plots comparing the number of components in each ICASSO partition and the (ordered) within-cluster similarity of all clusters for that partition are presented in Figure 3.2.3 for different dimensionality of the *RS* and *RS+5S* data sets from the simulation described above. In these plots, the color scale from blue to dark red indicates increasing similarity from 0 to 1, the number of components in each partition is reported on the x-axis and the cluster indices (after reordering according to decreasing similarity values) are reported on the y axis. For instance, the similarity value at position (10, 20) corresponds to the intracluster similarity (or compactness) of the 20th cluster in a partition with 10 components per cluster.

Based on these plots, it is possible to observe how considering more than 30 dimensions (e.g., 40, 60, 80) seems to produce not more than 30 highly reliable ICs, whereas for 20 and 30 dimensions there are equally stable components up to the number of dimensions (which corresponds to the number of independent components extracted by each repeated decomposition). This indicates that using 30 dimensions would be the most parsimonious choice for recovering the highest number of reliable independent components from this data set while minimizing the number of unreliable components. On the other hand, it is also clear that using more dimensions is still a valid choice although it presents the drawback of producing many more "unreliable" components, which might render the selection more difficult.

Comparing the lowest right part of the plots for *RS* (upper panel) and *RS+5S* (lower panel) data sets at 30 dimensions (second column) it is possible to observe the presence of relatively more reliable components at this dimensionality for the *RS+5S* data set. This observation is consistent with the post hoc verification that only by selecting (at least) 28 dimensions (but not less) could all five injected sources be successfully recovered by ICA. These simulations have important implications for ICA in fMRI.

PCA remains the method-of-choice for selecting the dimension of the data before ICA decomposition. However, the search for an exact cut-off for PCA may be misleading, as ICA can extract reliably low-CNR sources. A reliability analysis using randomization and clustering like ICASSO

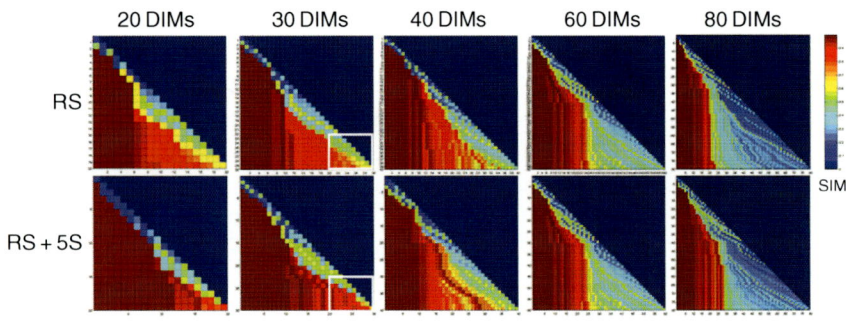

Figure 3.2.3. Image plots of intracluster centroid similarity vs. number of components per cluster (partition) at different dimensionality. Upper panels: resting-state data. Lower panels: resting-state data with 5 simulated sources added. The number of components in each partition is reported on the x-axis and the ordered cluster indices are reported on the y axis.

(Himberg et al., 2004) may be a useful and valid approach to decide the dimensionality before ICA. More in general, examining ICA results at multiple dimensionalities is important to gain confidence on the stability of the results (van de Ven et al., 2008).

Component Characterization and Classification: The IC-fingerprint

After the ICA decomposition has been performed, interesting components need to be selected for further analysis and interpretation. The simplest approach to this selection relies on the visual inspection of IC–spatial maps/time courses (Calhoun et al., 2001c; Bartels and Zeki, 2005). Selection of ICs based on their visual inspection, however, is very time consuming and highly dependent on the experience of the researcher. In most cases, ICs have been selected according to the amount of linear correlation of their time course with a model of the expected responses (McKeown et al., 1998a; Schmithorst and Brown, 2004; Moritz et al., 2005) or related measures in the temporal frequency domain (Moritz et al., 2003).

These approaches, however, appear to contrast with the data-driven nature of ICA. As an explorative tool, ICA may be particularly useful for detecting patterns of activity whose temporal dynamics cannot be easily modeled, such as in the case of hallucinations (van de Ven et al., 2005), epileptic seizures, or in sensory or cognitive paradigms in which expected hemodynamic responses may be very diverse (Castelo-Branco et al., 2002; Duann et al., 2002; Formisano et al., 2004). Furthermore, ICA is being increasingly used for the study of "resting-state" functional connectivity (Greicius et al., 2003; Greicius et al., 2004; van de Ven et al., 2004) or as a denoising step, which requires the selection of components reflecting noise and artifacts (Thomas et al., 2002). In all these cases, selection of ICs based on strong expectations on the profile of the IC–time courses is insufficient.

Alternatively, selection of ICs has been performed using strong a priori assumptions on the spatial layout of the activation (Castelo-Branco et al., 2002; van de Ven et al., 2004). In this approach, distributed brain networks are detected by selecting ICA components that load heavily in predefined regions of interest (ROIs). A priori expectation on one or more ROIs, however, is not always available and, as in ROI-based univariate analysis, interesting processes occurring outside the predefined ROIs are ignored.

Other, post hoc measures obtained from estimated ICs have been used for their sorting/selection. In analogy to PCA, McKeown et al. (1998a) sorted the ICs according to their variance contribution to the original mixture. In fMRI data, however, neurophysiologically interesting phenomena are usually weaker than some of the sources representing structured noise. Thus, ranking of the ICs in this way may not be informative. Formisano and colleagues (2002) characterized the ICs using a combination of three descriptive measures

(kurtosis of the spatial distribution, one-lag autocorrelation of the IC-time course and clustering of the IC's spatial layout). The underlying idea was that "meaningful" components aggregate in clustered regions in the three-dimensional space defined by these three measures. This heuristic criterion proved to be effective in isolating task-related components in a simple paradigm without using stimulus timing information.

De Martino et al. (2007) introduced the IC-*fingerprint*, a visual tool that aids the experimenter in displaying and characterizing the ICs. The IC-*fingerprint* is a representation of the component in a multidimensional space of descriptive measures, which can be visualized as a polar diagram (Figure 3.2.4). The underlying assumption is that ICs reflecting similar process types (e.g. BOLD activation, structured noise, movement) have similar *fingerprints*. To preserve the data-driven nature of ICA and the generality of the approach, the descriptive measures that define the space of the *fingerprints* are post hoc estimates of global properties of the ICs and do not rely on strong temporal or spatial hypotheses. In particular, values of eleven descriptive measures were derived from the IC's voxel values distribution (kurtosis, skewness, entropy), spatial layout (degree of clustering in the anatomical space), as well as their temporal (one-lag autocorrelation, entropy) and spectral (power contribution in five different frequency-bands) properties. For an exact definition of these measures and the rationale behind their inclusion see De Martino et al. (2007). An IC-*fingerprint* is thus a representation of an IC as a point of this eleven-dimensional space of parameters. IC-*fingerprints* are visualized using polar plots with eleven axes, each of them corresponding to one of the parameters normalized between 0 and 1.

Considering this type of representation, the problem of selecting "meaningful" components can be seen in the more general context of their (automatic) classification (see Figures 3.2.4 and 3.2.5). In fact, the selection problem can be formulated as subdividing the ICs in maximally disjoint classes and finding the optimal separating set of boundaries (hypersurfaces) in the multidimensional IC-fingerprint space.

In De Martino et al. (2007), a supervised learning algorithm (least-square support vector machine (Suykens et al., 2002) was trained by dividing the ICs from a small subset of data (one subject) into six classes of sources (see Figure 3.2.5). The trained algorithm classified automatically and with high correspondence to an expert classification the fMRI-ICs in all other subjects from the same experiment. Furthermore, the same classification algorithm has been successfully applied, without re-training, to fMRI collected using magnetic field, acquisition parameters, stimulation modality (auditory vs. visual) and timing (event-related vs. block design) considerably different from the experiment used for training (De Martino et al. 2007) and even in the clinical context of patients with focal epilepsy (Rodionov et al., 2007).

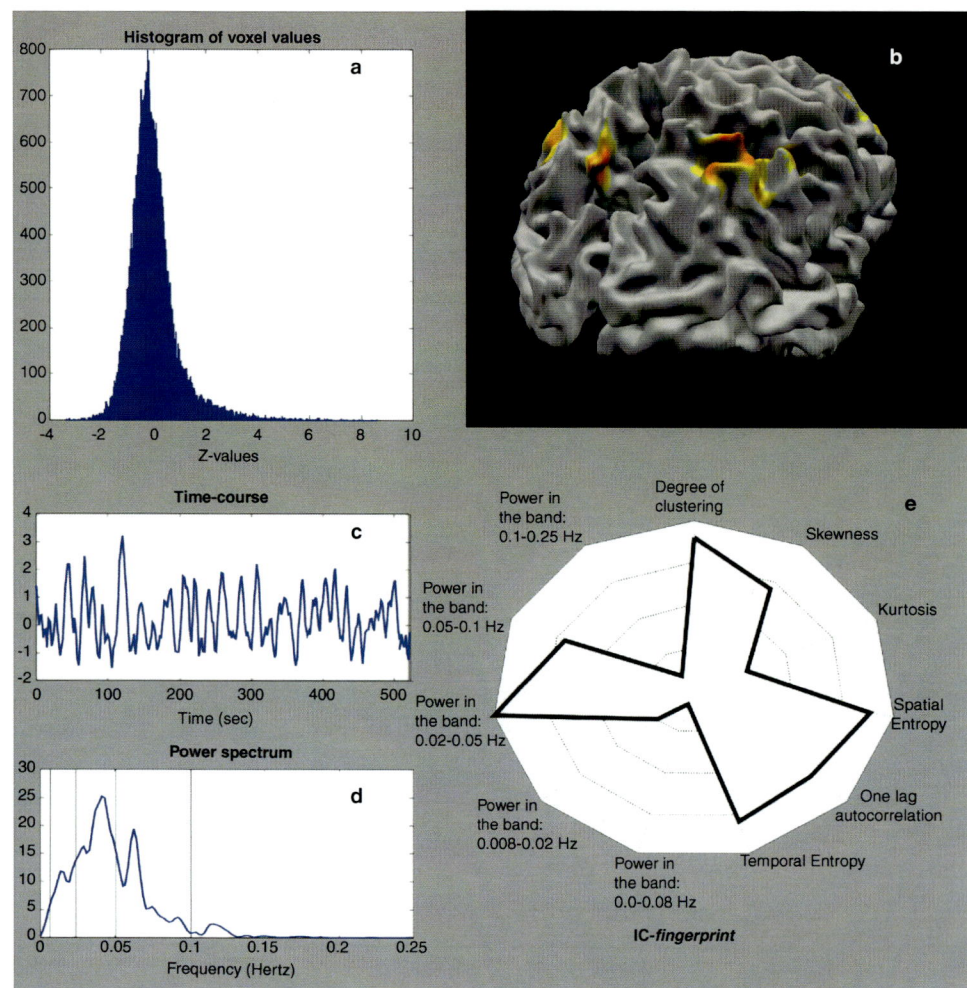

Figure 3.2.4. Characterization of one representative component in terms of its: a) histogram of voxel values; b) map layout (projected on the reconstructed cortical surface of the subject); c) time course; d) power spectrum; e) IC-*fingerprint*. Each axis in the polar plot corresponds to one of the normalized spatial, temporal, or spectral parameters. (From De Martino et al. (2007)).

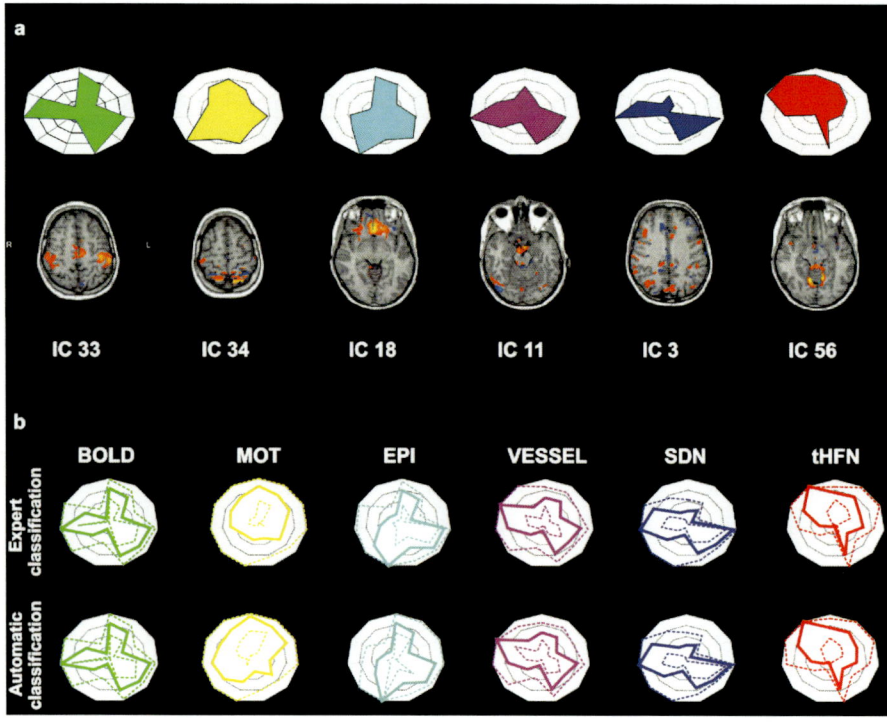

Figure 3.2.5. IC-*fingerprints* classes used in De Martino et al. (2007): BOLD class: components that are thought to reflect consistently task-related, transiently task-related, and non task-related (e.g., default state) neuronal activity; MOT: residual motion artifacts; EPI: typical EPI-susceptibility artifact, which is maximal in the frontal part of the brain; VESSEL: physiological noise with highly localized peaks (e.g., large vessels); SDN (spatially distributed noise): Noise at high spatial frequency; tHFN (temporal high frequency noise): Noise at high temporal frequency.

Tailoring ICA to fMRI

ICA algorithms (see "Algorithms and Performance," above) have been designed to decompose a set of observed signals X into a linear combination of statistically independent sources S. When used in fMRI, however, these algorithms do not consider the specific properties of this type of data, such as those deriving from the neuroanatomical and neurophysiological origins of the time series. Therefore several approaches have been proposed in order to optimize ICA for fMRI data analysis

Cortex-based ICA

In the sICA, as proposed in McKeown et al. (1998a), the entire matrix of the fMRI time-series is blindly decomposed. This matrix includes not only signals from the cerebral cortex, but also from other parts of the brain, including subcortical structures, white matter, and ventricles. The resulting decomposition, thus, also models the dynamics of the signal in these other structures.

In the cortex-based ICA (or cbICA; Formisano et al., 2004) sICA is combined with methods of cortex segmentation and reconstruction and the sICA decomposition is restricted to the "cortical" subregion of the matrix, improving the separation and anatomical accuracy of the ICs that represent cortical cognitive activations. As the number of voxels included in the data matrix does not affect the maximal number of spatial components which can be obtained (it equals the number of

time samples, i.e., functional scans), the exclusion of extra-cortical contributions to the signal data set allows using the same number of components, otherwise used to separate noninteresting processes (e.g., signal changes in the ventricles, near the eyes, imaging artifacts), only for the processes occurring on the cortical surface. Moreover, improvements are also observed because the measured spatial mixtures are influenced by the "nature" of the included signals. Signals from, e.g., the ventricles or near the eyes are "uninformative" with respect to the signals on the cortex. Thus, their inclusion in the data matrix leads to an increase in the complexity of the mixtures (in terms of number of sources) but does not improve the estimation of the cortical sources. Conversely, the restricted (yet statistically acceptable) sample of spatial observations considered in the cortex-based approach is highly "informative" with respect to the "interesting" sources and may lead to a better estimation of their spatial distribution. The steps of the cbICA are schematically illustrated in Figure 3.2.6. Input data sets consist of a high spatial resolution 3D anatomical volume and a functional time-series of the same subject, which have been previously co-registered.

Crucial to the application of the cbICA approach is the availability of an accurate reconstruction of each individual cortex and of an accurate coregistration between functional and anatomical data. In practice, this ensures an adequate selection of grey matter voxels. Due to partial volume effects and to the different resolution of functional and anatomical images, however, uncertainty can arise for the functional voxels at the border of the cortex. Alternatively, voxels may be treated using a probabilistic approach in which a voxel's contribution to the data set is weighted according to its

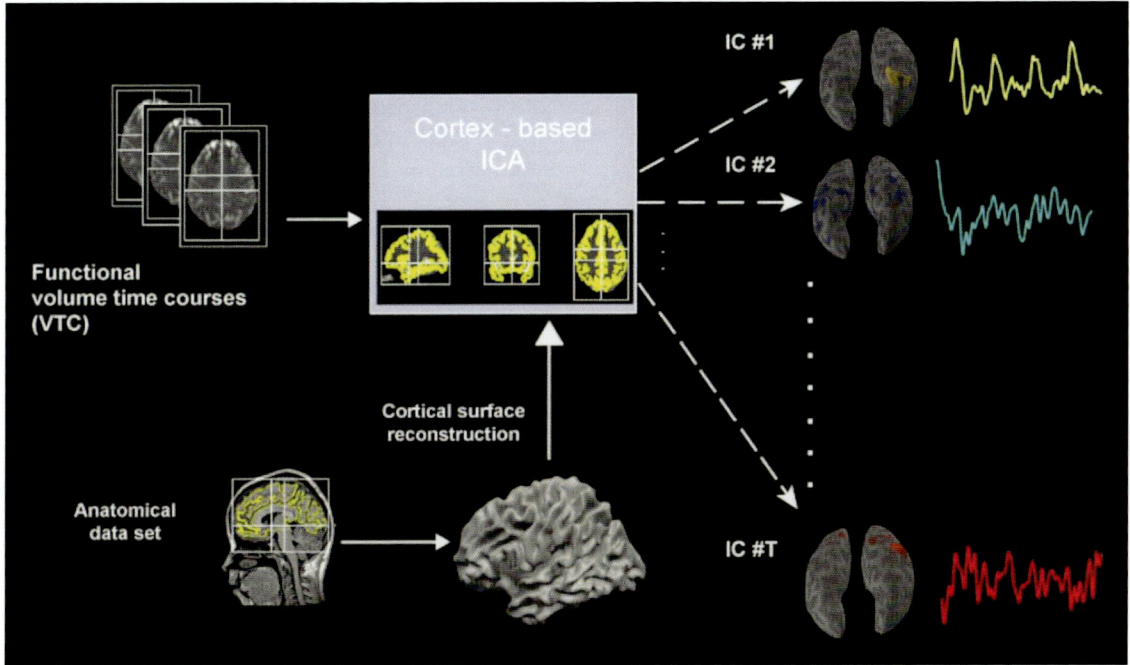

Figure 3.2.6. Schematic representation of the cortex-based ICA approach. (From Formisano et al., 2004).

likelihood to be "gray matter" (Beckmann and Smith, 2004). However, because voxels at the gray matter/white matter border only represent a small proportion of the data no great differences in the results are expected.

Optimizing the Contrast Function

Another possibility of tailoring ICA to fMRI is to optimize the contrast function used in the algorithm based on specific properties of the expected signal. Suzuki et al. (2002) conducted a study on contrast functions for the FastICA algorithm (Hyvarinen, 1999) and suggested that a skewed contrast function may improve accuracy in retrieving task-related components. Stone et al. (2002) combined skewed contrast functions with spatiotemporal independence (obtained maximizing a linear combination of spatial and temporal independence contrast functions).

In (Lu and Rajapakse, 2005) a "constrained ICA" approach has been developed where independence is maximized with an additional constraint imposed a priori. In particular, this approach makes it possible to include a reference function (i. e., an approximation of the time course of an experimental condition) into temporal ICA, extracting therefore only task-related sources. A complementary approach has been implemented in (Calhoun et al., 2005) to include this information in spatial ICA, by extracting all the sources together and performing a gradient optimization of independence together with a term influencing correlation between the selected source and the time course. The proposed method, named "semi-blind ICA," may be seen as an alternative to general linear model, whereas the prior information on the experimental paradigm lacks precision. Similarly, in Li et al. (2007) a framework to include specific templates of spatial activation into spatial ICA was developed.

Spatial Regularities in ICA

The approaches described above all consider specific (temporal or spatial) knowledge on the sources, which may limit the exploratory value of ICA. To preserve the "blindness" of

ICA while optimizing its performance, some more general assumptions besides (spatial) independence of the fMRI sources may be made for their optimal recovery. A physiologically plausible activation (in both spatial and temporal version) is expected to present spatial as well as temporal regularities. Classical ICA algorithms, however, do not pursue this objective while looking for independence. An illustrative example is presented in Figure 3.2.7, where three 2-dimensional maps have an identical histogram but completely different interpretation. In fact the first map (a) would be interpreted as a meaningful activation, while the others (b–c) would be associated with noise. For many of the ICA algorithms commonly employed in fMRI, the source of Figure 3.2.7 would look identical, as data are considered as "random variables" rather than "signals." This means that only their joint statistical distribution is considered while performing extraction regardless of their structure in space or in time.

Valente and colleagues (2009) included a regularity term in an ICA contrast function, whose optimization led to a decomposition of the mixtures accounting for both independence and prior knowledge.

This contrast function is formulated as:

$$F = J_G + \lambda H \tag{7}$$

where J_G, an estimate of negentropy, accounts for independence, H accounts for the spatial regularity of the sources, and λ weighs the two functions. The negentropy term is approximated as in Hyvarinen (1999), and, if the additional term λH is set to zero, the maximization of F leads to "classical" independent components extraction.

In Valente et al. (2009) the spatial regularity of the sources was accounted for in terms of their spatial autocorrelation. In particular, the evaluation of H_{sp} was divided into two steps: thresholding of spatial map and calculation of the spatial autocorrelation. The combination of map thresholding and autocorrelation evaluation (which involves a normalization of the thresholded map) makes the use of gradient-based optimization troublesome. Contrast function (7) was therefore optimized by means of Simulated

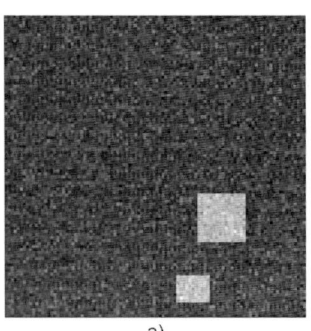 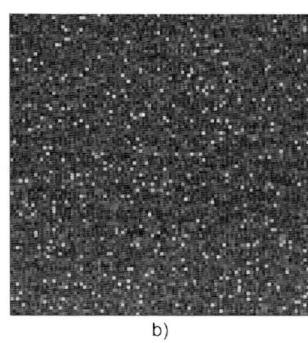  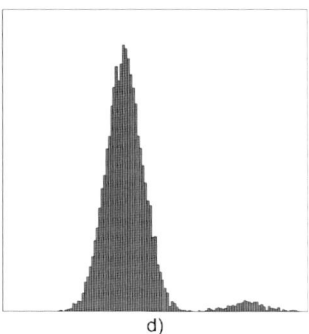

a)   b)   c)   d)

Figure 3.2.7. Three different spatial maps, (a)–(c), having the same histogram (d). An algorithm that only employs probability densities may discard the information of spatial regularity in map (a). (From Valente et al. (2009).)

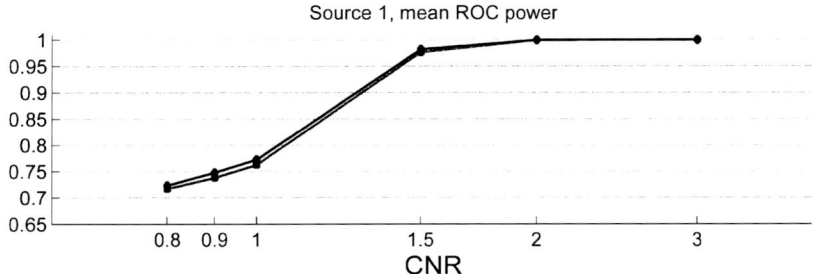

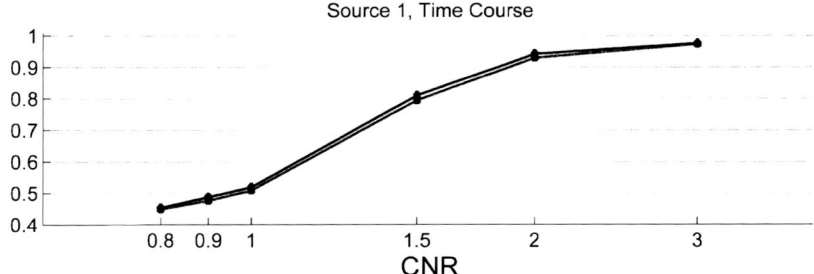

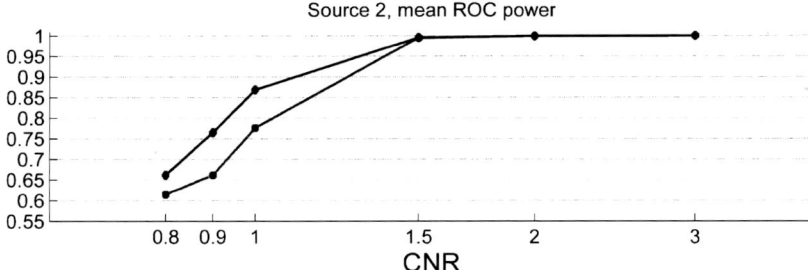

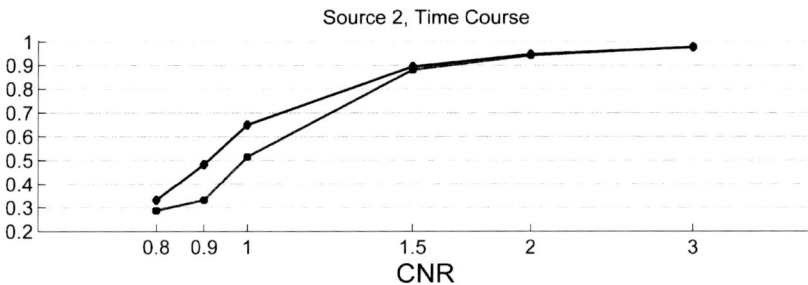

Figure 3.2.8. Analysis of performances at different contrast-to-noise ratios. FastICA values are indicated by a square (■) symbol, ICA with spatial autocorrelation by a diamond (♦) one. Left column: mean ROC power as a function of CNR. Right column: Correlation of the recovered time course with the original one. Results are presented in logarithmic scale with respect to X axis. (From Valente et al. (2009).)

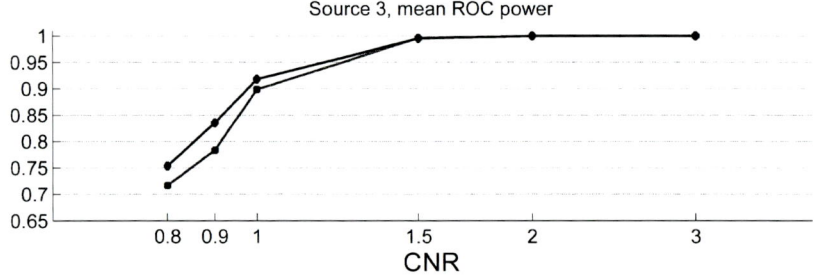

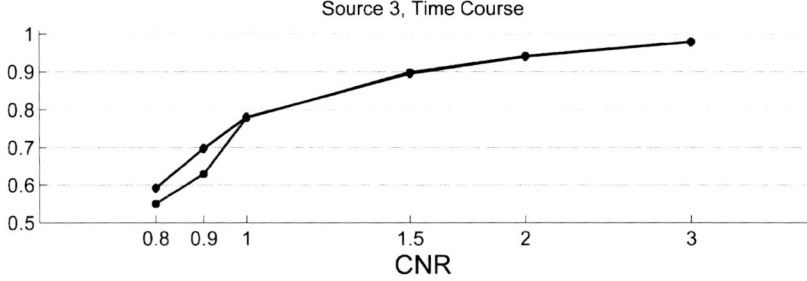

Figure 3.2.8. (Continued)

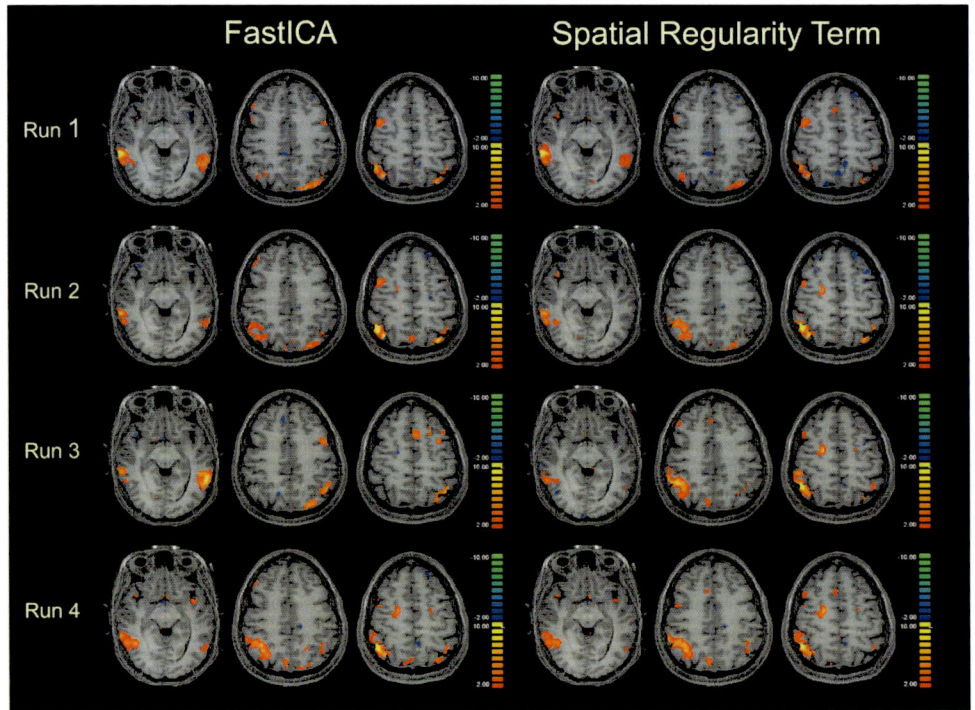

Figure 3.2.9. Comparison between the retrieved independent component associated with the late imagery processing stage for the two algorithms in the four runs of the experiment. (From Valente et al. (2009).)

Annealing (SA) (Kirkpatrick et al., 1983) that allows dealing with global nondifferentiable maximization (minimization) by means of a random search with a probabilistic acceptance criterion (note, however, that a simulated annealing optimization procedure is considerably slower than a gradient based one).

This optimized ICA algorithm was tested and validated on both simulated and real fMRI data set, and compared with a

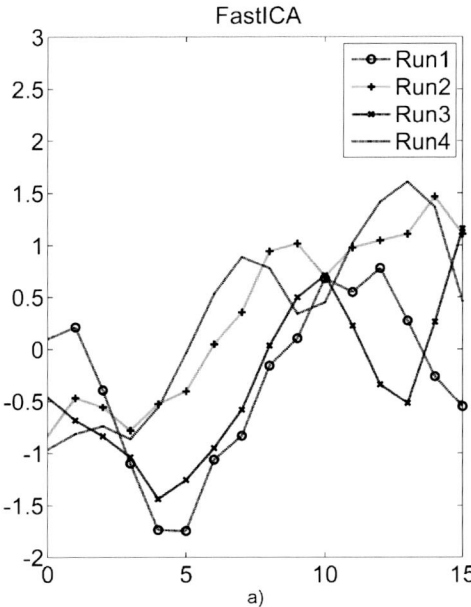
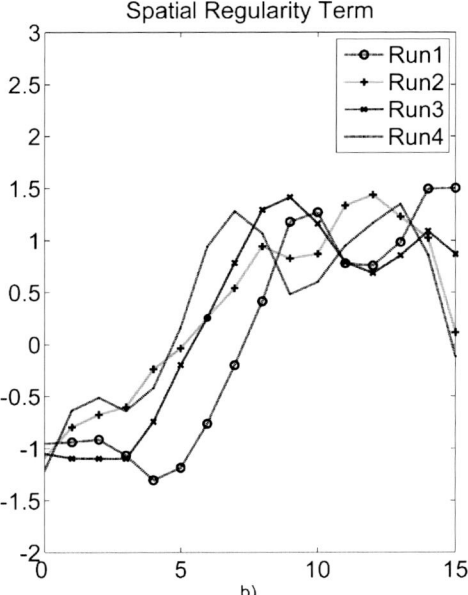

Figure 3.2.10. Average of the time courses of the components associated with the second imagery processing stage in the four runs of subject "CJ." The values are in normalized units. a) FastICA extraction, b) Negentropy with the additional spatial regularity term. (From Valente et al. (2009).)

traditional ICA model. The first simulation involved the use of a resting-state data set with superimposed artificial activations with associated time courses, at different CNRs, ranging from 0.8 to 3; for each level of noise, 20 extractions were performed for both algorithms. Performances were evaluated by means of ROC analysis (Sorenson and Wang, 1996; Skudlarski et al., 1999; Esposito et al., 2002) and the ROC power (i.e., the area under the curve) was considered as a single "figure of merit."

In Figure 3.2.8, left panel, the mean ROC powers of the three sources for the two algorithms, at CNR ranging from 0.8 to 3 are plotted. Not surprisingly, in low noise situations both algorithms were able to recover the sources with extremely good accuracy; in high noise situations, the spatial regularity term increased both spatial and temporal accuracy of the source extraction.

Furthermore, a comparison of the sources recovered with the optimized algorithm with those obtained with FastICA was performed using fMRI data collected during a visuospatial mental imagery task (Sack et al., 2008). Inclusion of the spatial autocorrelation term within the contrast function improved the across-run consistency of both spatial maps (Figure 3.2.9) and time courses (Figure 3.2.10) of a fronto-parietal component likely to be associated with the late processing stages of the imagery task (Sack et al., 2008; Valente et al. 2009).

Overall, these results indicate that the spatial regularity term renders the extraction of ICs more robust and it increases the consistency and neurophysiological plausibility of the "weak" components, which may not be detected by standard sICA.

ICA in Multisubject fMRI Studies

ICA has been successfully used for the decomposition of individual fMRI time-series. Since fMRI studies typically involve a statistical comparison of one or more groups of subjects (e.g., healthy people and patients), methods have been developed for extending the ICA framework to group and multigroup fMRI studies.

A natural way to proceed is to perform second-level analyses of the ICA-decompositions from individual data sets (Calhoun et al., 2001c; Seifritz et al., 2002). The main challenge in this approach has been to integrate ICA with a manual, semiautomatic or automatic matching of the estimated components across all subjects of the study. In order to generalize such an approach, an effective method for the subject- or group-level "matching" of components is necessary, otherwise the whole procedure remains prone to a loss of sensitivity caused by any possible mismatch of components that cannot be easily corrected.

Conventional model-driven univariate methods (e.g., regression analysis) have been naturally generalized from single- to multisubject methods by simple schemes of across-subject data aggregation based on matrix averaging and concatenation. For ICA similar schemes have been suggested that combine individual data sets into a single group data set prior to performing ICA. Three main (alternative) approaches have been proposed. Following up the matrix notation with time indexing the rows and space indexing the columns, column-wise (Calhoun et al.,

2001a) and row-wise (Svensen et al., 2002) data concatenation have been proposed. These methods have been reviewed and compared using artificial data sets with the simplest across-subject averaging by Schmithorst and Brown (2004). Beckmann and Smith (2005) introduced a tensorial extension to ICA in which a third dimension (besides time and space) has been added to the algebraic ICA problem formulation to account for subject-level variance in aggregated data sets. One common aspect to all the aggregate-data approaches is the assumption that a source exists as an "observable process" in all of (or most of) the subjects entering the analysis. Specifically, column-wise aggregation imposes a common space of observations for all the sources (the normalized anatomical space), although it allows different activation time-courses for the different subjects. Row-wise aggregation imposes a common time-course for a generic source to all of the subjects, although it allows "no activity" to occur in some subjects. Tensor-based group-level ICA introduces a new independent dimension in the factorization across subjects, thereby

allowing a direct inspection of between-subject variability in a given independent component. An important assumption of tensor ICA is that both the spatial layout and the temporal profile are unique to the entire cohort of subject and a co-linearity assumption for the pattern across subjects is implicit to the linear factorization.

Esposito et al. (2005) described the application of similarity measures to ICA patterns (Kherif et al., 2003; Himberg et al., 2004) to produce group inferences in multisubject studies. This approach starts from single-subject ICA runs and examines the grouping of independent components in the subject space using the intersubject pattern similarity (contrasted to the intrasubject similarity) as a mechanism for clustering. This approach was named "self-organizing group ICA" (sogICA; Esposito et al., 2005), since it extends ICA from individual to multisubject fMRI data sets without constraining a specific homology of the sources across subjects via some form of pre-aggregation of the data sets. SogICA searches for structures of the sources in the subject space

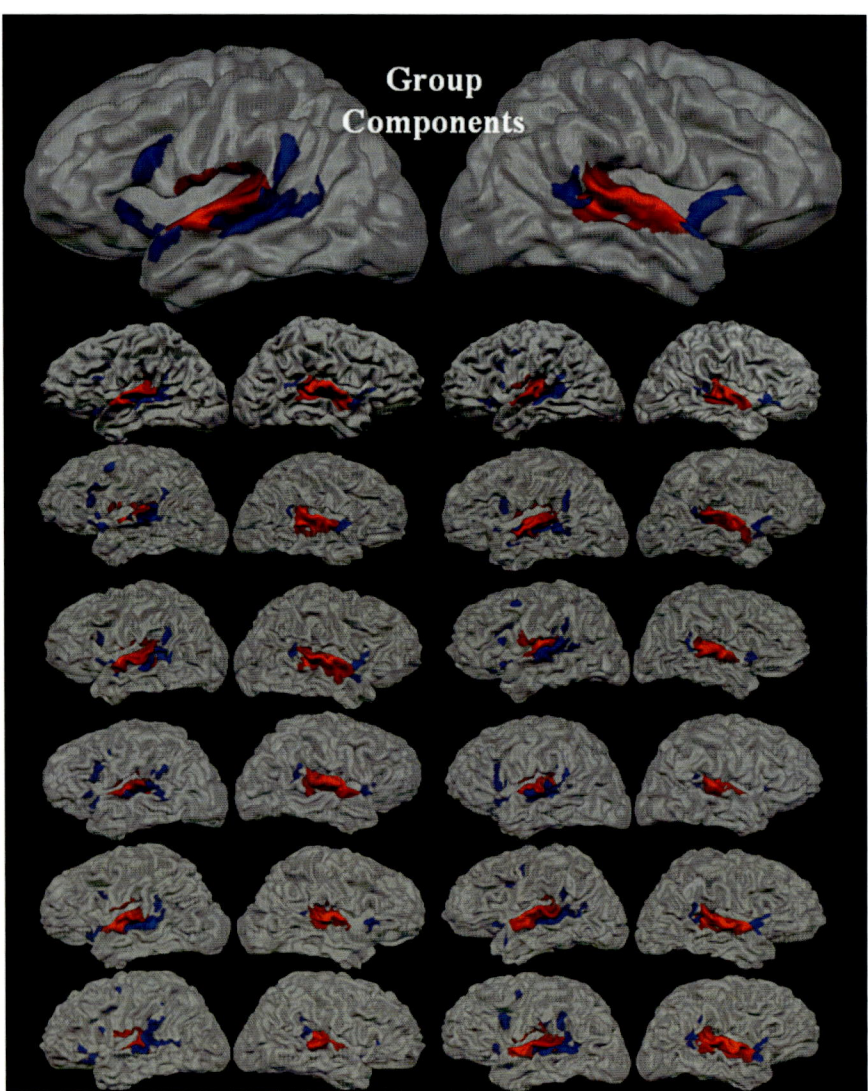

Figure 3.2.11. Self-organizing group-level ICA combined with cortex-based intersubject alignment. Two auditory components detected by individual cortex-based ICA in 12 separate subjects and successfully clustered by sogICA.

and has been applied in various studies (Esposito et al., 2006; Goebel et al., 2006; Mantini et al., 2007; Esposito et al., 2008; van de Ven et al., 2008).

In the sogICA algorithm, the ICs from each subject are organized in one single set of components, and a label preserving the link from the components to the original subject is assigned. All components are then clustered according to their mutual similarities (e.g., the absolute value of their mutual correlation coefficients in the space domain). A supervised hierarchical clustering algorithm is used to link the components to each other only when differently labeled (i.e., belonging to different subjects). For each cluster, the average component of a cluster is computed and assumed as the group-representative of the cluster. A random-effect group component can also be generated by dividing voxel-wise mean and variance across subjects of the cluster component values (Calhoun et al., 2001c). In population studies, the cluster partition can be used to define a within-subject factor (i.e., component I of subject J belonging "more" to cluster H than to cluster K) and a between-subject factor can be added to explore the significance of a given component for one cluster or the prevalence of one group (Esposito et al., 2008).

SogICA has also been combined with cortex-based inter-subject alignment (Goebel et al., 2006). The results of this combined application of sogICA and a cortex-based inter-subject alignment to an auditory stimulation experiment with repetition of sentences and/or speakers are illustrated in Figure 3.2.11. SogICA in the aligned cortex space was able to cluster two task-related components corresponding to those extracted using cbICA of the individual subjects. This application of group-level ICA is particularly powerful, since it allows a group representation of the ICs while preserving the natural spatial and temporal variability of the ICs at the level of individual subjects.

REFERENCES

Bartels A, Zeki S (2005) Brain dynamics during natural viewing conditions: a new guide for mapping connectivity in vivo. Neuroimage 24:339–349.

Baumgartner R, Scarth G, Teichtmeister C, Somorjai R, Moser E (1997) Fuzzy clustering of gradient-echo functional MRI in the human visual cortex. Part I: reproducibility. J Magn Reson Imaging 7:1094–1101.

Baumgartner R, Ryner L, Richter W, Summers R, Jarmasz M, Somorjai R (2000) Comparison of two exploratory data analysis methods for fMRI: fuzzy clustering vs. principal component analysis. Magn Reson Imaging 18:89–94.

Beckmann CF, Smith SM (2004) Probabilistic independent component analysis for functional magnetic resonance imaging. IEEE Trans Med Imaging 23:137–152.

Beckmann CF, Smith SM (2005) Tensorial extensions of independent component analysis for multisubject FMRI analysis. Neuroimage 25:294–311.

Bell AJ, Sejnowski TJ (1995) An information-maximization approach to blind separation and blind deconvolution. Neural Comput 7:1129–1159.

Biswal BB, Ulmer JL (1999) Blind source separation of multiple signal sources of fMRI data sets using independent component analysis. J Comput Assist Tomogr 23:265–271.

Calhoun VD, Adali T, Pearlson GD, Pekar JJ (2001a) A method for making group inferences from functional MRI data using independent component analysis. Hum Brain Mapp 14:140–151.

Calhoun VD, Adali T, Pearlson GD, Pekar JJ (2001b) Spatial and temporal independent component analysis of functional MRI data containing a pair of task-related waveforms. Hum Brain Mapp 13:43–53.

Calhoun VD, Adali T, McGinty VB, Pekar JJ, Watson TD, Pearlson GD (2001c) fMRI activation in a visual-perception task: network of areas detected using the general linear model and independent components analysis. Neuroimage 14:1080–1088.

Calhoun VD, Pekar JJ, McGinty VB, Adali T, Watson TD, Pearlson GD (2002) Different activation dynamics in multiple neural systems during simulated driving. Hum Brain Mapp 16:158–167.

Calhoun VD, Adali T, Stevens MC, Kiehl KA, Pekar JJ (2005) Semi-blind ICA of fMRI: A method for utilizing hypothesis-derived time courses in a spatial ICA analysis. Neuroimage 25:527–538.

Calhoun VD, Liu J, Adali T (2009) A review of group ICA for fMRI data and ICA for joint inference of imaging, genetic, and ERP data. Neuroimage 45:S163–172.

Castelo-Branco M, Formisano E, Backes W, Zanella F, Neuenschwander S, Singer W, Goebel R (2002) Activity patterns in human motion-sensitive areas depend on the interpretation of global motion. Proc Natl Acad Sci U S A 99:13914–13919.

Chicocki A, Amari S (2002) Adaptive blind signal and image processing: learning algorithms and applications. New York: John Wiley & Sons.

Comon P (1994) Independent component analysis: a new concept? Signal Process 36:287–314.

Cordes D, Nandy RR (2006) Estimation of the intrinsic dimensionality of fMRI data. Neuroimage 29:145–154.

Cover TM, Thomas JA (1991) Elements of information theory. New York: Wiley.

De Luca M, Beckmann CF, De Stefano N, Matthews PM, Smith SM (2006) fMRI resting state networks define distinct modes of long-distance interactions in the human brain. Neuroimage 29:1359–1367.

De Martino F, Gentile F, Esposito F, Balsi M, Di Salle F, Goebel R, Formisano E (2007) Classification of fMRI independent components using IC-fingerprints and support vector machine classifiers. Neuroimage 34:177–194.

Duann JR, Jung TP, Kuo WJ, Yeh TC, Makeig S, Hsieh JC, Sejnowski TJ (2002) Single-trial variability in event-related BOLD signals. Neuroimage 15:823–835.

Esposito F, Formisano E, Seifritz E, Goebel R, Morrone R, Tedeschi G, Di Salle F (2002) Spatial independent component analysis of functional MRI time-series: to what extent do results depend on the algorithm used? Hum Brain Mapp 16:146–157.

Esposito F, Scarabino T, Hyvarinen A, Himberg J, Formisano E, Comani S, Tedeschi G, Goebel R, Seifritz E, Di Salle F (2005)

Independent component analysis of fMRI group studies by self-organizing clustering. Neuroimage 25:193–205.

Esposito F, Bertolino A, Scarabino T, Latorre V, Blasi G, Popolizio T, Tedeschi G, Cirillo S, Goebel R, Di Salle F (2006) Independent component model of the default-mode brain function: assessing the impact of active thinking. Brain Res Bull 70:263–269.

Esposito F, Aragri A, Pesaresi I, Cirillo S, Tedeschi G, Marciano E, Goebel R, Di Salle F (2008) Independent component model of the default-mode brain function: combining individual-level and population-level analyses in resting-state fMRI. Magn Reson Imaging 26:905–913.

Formisano E, Goebel R (2003) Tracking cognitive processes with functional MRI mental chronometry. Curr Opin Neurobiol 13:174–181.

Formisano E, Esposito F, Kriegeskorte N, Tedeschi G, Di Salle F, Goebel R (2002) Spatial independent component analysis of functional magnetic resonance imaging time-series: characterization of the cortical components. Neurocomputing 49:241–254.

Formisano E, Esposito F, Di Salle F, Goebel R (2004) Cortex-based independent component analysis of fMRI time series. Magn Reson Imaging 22:1493–1504.

Friston KJ, Frith CD, Liddle PF, Frackowiak RS (1993) Functional connectivity: the principal-component analysis of large (PET) data sets. J Cereb Blood Flow Metab 13:5–14.

Goebel R, Esposito F, Formisano E (2006) Analysis of functional image analysis contest (FIAC) data with brainvoyager QX: From single-subject to cortically aligned group general linear model analysis and self-organizing group independent component analysis. Hum Brain Mapp 27:392–401.

Greicius MD, Krasnow B, Reiss AL, Menon V (2003) Functional connectivity in the resting brain: a network analysis of the default mode hypothesis. Proc Natl Acad Sci U S A 100:253– 258.

Greicius MD, Srivastava G, Reiss AL, Menon V (2004) Default-mode network activity distinguishes Alzheimer's disease from healthy aging: evidence from functional MRI. Proc Natl Acad Sci U S A 101:4637–4642.

Greicius MD, Flores BH, Menon V, Glover GH, Solvason HB, Kenna H, Reiss AL, Schatzberg AF (2007) Resting-state functional connectivity in major depression: abnormally increased contributions from subgenual cingulate cortex and thalamus. Biol Psychiatry 62:429–437.

Himberg J, Hyvarinen A, Esposito F (2004) Validating the independent components of neuroimaging time series via clustering and visualization. Neuroimage 22:1214–1222.

Hyvarinen A (1999) Fast and robust fixed-point algorithms for independent component analysis. IEEE Trans Neural Netw 10:626–634.

Hyvarinen A, Oja E (1997) A fast fixed-point algorithm for independent component analysis. Neural Comput 9: 1483–1492.

Hyvarinen A, Karhunen J, Oja E (2001) Independent component analysis. New York: John Wiley & Sons.

Kherif F, Poline JB, Meriaux S, Benali H, Flandin G, Brett M (2003) Group analysis in functional neuroimaging: selecting subjects using similarity measures. Neuroimage 20:2197–2208.

Kirkpatrick S, Gelatt CD, Jr., Vecchi MP (1983) Optimization by simulated annealing. Science 220:671–680.

Lange N, Strother SC, Anderson JR, Nielsen FA, Holmes AP, Kolenda T, Savoy R, Hansen LK (1999) Plurality and resemblance in fMRI data analysis. Neuroimage 10:282–303.

Lee TW, Girolami M, Sejnowski TJ (1999) Independent component analysis using an extended infomax algorithm for mixed sub-gaussian and supergaussian sources. Neural Comput 11:417–441.

Li YO, Adali T, Calhoun VD (2007) A feature-selective independent component analysis method for functional MRI. Int J Biomed Imaging 2007:15635.

Liao R, Krolik JL, McKeown MJ (2005) An information-theoretic criterion for intrasubject alignment of FMRI time series: motion corrected independent component analysis. IEEE Trans Med Imaging 24:29–44.

Lu W, Rajapakse JC (2005) Approach and applications of constrained ICA. IEEE Trans Neural Netw 16:203–212.

Mantini D, Perrucci MG, Del Gratta C, Romani GL, Corbetta M (2007) Electrophysiological signatures of resting state networks in the human brain. Proc Natl Acad Sci U S A 104:13170–13175.

McKeown MJ, Sejnowski TJ (1998) Independent component analysis of fMRI data: examining the assumptions. Hum Brain Mapp 6:368–372.

McKeown MJ, Makeig S, Brown GG, Jung TP, Kindermann SS, Bell AJ, Sejnowski TJ (1998a) Analysis of fMRI data by blind separation into independent spatial components. Hum Brain Mapp 6:160–188.

McKeown MJ, Jung TP, Makeig S, Brown G, Kindermann SS, Lee TW, Sejnowski TJ (1998b) Spatially independent activity patterns in functional MRI data during the stroop color-naming task. Proc Natl Acad Sci U S A 95:803–810.

Moritz CH, Rogers BP, Meyerand ME (2003) Power spectrum ranked independent component analysis of a periodic fMRI complex motor paradigm. Hum Brain Mapp 18:111–122.

Moritz CH, Carew JD, McMillan AB, Meyerand ME (2005) Independent component analysis applied to self-paced functional MR imaging paradigms. Neuroimage 25:181– 192.

Papoulis A (1991) Probability, random variables, and stochastic processes, 3rd Edition. New York: McGraw-Hill.

Petersson KM, Nichols TE, Poline JB, Holmes AP (1999) Statistical limitations in functional neuroimaging. I: Non-inferential methods and statistical models. Philos Trans R Soc Lond B Biol Sci 354:1239–1260.

Quigley MA, Haughton VM, Carew J, Cordes D, Moritz CH, Meyerand ME (2002) Comparison of independent component analysis and conventional hypothesis-driven analysis for clinical functional MR image processing. AJNR Am J Neuroradiol 23:49–58.

Rodionov R, De Martino F, Laufs H, Carmichael DW, Formisano E, Walker M, Duncan JS, Lemieux L (2007) Independent component analysis of interictal fMRI in focal epilepsy: comparison with general linear model-based EEG-correlated fMRI. Neuroimage 38:488–500.

Ross S (1997) Introduction to probability models, 6th Edition. New York: Academic Press.

Sack AT, Jacobs C, De Martino F, Staeren N, Goebel R, Formisano E (2008) Dynamic premotor-to-parietal interactions during spatial imagery. J Neurosci 28:8417–8429.

Schmithorst VJ, Brown RD (2004) Empirical validation of the triple-code model of numerical processing for complex math operations using functional MRI and group Independent

Component Analysis of the mental addition and subtraction of fractions. Neuroimage 22:1414–1420.

Seifritz E, Esposito F, Hennel F, Mustovic H, Neuhoff JG, Bilecen D, Tedeschi G, Scheffler K, Di Salle F (2002) Spatiotemporal pattern of neural processing in the human auditory cortex. Science 297:1706–1708.

Skudlarski P, Constable RT, Gore JC (1999) ROC analysis of statistical methods used in functional MRI: individual subjects. Neuroimage 9:311–329.

Sorenson JA, Wang X (1996) ROC methods for evaluation of fMRI techniques. Magn Reson Med 36:737–744.

Stone JV, Porrill J, Porter NR, Wilkinson ID (2002) Spatiotemporal independent component analysis of event-related fMRI data using skewed probability density functions. Neuroimage 15:407–421.

Suykens JAK, Van Gestel T, De Barbanter J, De Moor B, Vanderwalle J (2002) Least squares support vector machines. River Edge, NJ: World Scientific Publishing.

Suzuki K, Kiryu T, Nakada T (2002) Fast and precise independent component analysis for high field fMRI time series tailored using prior information on spatiotemporal structure. Hum Brain Mapp 15:54–66.

Svensen M, Kruggel F, Benali H (2002) ICA of fMRI group study data. Neuroimage 16:551–563.

Thomas CG, Harshman RA, Menon RS (2002) Noise reduction in BOLD-based fMRI using component analysis. Neuroimage 17:1521–1537.

Valente G, De Martino F, Filosa G, Balsi M, Formisano E (2009) Optimizing ICA in fMRI using information on spatial regularities of the sources. Magn Reson Imaging 27:1110–1119.

van de Ven VG, Formisano E, Prvulovic D, Roeder CH, Linden DE (2004) Functional connectivity as revealed by spatial independent component analysis of fMRI measurements during rest. Hum Brain Mapp 22:165–178.

van de Ven VG, Formisano E, Roder CH, Prvulovic D, Bittner RA, Dietz MG, Hubl D, Dierks T, Federspiel A, Esposito F, Di Salle F, Jansma B, Goebel R, Linden DE (2005) The spatiotemporal pattern of auditory cortical responses during verbal hallucinations. Neuroimage 27:644–655.

van de Ven VG, Bledowski C, Prvulovic D, Goebel R, Formisano E, Di Salle F, Linden DE, Esposito F (2008) Visual target modulation of functional connectivity networks revealed by self-organizing group ICA. Hum Brain Mapp 29:1450–1461.

3.3 Markus Ullsperger

EEG-Informed fMRI Analysis

Introduction

Electroencephalography (EEG) and functional magnetic resonance imaging (fMRI) have been established as the most widely used non-invasive tools to map sensory, motor, cognitive, and emotional processes in the human brain. They provide complementary advantages with respect to temporal and spatial resolution, such that great hope lies in co-registration of EEG and fMRI to achieve both optimal spatiotemporal measures of brain activity and combined information of the electrical and metabolic activity.

Recent advances in hardware development have made it feasible to record multi-channel EEG data and fMRI signals simultaneously (cf. Chapters 2.1, 2.2). Similarly, off-line preprocessing tools to control for artifacts contaminating the EEG data are readily available (cf. Chapter 2.3). Currently, it appears most challenging to optimally integrate the multimodal data sets in order to (1) learn about the implementation of specific information processing functions in the human brain, its underlying anatomy as well as the dynamics of activity in these networks, and (2) gather knowledge about the sources and mutual relationship of the measured electrical and hemodynamic signals. The following chapters in this section elaborate on a number of different approaches to these problems. This chapter focuses on an approach that capitalizes on the extraction of functionally relevant signals from the EEG that are used to inform fMRI analysis. The preconditions, promises, and limitations of this approach will be discussed.

Mostly resulting from the technical difficulties that until quite recently were associated with simultaneous recordings, many researchers have tried to fuse EEG and fMRI data sets recorded in separate sessions. However, simultaneous recordings provide fundamental advantages over separate recording protocols. It is challenging to ensure identical sensory stimulation in the EEG and fMRI laboratories, even

when, e.g., the EEG is recorded with the participant in supine position and with simulated scanner noise. Differences in preparation time, task experience, and the recording environment, as well as in the general and private contexts in which the recording session is embedded are likely to affect the participant's mood, vigilance, compliance, and behavior, as well as fluctuations in ongoing brain activity. Even in well-established cognitive experiments with identical task presentation, the behavior of the same participant can vary substantially between EEG and fMRI recording sessions (Ullsperger and von Cramon, 2001). In addition, many cognitive processes, such as learning, novelty processing, or object identification, are not well suited for repeated testing. In sum, simultaneous recordings guarantee identical sensory stimulation, perception, behavior, and state of the participant. They allow data fusion approaches that take into account the temporal dynamics of brain activity and provide a way to study the interaction of intrinsic brain states with event-related, extrinsic processing.

The Relationship of EEG and fMRI Measures

The fundamental assumption of any integration approach is that the signals recorded in both modalities are produced by closely interacting, or at least partly overlapping, brain structures. The EEG is a selective measure of current source activity, whereas the hemodynamic fMRI signal is related to energy consumption of neuronal populations (see Chapters 1.1, 1.2). The major methodological differences between EEG and fMRI are, in principle, consistent with positive, negative, or no correlations between the signals (Rugg, 1998; Nunez and Silberstein, 2000; Horwitz and Poeppel, 2002; Debener et al., 2006; Ritter and Villringer, 2006). These considerations gave rise to the notion of fMRI-blind EEG sources and EEG-blind fMRI sources. For example, deep sources or neuronal populations arranged in "closed fields" may not be detected in the EEG, while making contributions to the fMRI signal. In contrast, changes in EEG signals can result from changes in synchronicity of neuronal activity, whereas the fMRI signal may be equally sensitive to synchronous and asynchronous activity. These concerns notwithstanding, a growing number of EEG-fMRI studies have reported correlations of the two measures (e.g., Goldman et al., 2002; Laufs et al., 2003b; Debener et al., 2005; Eichele et al., 2005; Feige et al., 2005; Bénar et al., 2007; Mulert et al., 2008; Ritter et al., 2008b). The interpretation of such correlations must take into account prior knowledge of the processes under investigation and anatomical constraints. A correlation in a certain brain area may indicate that at least part of the generators of the electrical and hemodynamic responses overlap in this region. However, forward modeling using source localization algorithms should be used to verify that a projection of electrical activity from the identified brain structure to the scalp is likely to produce the EEG phenomenon of interest. More generally, correlations of the fMRI signal with the EEG suggest that the sources of these signals are functionally coupled although not necessarily spatially overlapping. For example, positive correlations of alpha EEG activity with the hemodynamic response in the thalamus (Feige et al., 2005) may indicate a strong functional role in generating the alpha rhythm, while the scalp-recorded electrical signal is likely generated in the cortex.

It has been pointed out that correlations between the data modalities may also occur when the sources of the hemodynamic and electrical signals have neither functional nor anatomical overlap, for example as a result of a common influence of ongoing brain activity on both neuronal source ensembles or when the same noise influences both measures (Nunez and Silberstein, 2000; Debener et al., 2005). The likelihood of falsely interpreting such correlation as indicative of a functional relationship can be reduced by demonstrating that the correlating hemodynamic and/or electrical signals also predict behavioral measures, such as reaction times or accuracy (Debener et al., 2005).

Furthermore, it has been argued that correlations between EEG and fMRI signals do not need to be linear (Bledowski et al., 2007). While a linear model is a natural starting point for EEG-informed fMRI analysis, this method can be generalized to any non-linear relationship simply by constructing non-linear fMRI regressors from the EEG features of interest (Büchel et al., 1998).

EEG–fMRI Covariation Across Subjects and in Parametric Designs

A number of studies using separate EEG and fMRI recordings have investigated across-subjects correlations of event-related potentials and fMRI signal changes related to a cognitive process of interest (Mathalon et al., 2003; Ford et al., 2004),

sometimes combined with parametric task manipulation (Horovitz et al., 2002; Horovitz et al., 2004; Schicke et al., 2006). A similar approach has also been applied successfully to simultaneously recorded data with respect to early auditory ERPs and the mismatch negativity (Liebenthal et al., 2003; Mulert et al., 2005; Sabri et al., 2006).

This analysis approach helps to localize indirectly a cognitive process that is temporally defined using an ERP amplitude, without necessitating simultaneous recordings. However, the major advantage of high temporal resolution of EEG is not optimally used when focusing on the amplitude of a selected peak of the *average* waveform across trials, thereby ignoring information about dynamic changes over time. Moreover, areas with fMRI signal increases that correlate with mean ERP amplitudes may exhibit a different temporal activation profile than the neuronal population underlying the ERP. The relatively small number of conditions that can be implemented during recording and that still yield reliable ERPs implicates that the correlation analysis suffers from a mixture of within-subject and between-subjects effects. Given the usually quite low number of participants, the power of these correlation analyses is often low; and functionally irrelevant between-subjects factors (e.g., anatomical differences that may affect the propagation and attenuation of EEG but do not influence the fMRI signal) may reduce the sensitivity of the analyses. Thus, this analysis approach seems likely to miss correlations between hemodynamic and EEG signals.

Simultaneous EEG and fMRI of Ongoing Activity

Simultaneous EEG and fMRI measurements allow analyses on a purely temporal, within-subject basis. The core approach of EEG-informed fMRI analysis is to extract measures reflecting EEG phenomena along the time course of the experiment. Under the assumption that changes in the EEG measure are associated with hemodynamic responses following the same characteristics as fMRI responses to external events, the EEG measure is convolved with the hemodynamic response function and used as a regressor in fMRI analysis using the general linear model. In the second-level (group) analysis, voxelwise tests of the beta estimates for this regressor against zero reveal brain areas in which the EEG measure covaries with the hemodynamic response. Figure 3.3.1 illustrates processing steps that directly relate EEG and fMRI signals to each other at a within-subject level with high temporal (event-related) resolution.

The first approaches in this direction used high-amplitude EEG signals, such as the alpha rhythm. Goldman and colleagues showed that spontaneous fluctuations of EEG alpha power in a resting state covaried with simultaneously recorded regional fluctuations of the hemodynamic signal (Goldman et al., 2002). Further studies replicated and

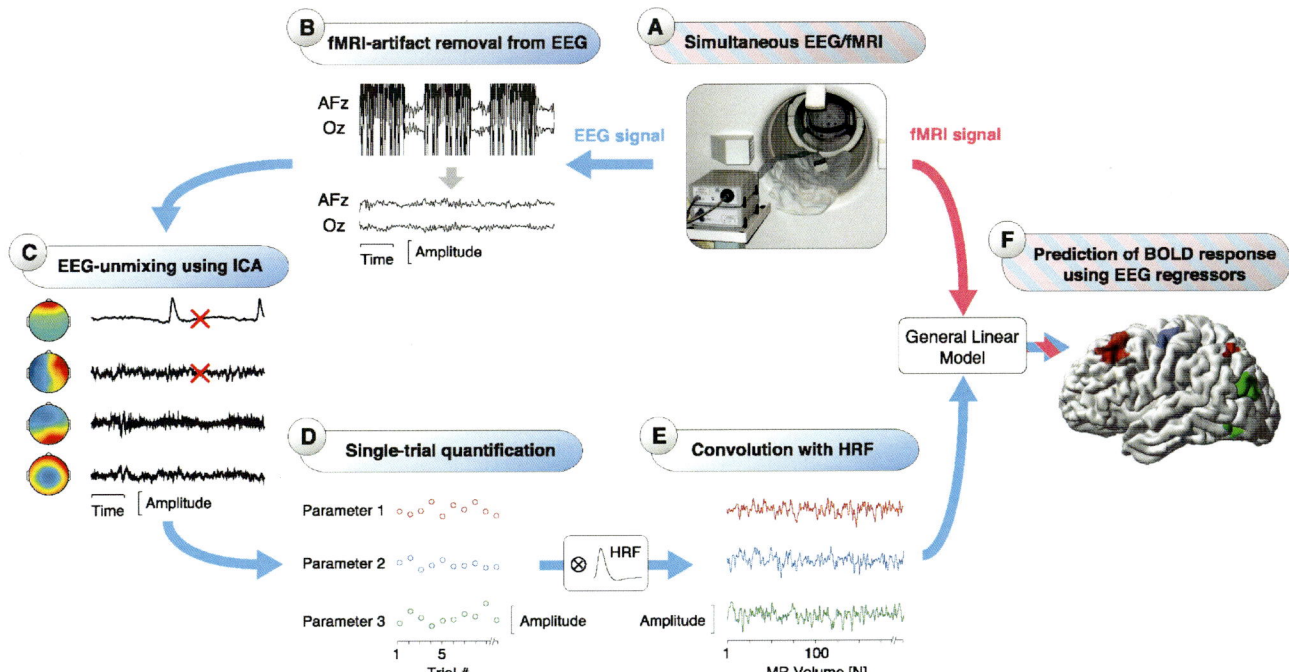

Figure 3.3.1. EEG-informed fMRI analysis. EEG (blue arrows) and fMRI (red arrow) can be recorded simultaneously (a), and, subsequently, EEG signals are corrected for fMRI artifacts. This is illustrated for two out of a larger set of EEG channels (b). Unmixing methods such as independent component analysis (ICA) applied to the EEG signal yields artifact-related and brain-activity-related component maps and activation time courses; typical to-be-removed artifact-related components are marked with red crosses (c). Selected components reflecting brain activity of interest can be used to obtain a measure for each recorded event, or, as in analyses of ongoing EEG analyses, for series of data epochs (d). After convolution with the hemodynamic response function (HRF), the single-event amplitudes yield EEG-based regressors (e) that parametrically predict the fMRI signal. Adapted from Figure 1 in Debener et al. (2006). Reproduced with permission.

extended this initial report (Laufs et al., 2003b; Laufs et al., 2003a; Moosmann et al., 2003; Martinez-Montes et al., 2004; Feige et al., 2005; Ritter et al., 2008a). Interestingly, the studies reported that the fMRI signal in the occipital cortex was negatively correlated with EEG alpha activity. This finding is consistent with the idea that large-scale synchronized activity in the alpha frequency range represents an "idling" rhythm and corresponds to cortical inactivation (Pfurtscheller and Lopes da Silva, 1999). This is an example demonstrating that generation of a large-amplitude EEG phenomenon does not necessarily require increased metabolic activity. Thus, simultaneous EEG-fMRI enables the identification of intrinsic states that reflect a "default mode" of brain activity expressed in both modalities (Gusnard and Raichle, 2001; Laufs et al., 2003a; Laufs et al., 2006). Interestingly, changes in other EEG frequency ranges, for example the theta band, correlate negatively with fMRI activity in the default mode network in resting state (Mantini et al., 2007; Sammer et al., 2007; Scheeringa et al., 2008). An interesting approach is to compare these within-subject correlations of ongoing EEG activity with the fMRI signal between subjects (Goncalves et al., 2006). Recently, not only the power of alpha band activity but also measures of global EEG synchronization has been used to inform fMRI analysis (Jann et al., 2009), thereby addressing the

question on the control of long-distance synchronization. Again, a covariation with activity in the default mode areas was found.

Event-Related Simultaneous EEG and fMRI

A logical further development of the EEG-informed fMRI analysis approach is to investigate trial-by-trial variations of EEG and fMRI signals in event-related designs. Two initial studies reported a positive correlation of the single-trial contingent negative variation (CNV) in the EEG with the fMRI response in the posterior medial frontal cortex and the thalamus (Nagai et al., 2004; Hinterberger et al., 2005). This was confirmed and extended by a study using independent-component analysis (ICA) for further improvement of signal-to-noise ratio of the EEG signal (Scheibe et al., 2007). Here, probability of the response in a two-stimulus paradigm was modulated prior to the imperative stimulus, which parametrically modulated the CNV (Scheibe et al., 2009) across conditions. Single-trial CNV amplitudes were used as a regressor for parametric fMRI analysis. Positive correlations of the fMRI signal with the CNV amplitude was found in the posterior medial frontal cortex with a maximum

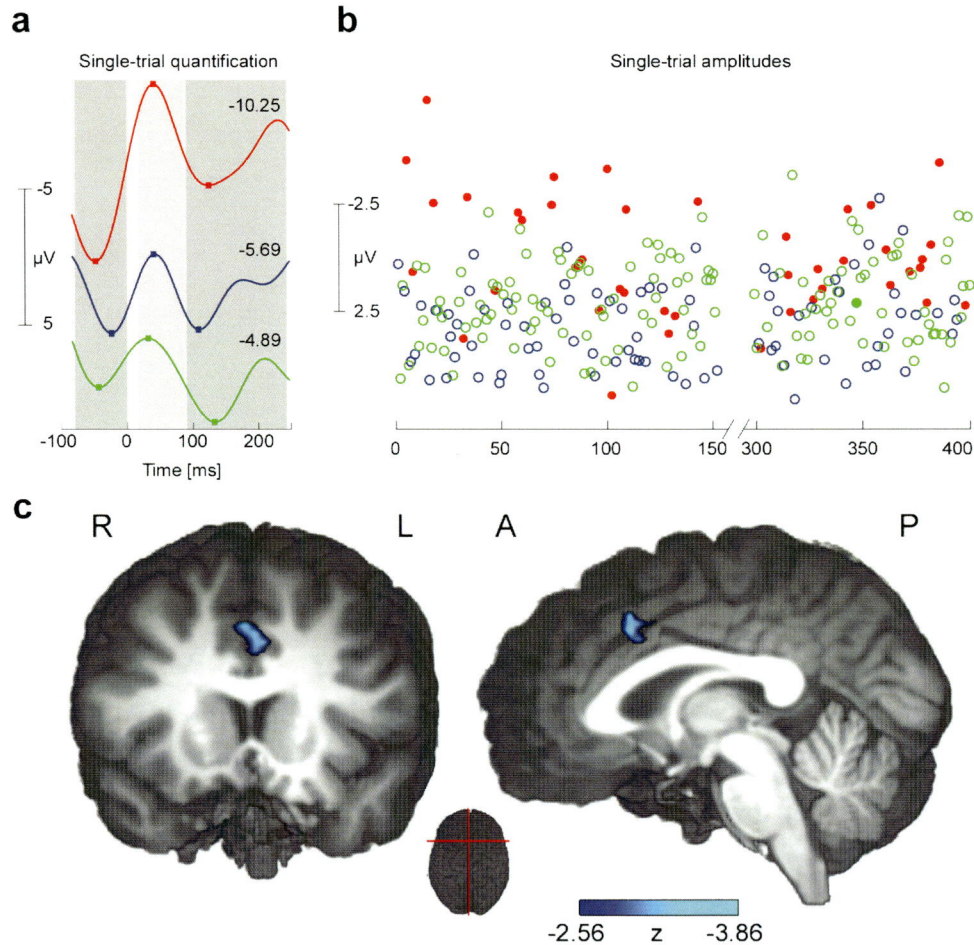

Figure 3.3.2. Example for EEG-informed fMRI analysis from Debener et al. (2005). After denoising of the EEG data, for each participant an independent component (IC) reflecting the error-related negativity (ERN) was obtained based on a selection criteria including a radial-central scalp topography, a differential waveform for erroneous responses as compared to correct responses in the time range 0–150 ms post-response in the single-subject average of the IC's activation time course, and an increased theta power in the time range of the erroneous response. At frontocentral electrodes, a single-trial quantification of the back-projected IC reflecting ERN activity was obtained for each response (a), yielding a vector of single-trial ERN amplitudes for each participant (b). After convolution with the hemodynamic response function, the single-trial ERN amplitude measures were used as predictors of the simultaneously recorded fMRI signal in the general linear model. The group analysis yielded a significant covariation of the single-trial ERN amplitude with the hemodynamic response in the rostral cingulate zone (c). Adapted from Figures 3 and 4 in Debener et al. (2006). Reproduced with permission.

in the supplementary motor area, the dorsal premotor cortex, the insula, and the intraparietal sulcus. Negative correlations were found in areas overlapping with the default-mode network, in particular the anterior medial frontal cortex and the posterior cingulate/precuneus. This is in line with findings that increases in activity in default mode areas are associated with reduced task-related activity and may reflect reduced preparation of the response (Weissman et al., 2006; Eichele et al., 2008).

In a performance-monitoring task yielding a sufficient number of erroneous responses, we used trial-by-trial event-related variations of the EEG reflecting the error-related negativity (ERN) to predict the hemodynamic response (Debener et al., 2005). The single-trial measure of the ERN correlated with the fMRI signal in the rostral

cingulate zone (RCZ) within the posterior medial frontal cortex (Figure 3.3.2). The direction of the correlation indicated that larger (i.e., more negative) ERN amplitudes were associated with greater fMRI signal increases. Electrical dipole localization analysis showed—in line with previous source localization studies of the ERN (Dehaene et al., 1994; Ullsperger and von Cramon, 2001)—that assuming the main generator in the RCZ is electrophysiologically plausible. Importantly, in accordance with current models of performance monitoring, the single-trial ERN amplitudes predicted the slowing of the subjects' reaction time on trials subsequent to errors. Similarly, it has been shown that variations in error-related RCZ activity measured with fMRI are predictive for post-error slowing (Kerns et al., 2004). This indicates that the variations of the EEG and fMRI measures underlying their correlation have a functional significance and cannot be attributed to shared noise. In other words, the correlation between the single-trial ERN and the fMRI signal in the RCZ strongly suggests that the ERN is generated in this brain area, and that the measured signals reflect performance monitoring.

Eichele and colleagues investigated trial-by-trial EEG modulations by systematically varying the sequence of target stimuli in an auditory oddball paradigm (Eichele et al., 2005). Single-trial amplitudes of ERP deflections in the latency ranges of the P200, N200, and P300 components, convolved with the hemodynamic response function, served as predictors in the fMRI analysis. Several spatiotemporal processing stages related to perceptual inference and pattern learning were identified. This study exemplifies a key benefit of EEG-fMRI integration, namely combining high spatial and temporal resolution. On a timescale of around 100 ms the EEG provided sufficient information to reveal several spatially separated regional activations that were differently modulated by the experimental manipulation. A further study investigating single-trial amplitude variations of the P300 in an auditory oddball task found a somewhat different pattern of correlations with the fMRI response (Bénar et al., 2007). At this stage, one can only speculate about the reasons for the discrepant findings, which may include differences in the paradigm as well as different methodological approaches in extracting the single-trial amplitudes. The study by Bénar and colleagues (Bénar et al., 2007) additionally extracted latencies of the single-trial P300 deflections and used those as predictors for the fMRI analysis. This analysis revealed a positive correlation with the fMRI signal in the precuneus and negative correlation with the fMRI response in the posterior medial frontal cortex. While correlations of latencies with the hemodynamic response cannot provide much information on the sources of the EEG activity, they are highly informative for functional interpretations. For example, the association of greater brain activity in the posterior medial frontal cortex with shorter P300 latencies is in line with the notion that this brain area is involved in performance monitoring and cognitive control as well as the allocation of effort (Ridderinkhof et al., 2004; Eichele et al., 2008). This interpretation is further supported by a trial-by-trial correlation of P300 latency and reaction time (Bénar et al., 2007). In a first EEG/fMRI study on an auditory oddball task single-trial EEG amplitude was extracted using a linear multivariate method for identifying task-discriminating components within specific stimulus- and response-locked windows (Goldman et al., 2009). The most surprising finding was a strong correlation of single-trial EEG activity with the hemodynamic activity in the lateral occipital complex in an auditory task. Taken together with a similar finding by Benár and colleagues (Bénar et al., 2007) in a visual oddball task, this finding suggests that this region serves a more general attention allocation function. A recent simultaneous EEG-fMRI study demonstrating single-trial effort-related variations of the N100 component

to be coupled with fMRI activity changes in the posterior medial frontal cortex lends further support to this interpretation (Mulert et al., 2008).

EEG-informed fMRI is, of course, not restricted to single-trial amplitude measures of classical ERP components. For example, Mizuhara and colleagues used phase coherence measures from the EEG to investigate fMRI signal changes associated with beta-band phase synchronization in a mental arithmetic task (Mizuhara et al., 2005). Such approaches may shed light on the metabolic changes associated with synchronizations of electrophysiological oscillation between different brain regions (see also Chapter 4.1). Trial-by-trial modulations in alpha and theta power in a working memory task were recently found to be negatively correlated with the fMRI signal in the primary visual cortex and the default mode areas, respectively, which again provides hints on the interactions between task-related and task-unrelated/ongoing brain activity (Scheeringa et al., 2009).

Recently, high-frequency population spikes in human EEG (around 600 Hz) elicited by median nerve stimulation have been recorded simultaneously with fMRI (Ritter et al., 2008b). Due to low signal-to-noise ratio of these high-frequency signals, trial-by-trial quantification was not feasible. Using a combinatorial algorithm, spontaneous fluctuations in the EEG signals of interest could be extracted in a blockwise fashion with reduced (three-class) amplitude resolution. Correlations with the hemodynamic response in the somatosensory cortex and the thalamus were found.

It is important to consider that scalp-recorded EEG reflects a mixture of activities that are generated by an unknown number of sources. Thus, EEG-informed fMRI analysis builds on extracting EEG features of interest and functional relevance. In other words, the EEG data need to be unmixed before portions are correlated with the fMRI signal. Unmixing methods, such as independent component analysis (ICA, cf. Chapters 3.2, 3.3, 3.5, 3.6) have been successfully used to deal efficiently with EEG artifacts and to unravel spatiotemporally overlapping brain activities (Debener et al., 2005; Eichele et al., 2005; Feige et al., 2005; Scheibe et al., 2007). While these EEG-fMRI studies propose, in part, different analysis strategies, they suggest that ICA helps to optimize signal-to-noise ratio of single-trial EEG estimates used to predict the fMRI signal.

Future Directions and Alternative Approaches

The goal of EEG-informed fMRI is to understand information processing in brain networks with high spatial and temporal resolution. Thus, it seems very promising not to restrict the analysis to one EEG feature or component alone, but rather to extract different portions of the EEG signal known to reflect different processing stages. EEG-informed fMRI can has the potential to provide information on interactions between brain structures underlying these processing steps on a real-time basis. Moreover, interactions of task-related and task-independent ongoing brain activity can be examined. When using more than one EEG parameter to predict fMRI data using the general linear model, it should be ensured that the different parameters vary orthogonally to each other (Ritter and Villringer, 2006). In cases where this cannot be achieved, other fusion methods such as joint or parallel ICA may be more appropriate (Chapters 3.5, 3.6). For example, parallel ICA approaches can be used to extract single-trial measures from the fMRI and EEG data and relate them to each other in further analysis steps. Finally, a number of fMRI-informed EEG analysis approaches have been developed. Usually, the fMRI results are used to constrain source modeling of EEG data (cf. Chapter 3.8). This approach rests on the assumption that the EEG generators overlap with the sources of the fMRI signal change, whereas correlative approaches such as EEG-informed fMRI do not require this strong assumption.

In sum, simultaneous EEG-fMRI recording protocols provide a promising non-invasive technique for directly relating electrical and hemodynamic signals. Direct, event-related correlations enable the identification of systematic fluctuations in brain activity thereby making it possible to study the dynamics of cognitive and ongoing processes at a previously unattained effective spatiotemporal resolution. EEG-informed fMRI analysis, particularly when verified by source modeling and linked to behavioral measures, currently provides the best non-invasive means to localize those structures that underlie temporally well resolved EEG-responses.

REFERENCES

Bénar CG, Schön D, Grimault S, Nazarian B, Burle B, Roth M, Badier JM, Marquis P, Liegeois-Chauvel C, Anton JL (2007) Single-trial analysis of oddball event-related potentials in simultaneous EEG-fMRI. Hum Brain Mapp 28:602–613.

Bledowski C, Linden DE, Wibral M (2007) Combining electrophysiology and functional imaging: different methods for different questions. Trends Cogn Sci 11:500–502.

Büchel C, Holmes AP, Rees G, Friston KJ (1998) Characterizing stimulus-response functions using nonlinear regressors in parametric fMRI experiments. NeuroImage 8:140–148.

Debener S, Ullsperger M, Siegel M, Fiehler K, von Cramon DY, Engel AK (2005) Trial-by-trial coupling of concurrent electroencephalogram and functional magnetic resonance imaging identifies the dynamics of performance monitoring. J Neurosci 25:11730–11737.

Debener S, Ullsperger M, Siegel M, Engel AK (2006) Single-trial EEG-fMRI reveals the dynamics of cognitive function. Trends Cogn Sci 10:558–563.

Dehaene S, Posner MI, Tucker DM (1994) Localization of a neural system for error detection and compensation. Psychol Sci 5:303–305.

Eichele T, Specht K, Moosmann M, Jongsma ML, Quiroga RQ, Nordby H, Hugdahl K (2005) Assessing the spatiotemporal evolution of neuronal activation with single-trial event-related potentials and functional MRI. Proc Natl Acad Sci U S A 102:17798–17803.

Eichele T, Debener S, Calhoun VD, Specht K, Engel AK, Hugdahl K, von Cramon DY, Ullsperger M (2008) Prediction of human errors by maladaptive changes in event-related brain networks. Proc Natl Acad Sci U S A 105:6173–6178.

Feige B, Scheffler K, Esposito F, Di Salle F, Hennig J, Seifritz E (2005) Cortical and subcortical correlates of electroencephalographic alpha rhythm modulation. J Neurophysiol 93:2864–2872.

Ford JM, Whitfield S, Mathalon DH (2004) The neuroanatomy of conflict and error: ERP and fMRI. In: Errors, conflicts, and the brain. Current opinions on performance monitoring (Ullsperger M, Falkenstein M, eds), pp 42–48. Leipzig: MPI for Human Cognitive and Brain Sciences.

Goldman RI, Stern JM, Engel J, Jr., Cohen MS (2002) Simultaneous EEG and fMRI of the alpha rhythm. Neuroreport 13:2487–2492.

Goldman RI, Wei CY, Philiastides MG, Gerson AD, Friedman D, Brown TR, Sajda P (2009) Single-trial discrimination for integrating simultaneous EEG and fMRI: identifying cortical areas contributing to trial-to-trial variability in the auditory oddball task. Neuroimage 47:136–147.

Goncalves SI, de Munck JC, Pouwels PJ, Schoonhoven R, Kuijer JP, Maurits NM, Hoogduin JM, Van Someren EJ, Heethaar RM, Lopes da Silva FH (2006) Correlating the alpha rhythm to BOLD using simultaneous EEG/fMRI: inter-subject variability. Neuroimage 30:203–213.

Gusnard DA, Raichle ME (2001) Searching for a baseline: functional imaging and the resting human brain. Nat Rev Neurosci 2:685–694.

Hinterberger T, Veit R, Wilhelm B, Weiskopf N, Vatine JJ, Birbaumer N (2005) Neuronal mechanisms underlying control of a brain-computer interface. Eur J Neurosci 21:3169–3181.

Horovitz SG, Skudlarski P, Gore JC (2002) Correlations and dissociations between BOLD signal and P300 amplitude in an auditory oddball task: a parametric approach to combining fMRI and ERP. Magn Reson Imaging 20:319–325.

Horovitz SG, Rossion B, Skudlarski P, Gore JC (2004) Parametric design and correlational analyses help integrating fMRI and electrophysiological data during face processing. Neuroimage 22:1587–1595.

Horwitz B, Poeppel D (2002) How can EEG/MEG and fMRI/PET data be combined? Hum Brain Mapp 17:1–3.

Jann K, Dierks T, Boesch C, Kottlow M, Strik W, Koenig T (2009) BOLD correlates of EEG alpha phase-locking and the fMRI default mode network. Neuroimage 45:903–916.

Kerns JG, Cohen JD, MacDonald III AW, Cho RY, Stenger VA, Carter CS (2004) Anterior cingulate conflict monitoring and adjustments in control. Science 303:1023–1026.

Laufs H, Krakow K, Sterzer P, Eger E, Beyerle A, Salek-Haddadi A, Kleinschmidt A (2003a) Electroencephalographic signatures of attentional and cognitive default modes in spontaneous brain activity fluctuations at rest. Proc Natl Acad Sci U S A 100:11053–11058.

Laufs H, Kleinschmidt A, Beyerle A, Eger E, Salek-Haddadi A, Preibisch C, Krakow K (2003b) EEG-correlated fMRI of human alpha activity. Neuroimage 19:1463–1476.

Laufs H, Holt JL, Elfont R, Krams M, Paul JS, Krakow K, Kleinschmidt A (2006) Where the BOLD signal goes when alpha EEG leaves. Neuroimage 31:1408–1418.

Liebenthal E, Ellingson ML, Spanaki MV, Prieto TE, Ropella KM, Binder JR (2003) Simultaneous ERP and fMRI of the auditory cortex in a passive oddball paradigm. Neuroimage 19:1395–1404.

Mantini D, Perrucci MG, Del Gratta C, Romani GL, Corbetta M (2007) Electrophysiological signatures of resting state networks in the human brain. Proc Natl Acad Sci U S A 104:13170–13175.

Martinez-Montes E, Valdes-Sosa PA, Miwakeichi F, Goldman RI, Cohen MS (2004) Concurrent EEG/fMRI analysis by multiway Partial Least Squares. Neuroimage 22:1023–1034.

Mathalon DH, Whitfield SL, Ford JM (2003) Anatomy of an error: ERP and fMRI. Biol Psychol 64:119–141.

Mizuhara H, Wang LQ, Kobayashi K, Yamaguchi Y (2005) Long-range EEG phase synchronization during an arithmetic task indexes a coherent cortical network simultaneously measured by fMRI. Neuroimage 27:553–563.

Moosmann M, Ritter P, Krastel I, Brink A, Thees S, Blankenburg F, Taskin B, Obrig H, Villringer A (2003) Correlates of alpha rhythm in functional magnetic resonance imaging and near infrared spectroscopy. Neuroimage 20:145–158.

Mulert C, Jager L, Propp S, Karch S, Stormann S, Pogarell O, Moller HJ, Juckel G, Hegerl U (2005) Sound level dependence of the primary auditory cortex: Simultaneous measurement with 61-channel EEG and fMRI. Neuroimage 28:49–58.

Mulert C, Seifert C, Leicht G, Kirsch V, Ertl M, Karch S, Moosmann M, Lutz J, Moller HJ, Hegerl U, Pogarell O, Jager L (2008) Single-trial coupling of EEG and fMRI reveals the involvement of early anterior cingulate cortex activation in effortful decision making. Neuroimage 42:158–168.

Nagai Y, Critchley HD, Featherstone E, Fenwick PB, Trimble MR, Dolan RJ (2004) Brain activity relating to the contingent negative variation: an fMRI investigation. Neuroimage 21:1232–1241.

Nunez PL, Silberstein RB (2000) On the relationship of synaptic activity to macroscopic measurements: does co-registration of EEG with fMRI make sense? Brain Topogr 13:79–96.

Pfurtscheller G, Lopes da Silva FH (1999) Event-related EEG/MEG synchronization and desynchronization: basic principles. Clin Neurophysiol 110:1842–1857.

Ridderinkhof KR, Ullsperger M, Crone EA, Nieuwenhuis S (2004) The role of the medial frontal cortex in cognitive control. Science 306:443–447.

Ritter P, Villringer A (2006) Simultaneous EEG-fMRI. Neurosci Biobehav Rev 30:823–838.

Ritter P, Moosmann M, Villringer A (2008a) Rolandic alpha and beta EEG rhythms' strengths are inversely related to fMRI-BOLD signal in primary somatosensory and motor cortex. Hum Brain Mapp 30:1168–1187.

Ritter P, Freyer F, Curio G, Villringer A (2008b) High-frequency (600 Hz) population spikes in human EEG delineate thalamic and cortical fMRI activation sites. Neuroimage 42:483–490.

Rugg MD (1998) Convergent approaches to electrophysiological and hemodynamic investigations of memory. Hum Brain Mapp 6:394–398.

Sabri M, Liebenthal E, Waldron EJ, Medler DA, Binder JR (2006) Attentional modulation in the detection of irrelevant deviance: a simultaneous ERP/fMRI study. J Cogn Neurosci 18:689–700.

Sammer G, Blecker C, Gebhardt H, Bischoff M, Stark R, Morgen K, Vaitl D (2007) Relationship between regional hemodynamic activity and simultaneously recorded EEG-theta associated with mental arithmetic-induced workload. Hum Brain Mapp 28:793–803.

Scheeringa R, Bastiaansen MC, Petersson KM, Oostenveld R, Norris DG, Hagoort P (2008) Frontal theta EEG activity correlates negatively with the default mode network in resting state. Int J Psychophysiol 67:242–251.

Scheeringa R, Petersson KM, Oostenveld R, Norris DG, Hagoort P, Bastiaansen MC (2009) Trial-by-trial coupling between EEG and BOLD identifies networks related to alpha and theta EEG power increases during working memory maintenance. Neuroimage 44:1224–1238.

Scheibe C, Ullsperger M, Sommer W, Heekeren HR (2007) FMRI and EEG data: Combined evidence for the influence of prior probability on decision making. In: 13th annual Human Brain Mapping. Chicago.

Scheibe C, Schubert R, Sommer W, Heekeren HR (2009) Electrophysiological evidence for the effect of prior probability on response preparation. Psychophysiology 46:758–770.

Schicke T, Muckli L, Beer AL, Wibral M, Singer W, Goebel R, Rosler F, Roder B (2006) Tight covariation of BOLD signal changes and slow ERPs in the parietal cortex in a parametric spatial imagery task with haptic acquisition. Eur J Neurosci 23:1910–1918.

Ullsperger M, von Cramon DY (2001) Subprocesses of performance monitoring: a dissociation of error processing and response competition revealed by event-related fMRI and ERPs. Neuroimage 14:1387–1401.

Weissman DH, Roberts KC, Visscher KM, Woldorff MG (2006) The neural bases of momentary lapses in attention. Nat Neurosci 9:971–978.

3.4 ⬛ Vince D. Calhoun and Tom Eichele

Fusion of EEG and fMRI by Parallel Group ICA

⬛ Introduction and Background

Independent component analysis (ICA) is increasingly utilized as a tool for evaluating the hidden spatiotemporal structure contained within brain imaging data. In this chapter, we first provide a brief overview of ICA and how ICA is applied to functional magnetic resonance imaging (fMRI) data. Next, we discuss group ICA and then the application of group ICA for data fusion with an emphasis on the methods developed within our group. We also discuss within a larger context the many alternative approaches that are feasible and currently in use.

ICA is a statistical method used to discover hidden factors (sources or features) from a set of measurements or observed data such that the sources are maximally statistically independent. Note that independence is more general than uncorrelatedness in that two independent variables are uncorrelated, but the reverse is not generally true. Typically, ICA assumes a generative model, where observations are assumed to be linear mixtures of independent sources, and unlike principal component analysis (PCA), which decorrelates the data using second-order statistics, ICA works with higher-order statistics to achieve independence. An intuitive example of ICA can be given by a scatter-plot of two independent signals s_1 and s_2. Figure 3.4.1a (left, middle) shows the projections for PCA and ICA, respectively, for a linear mixture of s_1 and s_2 and Figure 3.4.1a (right) a plot of the two independent signals (s_1, s_2) in a scatter-plot. PCA finds the orthogonal vectors u_1, u_2, but cannot identify the independent vectors. In contrast, ICA is able to find the independent vectors $\mathbf{a}_1, \mathbf{a}_2$ of the linearly mixed signals (s_1, s_2), and is thus able to restore the original sources.

A typical ICA model assumes that the source signals are not observable, statistically independent and non-Gaussian, with an unknown, but linear, mixing process. Consider an observed M–dimensional random vector denoted by $\mathbf{x} = [x_1, x_2, \ldots, x_M]^T$, which is generated by the ICA model:

$$\mathbf{x} = \mathbf{As} \tag{1}$$

where $\mathbf{s} = [s_1, s_2, \ldots, s_N]^T$ is an N-dimensional vector whose elements are the random variables that refer to the independent sources and $\mathbf{A}_{M \times N}$ is an unknown mixing matrix. Typically we assume more sensors than components, hence $M \geq N$, so that $\mathbf{A}$ is usually of full rank. The goal of ICA is to estimate an unmixing matrix $\mathbf{W}_{N \times M}$ such that $\mathbf{y}$ given by

$$\mathbf{y} = \mathbf{Wx} \tag{2}$$

is a good approximation to the "true" sources $\mathbf{s}$. Many ICA algorithms also assume that $M = N$, often introducing PCA as a data reduction step prior to ICA.

Since to achieve ICA, statistical information higher than second order is needed, it can either be generated using non-linear functions applied to the data or can be explicitly calculated. Algorithms that use non-linear functions to generate higher-order statistics have been the most popular ICA approaches and there are a number of algorithms derived based on maximum likelihood estimation, maximization of information transfer, mutual information minimization, and maximization of non-Gaussianity. The first three approaches are equivalent to each other, and they coincide with maximization of non-Gaussianity when the unmixing matrix $\mathbf{W}$ is constrained to be orthogonal (Adali et al., 2008). The algorithms derived within these formulations have optimal large sample properties in the maximum likelihood sense when the nonlinearity within each algorithm is chosen to match the source density. Two commonly used ICA algorithms derived within these formulations are Infomax (Bell and Sejnowski, 1995; Lee et al., 1999) and FastICA (Hyvarinen and Oja, 1997). A newer computationally efficient algorithm based on FastICA is EFICA (Tichavsky et al., 2006). Another popular algorithm

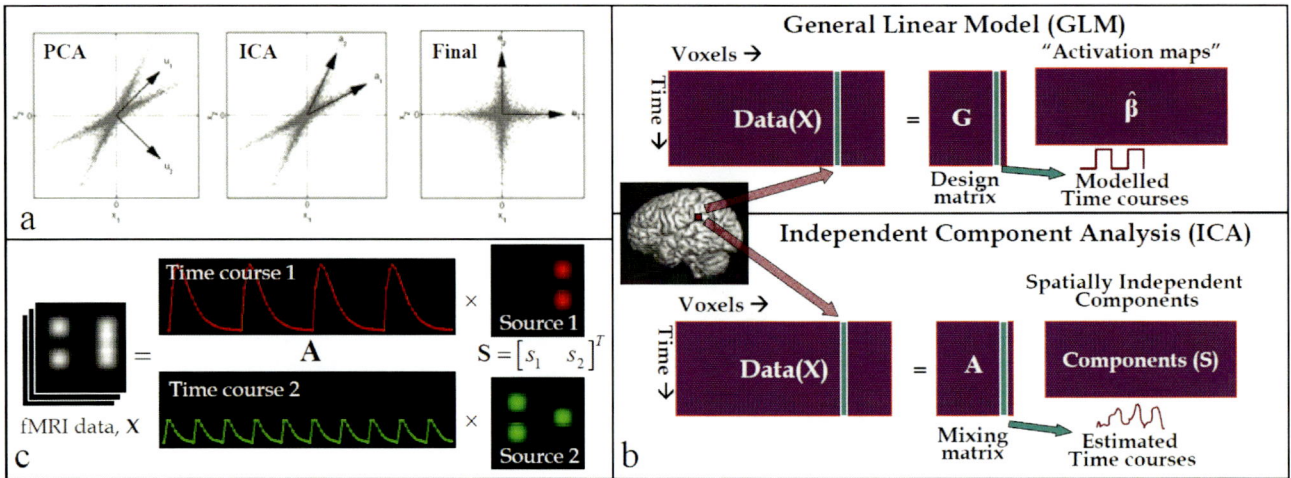

Figure 3.4.1. a) Illustration of the need for higher order statistics, b) Comparison of GLM and ICA for fMRI data, and c) Illustration of spatial ICA of fMRI data.

a) Illustration of the need for higher order statistics: principle component analysis (PCA) identifies orthogonal directions that capture the most variance (a second-order statistic), whereas ICA finds maximally independent directions using higher order statistics; b) Comparison of GLM and spatial ICA for fMRI data: the GLM requires the specification of the temporal model in the design matrix, whereas ICA estimates the time courses from the data by maximizing independences between the component images; and c) Illustration of spatial ICA of fMRI data: the fMRI data is assumed to be comprised of linearly mixed sources, which are extracted via ICA along with their corresponding time courses.

is joint approximate diagonalization of eigenmatrices (JADE) (Cardoso and Souloumiac, 1993), which relies on explicit computation of fourth-order statistical information. Both Infomax and FastICA typically work with a fixed non-linearity or one that is selected from a small set, e.g., two in the case of extended Infomax (Bell and Sejnowski, 1995; Lee et al., 1999). These algorithms typically work well for symmetric distributions and are less accurate for skewed distributions and for sources close to Gaussian. Since optimality condition requires the non-linearities to match the form of source distributions, there are a number of adaptation strategies that are developed. For example, a flexible ICA using a generalized Gaussian density model method is introduced in (Choi et al., 2000). Other flexible extensions of ICA include nonparametric ICA (Boscolo et al., 2001) and kernel ICA (Bach and Jordan, 2002) as well as approaches introduced in Vlassis and Motomura (2001) and Hong et al. (2005). The variety of recent approaches for performing ICA and its applications in areas as diverse as biomedicine, astrophysics, and communications demonstrates the vitality of research in this area.

ICA of fMRI Data

Following its first application to fMRI (McKeown et al., 1998), ICA has been successfully utilized in a number of exciting fMRI applications and especially in those that have proven challenging with the standard regression-type approaches (for a recent collection of examples see McKeown et al., 2003; Calhoun and Adali, 2006). Spatial ICA finds systematically non-overlapping, temporally

coherent brain regions without constraining the shape of the temporal response. The temporal dynamics of many fMRI experiments are difficult to study with traditional GLM-based analyses because of the lack of a well-understood brain-activation model, whereas ICA can reveal intersubject and interevent differences in the temporal dynamics. A strength of ICA is its ability to reveal dynamics for which a temporal model is not available (Calhoun et al., 2002; Eichele et al., 2008a). A comparison of the GLM approach and ICA as applied to fMRI analysis is shown in Figure 3.4.1b.

Independent component analysis is used in fMRI modeling to study the spatiotemporal structure of the signal, and it can be used to discover either spatially or temporally independent components (Jung, 2001). Most applications of ICA to fMRI use the former approach and seek components that are maximally independent in space. In such a setting, we let the observation data matrix be $\mathbf{X}$, an $N \times M$ matrix (where N is the number of time points and M is the number of voxels) as shown in Figure 3.4.1b. The aim of fMRI component analysis is then to factor the data matrix into a product of a set of time courses and a set of spatial patterns. An illustration of how ICA decomposes the data into a parsimonious summary of images and time courses is shown in Figure 3.4.1c. The number of components is a free parameter, which has previously been either empirically determined or estimated. There are a number of approaches for estimating the number of components using information theoretic approaches (Akaike, 1974; Rissanen, 1983) that have been shown to work well with fMRI data (Beckmann and Smith, 2004; Li et al., 2007).

Since the introduction of ICA for fMRI analysis, the choice of spatial or temporal independency has been controversial (Calhoun et al., 2001a). However, the two options are merely two different modeling assumptions. McKeown et al. argued that the sparse distributed nature of the spatial pattern for typical cognitive activation paradigms would work well with spatial ICA (sICA). Furthermore, since the prototypical confounds are also sparse and localized, e.g., vascular pulsation (signal localized to larger veins that are moving as a result of cardiac pulsation), CSF flow signals in the ventricles, or breathing-induced motion (signal localized to strong tissue contrast near discontinuities: "tissue edges"), the Infomax algorithm with a sparse prior is very well suited for spatial analysis (Petersen et al., 2000) and has also been used for temporal ICA (Calhoun et al., 2001a) as have decorrelation-based algorithms (Petersen et al., 2000). Stone et al. (1999) proposed a method that attempts to maximize both spatial and temporal independence. An interesting combination of spatial and temporal ICA was pursued by Seifritz et al. (2002); they used an initial sICA to reduce the spatial dimensionality of the data by locating a region of interest in which they then subsequently performed temporal ICA to study in more detail the structure of the nontrivial temporal response in the human auditory cortex.

Group ICA of fMRI Data

Unlike univariate methods (e.g., regression analysis, Kolmogorov-Smirnov statistics), ICA does not naturally generalize to a method suitable for drawing inferences about observations from multiple subjects. For example, when using the general linear model, the investigator specifies the regressors of interest, and so drawing inferences about group data comes naturally, since all individuals in the group share the same regressors. In ICA, by contrast, different individuals in the group will have different time courses and component maps, and components will appear in a different order across decompositions, so it is not immediately clear how to draw inferences about group data using ICA. Despite this, several ICA multisubject analysis approaches have been proposed for fMRI (Calhoun et al., 2001c; Calhoun et al., 2001b; Lukic et al., 2002; Svensen et al., 2002; Calhoun et al., 2004a; Schmithorst and Holland, 2004; Beckmann and Smith, 2005; Esposito et al., 2005; Guo and Giuseppe, 2008). The various approaches differ in terms of how the data is organized prior to the ICA analysis, what types of output are available (e.g., single-subject contributions, group averages, etc.), and how the statistical inference is made.

A summary of several group ICA approaches is provided in Figure 3.4.2. Approaches can be grouped into five categories. Figure 3.4.2a illustrates approaches that perform

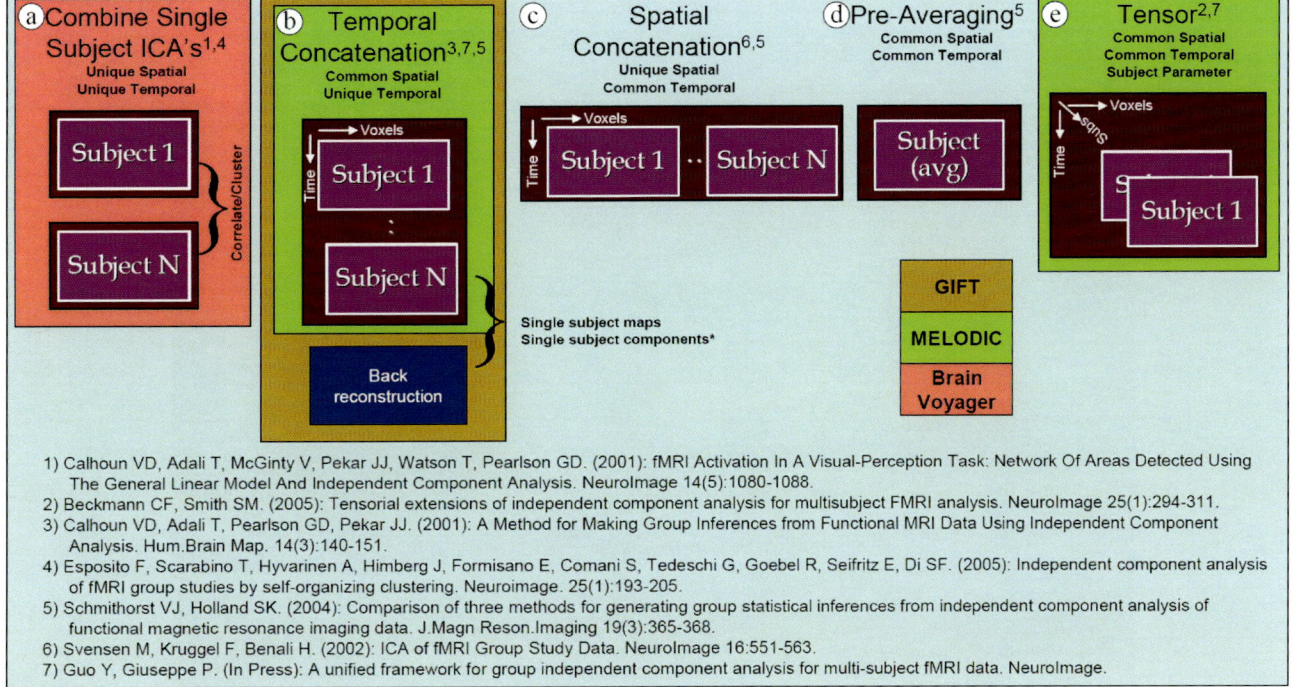

Figure 3.4.2. Several group ICA approaches.

A comparison of 5 group ICA approaches and some of the software packages that implement these methods as a primary pipeline. a) separate ICA analyses run on each subjects, followed by correlation or clustering to enable group interference, b) temporal concatenation followed by an aggregate ICA analysis is a popular approach that also can include a back-reconstruction step to compute single subject maps and time courses, c) spatial concatenation, or d) pre-averaging prior to ICA have also been proposed. Finally, e) tensor-based approaches stack the data into a cube.

single-subject ICA and then attempt to combine the output into a group post hoc by using approaches such as self-organized clustering or spatial correlation of the components (Calhoun et al., 2001c; Esposito et al., 2005). This has the advantage of allowing for unique spatial and temporal features, but has the disadvantage that since the data are noisy the components are not necessarily unmixed in the same way for each subject. The other four approaches involved an ICA computed on condensed group data directly. Temporal concatenation, Figure 3.4.2b, and spatial concatenation, Figure 3.4.2c, have both been examined. The advantage of these approaches is that they perform one ICA, which can then be divided into subject-specific parts, hence the comparison of subject differences within a component is straightforward. The temporal concatenation approach allows for unique time courses for each subject, but assumes common group maps, whereas the spatial concatenation approach allows for unique maps but assumes common time courses. Although they are really just two different approaches for organizing the data, temporal concatenation appears to work better for fMRI data (Schmithorst and Holland, 2004), most likely because the temporal variations in the fMRI signal are much larger than the spatial variations, and has been widely used for group ICA of fMRI data.

The temporal concatenation approach is implemented in the MELODIC software (http://www.fmrib.ox.ac.uk/fsl/) and also the GIFT Matlab software (http://icatb.source-forge.net/). The GIFT software additionally implements a back-reconstruction step, which produces subject specific images (Calhoun et al., 2001b). This enables a comparison of both the time courses and the images for one group or multiple groups (Calhoun et al., 2008b). The simulation in Calhoun et al. (2001b) shows that ICA with temporal concatenation plus back-reconstruction can capture variations in subject-specific images. The approach implemented in GIFT thus trades-off the use of a common model for the spatial maps against the difficulties of combining single subject ICA. An in-between approach would be to utilize temporal concatenation separately for each group (Celone et al., 2006), although in this case matching the components post hoc becomes again necessary. The approach in Figure 3.4.2d involves averaging the data prior to performing ICA. This approach is less computationally demanding, but makes a more stringent assumption that requires a common time course and a common spatial map. Finally, the tensorial approach in Figure 3.4.2e (implemented in MELODIC) involves estimating a common time course and a common image for each component but allows for a subject-specific parameter to be estimated.

Higher-order tensor decompositions (also known as multi-dimensional, multi-way, or n-way), one of the first class of algorithms that performed ICA successfully (Cardoso, 1989), have received renewed interest recently, although their adaptation to group and multigroup fMRI data is still being explored. Figure 3.4.2e shows an approach based on a three-dimensional tensor that has been developed to estimate a single spatial, temporal, and subject-specific "mode" for each component to attempt to capture the multidimensional structure of the data in the estimation stage (Beckmann and Smith, 2005). This approach however may not work as well (without additional

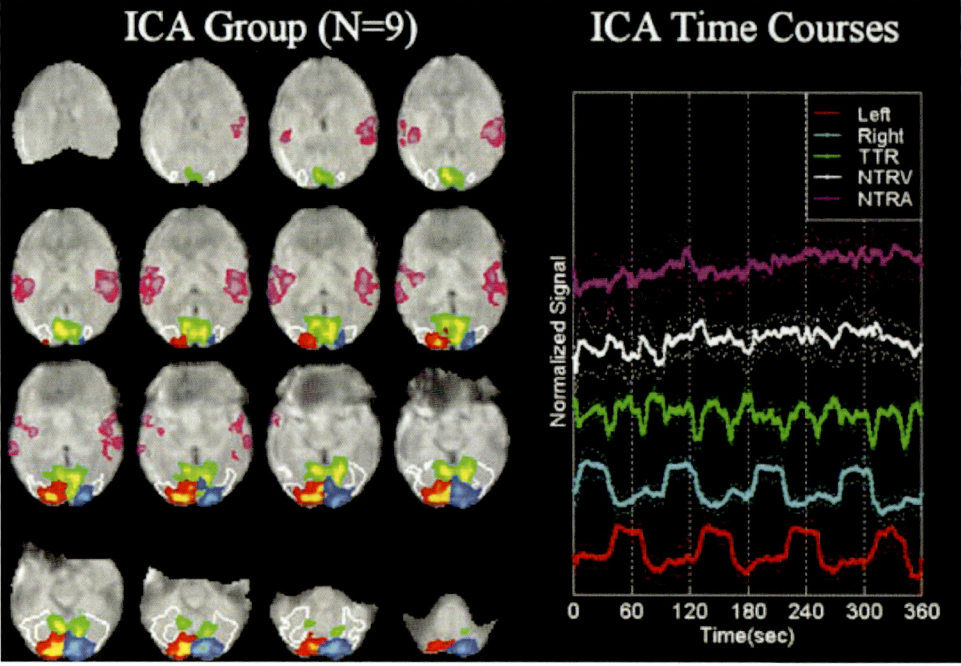

Figure 3.4.3. fMRI group ICA results from Calhoun et al., (2001).

Group ICA identifies temporally coherent networks that are spatially distinct. In a relatively simple visual stimulation paradigm ICA identified strongly task-related networks as well as transient and non–task related networks.

preprocessing) if the time courses between subjects share no commonalities, such as in resting-state studies. A detailed comparison of several group ICA approaches including temporal concatenation and tensor ICA by an independent group is provided in a recent paper (Guo and Giuseppe, 2008).

In the remainder of this paper, we focus on the group ICA approach implemented in the GIFT software which is available at http://icatb.sourceforge.net (Calhoun et al., 2001b). GIFT uses multiple data reduction steps following data concatenation to reduce the computational load, along with back-reconstruction and statistical comparison of individual maps and time courses following ICA estimation. An example group ICA analysis of nine subjects performing a four cycle alternating left/right visual stimulation task is presented in Figure 3.4.3 (from Calhoun et al., 2001b). Separate components for primary visual areas in the left and the right visual cortex (depicted in red and blue, respectively) were consistently task-related with respect to the appropriate stimulus. A large region (depicted in green) including occipital areas and extending into parietal areas appeared to be sensitive to changes in the visual stimuli. Additionally, some visual association areas (depicted in white) had time courses that were not task related. As we discuss later, one-sample group inference or two-sample comparison of groups can be performed by computing typical second-level random effects statistics on either the ICA maps or the time courses. Similarly, the coupling between the component timecourses can be estimated (Jafri et al., 2008)

ICA for Data Fusion

Many studies are currently collecting multiple types of imaging data from the same participants, often in settings where relatively large groups of participants are sampled (n > 100). Each imaging method reports on a limited domain and typically provides both common and unique information about the problem in question. Approaches for combining or fusing data in brain imaging can be conceptualized as having a place on an analytic spectrum with meta-analysis (highly distilled data) to examine convergent evidence at one end and large-scale computational modeling (highly detailed theoretical modeling) at the other end (Husain et al., 2002). In between are methods that attempt to perform a direct data fusion (Horwitz and Poeppel, 2002). One promising data fusion approach is to first process each image type and extract features from different modalities. These features are then examined for relationships among the data types at the group level (i.e., variations among individuals or between patients and controls). This approach allows us to take advantage of the "cross"-information among data types and when performing multimodal fusion provides a natural link among different data types (Ardnt, 1996; Savopol and Armenakis, 2002; Calhoun et al., 2006a).

A natural set of tools for performing data fusion include those that transform data matrices into a smaller set of modes or components. Such approaches include those

based on singular value decomposition (SVD) (Friston et al., 1996; McIntosh et al., 1996) as well as ICA (McKeown et al., 1998). An advantage of ICA over variance-based approaches like SVD or PCA is the use of higher-order statistics to reveal hidden structure. Here, we describe two approaches for data fusion, joint ICA and parallel ICA. We show two examples, the first one involving event-related potential (ERP) and fMRI data and a second one on fMRI and genetic data.

Theory

In this section, we review the methods behind group ICA, joint ICA, and parallel ICA.

Group ICA of fMRI

As we mentioned earlier, the group ICA approach implemented in GIFT incorporates temporal concatenation plus back-reconstruction. Figure 3.4.4 (top) provides a graphical representation of the GIFT approach that essentially involves estimating a mixing matrix which has partitions that are unique to each subject. Once the mixing matrix is estimated, the component maps for each subject can be computed by projecting the single-subject data onto the inverse of the partition of the mixing matrix that corresponds to that subject. In the end, this provides subject-specific time courses and images that can be used to make group and intergroup inferences.

An additional aspect to consider is that GIFT performs multiple data-reduction steps, primarily for computational reasons, but also for noise reduction. Mathematically, if we let $\mathbf{X}_i = \mathbf{F}_i^{-1}\mathbf{Y}_i$ be the $L \times V$ reduced data matrix from subject i, where $\mathbf{Y}_i$ is the $K \times V$ data matrix containing the preprocessed and spatially normalized data, $\mathbf{F}_i^{-1}$ is the $L \times K$ reducing matrix determined by the PCA decomposition, V is the number of voxels, K is the number of fMRI time points, and L is the size of the time dimension following reduction. Note that all matrix inverses are pseudo-inverses. The reduced data from all subjects is concatenated into a matrix and reduced using PCA to N dimensions the number of components to be estimated. The $N \times V$ reduced, concatenated matrix for the M subjects is

$$\mathbf{X} = \mathbf{G}^{-1}\begin{bmatrix} \mathbf{F}_1^{-1}\mathbf{Y}_1 \\ \vdots \\ \mathbf{F}_M^{-1}\mathbf{Y}_M \end{bmatrix} \qquad (3)$$

where $\mathbf{G}^{-1}$ is an $N \times LM$ reducing matrix (also determined by a PCA decomposition) and is multiplied on the right by the $LM \times V$ concatenated data matrix for the M subjects. Following ICA estimation, we can write $\mathbf{X} = \hat{\mathbf{A}}\hat{\mathbf{S}}$, where $\hat{\mathbf{A}}$ is the $N \times N$ mixing matrix and $\hat{\mathbf{S}}$ is the $N \times V$ component

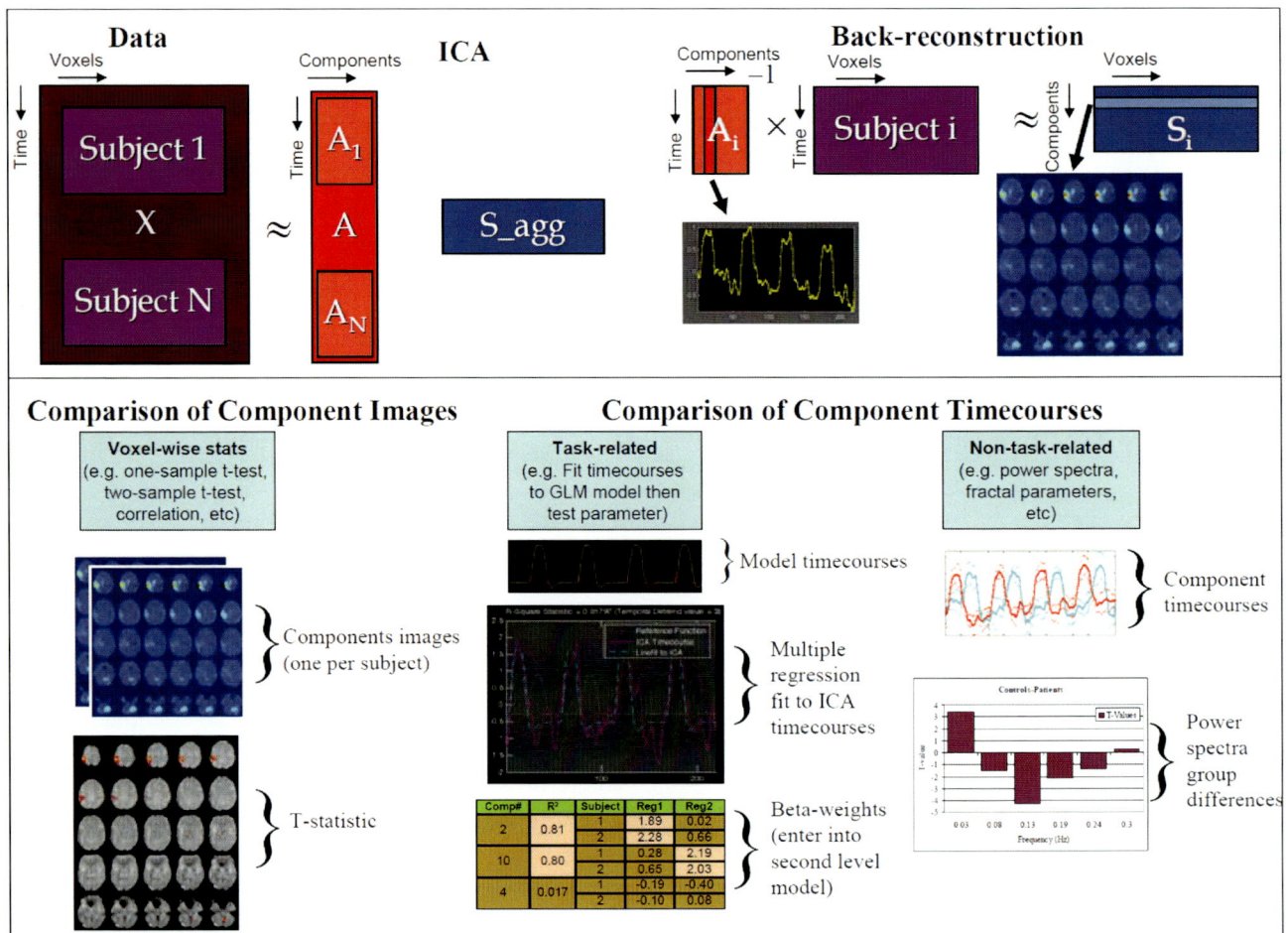

Figure 3.4.4. Graphical illustration of group ICA as implemented in GIFT.

Group. ICA as implemented in GIFT incorporates temporal concatenation plus a back-reconstruction step to produce single-subject maps and time courses. Which of these time courses is of interest depends on the question being asked, which can draw on comparisons of the component images or time courses (bottom panel).

map. Substituting this expression for $\mathbf{X}$ into Equation (3) and multiplying both sides by $\mathbf{G}$, we have

$$\mathbf{G}\hat{\mathbf{A}}\hat{\mathbf{S}} = \begin{bmatrix} \mathbf{F}_1^{-1}\mathbf{Y}_1 \\ \vdots \\ \mathbf{F}_M^{-1}\mathbf{Y}_M \end{bmatrix} \tag{4}$$

.

Partitioning the matrix $\mathbf{G}$ by subject provides the following expression

$$\begin{bmatrix} \mathbf{G}_1 \\ \vdots \\ \mathbf{G}_M \end{bmatrix} \hat{\mathbf{A}}\hat{\mathbf{S}} = \begin{bmatrix} \mathbf{F}_1^{-1}\mathbf{Y}_1 \\ \vdots \\ \mathbf{F}_M^{-1}\mathbf{Y}_M \end{bmatrix} \tag{5}$$

.

We then write the equation for subject i by working only with the elements in partition i of the above matrices such that

$$\mathbf{G}_i\hat{\mathbf{A}}\hat{\mathbf{S}}_i = \mathbf{F}_i^{-1}\mathbf{Y}_i \tag{6}$$

The matrix $\mathbf{S}_i$ in Equation 6 contains the single-subject maps for subject i and is calculated from the following equation:

$$\hat{\mathbf{S}}_i = (\mathbf{G}_i\hat{\mathbf{A}})^{-1}\mathbf{F}_i^{-1}\mathbf{Y}_i \tag{7}$$

We now multiply both sides of Equation (6) by $\mathbf{F}_i$ and write,

$$\mathbf{Y}_i \approx \mathbf{F}_i\mathbf{G}_i\hat{\mathbf{A}}\hat{\mathbf{S}}_i \tag{8}$$

which provides the ICA decomposition of the data from subject i, contained in the matrix $\mathbf{Y}_i$. The $N \times V$ matrix $\hat{\mathbf{S}}_i$ contains the N source maps and the $K \times N$ matrix $\mathbf{F}_i\mathbf{G}_i\hat{\mathbf{A}}$ is the single subject mixing matrix and contains the time course for each of the N components.

Group inferences can be made by analyzing the subject-specific time courses and spatial maps. Figure 3.4.4 (bottom) categorizes these analyses into three main areas. To evaluate spatial properties of a given component statistically, one can perform voxel-wise tests on the spatial maps, for example simple one-sample t-tests (Figure 3.4.4, bottom left). The time courses can be analyzed by fitting to a GLM (the same model one would use for a GLM analysis; e.g., multiple regression), but instead of fitting to the voxel-wise data the ICA time courses are the dependent variable (Figure 3.4.4, bottom middle). The estimated parameters can then be entered into a second-level statistical analysis to make inferences about how much each component is modulated by a given stimulus, whether one component is modulated more by one stimulus than another, whether one group shows a stronger task-modulation than another, etc. (Stevens et al., 2007). This provides a powerful way to make inferences about the components. Another way of probing how a component is related to an experiment is to deconvolve hemodynamic response functions (HRF) from the time course, and estimate the amplitude modulation of the HRF in a trial-by-trial analysis (Eichele et al., 2008a). The single-trial responses can then be sorted, averaged, and inspected for relevant effects for which a suitable temporal model is not available a priori. Finally, one may be interested in the properties of on-task-related components in block/event-related data, or components in resting-state data (Calhoun et al., 2008a). In this case, one can for example evaluate differences in the spectral power between groups (Garrity et al., 2007) or compute additional parameters such as the fractal dimension of the subject component time courses (Figure 3.4.4, bottom right). Also, resting-state time courses can be employed for functional connectivity analysis between components, yielding information that may have great diagnostic value (Sorg et al., 2007; Jafri et al., 2008)

Joint and Parallel ICA

Next, we introduce two approaches for performing data fusion with ICA, joint ICA and parallel ICA (both of which are implemented in the Matlab-based Fusion ICA Toolbox (FIT: http://icatb.sourceforge.net). In this section, we perform ICA at the second level and consider the "sensors" as subjects instead of fMRI time points.

Joint ICA

Joint ICA is an approach that enables us to jointly analyze multiple modalities that have all been collected in the same set of subjects. In our development, we primarily consider a set of extracted features from each subject's data, these data form the multiple observations—the vertical dimension in our group dataset. Given two sets of group data (can be more than two, for simplicity, we first consider two), $\mathbf{X}_F$ and $\mathbf{X}_G$, we concatenate the two datasets side-by-side to form $\mathbf{X}_J$ and write the likelihood as

$$L(\mathbf{W}) = \prod_{n=1}^{N} \prod_{v=1}^{V} p_{J,n}(u_{J,v}) \qquad (9)$$

where $\mathbf{u}_J = \mathbf{W}\mathbf{x}_J$. Here, we use the notation in terms of random variables such that each entry in the vectors $\mathbf{u}_J$ and $\mathbf{x}_J$ correspond to a random variable, which is replaced by the observation for each sample $n = 1, \ldots, N$ as rows of matrices $\mathbf{U}_J$ and $\mathbf{X}_J$. When posed as a maximum likelihood problem, we estimate a *joint* unmixing matrix $\mathbf{W}$ such that the likelihood $L(\mathbf{W})$ is maximized.

Let the two datasets $\mathbf{X}_F$ and $\mathbf{X}_G$ have dimensionality $N \times V_1$ and $N \times V_2$, then we have

$$L(\mathbf{W}) = \prod_{n=1}^{N} \left(\prod_{v=1}^{V_1} p_{F,n}(u_{F,v}) \prod_{v=1}^{V_2} p_{G,n}(u_{G,v}) \right), \qquad (10)$$

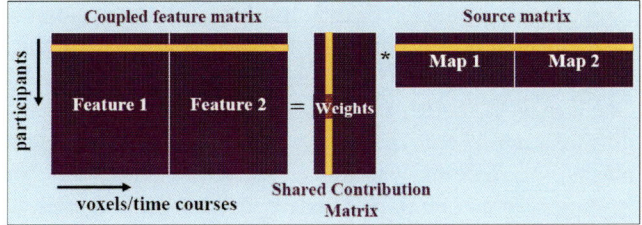

a Joint ICA
Shared Feature Profile

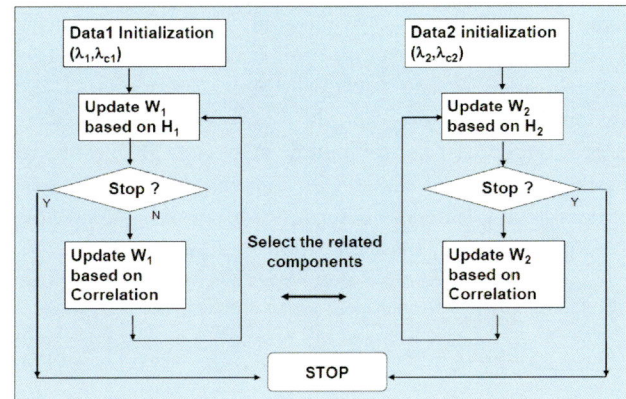

b Parallel ICA
Distinct but linked Feature Profile

Figure 3.4.5. Illustration of joint ICA and Parallel ICA models.

Joint ICA (left) assumes a shared contribution matrix for the two modalities. Parallel ICA (right) updates separate ICA processes using the correlation between the subject profiles for the two modalities.

Depending on the data types in question, the above formula can be made more or less flexible.

This formulation characterizes the basic jICA approach and assumes that the sources associated with the two data types (F and G) modulate the same way across N subjects (see Figure 3.4.5a). The assumption of the same linear covariation for both modalities is fairly strong, however it has the advantage of providing a parsimonious way to link multiple data types and has been demonstrated in a variety of cases with meaningful results (Calhoun et al., 2006c; Calhoun et al., 2006b; Calhoun et al., 2006a; Eichele et al., 2008b; Moosmann et al., 2008). In the case when the two modalities do not covary linearly across subjects the joint ICA model can still capture this such that the component weights for one of the modalities would be close to zero.

There are different ways to relax the assumptions made in the formulation above, such as instead of constraining the two types of sources to share the same mixing coefficients, i.e., to have the same modulation across N samples, we can require that the form of modulation across samples for the sources from two data types to be correlated but not necessarily the same (Correa et al., 2008). The approach we discuss next, called parallel ICA, provides this additional flexibility in modeling (Liu and Calhoun, 2006; Liu and Calhoun, 2007).

Parallel ICA

As noted earlier, the strong regularization imposed by the jICA framework can be relaxed in a number of ways to allow for more flexibility in the estimation. One such approach we developed is called parallel independent component analysis (paraICA). As a framework to investigate the integration of data from two imaging modalities, this method identifies components of both modalities and connections between them through enhancing intrinsic interrelationships (see Figure 3.4.5b). We have applied this approach to link fMRI/ERP data and also fMRI and genetic data (single nucleotide polymorphism arrays) (Liu and Calhoun, 2006; Liu and Calhoun, 2006; 2007; Liu et al., 2009). Results show that paraICA provides stable results and can identify the linked components with a relatively high accuracy.

In our initial application of paraICA, we defined a genetic independent component as a specific SNP association, i.e., a group of SNPs with various degrees of contribution, which partially determines a specific phenotype or endophenotype. This association can be modeled as a linear combination of SNP genotypes (Lee and Batzoglou, 2003; Dawy et al., 2005),

$$s = \beta_1 \cdot snp_1 + \beta_2 \cdot snp_2 + \ldots + \beta_{n1} \cdot snp_n; \quad (11)$$

where snp is a genotype at a given locus and β is a weight contributed from a SNP to the genetic association. Beside the independent component, the weight itself is also of interest, implying the influence factor and type, i.e., inhibitory or

excitatory to a phenotype. With the assumption that each component has an independent distribution pattern in 367 SNPs, we constructed the SNP data matrix, X, in a participant-by-SNP direction. The mixing process is presented in Equation 12,

$$
\begin{aligned}
\mathbf{X}_s &= \left[x_{s1}, x_{s2}, x_{s3}, \ldots, x_{sn} \right]^T, \\
\mathbf{S}_s &= \left[x_{s1}, x_{s2}, x_{s3}, \ldots, x_{sm} \right]^T; \\
\mathbf{S}_s &= \mathbf{W}_s \mathbf{X}_s; \\
\mathbf{A}_s &= \mathbf{W}_s^{-1}; \quad \mathbf{A}_s = \left[a_{s1}, a_{s2}, a_{s3} \ldots a_{sn} \right]^T
\end{aligned}
\quad (12)
$$

where, n is the number of participants and m is the number of components. x_{si} is a vector of 367 SNP genotypes for one participant. s_{si} is a vector of 367 SNP weights for one genetic component. A_s is the matrix of the loading parameters, presenting the influence of each SNP component on participants.

In our current formulation, the relationship between brain function and the genetic component is calculated as the correlation between the columns of the fMRI A_f matrix and the SNP A_s matrix (note this can also be defined using other criteria such as mutual information, to identify nonlinear coupling between fMRI and SNP data). Thus, we have the correlation term and the maximization function based on entropy, where data 1 is the fMRI data and data 2 is the SNP data. The procedure of parallel ICA is illustrated in Figure 3.4.5b. The algorithm proceeds such that two demixing matrices $\mathbf{W}$ are updated separately, during which the component with highest correlation from each modality is selected and used to modify the update of the demixing matrix based on the correlation value using appropriate stopping criteria.

Examples

In this section, we present examples of results from previous work using group ICA, joint ICA, and parallel ICA. The first example shows an analysis of a simulated driving paradigm, a case in which ICA is particularly useful as it is a naturalistic task that is difficult to parameterize for use in a traditional GLM analysis. fMRI data from 15 subjects were collected during a 10-minute paradigm with alternating 1-minute blocks of fixation, simulated driving, and watching (Calhoun et al., 2002). ICA time courses were first analyzed to evaluate task-relatedness. Six components were identified and entered into a voxel-wise one-sample t-test. A total of six components are presented showing different dynamics in response to simulated driving. In this case, ICA has proven to be a very powerful approach for analysis and enabled us to develop a model for the neural correlates of simulated driving that is nicely related to existing models based on behavioral data (Calhoun et al., 2002; Calhoun et al., 2004b; Calhoun et al., 2005; Meda et al., 2009).

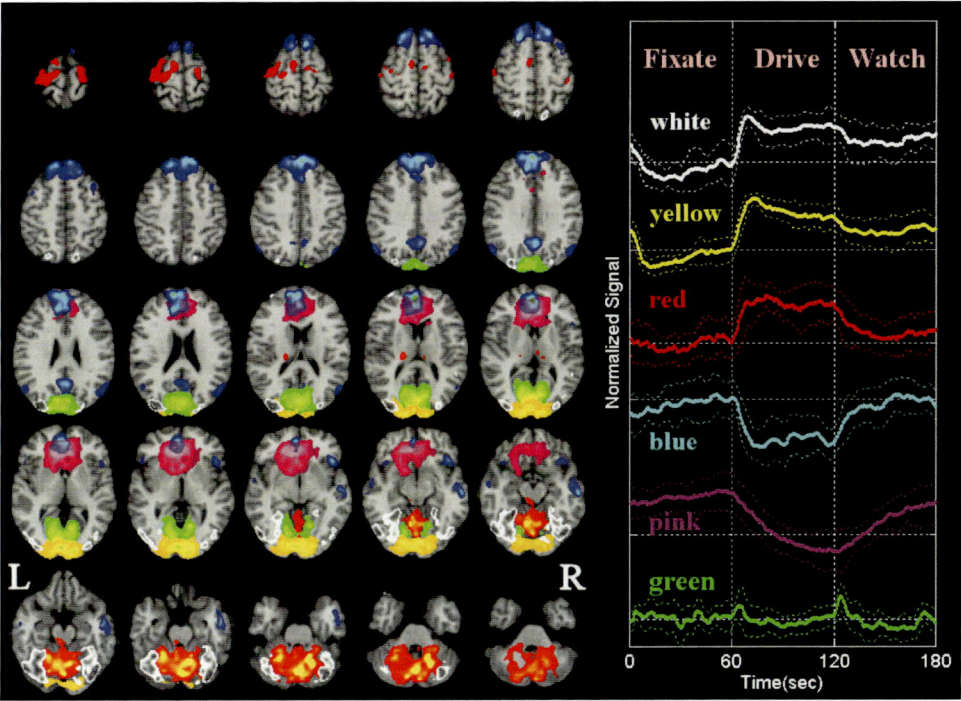

Figure 3.4.6. Naturalistic driving (from Calhoun et al., 2002).

Multiple networks identified during simulated driving. ICA enables us to study the complex and overlapping dynamics that occur during a naturalistic task.

The second example we present is an analysis of fMRI data collected from an auditory oddball task for two patients groups as well as healthy controls. Back-reconstructed component maps were entered into two sample t-tests to evaluate pair-wise differences between the three groups. Results are presented for each group for two components, one in temporal lobe and also the default mode (Figure 3.4.6, left). We performed a multiple regression including the target, novel, and standard stimuli and the mean of the estimated beta parameters is shown in Figure 3.4.6 (right). We were also able to utilize these results to accurately differentiate healthy controls, schizophrenia patients, and patients with bipolar disorder. This example illustrates the ability of group ICA to differentiate groups and also shows both a comparison of the spatial maps and the time courses.

The next example involves data fusion of event related EEG and fMRI data using parallel ICA. The fMRI data and the 32-channel ERP data are entered into a parallel ICA analysis. This provides us with not only a temporal ERP profile and a spatial fMRI profile, but the topography and average time course from the ERP data provides additional information for interpretation (see Figure 3.4.7). We

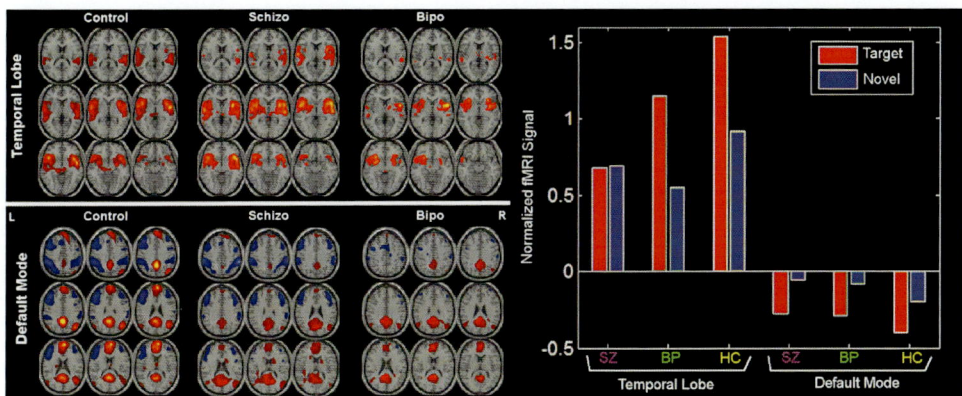

Figure 3.4.7. Pair-wise comparisons of the control, schizophrenia, and bipolar groups (from Calhoun et al., 2008b).

Two-sample t-tests were performed to illustrate most significant differences for each pair-wise comparison (left). Note that these maps are generated from all subjects and actual classification regions will be slightly different due to the leave-one-out approach. On the right is plotted the average beta weights for the stimuli broken out by group.

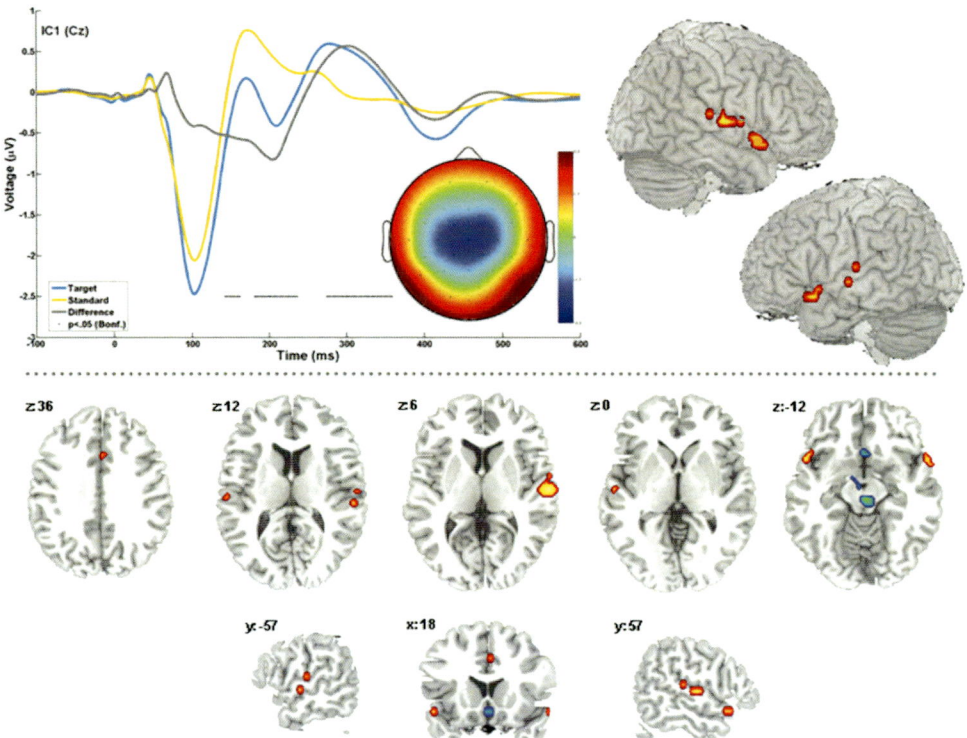

Figure 3.4.8. Fusion of ERP and fMRI data (from Eichele et al., 2008b).

Time course and topography for EEG-tIC1 for standard and target epochs as well as the difference wave between them. The difference wave was subjected to a pointwise one-sample t-test, black dots indicate time frames with significant difference from zero at p <.05, bonferroni corrected for 512 tests (t > 6.93). The bilateral temporal activation in the linked fMRI component is shown as a surface rendering (top right). Additional slices in the lower half illustrate the overall spatial pattern (see also Table 3.4.1). The maps are thresholded at 1% false discovery rate, cluster extent 5 voxels. Positive correlation is plotted in red, inverse correlation in blue.

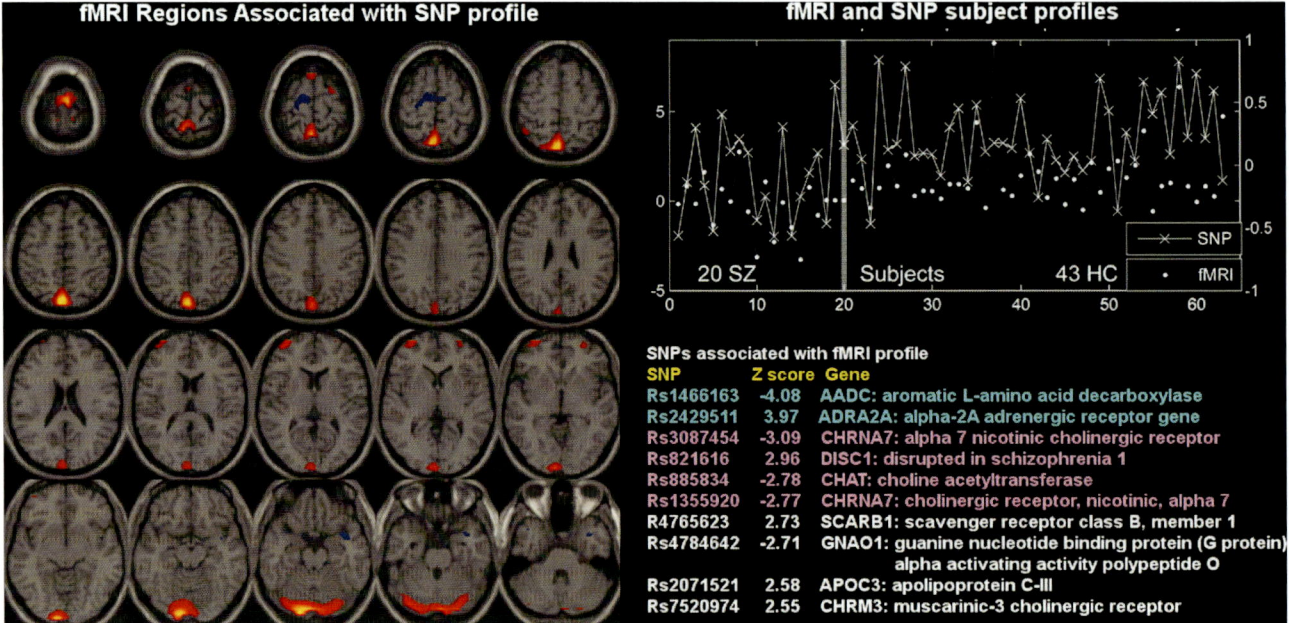

Figure 3.4.9. Fusion of fMRI and genetic (SNP) data (from Liu et al., 2009).

Parallel ICA provides an fMRI part (left) and a SNP part (bottom right) in addition to a correlated subject profile for both fMRI and SNP data (top right).

developed a method for parallel spatial and temporal independent component analysis for concurrent multisubject single-trial EEG-fMRI that addresses the mixing problem in both modalities, and integrates the data via correlation of the trial-to-trial modulation of the recovered fMRI maps and EEG time courses. The method affords extraction of a previously undetected spatiotemporal process from a concurrent EEG-fMRI dataset (Eichele et al., 2005), corresponding to the auditory onset response and subsequent low-level orienting/change detection. For full details please see Eichele et al. (2008b).

Our final example shows results from a parallel ICA analysis of auditory oddball fMRI data and 367 SNPs from schizophrenia patients and healthy controls (Liu et al., 2009). When 43 healthy controls and 20 schizophrenia patients, all Caucasian, were studied, we found a correlation of 0.38 between one fMRI component and one SNP component. This fMRI component consisted of regions in parietal lobe, right temporal lobe, and bilateral frontal lobe. The relevant SNP component was contributed to significantly by 10 SNPs located in genes including those coding for the nicotinic alpha-7cholinergic receptor, aromatic amino acid decarboxylase, disrupted in schizophrenia 1, among others. Both fMRI and SNP components showed significant differences in loading parameters between the schizophrenia and control groups (p < 0.001 for the fMRI component; p = 0.001 for the SNP component). The parallel ICA framework enabled us to identify interactions between brain functional and genetic information; our findings provide a proof-of-concept that genomic SNP factors can be investigated by using endophenotypic imaging findings in a multivariate format.

Summary

ICA is a powerful, data-driven approach that can be used to analyze group fMRI data or to analyze multimodal data including fMRI, EEG/ERP, and genetic data. The examples demonstrate the utility and diversity of ICA-based approaches for the analysis of brain imaging data.

ACKNOWLEDGMENTS

This research was supported in part by the National Institutes of Health, under grants 1 R01 EB 000840, 1 R01 EB 005846, and 1 R01 EB 006841.

REFERENCES

Adali T, Novey M, Cardoso JF (2008) Complex ICA using nonlinear functions. IEEE Trans Signal Processing 56:4536–4544.

Akaike H (1974) A new look at statistical model identification. IEEE Transon Automatic Control 19:716–723.

Arndt C, Loffeld, O (1996) Information gained by data fusion. Proc. SPIE 2784:32–40.

Bach F, Jordan M (2002) Kernel independent component analysis. J Mach Learn Res 3:1–48.

Beckmann CF, Smith SM (2004) Probabilistic independent component analysis for functional magnetic resonance imaging. IEEE T Med Imaging 23:137–152.

Beckmann CF, Smith SM (2005) Tensorial extensions of independent component analysis for multisubject FMRI analysis. NeuroImage 25:294–311.

Bell AJ, Sejnowski TJ (1995) An information maximisation approach to blind separation and blind deconvolution. Neural Comput 7:1129–1159.

Boscolo RH, Pan H, Roychowdhury VP (2001) Non-parametric ICA. In: Proceedings of the Third International Symposium on Independent Component Analysis and Blind Signal Separation. San Diego, CA.

Calhoun VD, Adali T (2006) "Unmixing" functional magnetic resonance imaging with independent component analysis. IEEE Eng Med Biol 25:79–90.

Calhoun VD, Adali T, Pearlson GD, Pekar JJ (2001a) Spatial and temporal independent component analysis of functional MRI data containing a pair of task-related waveforms. HumBrain Map 13:43–53.

Calhoun VD, Adali T, Pearlson GD, Pekar JJ (2001b) A method for making group inferences from functional MRI data using independent component analysis. HumBrain Map 14:140–151.

Calhoun VD, Adali T, McGinty V, Pekar JJ, Watson T, Pearlson GD (2001c) fMRI activation in a visual-perception task: network of areas detected using the general linear model and independent component analysis. NeuroImage 14:1080–1088.

Calhoun VD, Pekar JJ, McGinty VB, Adali T, Watson TD, Pearlson GD (2002) Different activation dynamics in multiple neural systems during simulated driving. HumBrain Map 16:158–167.

Calhoun VD, Adali T, Pekar JJ (2004a) A method for testing conjunctive and subtractive hypotheses on group fMRI data using independent component analysis. MagResImag 22:1181–1191.

Calhoun VD, Pekar JJ, Pearlson GD (2004b) Alcohol intoxication effects on simulated driving: exploring alcohol-dose effects on brain activation using functional MRI. Neuropsychopharmacology 29:2097–2107.

Calhoun VD, Carvalho K, Astur RS, Pearlson GD (2005) Using virtual reality to study alcohol intoxication effects on the neural correlates of simulated driving. Appl Psychophys Biof 30:285–306.

Calhoun VD, Pearlson GD, Kiehl KA (2006a) Neuronal chronometry of target detection: fusion of hemodynamic and event-related potential data. NeuroImage 30:544–553.

Calhoun VD, Adali T, Kiehl KA, Astur RS, Pekar JJ, Pearlson GD (2006b) A method for multi-task fMRI data fusion applied to schizophrenia. Hum Brain Mapp 27:598–610.

Calhoun VD, Adali T, Giuliani N, Pekar JJ, Pearlson GD, Kiehl KA (2006c) A method for multimodal analysis of independent source differences in schizophrenia: combining gray matter structural and auditory oddball functional data. Hum Brain Mapp 27:47–62.

Calhoun VD, Kiehl KA, Pearlson GD (2008a) Modulation of temporally coherent brain networks estimated using ICA at rest and during cognitive tasks. Hum Brain Mapp 29:828–838.

Calhoun VD, Pearlson GD, Maciejewski P, Kiehl KA (2008b) Temporal lobe and "default" hemodynamic brain modes discriminate between schizophrenia and bipolar disorder. Hum Brain Mapp 29:1265–1275.

Cardoso JF (1989) Source separation using higher order moments. In: Proceedings of the IEEE International Conference on Acoustics, Speech, and Signal Processing, vol 4, pp 2109–2112. Glasgow, Scotland.

Cardoso JF, Souloumiac A (1993) Blind beamforming for non gaussian signals. IEE-Proceeding-F 140:362–370.

Celone KA, Calhoun VD, Dickerson BC, Atri A, Chua EF, Miller S, DePeau K, Rentz DM, Selkoe D, Albert MS, Sperling RA (2006) Alterations in memory networks in mild cognitive impairment and Alzheimer's disease: an independent component analysis. J Neurosci 26:10222–10231.

Choi S, Cichocki A, Amari SI (2000) Flexible independent component analysis. J VLSI Signal Proc 26:25–38.

Correa N, Adali T, Li Y, Calhoun VD (2008) Examining associations between fMRI and EEG data using canonical correlation analysis. In: Proc ISBI, pp 1251–1254.

Dawy A, Sarkis M, Hagenauer J, Mueller J (2005) A novel gene mapping algorithm based on independent component analysis. In: Proceedings of the IEEE International Conference on Acoustics, Speech, and Signal Processing, pp 381–384. Philadelphia, PA.

Eichele T, Specht K, Moosmann M, Jongsma ML, Quiroga RQ, Nordby H, Hugdahl K (2005) Assessing the spatiotemporal evolution of neuronal activation with single-trial event-related potentials and functional MRI. Proc Natl Acad Sci U S A 102:17798–17803.

Eichele T, Debener S, Calhoun VD, Specht K, Engel AK, Hugdahl K, von Cramon DY, Ullsperger M (2008a) Prediction of human errors by maladaptive changes in event-related brain networks. Proc Natl Acad Sci U S A 105:6173–6178.

Eichele T, Calhoun VD, Moosmann M, Specht K, Jongsma M, Quiroga R, Nordby H, Hugdahl K (2008b) Unmixing concurrent EEG-fMRI with parallel independent component analysis. Int J Psych 67:222–234.

Esposito F, Scarabino T, Hyvarinen A, Himberg J, Formisano E, Comani S, Tedeschi G, Goebel R, Seifritz E, Di SF (2005) Independent component analysis of fMRI group studies by self-organizing clustering. Neuroimage 25:193–205.

Friston K, Poline JP, Strother S, Holmes A, Frith CD, Frackowiak RS (1996) A Multivariate analysis of PET activation studies. Hum Brain Mapp 4:140–151.

Garrity A, Pearlson GD, McKiernan K, Lloyd D, Kiehl KA, Calhoun VD (2007) Aberrant "default mode" functional connectivity in schizophrenia. Am J Psych 164:450–457.

Guo Y, Giuseppe P (2008) A unified framework for group independent component analysis for multi-subject fMRI data. NeuroImage 42:1078–1093.

Hong B, Pearlson GD, Calhoun VD (2005) Source-Density driven independent component analysis approach for fMRI data. Hum Brain Mapp 25:297–307.

Horwitz B, Poeppel D (2002) How can EEG/MEG and fMRI/PET data be combined? Hum Brain Mapp 17:1–3.

Husain FT, Nandipati G, Braun AR, Cohen LG, Tagamets MA, Horwitz B (2002) Simulating transcranial magnetic stimulation during PET with a large-scale neural network model of the prefrontal cortex and the visual system. NeuroImage 15:58–73.

Hyvarinen A, Oja E (1997) A fast fixed-point algorithm for independent component analysis. Neural Comput 9:1483–1492.

Jafri MJ, Pearlson GD, Stevens M, Calhoun VD (2008) A method for functional network connectivity among spatially independent resting-state components in schizophrenia. Neuroimage 39:1666–1681.

Jung A (2001) An introduction to a new data analysis tool: Independent Component Analysis. In: Proceedings of Workshop GK "Nonlinearity." Regensburg, Germany.

Lee SI, Batzoglou S (2003) Application of independent component analysis to microarrays. Genome Biol 4:R76.

Lee TW, Girolami M, Sejnowski TJ (1999) Independent component analysis using an extended infomax algorithm for mixed sub-gaussian and supergaussian sources. Neural Comput 11:417–441.

Li Y, Adali T, Calhoun VD (2007) Estimating the number of independent components for fMRI data. Hum Brain Mapp 28:1251–1266.

Liu J, Calhoun VD (2006) A novel approach to analyzing fMRI and SNP data via parallel independent component analysis. In: Proc SPIE 6511:1301–1311.

Liu J, Calhoun VD (2007) Parallel independent component analysis for multimodal analysis: Application to fMRI and EEG Data. In: Proc ISBI, pp 1028–1031.

Liu J, Pearlson GD, Windemuth A, Ruano G, Perrone-Bizzozero NI, Calhoun VD (2009) Combining fMRI and SNP data to investigate connections between brain function and genetics using parallel ICA. Hum Brain Mapp 30:241–255.

Lukic AS, Wernick MN, Hansen LK, Strother SC (2002) An ICA algorithm for analyzing multiple data sets. In: Proceedings of International Conference on Image Processing (ICIP), pp 821–824. Rochester, NY.

McIntosh AR, Bookstein FL, Haxby JV, Grady CL (1996) Spatial pattern analysis of functional brain images using partial least squares. NeuroImage 3:143–157.

McKeown MJ, Makeig S, Brown GG, Jung TP, Kindermann SS, Bell AJ, Sejnowski TJ (1998) Analysis of fMRI data by blind separation into independent spatial components. Hum Brain Mapp 6:160–188.

McKeown MJ, Hansen LK, Sejnowsk TJ (2003) Independent component analysis of functional MRI: what is signal and what is noise? Curr Opin Neurobiol 13:620–629.

Meda S, Calhoun VD, Astur R, Turner B, Ruopp K, Pearlson GD (2009) Alcohol dose effects on brain circuits during simulated driving: An fMRI study. Hum Brain Mapp 30:1257–1270.

Moosmann M, Eichele T, Nordby H, Hugdahl K, Calhoun VD (2008) Joint independent component analysis for simultaneous EEG-fMRI: principle and simulation. Int J Psych 67:212–221.

Petersen KS, Hansen LK, Kolenda T, Rostrup E, Strother SC (2000) On the independent components of functional neuroimages. In: Proceedings of the Third International Conference on Independent Component Analysis and Blind Source Separation, pp 615–620. Helsinki, Finland.

Rissanen J (1983) A universal prior for integers and estimation by minimum description length. Ann Stat 11:416–431.

Savopol F, Armenakis C (2002) Mergine of heterogeneous data for emergency mapping: data integration or data fusion? In: Proceedings of ISPRS, pp 615–620. Buenos Aires, Argentina.

Schmithorst VJ, Holland SK (2004) Comparison of three methods for generating group statistical inferences from independent component analysis of functional magnetic resonance imaging data. JMRI-J Magn Reson Im 19:365–368.

Seifritz E, Esposito F, Hennel F, Mustovic H, Neuhoff Jg, Bilecen D, Tedeschi G, Scheffler K, Salle FD (2002) Spatiotemporal pattern of neural processing in the human auditory cortex. Science 297 1706–1708.

Sorg C, Riedl V, Muhlau M, Calhoun VD, Eichele T, Laer L, Drzezga A, Forstl H, Kurz A, Zimmer C, Wohlschlager AM (2007) Selective changes of resting-state networks in individuals at risk for Alzheimer's disease. Proc Natl Acad Sci U S A 104:18760–18765.

Stevens M, Kiehl KA, Pearlson GD, Calhoun VD (2007) Functional neural circuits for mental timekeeping. Hum Brain Mapp 28:394–408.

Stone JV, Porrill J, Buchel C, Friston K (1999) Spatial, temporal, and spatiotemporal independent component analysis of fMRI data. In: Proceedings of Leeds Statistical Research Workshop, pp 1–4. Leed, UK.

Svensen M, Kruggel F, Benali H (2002) ICA of fMRI group study data. NeuroImage 16:551–563.

Tichavsky P, Koldovski Z, Oja E (2006) Efficient variant of algorithm FastICA for independent component analysis attaining the Cramer-Rao lower bound. IEEE Trans Neural Netw 17:1265–1277.

Vlassis N, Motomura Y (2001) Efficient source adaptivity in independent in independent component analysis. IEEE Trans Neural Netw 12:559–566.

3.5 Tom Eichele and Vince D. Calhoun

Parallel EEG-fMRI ICA Decomposition

Introduction

How Can EEG and fMRI Data be Combined with Group ICA?

Processing of simple stimuli and tasks produces spatially and temporally extensive event-related responses in the brain (Baudena et al., 1995; Halgren et al., 1995a; Halgren et al., 1995b; Halgren and Marinkovic, 1995; Kiehl et al., 2005). These responses can be observed across scales and modalities from single-unit recordings to intracranial and scalp electrophysiology, as well as metabolic and hemodynamic signals. However, no single technique provides a full view of all the temporal, spatial, and functional aspects of these responses. It has been proposed that visibility can be improved with techniques that integrate data across different neuroimaging modalities (Debener et al., 2006; Hopfinger et al., 2005; Horwitz and Poeppel, 2002; Makeig, 2002). In the case of concurrent EEG-fMRI recordings, one important prospect is to complement the temporal resolution provided by scalp electrophysiology with the spatial precision of fMRI (Eichele et al., 2005).

Typical state-of-the-art concurrent experiments generate a multidimensional data set consisting of about 10^4 to 10^5 volume elements by 10^2 to 10^3 time points sampled in the fMRI, by 10^2 to 10^3 time points by 10^2 to 10^3 trials by 32–128 scalp channels sampled in the EEG, by a number of participants that constitute a group study, providing a complex and enormously rich source of information. Generally, the utility of blind methods such as independent component analysis (ICA) lies in exploratory assessment of such data. One aspect is that ICA provides a means to visualize the data, another is that these methods are appropriate when detailed hypotheses regarding spatial and temporal relationships are lacking. In other words, ICA is useful when a traditional inference test,

and its implementation in the statistical parametric mapping framework (Friston et al., 1995), is not justifiable, or is too insensitive due to ensuing conservative significance thresholds in the presence of multiple tests. However, ICA trades in the "localizing power" afforded by mass-univariate testing (Friston, 2003; Kiebel and Friston, 2004), i.e., the possibility of drawing inferences from the sizes of the correlation of a time-series model with particular voxels in the fMRI and time points/channels in the EEG.

There are a variety of possible ways in which EEG and fMRI can be combined, each with somewhat different backgrounds, concepts, strategies for data reduction, inferences, and areas of application (Hopfinger et al., 2005). These can be grouped into three basic approaches to multimodal integration: *(1)* through *fusion*, usually referring to the use of a common forward or generative model that can explain both the EEG and fMRI data (Calhoun et al., 2006; Daunizeau et al., 2007; Martinez-Montes et al., 2004); *(2)* through *constraints*, where spatial information from the fMRI is used for a spatiotemporal source reconstruction of the EEG (Bledowski et al., 2004; Liu et al., 1998); and *(3)* through *prediction*, where the fMRI signal is modeled as some measure of the EEG convolved with a hemodynamic response function. Here we focus on "integration-by-prediction", i.e. using the covariation between EEG and fMRI activity over time to make inferences about when and where the modalities are coupled (Debener et al., 2006).

Integration-by-prediction is based on the assumption that the hemodynamic response is linearly related to local changes in neuronal activity, in particular local field potentials (Heeger and Ress, 2002; Lauritzen and Gold, 2003; Logothetis et al., 2001). Large-scale synchronous LFPs are the basis for the scalp EEG and ERP (Nunez, 1995), such that spatiotemporal data integration can be achieved by investigating correlations between BOLD and scalp EEG/ERP. This can be done either continuously over time, as in the study of background rhythms and epileptic discharges in the EEG (for a review see Laufs et al., 2008), or in the context of inducing variation in some cognitive operation (Debener et al., 2006; Debener et al., 2005; Eichele et al., 2005). A similar approach is to estimate hemodynamic responses from EEG features through deconvolution, such as the fluctuations in EEG alpha power (de Munck et al., 2008; de Munck et al., 2007). When a consistent relationship is detected, one can infer that the corresponding fMRI activations either directly represent the electric source, or modulate remote generators.

We have previously examined the correlations between single-trial modulations at various latencies in the event-related EEG and regional activations in the fMRI volume employing mass univariate voxel-by-voxel analysis (Eichele et al., 2005). Implicit in this approach is the assumption that the scalp EEG data from a selected channel and latency can predict the fMRI activation in single voxels (Friston, 2005a; Friston et al., 1995). This is imposed by the sampling properties of the recordings, and the way fMRI time-series data are commonly analyzed. While this assumption provides a working solution to integration-by-prediction, one needs to consider that it is not necessarily physiologically plausible for many of the samples from both modalities. The reason for this is that a salient event can induce multiple, simultaneously active, regionally overlapping responses that add to existing background activity. In other words, it is more likely that event-related processes are spatially and temporally mixed across the brain than being separable entities. The scalp EEG samples a volume-conducted, spatially degraded version of the responses, where the potential at any location and latency can be considered a mixture of multiple independent time courses that stem from large-scale synchronous field potentials (Makeig et al., 2004a; Onton et al., 2006). Similarly, the neurovascular transformation of the distributed neuronal activity into hemodynamic signals (Lauritzen and Gold, 2003; Logothetis, 2003) affords detection of blood oxygenation level dependent (BOLD) responses (BOLD, Ogawa et al., 1990) that are temporally degraded and spatially mixed across the fMRI volume (Calhoun and Adali, 2006; McKeown et al., 2003).

The spatial and temporal mixing in both modalities can create situations in which prediction of fMRI activity by EEG features may be difficult, since neither the predictor, nor the response variables are likely to represent single and corresponding sources of variability. For example, the point-to-point correlation between the two data mixtures might fail when the trial-to-trial modulation in the EEG receives different contributions from several function-relevant spatially separate sources such that no single regional fMRI response represents the predicted signal.

A partial solution to this problem was achieved through temporal unmixing of the EEG into independent factors (Debener et al., 2005; Feige et al., 2005; Scheeringa et al., 2008). In these studies, ICA was used to separate processes of interest, i.e., the ERN (Debener et al., 2005), alpha (Feige et al., 2005), and theta (Scheeringa et al., 2008) rhythms from other

sources in the EEG. However, although the mixing problem in the EEG was addressed, this was not extended to the treatment of the fMRI data. Likewise, a similarly incomplete solution was a decomposition of resting-state fMRI (Mantini et al., 2007) and event-related data from a target detection experiment (Mantini et al., 2008) into spatially independent factors, which were then correlated with power/amplitude fluctuations in the (mixed) EEG. Both approaches certainly solve parts of the problem and make way for refined spatiotemporal mapping. However, the choice to unmix one modality but not the other is somewhat inconsistent with the reasoning that led one to use ICA on the data.

Thus, one improvement to achieve a more symmetric treatment of the data is to unmix both modalities in parallel. We have developed such an analysis framework for group data that employs Infomax ICA (Bell and Sejnowski, 1995; Lee et al., 1999; for an overview see Stone, 2002) to recover a set of statistically independent maps from the fMRI (sICA), and independent time courses from the EEG (tICA) separately, and match these components across modalities by correlating their trial-to-trial modulation (Eichele et al., 2008a). We utilized the group-level approach that is described in the previous chapter, i.e., we created aggregate data containing observations from all subjects, estimated a single set of ICs, and then back-reconstructed these in the individual data (Calhoun et al., 2001; Schmithorst and Holland, 2004). The analysis is done on single-trial level rather than averaged data (cf. Calhoun et al., 2006), and it does not assume a joint mixing matrix for both modalities (cf. Calhoun et al., 2006; cf. Moosmann et al., 2008).

Parallel group ICA provides a means to disentangle and visualize large-scale networks both in their spatial and temporal form (Calhoun and Adali, 2006; Debener et al., 2006; Makeig et al., 2004a; McKeown et al., 2003; Onton et al., 2006), and can identify coherent neuronal sources that jointly express scalp electrophysiological and hemodynamic features. Here, we provide an example of how the method can be used. We examine the question whether error precursors can be detected in the scalp EEG, and if so, how they relate to those detected in the fMRI.

Are there Error Precursors in the EEG and How do They Relate to fMRI?

Research of human performance monitoring typically investigates brain activity evoked by, and occurring *after* behavioral errors, and the ensuing adaptive, compensatory mechanisms (Debener et al., 2005; Ridderinkhof et al., 2004; Rushworth et al., 2007; Ullsperger and von Cramon, 2004). However, some EEG and fMRI evidence exists suggesting that activity in the preceding trial foreshadows subsequent errors, but not clearly any earlier than that (Allain et al., 2004; Hajcak et al., 2005; Li et al., 2007; Ridderinkhof et al., 2003). We have recently explored whether brain activity patterns foreshadow the outcome in some systematic way using fMRI. In particular, we focused on the identification of components that show changes of activity preceding errors (Eichele et al., 2008b). This was challenging since it was not possible to specify a model regarding the actual timing and modulation of the assumed precursor signals, and adequate parameters of the associated hemodynamic response function (HRF). Therefore, we used a spatial ICA decomposition of the fMRI data, followed by deconvolution of hemodynamic response functions from the IC time courses (Aguirre et al., 1998; Handwerker et al., 2004), and then estimated single-trial responses. This analysis yielded set of brain regions in which the temporal evolution of hemodynamic activation predicted performance errors at least six seconds ahead in time, with linear trends starting as early as 30 seconds before an erroneous response. A coincident decrease of deactivation in regions of the default mode network (Raichle et al., 2001; Raichle and Snyder, 2007), together with a decline of activation in frontal regions associated with resource allocation and maintaining task effort, raised the probability of future errors.

An important outstanding question, with relevance to the possible applicability of the finding in real-world scenarios is obviously whether such precursors can also be detected in the concurrent scalp EEG. And, if they can be detected, how do they relate to those found in the fMRI? We examined this question using group tICA for decomposition of the EEG data and found two components that displayed significant slow trends with the same slope across trials as previously seen in the fMRI, in addition to a number of error-related signals. Correlations between EEG and fMRI components were ubiquitous, and also present for the EEG components displaying the error precursors which were correlated to corresponding fMRI components.

In the following, we will lay out in detail the relevant methodology, present the EEG and fMRI components and the covariation between EEG and fMRI, and discuss the utility of the method in light of these findings.

Methods

Participants

Concurrent EEG-fMRI data from 13 healthy participants, eight females and five males (22–29 years), were analyzed here (Debener et al., 2005). Written informed consent was obtained from each participant according to the declaration of Helsinki prior to the start of the experiment.

Behavioral Task

Stimuli were presented on a back-projection screen mounted inside the scanner behind the participants' head. A speeded flanker task was used: participants were presented with a fixation mark in the center of the screen, after which four horizontal flanker arrows occurred for a total 110 ms. After an 80 ms delay, the target arrow was presented for 30 ms in the center of the flanker arrows. In half of the trials the flankers were compatible, i.e, they pointed in the same direction as the target; in the other half of the trials the target pointed in the opposite direction (incompatible trials). Compatible and incompatible trials appeared in randomized order. Participants were instructed to respond as fast and as accurately as possible to the target arrow with the response hand indicated by the arrow direction. A symbolic feedback was presented for 1400 ms after target onset, instructing participants to speed up whenever they failed a dynamically adapting response deadline. The average intertrial interval amounted to 6 s.

EEG Recording

Continuous EEG data were collected from 30 standard scalp sites using the BrainAmps MR plus, a high-input impedance amplifier specifically designed for recordings in high magnetic fields (BrainProducts, Munich, Germany). Sintered Ag/AgCl ring electrodes with built-in 5 kOhm resistors were used and mounted into an electrode cap according to the 10–20 system (Falk Minow Services, Herrsching, Germany). Two additional electrodes were placed below the left eye and on the back to monitor eye blinks and electrocardiogram, respectively. Electrode impedances were kept below 10 kOhms. Participants' heads were immobilized using vacuum cushions and sponge pads. All 32 channels were recorded with FCz as reference and a passband of 0.016 to 250 Hz. The data were digitized with 5000 samples/second at 16 bit with 0.5 μV resolution.

EEG Preprocessing

EEG data were corrected for MR gradient and ballistocardiac artifacts by applying modified versions of the algorithms proposed by Allen and colleagues (Allen et al., 1998; Allen et al., 2000). Gradient artifacts were removed as implemented in the software Vision Analyzer 1.04 (BrainProducts, Munich, Germany), by subtracting an artifact template from the 40 Hz low pass filtered data, using a baseline-corrected sliding average of 20 consecutive volumes. Further preprocessing of the 250 Hz downsampled data was performed using Matlab 6.5 (The Mathworks) and EEGLAB (Delorme and Makeig, 2004). A modified version of the algorithm (Kim et al., 2004) as implemented in the EEGLAB-plugin FMRIB 1.0 (Niazy et al., 2005); FMRIB EEGLAB plug-in for removal of fMRI-related artifacts, http://www.fmrib.ox.ac.uk/~arami/fmribplugin) was used on 0.4–35 Hz finite impulse response (FIR) filtered data to remove cardioballistic artifacts.

After correction for gradient and cardioballistic artifacts, the data were epoched from −400 to 600 ms around stimulus onsets, and separately from −600 to 400 ms around button press responses. The concatenated single sweeps of each participant were decomposed with an individual tICA as implemented in EEGLAB (Delorme and Makeig, 2004). This step was used to identify and remove residual pulse and eye movement artifacts from the data (cf. Debener et al., 2007; Jung et al., 2000), retaining minimally 20 out of 30 components. Single trials were then wavelet-denoised (Quian Quiroga and Garcia, 2003), constraining the single-trial EEGs to the time-frequency features relevant for the evoked activity around stimulus and response onsets, respectively.

Group Temporal ICA of Event-Related EEG

We have recently presented a group ICA method for parallel as well as joint decompositions of concurrent EEG-fMRI recordings (Eichele et al., 2008a; Moosmann et al., 2008). ICA has general applicability to two-dimensional mixtures of different sources, and regarding psychophysiological data it has been used for decomposition of averaged ERPs (Makeig et al., 1997), single-trial EEG (Makeig et al., 2004b; Onton et al., 2006), fMRI (Calhoun and Adali, 2006), and EEG-fMRI (Calhoun et al., 2006; Debener et al., 2005; Feige et al., 2005; Scheeringa et al., 2008). ICA can be used for EEG-fMRI integration assuming that the different recording modalities faithfully sample features from the same set of sources, expressed in the covariation between single trials (Debener et al., 2005) or subjects (Calhoun et al., 2006). The basic ICA model applies to single subject data, thus one inherent limitation to the use of ICA in typical multisubject/session EEG studies is that this method is not naturally suited to generalize results from a group of subjects, since different subjects in a group will have different scalp maps and time courses across decompositions, and so it is not immediately clear how to draw population inferences using ICA. Here, we present in detail the group-level temporal ICA based on the rationale proposed by Calhoun (Calhoun et al., 2001) for single-trial analysis of event related EEG. This method is implemented in the EEGIFT toolbox which is available at http://icatb.sourceforge.net/. EEGIFT runs in Matlab (The Mathworks, Natick, MA), and employs preprocessed data from EEGLAB (Delorme and Makeig, 2004). It supports group analysis with a number of ICA algorithms, e.g., infomax (Bell and Sejnowski, 1995), fastICA (Hyvarinen and Oja, 1997), JADE (Cardoso and Souloumiac, 1993), and others.

Due to aggregation and data reduction with PCA preceding component estimation, and concatenation across subjects, group tICA of EEG time domain data is preferentially suited to the detection of components that contribute to event-related potentials. Processes that are not well time/phase-locked within and across subjects, such as background rhythms, cannot be satisfyingly reconstructed. It follows also that the accuracy of component detection and back-reconstruction with this group model is dependent on the degree of intra- and interindividual latency jitter of event-related EEG processes. Similar to findings in early studies of PCA decomposition of ERP averages (Donchin

and Heffley, 1978; Mocks, 1986), excess latency jitter results in splitting of a single source into two (or more) independent components representing the source and its approximate time derivative (see also Moosmann et al., 2008). Additionally, in the data set we analyzed here there was a substantial overlap of stimulus-locked and response-locked potentials, and we therefore processed the data separately, once for the stacked stimulus-locked and once for response-locked epochs.

For the group ICA, all subjects were analyzed at once, and principal component analysis (PCA) was used for compression to allow the datasets to be processed together. In the PCA steps, data from each data set was reduced over the spatial dimension, i.e., from the number of channels to 20 principal components, concatenated across subjects, and again reduced to 20 components. Temporal ICA was then performed using the infomax algorithm (Bell and Sejnowski, 1995) with subsequent back-reconstruction into single subjects.

The group ICA model is divided into the underlying data generation and mixing process, recording, preprocessing, reduction, component estimation, and back-reconstruction, and is schematically illustrated in Figure 3.5.1.

We assume that the scalp EEG signal is a Gaussian mixture containing statistically independent non-Gaussian source time-series

$$s(t) = \left[s_1(t), s_2(t), \ldots, s_i(t) \right]^T \qquad (1)$$

indicated by $s_i(t)$ at time t for the ith source. The sources have weights that specify the contribution to each time point. The weights are multiplied by each source's fixed topography. Secondly, it is assumed that the N sources are linearly mixed so that a given time point contains a weighted mixture of the sources. The linear combination of sources is represented by the unknown mixing system A, and yields

$$u(t) = \left[u_1(t), u_2(t), \ldots, u_N(t) \right]^T \qquad (2)$$

representing N ideal samples of the signals $u_n(t)$ at time t, for the ith source in the brain. The sampling of the electric activity on the scalp results in

$$y(i) = \left[y_1(i), y_2(i), \ldots, y_k(i) \right]^T \qquad (3)$$

where the EEG is sampled at T time points indicated by $i = 1, 2, \ldots, T$. A set of possible transformations during preprocessing, such as downsampling and filtering determine the effective sampling such that

$$y(j) = [y_l(j), y_2(j)m, \ldots, y_k(j)]^T \qquad (4)$$

Data Reduction

Principal component analysis (PCA) preconditions the data and simplifies ICA estimation due to the orthogonal

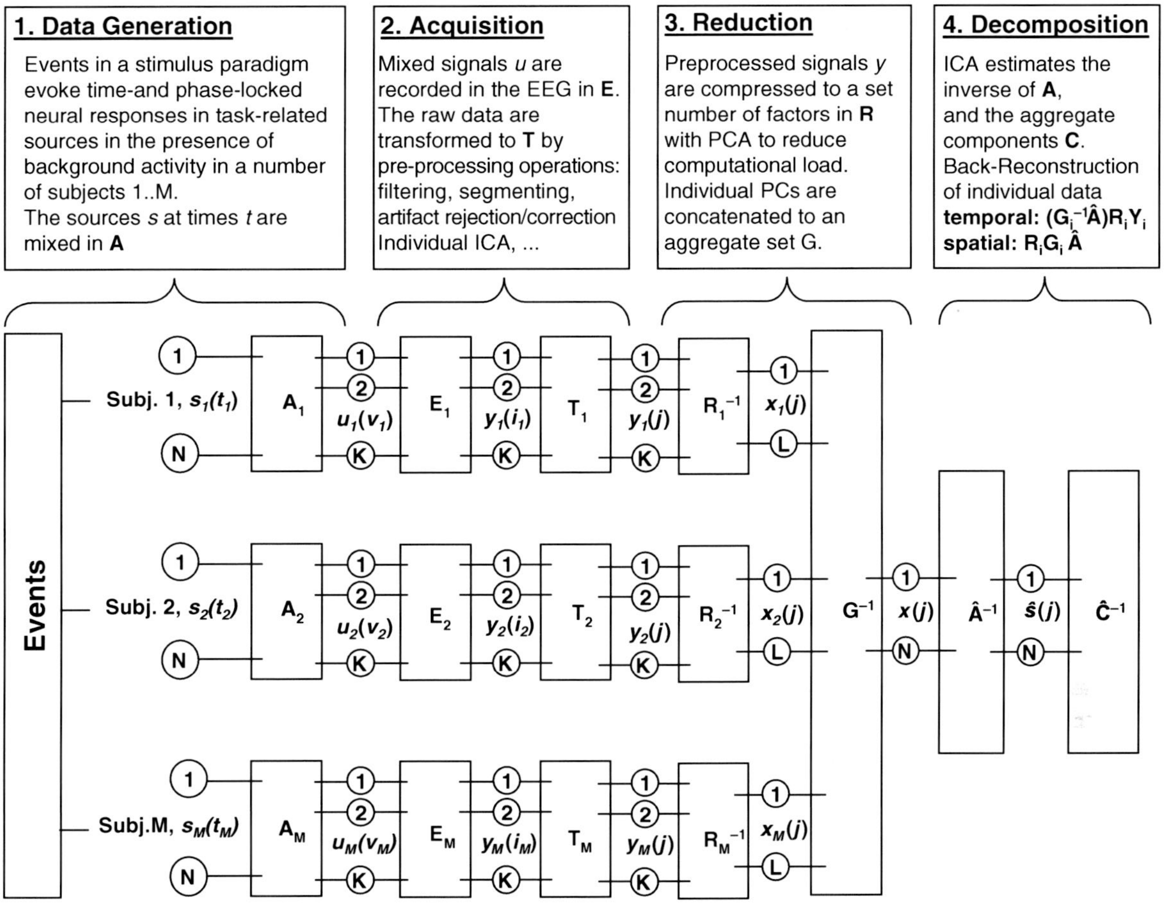

Figure 3.5.1. Group temporal ICA of event related EEG data. In the group ICA model, we assume that the EEG is a linear mixture of temporally independent sources in each subject s(t). The linear combination of sources is represented by the unknown mixing matrix A, and yields the ideal samples of brain activity u(t), and the signals recorded with the EEG amplifier (E). Transformations (T) during preprocessing contain filtering, epoching, artifact rejection, individual ICA for additional artifact reduction, and so forth, altering the effective temporal sampling and dimensionality of the data y(i). For each individual separately, the preprocessed single trial data are prewhitened and reduced to R via PCA. Group data is generated by concatenating individual principal components in the aggregate data set G. Temporal ICA is performed in this set, estimating aggregate components (C). From the aggregate components, the individual data are reconstructed (see text for details)

projection, reduction of complexity, and denoising, as well as compressing the data and thus reducing the computational load. We compute a temporal PCA, and reduce EEG data in the spatial dimension for each dataset. Individual principal components are concatenated across the reduced spatial dimension, the aggregate is a "tall and skinny" [components, subjects]-by-[time points, trials] matrix, and the second reduction step compresses again the concatenated components. For each individual separately, the preprocessed single-trial data $y(j)$ are prewhitened and reduced (Figure 3.5.1, $R_1^{-1} \ldots R_M^{-1}$) containing the major proportion of variance in the N uncorrelated time courses of

$$x(j) = \left[x_l(j_1), x_2(j) \ldots, x_N(j) \right] T \qquad (5)$$

Group data is generated by concatenating the components in the aggregate data set G. In detail, let $X_i = R_i^{-1} Y_i$ be the

L-by-V reduced data matrix from subject i where Y_i is the K-by-V data matrix containing preprocessed EEG epochs from all channels, R_i^{-1} is the L-by-K reducing matrix from the principal component decomposition, V is the number of time points, K is the number of scalp channels, and L is the size of the channel dimension following reduction. The next step is to concatenate the reduced data from all subjects into a matrix and reduce this matrix to N, the number of components to be estimated. The N-by-V reduced, concatenated matrix for the M subjects is

$$X = G^{-1} \begin{bmatrix} R_1^{-1} Y_1 \\ \vdots \\ R_M^{-1} Y_M \end{bmatrix} \qquad (6)$$

where G^{-1} is an N-by-LM reducing matrix from a second PCA decomposition and is multiplied on the right by the *LM-by-V* concatenated data matrix for the *M* subjects.

ICA Estimation

After concatenation of individual principal components in the aggregate data set G, this matrix is decomposed by ICA, estimating the optimal inverse of the mixing matrix $\hat{A}$, and a single set of component timecourses ($\hat{s}$). Following ICA estimation, we can write $X = \hat{A}\hat{S}$, where $\hat{A}$ is the *N-by-N* mixing matrix and $\hat{S}$ are the N-by-V component time courses. Substituting this expression for X into Equation 1 and multiplying both sides by G results in

$$G\hat{A}\,\hat{S} = \begin{bmatrix} R_1^{-1}Y_1 \\ \vdots \\ R_M^{-1}Y_M \end{bmatrix} \qquad (7)$$

Partitioning and Single-Subject Reconstruction

Partitioning the matrix G by subject provides the following expression:

$$\begin{bmatrix} G_1 \\ \vdots \\ G_M \end{bmatrix} \hat{A}\,\hat{S} = \begin{bmatrix} R_1^{-1}Y_1 \\ \vdots \\ R_M^{-1}Y_M \end{bmatrix} \qquad (8)$$

We then write the equation for subject *i* by working only with the elements in partition *i* of the above matrices such that

$$G_i\hat{A}\,\hat{S}_i = \begin{bmatrix} R_i^{-1}Y_i \end{bmatrix} \qquad (9)$$

The matrix $\hat{S}_i$ in Equation 4 contains the single-subject component time courses for subject *i*, calculated from the following equation:

$$\hat{S}_i = (G_i\hat{A})^{-1}R_i^{-1}Y_i \qquad (10)$$

We now multiply both sides of Equation 4 by R_i and write,

$$Y_i \approx F_iG_i\hat{A}\,\hat{S}_i \qquad (11)$$

yielding the ICA decomposition of the data from subject *i* contained in the matrix Y_i. The *N-by-V* matrix $\hat{S}_i$ contains the N component time courses, and the *K-by-N* matrix $F_iG_i\hat{A}$ is the single-subject mixing matrix, yielding the scalp maps for N components. The back-reconstructed time courses and topographies are a function primarily of the variability within subjects, as opposed to being a representation of the average across subjects.

EEG Component Selection and Inference

Components were selected for further processing based on the spatial and temporal statistics. In order to quantify the significance of the scalp maps, the IC weights at each channel were entered into zero-mean t-tests, and considered significant at p < 0.01. Similarly, the average activation time courses of each component were tested for significance at each time point, and considered significant when passing a p < 0.01 threshold across at least 10 adjacent samples. Five components from each decomposition were jointly significant in the spatial and temporal domain, i.e., the IC maps passed the threshold at the maxima and were considered robust reflections of the single subjects in the sample, and the activations at peak latencies of all components passed the threshold. The remaining 15 components captured non-event-related activity, background activity as suggested by some topographies. Also components that were present only in a subsample of the subjects, and residual artifacts were reflected here.

In the selected components, we estimated and removed the variability associated with the response-to-trial compatibility and response time modulation from the amplitudes, using multiple linear regression, and used the residual data for estimating the error precursors and the EEG-fMRI correlation, in order to ensure that the inferences about coupling were specific to trial-by-trial variability rather than categorical effects and possible common confounds.

After removal of the variability associated with the aforementioned predictors we used the residual tIC data to check for the presence of error-preceding activity at the peak latency of the stimulus-locked IC's; in the response-locked IC's two time-windows from 20–80ms and 120–200ms post-response were used. This was done by generating averages from the residuals for sequences from six trials before to three trials after errors. Based on our previous results (Eichele et al., 2008b), we generated a design matrix with two regressors, one modeling the precursor signal, an error-preceding gradient with a reset at the error trial, and the other modeling error signals per se, i.e., activity increases at the error trial. This model was tested in the individual sequences with the trial-by-trial amplitude modulation around errors. Individual β-estimates were entered into one-sample t-tests and effects were considered significant at p < 0.01.

fMRI Recording

Imaging was performed at 3 Tesla on a Siemens (Erlangen, Germany) Trio system equipped with the standard bird cage head coil. Twenty-two functional slices were obtained parallel to the anterior commissure–posterior commissure (AC–PC) line (thickness, 4 mm; interslice gap, 1 mm) using a gradient-echo EPI sequence with a TE of 30 ms, a flip angle of 90 degrees, a TR of 2000 ms, and an acquisition bandwidth of 100 kHz. Acquisition of the slices was arranged such that they all were acquired within 1500 ms, and followed by a 500 ms no acquisition period to complete the TR. This was done to monitor visually proper recording of the EEG signal during MR scanning, and to include for each TR a nongradient contaminated baseline period into the EEG recordings. The fMRI matrix acquired was 64×64 with a FOV of 19.2cm, resulting in an in-plane resolution of 3×3 mm^3. A total of 1309 volumes were acquired, the three first volumes were rejected. Functional data were motion-corrected offline with the Siemens motion correction protocol (Siemens, Erlangen, Germany). Before the functional runs, anatomical modified driven equilibrium Fourier transform (MDEFT) and EPI-T1 slices in the plane with functional images were collected.

fMRI Preprocessing

All images were realigned to the first image in the time-series to correct for head movement and then normalized to the MNI (Montreal Neurological Institute) reference space using SPM2 (http://www.fil.ion.ucl.ac.uk/spm). Normalized data were resliced to a cubic voxel size of 2mm^3 and smoothed with a Gaussian kernel with 8mm FWHM.

Group Spatial ICA of fMRI Data

For estimation of the group spatial ICA we employed the rationale proposed by Calhoun and colleagues (Calhoun and Adali, 2006; Calhoun et al., 2001), and extended it with deconvolution of hemodynamic response functions and subsequent single-trial estimation to recover the single-trial amplitude modulation (Eichele et al., 2008b). The fMRI data were first partitioned into eight spatially redundant sets by sampling the volume at every other voxel of the x, y, and z directions starting from the first or second voxel, respectively, for computational feasibility, and in order to control the consistency of component estimates in nonidentical subsets of the data. The replicability of IC results was assessed by measuring the spatial correlation between the results of the first analysis and the following runs, and aggregate ICs with spatial correlation exceeding $r > 0.8$ across all replications were further analyzed.

Group ICA requires that all subjects be analyzed at once, and a method for data compression using principal component analysis (PCA) was used to allow the data sets to be processed together. In the PCA step, data from each subject were reduced from the number of time points within the experiment (n = 1306) to 52 dimensions, retaining more than 95% of the non-zero eigenvalues. We adjusted the number of dimensions that were estimated in this study heuristically to accommodate extraction of the maximum number of components that was computationally feasible and yield a high replicability of ICs across runs while consistently separating sources representing artifacts and known components of interest (Damoiseaux et al., 2006; Malinen et al., 2007). A group spatial ICA was then performed using the infomax algorithm (Bell and Sejnowski, 1995), with subsequent back-reconstruction into single subjects. The resulting output is an independent component map and an associated IC time course for every component and subject. The maps were entered into second-level random effects analyses, and the time courses were used further for deconvolution and single trial estimation.

Replicable ICs were inspected to identify and discard those primarily associated with artifacts such as motion, flow, and susceptibility. From the remaining ICs, only those with significant random effects t-statistics of their maps, adjusted for multiple comparisons at 1% false positive discovery rate (FDR) and cluster extent of at least 27 contiguous voxels were considered further. For these ICs, the individual time courses were high pass filtered at 72 seconds, averaged across replications, and normalized to unit variance.

Deconvolution

The event-related hemodynamic response function for the ICs was then deconvolved from the time courses by forming the convolution matrix of the stimulus onsets with an assumed kernel length of 20 seconds, and multiplying the pseudoinverse of this matrix with the IC time course. Single-trial estimation was only performed in ICs where consistent event-related HRFs were present, i.e., where yielding a mono-/biphasic form with a peak-latency between 3 and 12 seconds in all subjects. Single-trial response amplitudes were then recovered by fitting a design matrix (X) containing separate predictors for the onset times of each trial convolved with the estimated HRF onto the IC time course, estimating the scaling coefficients (β) in the multiple linear regression model $y = \beta \cdot X + \varepsilon$ using least squares. Single-trial β estimates were subsequently entered into within-subjects one-sample t-tests, and nine components with significant ($p < 0.01$) differences from zero magnitude in all participants were considered further here (see Figure 3.5.2).

In the selected components, we estimated and removed the variability associated with the response to trial compatibility, feedback, and response time modulation using multiple linear regression and used the residual data for predicting the EEG amplitude modulation, in order to ensure that the EEG-fMRI coupling was specific to trial-by-trial variability rather than categorical effects and possible common confounds.

tIC-sIC Integration

Previously, we used the single trial variability of the event related EEG components convolved with a canonical HRF to predict the time courses of the fMRI components (Eichele et al., 2008a). Since the necessity to compensate for the HRF delay and shape is effectively removed by the combination of

Stimulus-locked EEG decomposition

Component scalp maps

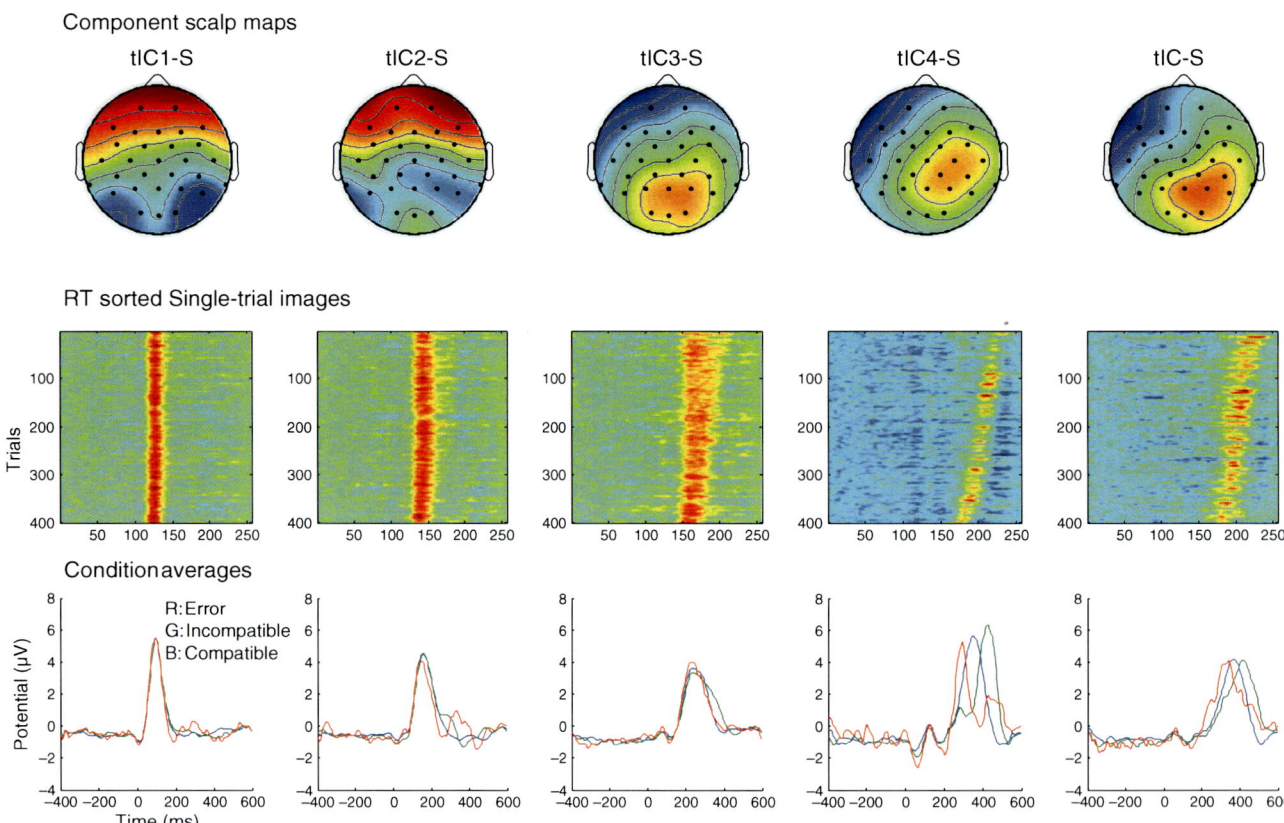

Figure 3.5.2. Trial-by-trial modulation of EEG-ICs around behavioral errors. In order to assess error precursors and other error-related signals here group trial sequences from -6 to +3 around response errors were analyzed and the group averages (±1 S.E.M) are plotted in the top row for the 120–180 ms post-stimulus time window in the stimulus-locked components. In the middle row, the early post-response period from 20 to 80 ms in the response-locked components is plotted, the bottom row shows the 120–180 ms window for the same components. In the components where the random effects statistic of precursor and error signals was significant ($p < 0.01$), the average model fit was plotted over the average data; the precursor signals are shown in light blue, the error related response in orange. These plots represent the residual data after removal of variability accounted for by trial category and response times. Significant precursors were present in tIC4-R (early), and in tIC1-R (late); large error responses were seen in the early period of tIC2-R and tIC5-R, as well as in tIC3-S and tIC3-R at both latencies.

deconvolution and single-trial estimation (Eichele et al., 2008b), we use here the modulation of the fMRI IC's as predictors of EEG activity. A schematic illustration of the EEG-fMRI integration is provided in Figure 3.5.3.

Separately for the nine sICSs we formed a design matrix with two predictors that contained the mean over all sICs and the residual single trial weights from one sIC. The predictors were decorrelated (Schmidt-Gram orthogonalization) to ensure that the correlation between the respective fMRI sIC and the EEG tIC was not confounded by variations of the global mean. These predictors were then regressed onto the trial-by-trial activity in all peri-stimulus/response time points in all EEG tICs. This analysis was repeated with the approximated differentials of the sICs and tICs, respectively. The two former analyses measured the correlation of EEG and fMRI across all trials, implicitly assuming that the relationship is fixed over time and trial categories. Inspection of the tIC activity in trial sequences surrounding errors suggested a

different behavior of fMRI and EEG before and after errors we also estimated the coupling separately for trial sequences preceding and succeeding errors, respectively. On group level, random effects analyses were performed by entering the individual β-weights from the regression between each EEG-tIC and fMRI-sIC into one-sample t-tests. The coupling between the trial-to-trial time courses from the two modalities was considered significant at $p < 0.01$.

Results

fMRI Components

Nine spatially independent components were selected in the fMRI and are shown in Figure 3.5.3 along with their HRF.

Response-locked EEG decomposition

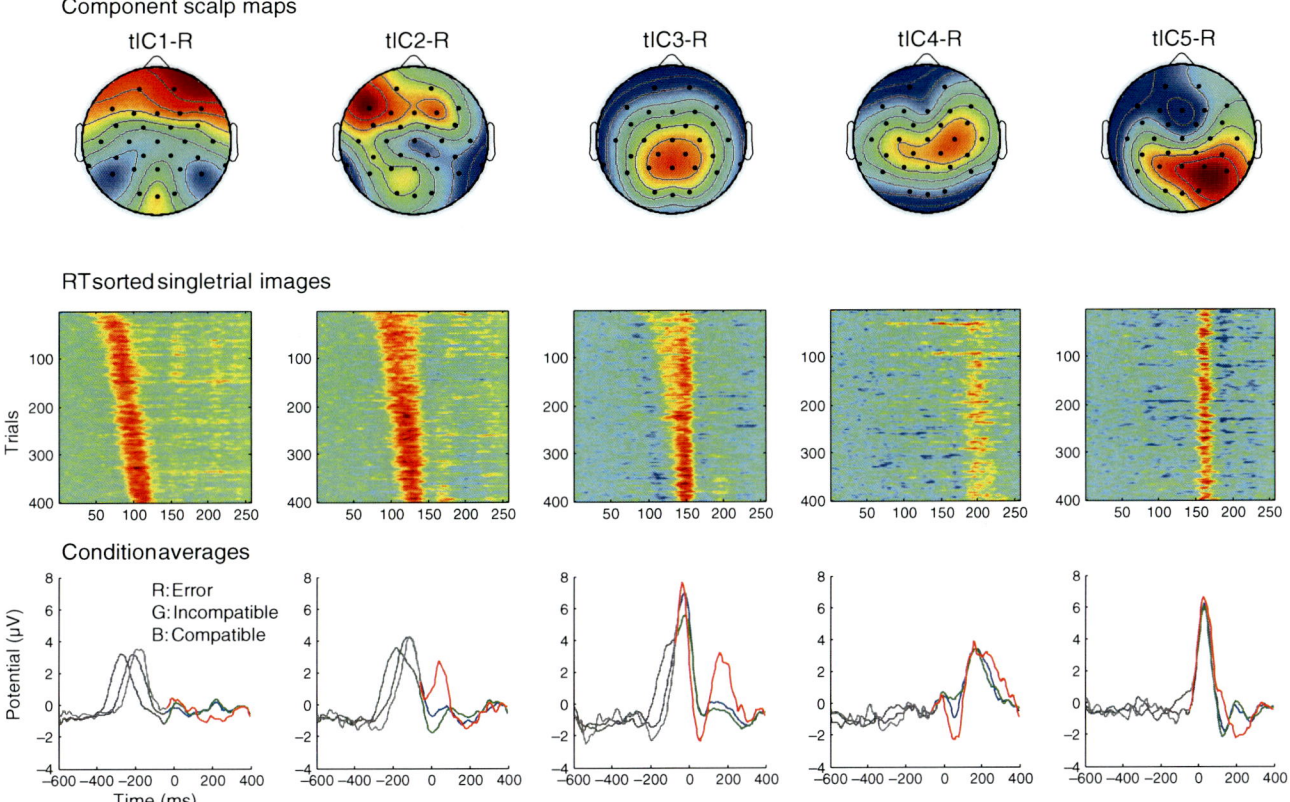

Figure 3.5.3. Response-locked EEG-ICs. As in the previous figure, the top row shows the group mean topographies of the five components with positive weights in red, and negative weights in blue. The component topographies were sorted such that they correspond to the stimulus-locked ICs. Note, however, that the reconstructed topographies and time courses are somewhat variable due to the different decompositions. TIC1-R and tIC2-R correspond to the stimulus-locked negativities parieto-occipital negativities, with shifts of the peak latency by the average response time of the three conditions (errors < compatible < incompatible) before the response (0 ms). tIC3-R, tIC4-R, and tIC5-R constitute response-locked processes with complex transient waveforms in the peri-response interval. tIC2-R, tIC3-R and tIC4-R show error-related signals in the early late post-response interval from about 20 to 80 ms, while tIC5-R produces an overall larger medial frontal negativity with somewhat smaller differences between the conditions.

The figure shows the activation maps of the components at representative transverse slices. IC activations were considered significant at $p < 0.01$ (FDR corrected) when exceeding a cluster extent of at least 27 contiguous voxels.

Since the focus of this chapter is not on the spatial analysis of the IC maps, we provide just a short overview of the main locations in each component: sIC1 represented an event-related deactivation in the inferior portion of the precuneus, adjacent PCC, retrosplenial cortex, extending into the cuneus. sIC2 was localized to the lingual gyri, extending upward into the calcarine and superior occipital gyri bilaterally. sIC3 encompassed left-dominant sensorimotor activity in pre/post-central gyri and SMA. sIC4 showed activations in the superior parietal lobes bilaterally with a rightward dominance. sIC5 showed bilateral activation in the inferior and middle occipital gyri, in the right hemisphere also extending into the fusiform gyrus. sIC6 was a deactivation localized to the anterior medial wall of the frontal lobes, covering parts of the anterior cingulate gyri, as well as the medial superior frontal gyri, and bordering on the gyrus rectus. sIC7 was a right fronto-parietal network with activations in the inferior frontal and angular gyri. sIC8 was composed of two regions, the orbital part of the right inferior frontal gyrus, posterior orbital gyrus (orbitofrontal cortex, OFC), extending into the adjacent inferior anterior insula, and the superior pMFC (pre-SMA, BA 8m). sIC9 represented a pattern of activation in the pMFC encompassing the rostral cingulate zone and presupplementary motor area, with additional activation in the dorsal premotor cortex, the right inferior frontal junction and the anterior insula bilaterally.

Note that sIC1 and sIC8 show gradual changes of their activity prior to errors, which can be seen in our recent report (Eichele et al., 2008b), where these components were labeled "IC4" and "IC3," respectively. Also, sIC4 corresponds to "IC2," and sIC9 to "IC1."

EEG Components

The group tICA decomposition of the stimulus- and response-locked EEG each yielded five robust components with event-related responses. The group average maps, RT-sorted single trial images, and average timecourses of the stimulus-locked components are shown in Figure 3.5.4, and the response-locked components in Figure 3.5.5. The results from the separate decompositions were matched by their topography and time course, such that, e.g., tIC1-S and tIC1-R are thought to reflect essentially the same processes, the differences between the components in terms of the functional modulation around errors, and correlations with the fMRI sICs are considered to arise mainly from response timing, and to some degree also from the separated decompositions, here mainly due to the fact that the input data to the two group ICAs are not identical.

tIC1 and tIC2 correspond mainly to stimulus-related posterior negativities in the time window from about 100 to 200 ms. The peak latency of tIC1 was at 95 ms after target onset, tIC2 peaked at 160 ms; both peaks were unaffected by response times, and did not show relevant differences between the conditions at their peak latencies. Apart from the large peaks related to the visual stimulation, the response-locked decomposition revealed an a linear trend preceding errors signal in the late post-response period of tIC1 (Figure 3.5.6, bottom left), and a large error related response in the early post-response interval in tIC2 (Figure 3.5.6, middle, second from left), which can also be seen the response-locked average (Figure 3.5.5).

The stimulus-locked portions of tIC3, tIC4, and tIC5 yield parietal positivities from about 200 to 500 ms after stimulus onset. The response-locked portion of tIC5 additionally shows negative loadings at midline frontal sites, producing a prominent negativity at 30 ms post-response. In tIC4 and tIC5, the peaks are shifted by the response latency and yield the earliest peaks for errors, followed by compatible and

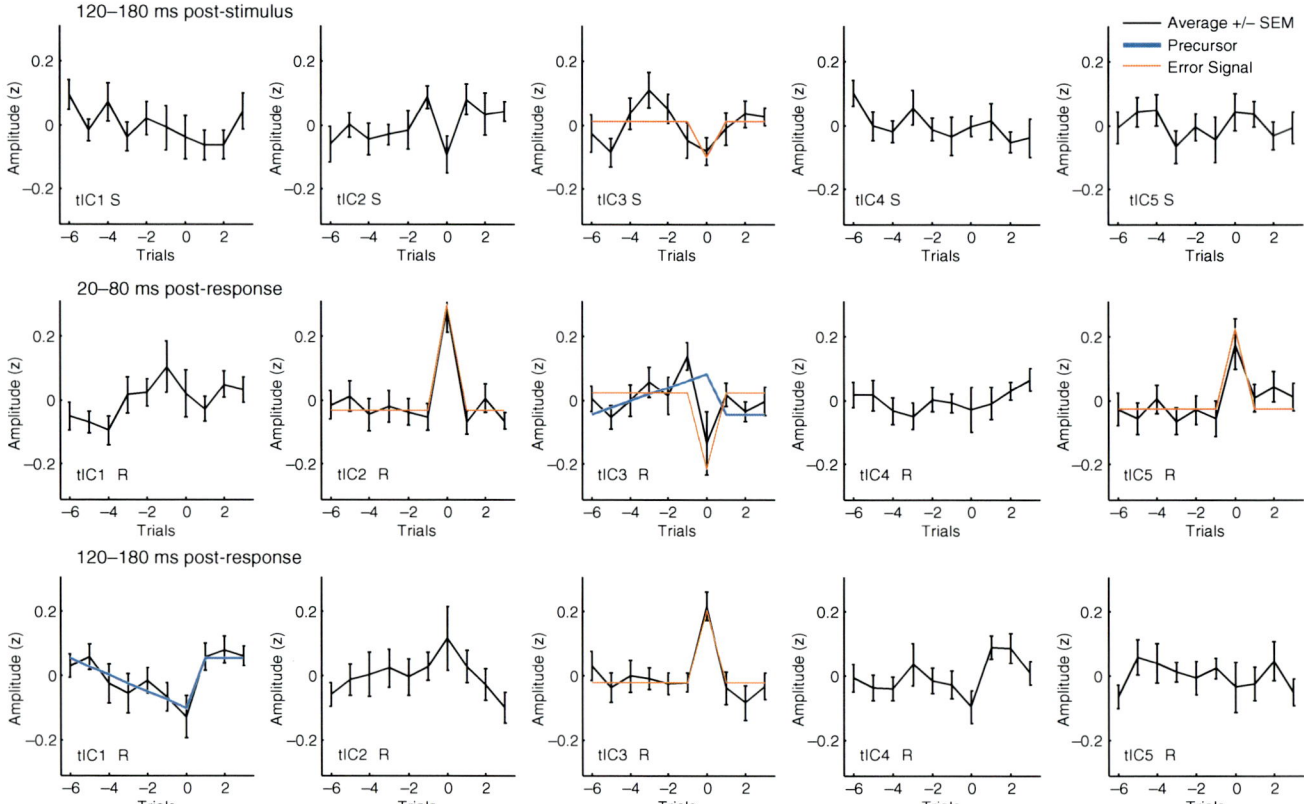

Figure 3.5.4. EEG-fMRI integration. The spatial ICA of the fMRI data results in individual maps and time courses. The Single-Trial HRF amplitude modulation estimated from the IC time courses are used for prediction of EEG activity. In order to recover the amplitude modulation (AM), the pseudoinverse of a convolution matrix generated from the stimulus timing and a assumed HRF length of 20 seconds is multiplied with the IC time course, yielding individually and regionally specific HRFs. These HRFs are then convolved separately with each stimulus onset, yielding a design matrix (X) with predictors for each trial 1..n. The regression of the design onto the IC time course (y) yields the single trial amplitude modulation for this IC (β_1.. β_n). After removal of the variability associated with trial compatibility, feedback, and response time modulation, the residual data are used for predicting the EEG tIC amplitude modulation.

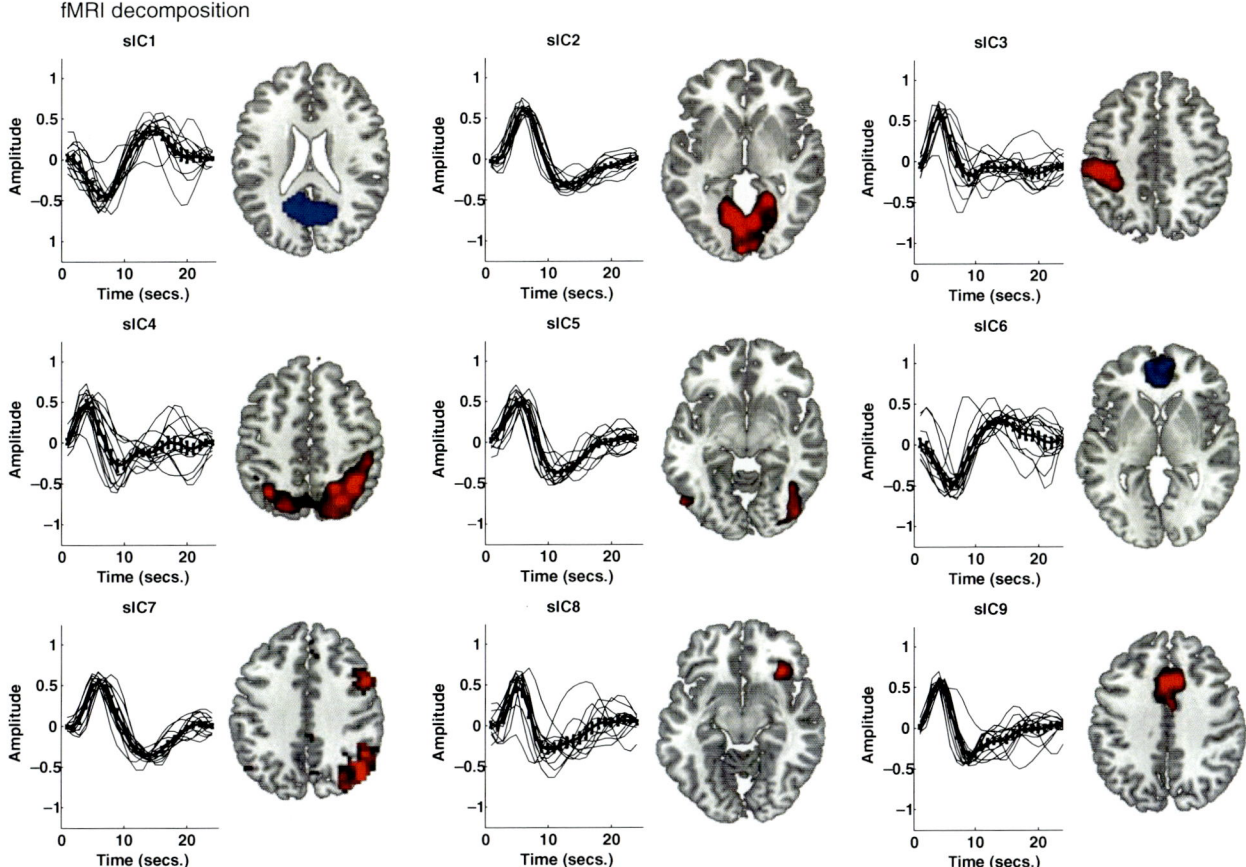

Figure 3.5.5. Independent components in the fMRI. The figure shows the activation maps of the nine independent components rendered onto the MNI template at representative transverse slices. The maps are shown in neurological convention (left hemisphere is on the left). IC areas were considered significant when exceeding a cluster extent of at least 27 contiguous volume elements (voxels), and at 1% false positive discovery rate. Activations are plotted in red, deactivations in blue. To the left of each map, the hemodynamic response functions within the respective ICs as estimated via deconvolution from 1–20 seconds after stimulus onset, in arbitrary (range-scaled) amplitude units are displayed. The group average from the 13 participants is plotted as a solid line, error bars indicate ±1 S.E.M., dotted lines represent all individual estimates. The empirical HRFs were used to estimate single trial amplitudes in the fMRI data (not shown).

incompatible trials, respectively (Figure 3.5.4, bottom right); this effect is not clearly visible in tIC3-S. In the response-locked group ICA result (Figure 3.5.5), the average time course of tIC3-R to errors yields a larger positivity at 40 ms prior to the response, followed by a negativity at 50 ms, and a positivity at about 160 ms after the response. The trial sequences around errors (Figure 3.5.6) show that this component can be modeled as the sum of a precursor (decreasing negativity from t_{-6} to t_0) and an error signal (increased negativity at t_0) early after the response, as well as showing an error related increase of the positivity later. No such modulations were seen in tIC4, but the early post-response period in tIC5-R hosts an error-related increase of activity.

EEG Error Precursors

The group averaged trial-by-trial modulation of EEG-ICs around behavioral errors is shown in Figure 3.5.6. In order to assess error precursors and error-related signals sequences from −6 to +3 trials around response errors were analyzed. In the components where the random effects statistic of precursor and error signals was significant (p < 0.01), the average model fit was plotted over the average data; the precursor signals are shown in light blue, the error-related response in orange. Significant precursors were present in tIC4-R (early), and in tIC1-R (late); large error-related responses were seen in the early period of tIC2-R and tIC5-R, as well as in tIC3-S and tIC3-R at both latencies.

EEG-fMRI Coupling

The averaged modulations (Figure 3.5.6) suggest that tIC1 and tIC3 should relate to the error precursors in sIC1 and sIC8 (IC3 and IC4 in Eichele et al., 2008b), and also that the error-related signals in tIC2, tIC3, and tIC5 should be

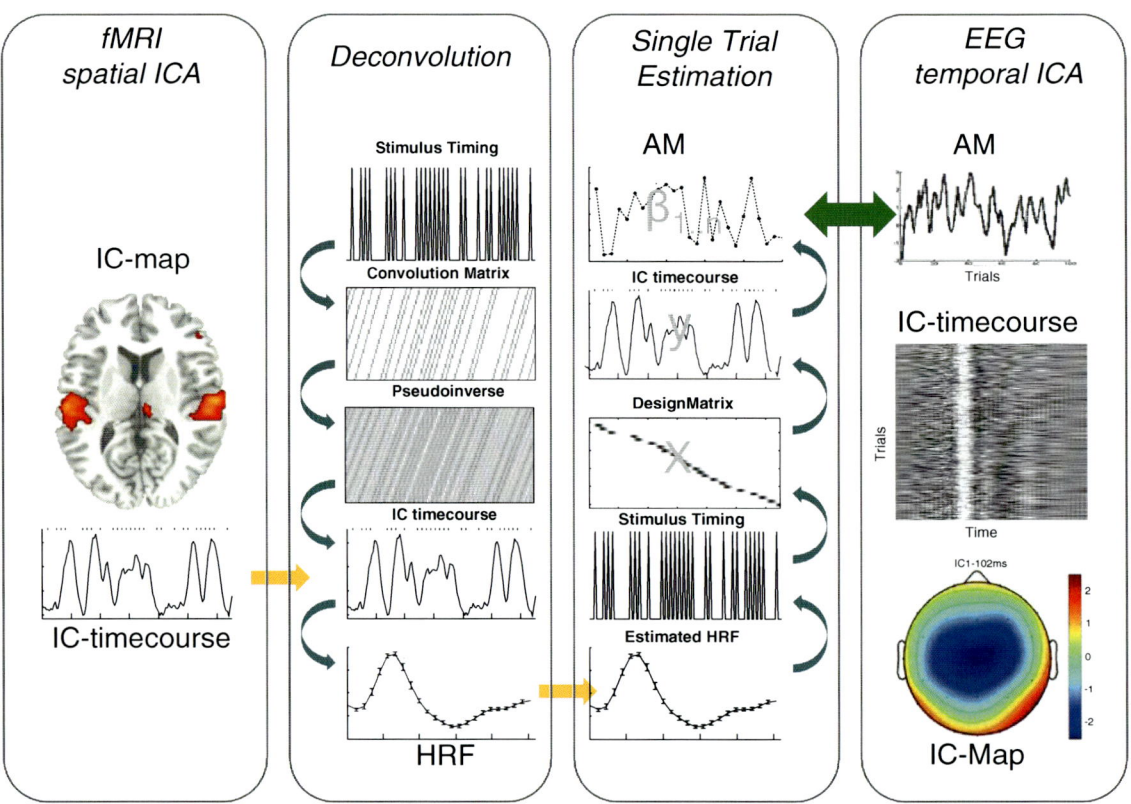

Figure 3.5.6. Stimulus-locked EEG-ICs. The top row shows the group mean topographies of the five components. The colormap indicates positive weights in red, and negative weights in blue. tIC1-S and tIC2-S correspond to parieto-occipital negativities in the latency range from about 100 to 200ms; tIC3-S, tIC4-S, and tIC5-S yield parietal positivities at 250 to 500 ms. In the middle row, the group-averaged single-trial images sorted by response time are plotted, showing no clear RT dependence in the first three components; in the last two components the positive peaks from approximately 250 to 500 ms are shifted by the response latency, indicating an interdependency between response speed and peak latency. The bottom row shows the event related grand source time courses of the from −400 to 600ms, averaged by condition. Error trials are plotted in red, incompatible in green, and compatible in blue. There are no strong differences between the conditions at the peaks of first three components, the last two ICs again show a shift of the peak latency by the average response time of the three conditions (errors < compatible < incompatible).

linked with the activity in sIC9, which contains the anterior cingulate gyrus (Debener et al., 2005). However, the single-trial correlation results were somewhat less clear, and only partially consistent with these assumptions. Significant relationships (p < 0.01) between EEG and fMRI components are summarized in Tables 3.5.1–3.5.4; Table 3.5.1 shows the correlations between the stimulus-locked EEG components and the fMRI, as well as the trial-by-trial differential estimated in all trials, Table 3.5.2 shows the correlations for the response-locked EEG; see Table 3.5.3 for the EEG-fMRI correlation in trial sequences preceding errors, and Table 3.5.4 for trial sequences succeeding errors.

tIC1-R was indeed correlated with sIC1 (Table 3.5.2), however at an earlier latency (-18 ms) than expected from the latency of the error precursor in the EEG. tIC1-R was also coupled to sIC2, sIC4, and sIC9, while tIC1-S (Table 3.5.1) was related to sIC6, and in the differential also to sIC2 and sIC8. Surprisingly, tIC1 was not significantly related to any sIC in pre-error trials (Table 3.5.3), in

post-error trials, it was however linked to sIC2 and sIC6 (Table 3.5.4).

tIC2-R, showing an error-related activity increase in the early post-response window, was correlated to sIC8, but not sIC9 in the response-locked analysis (Table 3.5.2), and to sIC3 and sIC7 in the stimulus-locked analysis (Table 3.5.1), in pre-error trials tIC2-S related to sIC3, sIC6, sIC8, and sIC9, and tIC2-R was correlated with sIC2 and sIC3 (Table 3.5.3); post-error trials showed a relationship between tIC2-S and sIC3 (Table 3.5.4).

Consistent with our assumptions, tIC3-R was correlated with sIC1 in pre-error trials, and also with sIC4 and sIC5, but not sIC8 (Table 3.5.3). In post-error trials, tIC3-R was related to sIC3, sIC5, sIC6, and sIC9 (Table 3.5.4). Across all response-locked trials, there was however no significant correlation (Table 3.5.2), while the stimulus-locked analysis showed the strongest statistic at sIC9 at about 130 ms, as well as sIC4, sIC6, and sIC7.

tIC4 showed no particular amplitude modulation around errors but tIC4-S was correlated with sIC1, sIC8, and sIC9

Table 3.5.1.
Coupling between fMRI spatial ICs (sIC1-9) and stimulus-locked EEG temporal ICs (tICnS), and the corresponding trial-by-trial differentials (d), estimated in all single trials.

		fMRI								
		sIC1	sIC2	sIC3	sIC4	sIC5	sIC6	sIC7	sIC8	sIC9
	tIC1-S						131t=−2.79			
	tIC1-S d		155ms t=2.69						57mst=2.70	
	tIC2-S			319ms t=2.77				498ms t=−2.99		
EEG	tIC2-S d			362ms t=−2.95						
	tIC3-S				385ms t=−2.81		284ms t=−3.37	424ms t=−3.22		135ms t=3.58
	tIC3-S d									127ms t=3.79
	tIC4-S	178ms t=3.27					420ms t=−3.85		268ms t=3.97	159ms t=3.39
	tIC4-S d									163ms t=−2.81
	tIC5-S			225ms t=−2.77				245ms t=−2.70		
	tIC5-S d		405ms t=2.84	96ms t=2.87						237ms t=3.87

(Tables 3.5.1 and 3.5.3), as well as sIC4, sIC6, and sIC7 (Tables 3.5.2 and 3.5.4).

tIC5-S was related to sIC9 in the differential (Table 3.5.1), and tIC5-R was related to sIC1, sIC8, and sIC9 in post error trials (Table 3.5.4), but not in pre-error trials (Table 3.5.3), or as well as to sIC2, sIC3, and sIC7 (Tables 3.5.1 and 3.5.2), and to sIC1 in response-locked trials overall (Table 3.5.2).

Table 3.5.2.
Coupling between the fMRI spatial ICs (sIC1-9) and response-locked EEG temporal ICs (tICn-R), and the corresponding trial-by-trial differentials (d), estimated in all single trials.

		fMRI								
		sIC1	sIC2	sIC3	sIC4	sIC5	sIC6	sIC7	sIC8	sIC9
	tIC1-R	−18ms t=4.40	48ms t=4.92		123ms t=3.66					64ms t=2.78
	tIC1-R d		56ms t=3.87							
	tIC2-R								−22ms t=−2.72	
	tIC2-R d									
EEG	tIC3-R									
	tIC3-R d					103ms t=3.13	−80ms t=−2.89		−2ms t=−3.70	
	tIC4-R				224ms t=−3.04		−45ms t=3.03	142ms t=3.28		
	tIC4-R d	25ms t=2.82			240ms t=−3.54		−49ms t=3.53			
	tIC5-R	127ms t=3.68						29ms t=−2.81		
	tIC5-R d			37ms t=−2.68						

Table 3.5.3.
Coupling between the fMRI spatial ICs (sIC1-9) and EEG temporal ICs (tICn-S/R)), estimated in the subsample of *pre*-error trials.

		fMRI								
		sIC1	sIC2	sIC3	sIC4	sIC5	sIC6	sIC7	sIC8	sIC9
EEG	tIC1-S									
	tIC2-S		409ms t=−3.49				471ms t=−3.27		413ms t=−2.95	327ms t=−2.87
	tIC3-S									
	tIC4-S			57ms t=3.19			131ms t=2.93		280ms t=2.99	159ms t=−3.17
	tIC5-S				256ms t=−2.91					
	tIC1-R		48ms t=4.03			213ms t=3.13	17ms t=−3.48	−10ms t=2.81		
	tIC2-R		189ms t=−2.95	127 t=2.71						
	tIC3-R	103ms t=−3.01			197ms t=−2.68	33ms t=3.59				
	tIC4-R				220ms t=−3.24				244ms t=3.70	
	tIC5-R						−61ms t=2.80			

Table 3.5.4.
Coupling between the fMRI spatial ICs (sIC1-9) and EEG temporal ICs (tICn-s/R), estimated in the subsample of *post*-error trial sequences.

		fMRI								
		sIC1	sIC2	sIC3	sIC4	sIC5	sIC6	sIC7	sIC8	sIC9
EEG	tIC1-S		346ms t=2.68				69ms t=3.42			
	tIC2-S			370ms t=−2.74						
	tIC3-S								88ms t=2.69	
	tIC4-S									159ms t=−3.36
	tIC5-S			217ms t=−2.86						
	tIC1-R		95ms t=3.19			107ms t=3.14			275ms t=3.29	
	tIC2-R									
	tIC3-R			−77ms t=3.43		162ms t=−2.87	−80ms t=−2.94			−65ms t=2.98
	tIC4-R						181ms t=−2.82			
	tIC5-R	158ms t=−2.77			197ms t=−3.47			267ms t=−3.11	220ms t=3.05	−77ms t=−2.89

Discussion

We presented an approach to perform a temporal independent component analysis on single-trial time domain EEG data for multiple subjects, and a parallel spatial decomposition of the fMRI data, in order to search for error-preceding activity in the EEG, and to integrate the EEG with the fMRI. The data are integrated via correlation of the estimated amplitude modulation of the fMRI sICs with the corresponding trial-by-trial dynamics of the EEG tICs. Our model uses a combination of principal component analysis for data reduction, subsequent independent component analysis on the aggregate data, and back-reconstruction of the aggregate mixing matrix to the individual subject, single-trial level (Calhoun et al., 2001; Eichele et al., 2008a). The reconstructed time courses and topographies are a function primarily of the variability within subjects, as opposed to being a representation of the average across subjects. From testing the performance of this model extensively in simulated, hybrid, and real data sets with different algorithms we believe that this approach offers a straightforward and computationally tractable solution to the task of multisubject analysis of EEG, fMRI, and particularly concurrent EEG-fMRI with ICA. In the following, we will discuss some methodological aspects, and then present some thoughts on the error precursors.

Jitter

Group ICA works well for sources that are consistent across a number of subjects, and will readily detect such sources when present in about 10% of the sampled population (Schmithorst and Holland, 2004). For the sICA on fMRI data this means that regional activity that overlaps across subjects can yield group-relevant components, which is the same criterion that applies to group (second-level) statistics of fMRI contrast images or simple averaging. Processes that are spatially variable cannot be captured by this implementation. Correspondingly, the group tICA on EEG single-trial time domain data is preferentially suited to detect components that represent event-related responses visible in averaged data. With respect to decomposition of EEG time domain data, the critical determinant for the success of a group model is intra- and intersubject latency jitter. There is considerable difficulty in reliably estimating latency jitter of event-related responses in real EEG data. However, if we assume that physiologic jitter is roughly on the order of the full width at half maximum of component peaks (Spencer, 2005), the group model reaches about 90% accuracy in reconstructing sources from mixed hybrid data. The limitation of the current method is that responses with poor time/phase-locking are not satisfyingly reconstructed (Donchin and Heffley, 1978; Mocks, 1986; Moosmann et al., 2008), which is a consequence of the data reduction and aggregation, which inherently limits the visibility of this method to event-related activity when EEG time domain data is used. This is in clear contradistinction to the performance of single subject temporal ICA on EEG data, which is insensitive to trial-to-trial phase/latency variability of sources. Individual ICA with subsequent ordering of components across subjects can thus achieve optimal accuracy with an ideal clustering technique, or a clearly specified criterion as, e.g., in Debener's work (2005). Correspondingly, one could then employ single-subject spatial ICA on the fMRI data and cluster components manually or (semi-)automatically (De Martino et al., 2007; Esposito et al., 2005). This would be useful when interindividual variability and its impact on the EEG-fMRI relationship is of interest (cf. Goncalves et al., 2006).

Deconvolution

Most previous concurrent EEG-fMRI studies convolved the EEG with a generic hemodynamic response function (e.g. derived from Boynton et al., 1996) to model the hemodynamic activation, whereby the parameters of the HRF such as shape and latency of the peak and undershoot are implicitly assumed to be fixed across the brain and across subjects. As can be seen in our data and in the previous literature there is, however, quite some variability of the HRF across regions and subjects (Aguirre et al., 1998; Glover, 1999; Handwerker et al., 2004; Hinrichs et al., 2000). Inclusion of derivative terms of the HRF into the model can alleviate such differences on the first level. However, it ignores the potential for amplitude bias induced by model mismatches due to variable hemodynamic delays and is not helpful for second-level random effects analyses (Calhoun et al., 2004). Therefore, in order to achieve a more sensitive and less biased analysis toward the particular parameters of the canonical HRF, it is desirable to estimate subject- and region-specific HRFs and employ these for convolution of the EEG measures. In our approach, the HRF is estimated and then effectively removed from the hemodynamic data, leaving just the amplitude modulation across trials, which has the same resolution as the EEG trial-by-trial dynamics. Here, we simply used the stimulus timing as input for deconvolution. Estimation of HRFs directly from concurrent EEG data is another powerful option to investigate the relationship between EEG and fMRI signals (de Munck et al., 2008; de Munck et al., 2007).

Integration

We used linear regression between each fMRI-sIC and each EEG-tIC separately to find IC-pairs across modalities that represent coherent neuronal sources that jointly express scalp electrophysiologic and hemodynamic features. In searching exclusively for such one-to-one mappings we assume that an EEG tIC is related to a single fMRI sIC. Although this is justifiable since both the sIC and tIC topographies are different from each other and stationary, it appears oversimplified in the face of the results (Tables 3.5.1–3.5.4), where several fMRI sICs affect several EEG tICs. One explanation might be that one sIC is a generator if scalp potentials (e.g., sIC4 and sIC7) with a large open field configuration; other sICs may transiently and remotely modulate this source, while being electrophysiologically silent on the scalp. This explanation already implies that the sICs are coupled with each other, which is reflected in their functional connectivity (Eichele et al., 2008b; Jafri et al., 2008), and effective connectivity (Stevens et al., 2007). Another related explanation is that the sICs might be considered spatially independent nodes in regionally distributed, functionally coherent source networks, such that many nodes can contribute directly or indirectly to the scalp potentials in a given paradigm/task. Here, the EEG-tICs, although temporally independent on the scalp, would not represent a single source but still a weighted average of multiple regional sources. Both these explanations are physiologically plausible (Baudena et al., 1995; Halgren et al., 1995a; Halgren et al., 1995b; Halgren and Marinkovic, 1995). Although it is typically not the aim of integration-by-prediction to solve the inverse problem but rather to bypass it, it is helpful to consider in which way the topographies and timecourses of sICs and tICs relate to each other, in order to come to a suitable way of statistically testing the relationship between them. If we assume that many sICs affect one tIC as seen in our results, one simple way of going about is to employ multiple regression with a design that contains all sIC time courses for prediction of EEG activity. The problem of collinearity between regressors would need to be addressed by orthogonalization (Andrade et al., 1999), stepwise selection, or a decomposition of the sIC time courses into set of unrelated factors by means of, e.g., PCA or ICA (similar to the procedure in Seifritz et al., 2002). However, such a treatment also means that the interpretation of the results becomes more difficult. Other options include canonical correlation analysis (CCA) in order to treat the problem. Here however, second-level inference is less well defined. Also, a joint (temporal) ICA of the sIC and tIC trial-by-trial modulations appears feasible (Calhoun et al., 2006; Moosmann et al., 2008), but has as yet not been explored in this context. A conceptually more advanced approach that, however, needs detailed specifications would be to adapt dynamic causal models that explain the EEG/ERP responses as changes in the effective connectivity between independent sources (Friston, 2005b; Friston et al., 2003; Garrido et al., 2007).

It remains to be determined which of the currently available analytic strategies is preferable under given conditions, i.e., yields robust results under minimal assumptions and methodological complexity and makes most effective use of the possible spatial and temporal resolution in each modality.

Error Precursors

The trial-by-trial modulation of the EEG components revealed error precursors in tIC1-R and tIC3-R, which corresponded to the average error-preceding activity observed in our recent report (Eichele et al., 2008b), and which were among others correlated with the event-related deactivation in the precuneus (sIC1) on a trial-by-trial level. The present results demonstrate that slow activity changes preceding errors extending across approximately 30 seconds can be detected in the EEG as well as in the fMRI, extending previous EEG studies reporting a reduced medial frontal negativity time-locked to correct responses on trials immediately preceding errors (Allain et al., 2004; Hajcak et al., 2005; Ridderinkhof et al., 2003). Moreover, the contingent negative variation (CNV) reflecting the preparatory action in a prefrontal-extrastriate network has been found to be reduced

from about 100 ms prior to the actual error (Padilla et al., 2006). The linear trends in the even related components suggest that changes in brain states eventually leading to task errors may start many seconds prior to the actual erroneous response. On the other hand, committing (and detecting) the error seems to induce increased activity in the components. It is interesting to note that in tIC3 the precursor and the error signal coexisted. The error signals apparently lead to a reset and enhanced activity in the areas associated with effort in cognitive tasks (Ridderinkhof et al., 2004). The monitoring system reflected in sIC9 was also related to the components that showed precursors and error signals, which is consistent with previous studies implicating the pMFC in monitoring of errors (Holroyd et al., 2004; Ridderinkhof et al., 2004; Ullsperger and von Cramon, 2001). Previous EEG and neuroimaging studies did not find much evidence for error-predicting activity changes more than one trial ahead in time. Our findings suggest that brain activity changes gradually over longer time toward an error-prone pattern. Whenever the performance monitoring system encounters an event indicating a performance problem—such as an overt error, this activity pattern is reset to a state supporting the recruitment of cognitive control.

The results reported here focused on identification error precursors in event-related activity. One line of future research should inquire if features in the ongoing EEG also carry similar precursors. In particular, it is prudent to assume that the modulation of the power in theta and alpha band can provide complementary predictive information. In situations where events are occurring very sparsely, but also where performance is continuous, and not defined by discrete stimulus/response onsets, features from the ongoing EEG would provide a better moment-to-moment description of the state of the system. In a refined experimental design, a joint assessment of ongoing and event-related activity can help to elucidate the question of how ongoing and event-related activity shape behavioral variability and how these types of of activity interact in EEG and fMRI (Arieli et al., 1996; Fox and Raichle, 2007).

Summary

This chapter introduced and applied the concept of parallel spatial and temporal unmixing with group ICA for concurrent EEG-fMRI. We used HRF deconvolution and single-trial estimation in the fMRI data, and used the single-trial weights as predictors for the amplitude modulation in the EEG. For illustration, data from a previously published performance monitoring experiment were analyzed to identify error-preceding activity in the EEG modality (Debener et al., 2005; Eichele et al., 2008b). We described EEG components that displayed such slow trends and that were coupled to the corresponding fMRI components. We believe that parallel ICA for analysis of concurrent EEG-fMRI on a trial-by-trial basis is a very useful addition to the toolbelt of researchers interested in multimodal integration.

ACKNOWLEDGMENT

We wish to express our sincere gratitude to Stefan Debener and Markus Ullsperger for sharing their experience, thoughts, time, and data with us in this effort. We also greatly appreciate the helpful discussions with Julie Onton and Jan C. de Munck. This work was supported by a grant from the L. Meltzer university fund (801616) to TE, and by the National Institutes of Health, under grants 1 R01 EB 000840, 1 R01 EB 005846, and 1 R01 EB 006841 to VDC. The data were collected at the Max-Planck Institute for Human Cognitive Brain Science, Leipzig, Germany, under a grant from the Deutsche Forschungsgemeinschaft to Markus Ullsperger. The fMRI data are publicly available from the Mind Research Network Database http://portal.mind.unm.edu/dcon/.

REFERENCES

Aguirre, G.K., Zarahn, E., D'Esposito, M., (1998). The variability of human, BOLD hemodynamic responses. Neuroimage 8, 360–369.

Allain, S., Carbonnell, L., Falkenstein, M., Burle, B., Vidal, F., (2004). The modulation of the Ne-like wave on correct responses foreshadows errors. Neurosci Lett 372, 161–166.

Allen, P.J., Josephs, O., Turner, R., (2000). A method for removing imaging artifact from continuous EEG recorded during functional MRI. NeuroImage 12, 230–239.

Allen, P.J., Polizzi, G., Krakow, K., Fish, D.R., Lemieux, L., (1998). Identification of EEG events in the MR scanner: the problem of pulse artifact and a method for its subtraction. NeuroImage 8, 229–239.

Andrade, A., Paradis, A.L., Rouquette, S., Poline, J.B., (1999). Ambiguous results in functional neuroimaging data analysis due to covariate correlation. Neuroimage 10, 483–486.

Arieli, A., Sterkin, A., Grinvald, A., Aertsen, A., (1996). Dynamics of ongoing activity: explanation of the large variability in evoked cortical responses. Science 273, 1868–1871.

Baudena, P., Halgren, E., Heit, G., Clarke, J.M., (1995). Intracerebral potentials to rare target and distractor auditory and visual stimuli. III. Frontal cortex. Electroencephalogr Clin Neurophysiol 94, 251–264.

Bell, A.J., Sejnowski, T.J., (1995). An information-maximization approach to blind separation and blind deconvolution. Neural Comput 7, 1129–1159.

Bledowski, C., Prvulovic, D., Hoechstetter, K., Scherg, M., Wibral, M., Goebel, R., Linden, D.E., (2004). Localizing P300 generators in visual target and distractor processing: a combined event-related potential and functional magnetic resonance imaging study. J Neurosci 24, 9353–9360.

Boynton, G.M., Engel, S.A., Glover, G.H., Heeger, D.J., (1996). Linear systems analysis of functional magnetic resonance imaging in human V1. J Neurosci 16, 4207–4221.

Calhoun, V., Adali, T., (2006). Unmixing fMRI with independent component analysis. IEEE Engineering in Medicine and Biology Magazine 25, 79–90.

Calhoun, V.D., Adali, T., Pearlson, G.D., Kiehl, K.A., (2006). Neuronal chronometry of target detection: fusion of hemodynamic and event-related potential data. Neuroimage 30, 544–553.

Calhoun, V.D., Adali, T., Pearlson, G.D., Pekar, J.J., (2001). A method for making group inferences from functional MRI data using independent component analysis. Hum Brain Mapp 14, 140–151.

Calhoun, V.D., Stevens, M.C., Pearlson, G.D., Kiehl, K.A., (2004). fMRI analysis with the general linear model: removal of latency-induced amplitude bias by incorporation of hemodynamic derivative terms. Neuroimage 22, 252–257.

Cardoso, J.F., Souloumiac, A., (1993). Blind Beamforming for Non Gaussian Signals. IEE-Proceeding-F 140, 362–370.

Damoiseaux, J.S., Rombouts, S.A., Barkhof, F., Scheltens, P., Stam, C.J., Smith, S.M., Beckmann, C.F., (2006). Consistent resting-state networks across healthy subjects. Proc Natl Acad Sci U S A 103, 13848–13853.

Daunizeau, J., Grova, C., Marrelec, G., Mattout, J., Jbabdi, S., Pelegrini-Issac, M., Lina, J.M., Benali, H., (2007). Symmetrical event-related EEG/fMRI information fusion in a variational Bayesian framework. Neuroimage 36, 69–87.

De Martino, F., Gentile, F., Esposito, F., Balsi, M., Di Salle, F., Goebel, R., Formisano, E., (2007). Classification of fMRI independent components using IC-fingerprints and support vector machine classifiers. Neuroimage 34, 177–194.

de Munck, J.C., Goncalves, S.I., Faes, T.J., Kuijer, J.P., Pouwels, P.J., Heethaar, R.M., Lopes da Silva, F.H., (2008). A study of the brain's resting state based on alpha band power, heart rate and fMRI. Neuroimage.

de Munck, J.C., Goncalves, S.I., Huijboom, L., Kuijer, J.P., Pouwels, P.J., Heethaar, R.M., Lopes da Silva, F.H., (2007). The hemodynamic response of the alpha rhythm: an EEG/fMRI study. Neuroimage 35, 1142–1151.

Debener, S., Strobel, A., Sorger, B., Peters, J., Kranczioch, C., Engel, A.K., Goebel, R., (2007). Improved quality of auditory event-related potentials recorded simultaneously with 3-T fMRI: removal of the ballistocardiogram artefact. Neuroimage 34, 587–597.

Debener, S., Ullsperger, M., Siegel, M., Engel, A.K., (2006). Single-trial EEG-fMRI reveals the dynamics of cognitive function. Trends Cogn Sci 10, 558–563.

Debener, S., Ullsperger, M., Siegel, M., Fiehler, K., von Cramon, D.Y., Engel, A.K., (2005). Trial-by-trial coupling of concurrent electroencephalogram and functional magnetic resonance imaging identifies the dynamics of performance monitoring. J Neurosci 25, 11730–11737.

Delorme, A., Makeig, S., (2004). EEGLAB: an open source toolbox for analysis of single-trial EEG dynamics including independent component analysis. J Neurosci Methods 134, 9–21.

Donchin, E., Heffley, E.F., (1978). Multivariate analysis of event-related potential data: A tutorial review. In: Otto, D. (Ed.), Multidisciplinary perspectives in event-related potential research. U.S. Government Printing Office, Washington, DC.

Eichele, T., Calhoun, V.D., Moosmann, M., Specht, K., Jongsma, M.L., Quiroga, R.Q., Nordby, H., Hugdahl, K., (2008a). Unmixing concurrent EEG-fMRI with parallel independent component analysis. Int J Psychophysiol 67, 222–234.

Eichele, T., Debener, S., Calhoun, V.D., Specht, K., Engel, A.K., Hugdahl, K., von Cramon, D.Y., Ullsperger, M., (2008b). Prediction of human errors by maladaptive changes in event-related brain networks. Proc Natl Acad Sci U S A 105, 6173–6178.

Eichele, T., Specht, K., Moosmann, M., Jongsma, M.L., Quiroga, R.Q., Nordby, H., Hugdahl, K., (2005). Assessing the spatiotemporal evolution of neuronal activation with single-trial event-related potentials and functional MRI. Proc Natl Acad Sci U S A 102, 17798–17803.

Esposito, F., Scarabino, T., Hyvarinen, A., Himberg, J., Formisano, E., Comani, S., Tedeschi, G., Goebel, R., Seifritz, E., Di Salle, F., (2005). Independent component analysis of fMRI group studies by self-organizing clustering. Neuroimage 25, 193–205.

Feige, B., Scheffler, K., Esposito, F., Di Salle, F., Hennig, J., Seifritz, E., (2005). Cortical and subcortical correlates of electroencephalographic alpha rhythm modulation. J Neurophysiol 93, 2864–2872.

Fox, M.D., Raichle, M.E., (2007). Spontaneous fluctuations in brain activity observed with functional magnetic resonance imaging. Nat Rev Neurosci 8, 700–711.

Friston, K.J., (2003). Human Brain Function, 2nd ed. Elsevier.

Friston, K.J., (2005a). Models of brain function in neuroimaging. Annu Rev Psychol 56, 57–87.

Friston, K.J., (2005b). A theory of cortical responses. Philos Trans R Soc Lond B Biol Sci 360, 815–836.

Friston, K.J., Harrison, L., Penny, W., (2003). Dynamic causal modelling. Neuroimage 19, 1273–1302.

Friston, K.J., Holmes, A.P., Poline, J.B., Grasby, P.J., Williams, S.C., Frackowiak, R.S., Turner, R., (1995). Analysis of fMRI time-series revisited. Neuroimage 2, 45–53.

Garrido, M.I., Kilner, J.M., Kiebel, S.J., Friston, K.J., (2007). Evoked brain responses are generated by feedback loops. Proc Natl Acad Sci U S A 104, 20961–20966.

Glover, G.H., (1999). Deconvolution of impulse response in event-related BOLD fMRI. Neuroimage 9, 416–429.

Goncalves, S.I., de Munck, J.C., Pouwels, P.J., Schoonhoven, R., Kuijer, J.P., Maurits, N.M., Hoogduin, J.M., Van Someren, E.J., Heethaar, R.M., Lopes da Silva, F.H., (2006). Correlating the alpha rhythm to BOLD using simultaneous EEG/fMRI: inter-subject variability. Neuroimage 30, 203–213.

Hajcak, G., Nieuwenhuis, S., Ridderinkhof, K.R., Simons, R.F., (2005). Error-preceding brain activity: robustness, temporal dynamics, and boundary conditions. Biol Psychol 70, 67–78.

Halgren, E., Baudena, P., Clarke, J.M., Heit, G., Liegeois, C., Chauvel, P., Musolino, A., (1995a). Intracerebral potentials to rare target and distractor auditory and visual stimuli. I. Superior temporal plane and parietal lobe. Electroencephalogr Clin Neurophysiol 94, 191–220.

Halgren, E., Baudena, P., Clarke, J.M., Heit, G., Marinkovic, K., Devaux, B., Vignal, J.P., Biraben, A., (1995b). Intracerebral potentials to rare target and distractor auditory and visual stimuli. II. Medial, lateral and posterior temporal lobe. Electroencephalogr Clin Neurophysiol 94, 229–250.

Halgren, E., Marinkovic, K., (1995). General principles for the physiology of cognition as suggested by intracranial ERPs. In: Ogura, C., Koga, Y., Shimokochi, M. (Eds.), Recent Advances in Event-Related Brain Potential Research. Elsevier, Amsterdam, pp. 1072–1084.

Handwerker, D.A., Ollinger, J.M., D'Esposito, M., (2004). Variation of BOLD hemodynamic responses across subjects and brain regions and their effects on statistical analyses. Neuroimage 21, 1639–1651.

Heeger, D.J., Ress, D., (2002). What does fMRI tell us about neuronal activity? Nat Rev Neurosci 3, 142–151.

Hinrichs, H., Scholz, M., Tempelmann, C., Woldorff, M.G., Dale, A.M., Heinze, H.J., (2000). Deconvolution of event-related fMRI responses in fast-rate experimental designs: tracking amplitude variations. J Cogn Neurosci 12 Suppl 2, 76–89.

Holroyd, C.B., Nieuwenhuis, S., Yeung, N., Nystrom, L., Mars, R.B., Coles, M.G., Cohen, J.D., (2004). Dorsal anterior cingulate cortex shows fMRI response to internal and external error signals. Nat Neurosci 7, 497–498.

Hopfinger, J.B., Khoe, W., Song, A.W., (2005). Combining Electrophysiology with Structural and Functional Neuroimaging: ERPs, PET, MRI, and fMRI. In: Handy, T.C. (Ed.), Event Related Potentials. A Methods Handbook. The MIT Press, Cambridge, pp. 345–380.

Horwitz, B., Poeppel, D., (2002). How can EEG/MEG and fMRI/PET data be combined? Hum Brain Mapp 17, 1–3.

Hyvarinen, A., Oja, E., (1997). A fast fixed-point algorithm for independent component analysis. Neural Comput. 9, 1483–1492.

Jafri, M.J., Pearlson, G.D., Stevens, M., Calhoun, V.D., (2008). A method for functional network connectivity among spatially independent resting-state components in schizophrenia. Neuroimage 39, 1666–1681.

Jung, T.P., Makeig, S., Humphries, C., Lee, T.W., McKeown, M.J., Iragui, V., Sejnowski, T.J., (2000). Removing electroencephalographic artifacts by blind source separation. Psychophysiology 37, 163–178.

Kiebel, S.J., Friston, K.J., (2004). Statistical parametric mapping for event-related potentials: I. Generic considerations. Neuroimage 22, 492–502.

Kiehl, K.A., Stevens, M.C., Laurens, K.R., Pearlson, G., Calhoun, V.D., Liddle, P.F., (2005). An adaptive reflexive processing model of neurocognitive function: supporting evidence from a large scale (n = 100) fMRI study of an auditory oddball task. Neuroimage 25, 899–915.

Kim, K.H., Yoon, H.W., Park, H.W., (2004). Improved ballistocardiac artifact removal from the electroencephalogram recorded in fMRI. J Neurosci Methods 135, 193–203.

Laufs, H., Daunizeau, J., Carmichael, D.W., Kleinschmidt, A., (2008). Recent advances in recording electrophysiological data simultaneously with magnetic resonance imaging. Neuroimage 40, 515–528.

Lauritzen, M., Gold, L., (2003). Brain function and neurophysiological correlates of signals used in functional neuroimaging. J Neurosci 23, 3972–3980.

Lee, T., Girolami, M., Sejnowski, T., (1999). Independent Component Analysis Using an Extended Infomax Algorithm for Mixed Subgaussian and Supergaussian Sources. Neural Comput 11, 417–441.

Li, C.S., Yan, P., Bergquist, K.L., Sinha, R., (2007). Greater activation of the "default" brain regions predicts stop signal errors. Neuroimage 38, 640–648.

Liu, A.K., Belliveau, J.W., Dale, A.M., (1998). Spatiotemporal imaging of human brain activity using functional MRI constrained magnetoencephalography data: Monte Carlo simulations. Proc Natl Acad Sci U S A 95, 8945–8950.

Logothetis, N.K., (2003). The underpinnings of the BOLD functional magnetic resonance imaging signal. J Neurosci 23, 3963–3971.

Logothetis, N.K., Pauls, J., Augath, M., Trinath, T., Oeltermann, A., (2001). Neurophysiological investigation of the basis of the fMRI signal. Nature 412, 150–157.

Makeig, S., Debener, S., Onton, J., Delorme, A., (2004a). Mining event-related brain dynamics. Trends Cogn Sci 8, 204–210.

Makeig, S., Delorme, A., Westerfield, M., Jung, T.P., Townsend, J., Courchesne, E., Sejnowski, T.J., (2004b). Electroencephalographic brain dynamics following manually responded visual targets. PLoS Biol 2, e176.

Makeig, S., Jung, T.P., Bell, A.J., Ghahremani, D., Sejnowski, T.J., (1997). Blind separation of auditory event-related brain responses into independent components. Proc Natl Acad Sci U S A 94, 10979–10984.

Makeig, S., Jung, T-P-, Sejnowski, TJ, (2002). Having your voxels and timing them too? In: Sommer, F., Wichert, A. (Ed.), Exploratory Analysis and Data Modeling in Functional Neuroimaging. The MIT Press, Cambridge.

Malinen, S., Hlushchuk, Y., Hari, R., (2007). Towards natural stimulation in fMRI–issues of data analysis. Neuroimage 35, 131–139.

Mantini, D., Corbetta, M., Perrucci, M.G., Romani, G.L., Del Gratta, C., (2008). Large-scale brain networks account for sustained and transient activity during target detection. Neuroimage.

Mantini, D., Perrucci, M.G., Del Gratta, C., Romani, G.L., Corbetta, M., (2007). Electrophysiological signatures of resting state networks in the human brain. Proc Natl Acad Sci U S A 104, 13170–13175.

Martinez-Montes E., Valdes-Sosa, P.A., Miwakeichi, F., Goldman, R.I., Cohen, M.S., (2004). Concurrent EEG/fMRI analysis by multiway Partial Least Squares. Neuroimage 22, 1023–1034.

McKeown, M.J., Hansen, L.K., Sejnowski, T.J., (2003). Independent component analysis of functional MRI: what is signal and what is noise? Curr Opin Neurobiol 13, 620–629.

Mocks, J., (1986). The influence of latency jitter in principal component analysis of event-related potentials. Psychophysiology 23, 480–484.

Moosmann, M., Eichele, T., Nordby, H., Hugdahl, K., Calhoun, V.D., (2008). Joint independent component analysis for simultaneous EEG-fMRI: Principle and simulation. Int J Psychophysiol 67, 212–221.

Niazy, R.K., Beckmann, C.F., Iannetti, G.D., Brady, J.M., Smith, S.M., (2005). Removal of FMRI environment artifacts from EEG data using optimal basis sets. Neuroimage 28, 720–737.

Nunez, P.L., (1995). Neocortical dynamics and human EEG rhythms. Oxford University Press, New York.

Ogawa, S., Lee, T.M., Kay, A.R., Tank, D.W., (1990). Brain magnetic resonance imaging with contrast dependent on blood oxygenation. Proc Natl Acad Sci U S A 87, 9868–9872.

Onton, J., Westerfield, M., Townsend, J., Makeig, S., (2006). Imaging human EEG dynamics using independent component analysis. Neurosci Biobehav Rev 30, 808–822.

Padilla, M.L., Wood, R.A., Hale, L.A., Knight, R.T., (2006). Lapses in a prefrontal-extrastriate preparatory attention network predict mistakes. J Cogn Neurosci 18, 1477–1487.

Quian Quiroga, R., Garcia, H., (2003). Single-trial event-related potentials with wavelet denoising. Clin Neurophysiol 114, 376–390.

Raichle, M.E., MacLeod, A.M., Snyder, A.Z., Powers, W.J., Gusnard, D.A., Shulman, G.L., (2001). A default mode of brain function. Proc Natl Acad Sci U S A 98, 676–682.

Raichle, M.E., Snyder, A.Z., (2007). A default mode of brain function: a brief history of an evolving idea. Neuroimage 37, 1083–1090; discussion 1097–1089.

Ridderinkhof, K.R., Nieuwenhuis, S., Bashore, T.R., (2003). Errors are foreshadowed in brain potentials associated with action monitoring in cingulate cortex in humans. Neuroscience Letters 348, 1–4.

Ridderinkhof, K.R., Ullsperger, M., Crone, E.A., Nieuwenhuis, S., (2004). The role of the medial frontal cortex in cognitive control. Science 306, 443–447.

Rushworth, M.F., Buckley, M.J., Behrens, T.E., Walton, M.E., Bannerman, D.M., (2007). Functional organization of the medial frontal cortex. Curr Opin Neurobiol 17, 220–227.

Scheeringa, R., Bastiaansen, M.C., Petersson, K.M., Oostenveld, R., Norris, D.G., Hagoort, P., (2008). Frontal theta EEG activity correlates negatively with the default mode network in resting state. Int J Psychophysiol 67, 242–251.

Schmithorst, V.J., Holland, S.K., (2004). Comparison of three methods for generating group statistical inferences from independent component analysis of functional magnetic resonance imaging data. J Magn Reson Imaging 19, 365–368.

Seifritz, E., Esposito, F., Hennel, F., Mustovic, H., Neuhoff, J.G., Bilecen, D., Tedeschi, G., Scheffler, K., Di Salle, F., (2002). Spatiotemporal pattern of neural processing in the human auditory cortex. Science 297, 1706–1708.

Spencer, K.M., (2005). Averaging, Detection, and Classification of single-trial ERPs. In: Handy, T.C. (Ed.), Event Related Potentials. A Methods Handbook. The MIT Press, Cambridge, pp. 209–228.

Stevens, M.C., Kiehl, K.A., Pearlson, G.D., Calhoun, V.D., (2007). Functional neural networks underlying response inhibition in adolescents and adults. Behav Brain Res 181, 12–22.

Stone, J.V., (2002). Independent component analysis: an introduction. Trends Cogn Sci 6, 59–64.

Ullsperger, M., von Cramon, D.Y., (2001). Subprocesses of performance monitoring: a dissociation of error processing and response competition revealed by event-related fMRI and ERPs. Neuroimage 14, 1387–1401.

Ullsperger, M., von Cramon, D.Y., (2004). Neuroimaging of performance monitoring: error detection and beyond. Cortex 40, 593–604.

3.6

JC de Munck, SI Gonçalves, PJ van Houdt, R Mammoliti, P Ossenblok, and FH Lopes da Silva

The Hemodynamic Response of EEG Features

Introduction

Surface EEG represents time varying voltage differences measured from the human scalp. The generators of these signals consist of current sources formed by the postsynaptic currents associated with interacting neurons (Lopes da Silva and Van Rotterdam, 1982). During rest, when no stimulus is given to the subject, the EEG consists of several rhythms that give information about the subject's brain state and vigilance level. Although much is known about the meaning and (patho-) physiology of the EEG, the localization of brain regions that are involved in the generation of the different EEG components remains a central difficulty. For spontaneous EEG, many sources with different geometries are simultaneously active and therefore the underlying assumptions of inverse modeling techniques like dipole fitting (e.g., Mosher and Leahy, 1998; De Munck et al., 2001) and minimum norm estimation (e.g., Sarvas, 1987; Pascual-Marqui 1999) are easily violated, thereby severely restricting the applicability of these data analysis techniques.

Correlation analysis of simultaneously recorded EEG and fMRI, described elsewhere in this volume, provides a completely different way of addressing the source localization problem, without the need to rely on dipole models and volume conductor geometries. Briefly, reference functions are extracted from the EEG representing for instance the amount of alpha rhythm or the presence/absence of sleep spindle activity. If the reference function is correlated to the fMRI time-series, the underlying generators of the reference functions can be localized in much the same way as with standard fMRI analysis. This technique was developed initially to localize interictal spikes (e.g., Ives et al., 1993; Warach et al., 1996; Lemieux et al., 2001; Gotman et al., 2004; Liston et al., 2006a; Zijlmans et al., 2007), and later it was extended to studies on other EEG phenomena and the alpha band in particular (Goldman et al., 2002; Laufs et al., 2003a; Laufs

et al., 2003b; Moosmann et al., 2003; Gonçalves et al., 2006; Mantini et al., 2007).

Apart from the localization power of combined EEG/fMRI, these registrations may provide much more insight into the physiological meaning of spontaneous EEG and trial-by-trial variations of event-related responses (e.g., Debener et al., 2005; Eichele et al., 2005). For instance, the sign of the correlation coefficient provides information about the metabolism associated with the EEG features investigated. It has been found, in several independent EEG/fMRI studies, that the EEG alpha power correlates negatively to BOLD at cortical areas, whereas it correlates positively at the thalamus (Goldman et al., 2002; Laufs et al., 2003a; Laufs et al., 2003b; Gonçalves et al., 2006). In this way, it has been confirmed that the driving force of the alpha rhythm is located at the thalamus, whereas the cortical correlation areas decrease their metabolism due to decreased level of alertness, at the periods of increased alpha power.

In the first studies where EEG and fMRI were correlated (Goldman et al., 2002; Moosmann et al., 2003), the occurrence of epileptic spikes or the amplitude of the alpha rhythm was convolved with a canonical hemodynamic response function (HRF). This convolution was necessary to obtain a reference function that well describes the expected BOLD response on the observed EEG features. However, it has been demonstrated that HRFs tend to vary over subject, stimulus modality, and stimulus duration (Lemieux et al., 2001; Boynton et al., 1996; Aguirre et al., 1998; Glover, 1999), and therefore regional and intersubject differences might be masked by the use of a constant HRF model. In De Munck et al. (2007a) EEG/fMRI correlation analysis was performed in a more general way by estimating the HRF from the data (see also Hinrichs et al., 2000; Lu et al., 2006). The fMRI BOLD signals are then treated as the output of an unknown linear time invariant filter, with EEG reference function as input. At those voxels where the combined filter coefficients deviate significantly from zero, the shape of the estimated HRF provides information about the physiological processes underlying the EEG. In a study on the alpha rhythm where this approach was used (De Munck et al. 2007a), it was found that the HRF of the thalamus is biphasic and peaks several seconds earlier than the HRF at the cortex.

By adding filter coefficients corresponding to negative time shifts to the estimation model, it is possible to detect whether any BOLD activity precedes the EEG features. Such type of correlation might seem odd at first sight, but it should be realized that EEG only registers the effect of locally synchronous cells. Asynchronous activity consumes energy and may contribute to the BOLD signal, but does not result in a detectable EEG features. In case of epileptic spikes, anti-causal EEG/fMRI correlation could indicate that the observed spike is only "the tip of the iceberg," caused by a period of temporal neural synchronization of the network, in a stream of asynchronous pathological activity associated with epilepsy (Hawco et al., 2007).

In recent years, the study of the brain's resting state with fMRI alone has become quite popular (e.g., Greicius et al. 2003; Damoiseaux et al., 2006; Fox and Raichle, 2007), for instance because this paradigm is simple and therefore adequate for various patient studies. One of the difficulties of these types of studies is that the meaning of the BOLD signal is not physiologically unambiguous (Logothetis, 2007). The BOLD signal depends on the one hand on local factors, such as blood volume, blood flow, and blood oxygenation, and on the other hand on global factors such as heart beat (e.g., Glover et al., 2000; Liston et al., 2006b; Lund et al. 2006) and respiration (Windischberger et al., 2002). These multiple influences hamper the interpretation of BOLD as a pure neuronal signal. By analyzing simultaneously recorded EEG, fMRI, ECG, pulse oxygenation, and respiration, the contribution of different components to the BOLD can be identified, potentially resulting in a better understanding of the meaning of BOLD.

In Shmueli et al. (2007) and De Munck et al. (2007b; De Munck et al., 2008) the effect of heartbeat intervals on BOLD was investigated. Because no instantaneous correlation was anticipated, an impulse response model was developed, wherein the BOLD was modeled as output of a linear filter with the heart rate variations as input, similar to the estimation model for the HRF of the alpha band. In the present chapter, the HRF estimation problem is described in detail and its underlying assumptions are discussed. Furthermore, different variants of the method are applied using the data of a single subject that was chosen for illustrative purposes.

Methods

Extracting Reference Functions from EEG and Pulse Oxygenation

The main difficulty in extracting a reference function from the EEG that can be correlated to fMRI is that EEG and fMRI are recorded on completely different time scales. Furthermore, fMRI volumes are not measured instantaneously, but consist of different slices that are recorded sequentially. A simple and straightforward approach to the latter problem is to interpolate the BOLD signals in the time domain, in order to obtain a derived data set that can be considered as measured instantaneously. However, fMRI signals are typically undersampled because multiple EEG events may occur during a TR of 3 s. Therefore, temporal interpolation may cause aliasing of high-frequency components into low frequencies. In principal, a better approach is to derive slice-specific regressors from the EEG, which are adapted to the timings of the individual slices and to use these slice-specific regressors in the EEG/fMRI correlation analysis. Care should be taken that regression parameters extracted from different slices be mutually comparable.

One can globally distinguish two types of phenomena that one may wish to study with coregistered EEG/fMRI (Figure 3.6.1). One type consists of short events (like inter-ictal epileptic spikes) that occur at times $\tau_0, \tau_1, \ldots, \tau_k, \ldots$. The other type consists of a continuously varying parameter, like the amplitude of the alpha rhythm. For the first kind of phenomena it is assumed that each event results in a fixed HRF $h(t)$, which linearly adds to BOLD, independent of the other events. The reference function for the i-th slice can be expressed as

$$r^{(i)}\left(jT_V\right) = r^{(i)}\left(t_j\right) = \sum_k h\left(t_j + iT_S - \tau_k\right),$$

$$i = 0, \ldots, I - 1, \ j = 0, \ldots, J - 1 \qquad (1)$$

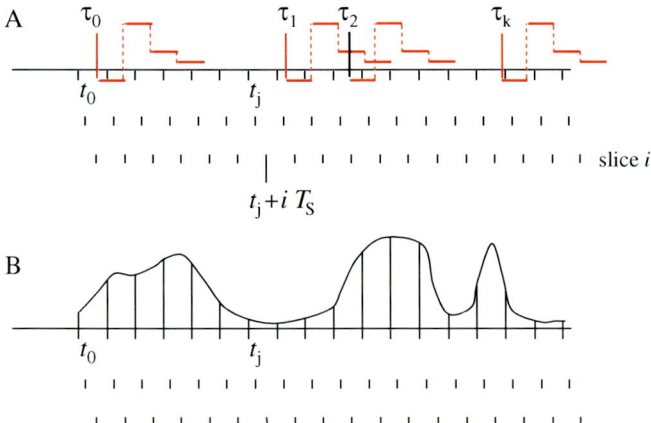

Figure 3.6.1. The derivation of slice time dependent regressors from EEG signals is described for a discrete (A) or a continuous (B) phenomenon. In case A, the contribution of each slice to a certain event depends on the relative timing of the events and the slice times. The case of a piecewise constant HRF interpolation is depicted. When the EEG phenomenon is (practically) continuous, like the alpha power computed with overlapping windows with a small time shift, the slice time corrected regressors are simply obtained by subsampling the continuous function.

where $t_j = j\,T_V$, are the times at which the first slice of each volume is recorded, T_V is the volume time TR, T_S is the slice time, I is the number of slices, and J the number of volumes.

When continuous phenomena are investigated, and the amplitude representative for the time window from $t_j + iT_S$ to $t_j + iT_S + T_\alpha$ is indicated with $\alpha^{(i)}(t_j)$, one obtains, assuming a linear and time-invariant response model,

$$r^{(i)}\left(t_j\right) = \int\limits_{-\infty}^{\infty} \alpha^{(i)}\left(t_j - T\right)h(T)\mathrm{d}T$$

$$\approx T_S \sum_m \alpha^{(i)}\left(t_j - mT_S\right)h(mT_S) \qquad (2)$$

In Equation 2 the summation extends over all times for which the argument of $h(t)$ is non-zero. So, for causal models, integration and summation start at 0 instead of $-\infty$. Furthermore, it assumes that the shortest time shifts over which the alpha power variations are computed equals T_S. When $\alpha(t)$ variations are slow, larger step sizes may be taken, like mT_V. In the sequel the step size factor T_S in Equation 2 will be omitted, or absorbed in $h(t)$.

In both Equations 1 and 2, slice time specific references are obtained and their presence in the BOLD signal can be tested statistically using a t-test. In this type of correlation analysis, the estimated parameter associated with the effect is unimportant; the only result that matters is its significance and the sign of correlation. When the goal is to estimate the HRF from the data, the meaning of the parameters becomes important and care must be taken that slice time effects are eliminated. Furthermore, a parameterization of $h(t)$ is needed because one needs to bridge the gap between the high temporal resolution with which the EEG events are known, and the low temporal resolution on which fMRI is recorded. A very general way to parameterize the HRF is to assume a base function $\xi(t)$, which is shifted over multiple volume times. For instance, $\xi(t)$ can be a hat-shaped function that varies linearly from 0 to 1 when $-T_V < t < 0$ and from 1 to 0 when $0 < t < T_V$, resulting in a piecewise linear representation of $h(t)$. Alternatively, one may choose $\xi(t)$ such that $\xi(t) = 1$ for $0 < t < T_V$ and $\xi(t) = 0$ otherwise, resulting in a piecewise constant representation. The parameterization can be expressed as

$$h(t) = \sum_n h_n\xi(t - t_n) \qquad (3)$$

Note that with this formulation, one has that $h_n = h(t_n)$ so that the interpretation of h_n is independent of the slice number. When Equation 3 is substituted in Equation 1, one obtains

$$r^{(i)}\left(t_j\right) = \sum_n h_n \sum_k \xi\left(t_j + iT_S - \tau_k - t_n\right)$$

$$= \sum_n h_n s^{(i)}\left(t_j - t_n\right) \qquad (4)$$

where

$$s^{(i)}(t) = \sum_k \xi(t + iT_S - \tau_k) \qquad (5)$$

is the slice time specific event density function. Equation 5 gives a recipe to attribute an event detected in the middle of a volume to different slice regressors. When $h(t)$ is interpolated with piecewise constant functions $\xi(t)$, the function $s^{(i)}(t)$ simply counts the number of events occurring in the time interval between $t_j + i\,T_S$ and $t_{j+1} + i\,T_S$. For piecewise linear interpolation Equation 5 provides a way to split the contribution of an event to two subsequent volumes, where the contribution depends in the slice time.

In case of the continuous variations, one obtains, if the alpha power is sampled every volume instead of every slice,

$$r^{(i)}\left(t_j\right) = \sum_n h_n \sum_m \alpha^{(i)}\left(t_j - t_m\right)\xi(t_m - t_n)$$

$$= \sum_n h_n\alpha^{(i)}\left(t_j - t_n\right) \qquad (6)$$

Here it has been used that at multiples of T_V, $\xi(t-t_n)$ is either 0 or 1.

It appears from Equations 4 and 6 that both the event-related and the continuous case lead to the same formulation of slice dependent regressors. The advantage of slice time dependent regressors is that the estimated parameters are intrinsically slice time corrected, but the disadvantage is that the regression model is slice dependent resulting in a slower performance of the correlation algorithm. An alternative method, which is more ad hoc, is to use the same regressors for different slices, and to shift the estimated HRFs afterward according to the slice time. In this chapter both approaches will be compared.

In De Munck et al. (2008) slice dependent heartbeat interval (HBI) regressors were derived from the coregistered pulse oxygenation signal. In this context, the regressor $\beta^{(i)}(t_j)$ indicates the average HBI in the time interval from $t_j + i\,T_S$ to $t_j + i\,T_S + T_{Ave}$ where T_{Ave} is an averaging time interval. Contrary to the heartbeat regressors proposed by Glover et al. (2000), which represent a non-linear function of the phase of the heart at the moment a slice is recorded, the HBI-regressor $\beta(t)$ gives information about the pumping speed of the heart. Changes herein may have a delayed effect on the BOLD signal, and because the effect size as a function of time delay is a priori not known, it is appealing to determine its effect on the basis of an unknown impulse response function. This approach leads to a formulation that is very similar to Equation 6.

Correlation Analysis

When the hemodynamic responses to events (Equation 4) or to the alpha power variations (Equation 6) are to be determined from an equidistantly sampled data set and a linear time invariant model is adopted, it may seem advantageous to perform the analysis in the frequency domain. For instance, taking the discrete Fourier transform of Equation 6 yields,

$$R^{(i)}(\omega_k) = H(\omega_k)A^{(i)}(\omega_k) \qquad (7)$$

where capitals indicate transformed variables and $\omega_k = 2\pi k/(J\,T_V)$. In principle, one could eliminate $H(\omega_k) = R^{(i)}(\omega_k)/A^{(i)}(\omega_k)$ and transform it back to the time domain yielding $h(t)$.

The problem with this approach is that the BOLD signal is contaminated with noise and slow trends related to subject motion, respiration, and the heart beat. These effects would have to be eliminated from $A^{(i)}(\omega_k)$ first. More difficult, there are often bad data points (e.g., caused by sudden motion) in both the BOLD-signal and the EEG-derived reference functions, in particular in the continuous case. These bad points render the assumption of equidistant sampling invalid. Finally, the DFT approach does not address the localization question: at which points is the BOLD signal explained by the response to the EEG derived reference function?

Most of the above mentioned problems are avoided when the correlation problem is formulated in the time domain as a general linear regression model (GLM). On the other hand, in the time domain additional assumptions need to be made concerning the onset and duration of the response function. With the standard HRF used in fMRI, the onset of the response is at $t = 0$. When a response function is extracted from the data one has the option to let the response start, before the EEG is observed, thus giving rise to a noncausal response. Here, onset time and duration are indicated with fixed parameters, which have to be set prior to data analysis. When slice indices (i) are omitted and continuous functions are sampled at T_V, $\alpha^{(i)}(t_j)$ can be simplified to α_j and the BOLD signal at time t_j can be modeled as

$$\text{BOLD}_j = \sum_{m=M_{Start}}^{M_{End}-1} h_m\alpha_{j-m} + \sum_{n=N_{Start}}^{N_{End}-1} b_n\beta_{j-n} + \sum_{k=0}^{K-1} c_k\gamma_{j,k} + \eta_j \qquad (8)$$

Here, the alpha band response starts at $t = M_{start}T_V$ (which may be negative) and ends at $t = (M_{end} - 1)T_V$ and similarly for the heartbeat response b_n. There are K regressors $\gamma_{j,k}$ added to the model that describe trends, motion (Friston et al., 1996), and effects related to the phase of the heartbeat (Glover et al., 2000). Finally, η_j is a Gaussian variable, which describes measurement noise in the fMRI data. The simplest assumption with regard to noise is that noise realizations on different time samples are uncorrelated. In that case the parameters (h_m, b_n, c_k) have a maximum likelihood estimator that can be computed with ordinary least squares (OLS). It has been argued that this assumption is false (e.g. Dale, 1999; Worsley et al., 2002) mainly because of physiological artifacts (respiration, cardiac activity) that influence the BOLD on time scales that

exceed fMRI sample time T_V and resulting in correlated noise. When both the noise correlation and the parameters are estimated from the data, the regression problem becomes much more involved and can only be solved approximately. Moreover, the more physiological effects are incorporated into the model as regressors, the less their effect on the noise and the less one has to worry about noise autocorrelation. Here, uncorrelated noise will be assumed, and parameters are estimated with OLS.

Although the number of time samples equals J, which amounts typically to a couple of hundreds, they cannot all be used in the parameter estimation procedure. One reason is that, depending on the choices made for M_{start}, N_{start}, M_{end}, and N_{end}, the indices of α and β of Equation 8 run out of their domain. For instance, when $M_{start} = -10$, there is not a complete model for the last 10 data points, and similarly, when $M_{end} = 20$, the first 19 data points must be skipped (the index of α exceed the range $0, \ldots, J-1$). A similar window of skipped data points must be accounted for when the reference function α_j contains isolated bad points (e.g., due to head motion). Isolated bad points in the BOLD signal have a much smaller impact on the data analysis because in those cases one can simply leave out the bad fMRI point while keeping its neighbors. Bad points, particularly in the EEG-reference function, occur very often, and therefore the equidistant assumption needed for frequency domain computations is generally violated.

As mentioned above, the parameters (h_m, b_n, c_k) are estimated using OLS, but that in itself does not address the question, e.g., as to which parts of the brain contribute to the alpha rhythm. One way to do this is to determine, for all brain voxels, whether the model that includes the α_j regressors in addition to β_j and γ_{kj} is a significant extension of the model consisting of the β_j and γ_{kj} regressors alone. If so, the BOLD signal in such a voxel correlates in a significant way to the EEG reference function and if not, the contribution of that voxel to the reference function is not known. Therefore, one has to decide whether the combined effect of $(h_{MStart}, \ldots, h_{MEnd-1})$ deviates from zero, thereby disregarding the results of the other parameters.

This goal fits precisely in the framework of the general linear regression model. When the fMRI data is represented by the N-dimensional column vector $\mathbf{d}$, and the regressors of Equation 8 are represented as

$$\mathbf{A} = \begin{pmatrix} \ldots \alpha_{-1} & \alpha_0 & \alpha_1 & \ldots \\ & \alpha_0 & \alpha_1 & \alpha_2 \\ \ldots \alpha_1 & \alpha_2 & \alpha_3 & \ldots \\ & \alpha_2 & \vdots & \vdots \end{pmatrix} \quad \text{and} \qquad (9)$$

$$\mathbf{S} = \begin{pmatrix} \ldots \beta_{-1} & \beta_0 & \beta_1 & \beta_2 & & \gamma_{00} & \gamma_{01} & \ldots \\ & \beta_0 & \beta_1 & \beta_2 & \beta_3 & & \gamma_{10} & \gamma_{11} \\ \ldots & \beta_1 & \beta_2 & \beta_3 & & \ldots & \gamma_{20} & \gamma_{21} & \ldots \\ & \beta_2 & \beta_3 & \ddots & \vdots & & \gamma_{30} & \gamma_{31} \end{pmatrix}$$

Equation 8 can be expressed more concisely as

$$\mathbf{d} = \mathbf{A}\theta + \mathbf{S}\varphi + \eta \qquad (10)$$

where θ is the vector of parameters of interest and φ is the vector of nuisance parameters. In Equation 9 the shifted HBI regressors and the standard regressors of noninterest are combined in $\mathbf{S}$. It appears that testing whether $\mathbf{A}\theta$ is a significant extension of the model consisting of $\mathbf{S}\varphi$ alone is equivalent to filtering the nuisance regressors from both the data and the model, and testing the significance of θ in the reduced model. Filtering the nuisance regressors must be done with the projection matrix $\mathbf{P_S}$, computed from

$$\mathbf{P_S} \equiv \mathbf{I} - \mathbf{S}\left(\mathbf{S}^T\mathbf{S}\right)^{inv}\mathbf{S}^T \qquad (11)$$

and the reduced data and model are $\mathbf{d'} = \mathbf{P_S}\mathbf{d}$ and $\mathbf{A'} = \mathbf{P_S}\mathbf{A}$, respectively. The projection operator has the properties that $\mathbf{P_S} = \left(\mathbf{P_S}\right)^T = \left(\mathbf{P_S}\right)^2$ and therefore the OLS estimator $\hat{\theta}$ of the parameters θ can, in the reduced mode, be expressed as

$$\hat{\theta} = \left(\mathbf{A'}^T\mathbf{A'}\right)^{inv}\mathbf{A'}^T\mathbf{d'} = \left(\mathbf{A}^T\mathbf{P_S}\mathbf{A}\right)^{inv}\mathbf{A}^T\mathbf{P_S}\mathbf{d} \qquad (12)$$

This is also the OLS estimator of Equation 10. Furthermore, the estimated covariance matrix of the estimated parameters is given by

$$\hat{C}_{\hat{\theta}} = \hat{\sigma}^2 \left(\mathbf{A}^T\mathbf{P_S}\mathbf{A}\right)^{inv} \qquad (13)$$

where $\hat{\sigma}^2$ is the estimated noise level. The diagonal elements of this matrix give the estimated variances of each of the estimated parameters. Note that, apart from the factor the $\hat{\sigma}^2$ the covariance matrix in Equation 13 is independent of the data and therefore the normalized parameter covariance matrix is identical for all voxels. Small off-diagonal elements indicate that the estimated parameters are mutually independent. This is not the case when the regressors of the GLM are (almost) linearly dependent, or when too long an impulse response window was taken.

The data predicted by $\hat{\theta}$ in the reduced model equals $\mathbf{P_S}\mathbf{A}\hat{\theta}$ and a measure of the quality of fit is provided by ρ^2, which is the correlation between predicted data and reduced data $\mathbf{P_S}\mathbf{d}$:

$$\rho^2 = \frac{\mathbf{d}^T\mathbf{P_S}\mathbf{A}\hat{\theta}}{\left(\mathbf{d}^T\mathbf{P_S}\mathbf{d}\right)\left(\hat{\theta}^T\mathbf{A}^T\mathbf{P_S}\mathbf{A}\hat{\theta}\right)} \qquad (14)$$

The significance of ρ^2 can be tested with an F-test using p and q degrees of freedom, where p is the number of components of $\hat{\theta}$ ($q = M_{end} - M_{start}$) and q is the number of good data points N minus the total number of parameters ($q = N - (M_{end} - M_{start} + N_{end} - N_{start} + K)$).

The F-test applied as described above tests whether the alpha band response is, in statistical sense, a necessary extension of the model consisting of heartbeat regressors and other nuisance effects. Since heart rate and alpha power are strongly correlated (e.g., Ehrhart et al., 2000; De Munck et al., 2008), the inclusion of heart rate nuisance parameters

avoids the detection of alpha-BOLD correlations that are an indirect effect of heart rate variations.

The idea of projecting away nuisance effects in order to obtain a better focus on parameters of interest can also be exploited when studying the generators of different EEG frequency bands using EEG/fMRI data. For instance, when a subject is instructed to stay in a resting state for half an hour, it is very likely that amplitude variations of different frequency bands are mutually correlated. One example is the beta band when it is chosen such that it includes the second harmonic of the alpha band. Another example is the delta band, which may be negatively correlated to the alpha band when the subject is falling asleep during the recordings. Therefore, when a single frequency band of interest is selected, one should preferably exclude the contribution of other rhythms by adding them to the model as regressors of noninterest.

Another use of nuisance effects is the study of anti-causal EEG/fMRI correlations. If one is interested in the contribution of future alpha band variations to present BOLD signals, one should account for the possible contribution of past alpha bands. This problem perfectly fits the GLM formulation presented in Equation 10. By using Equation 8 as model description of the BOLD signal, and using positive shifts of the EEG reference function as nuisance parameters and negative shifts as parameters of interest, the rejection of the NULL-hypothesis using the F-test can be interpreted as the statistical necessity of including negative time shifts into the model. When statistical significant anti-causal correlation is found this indicates that "something" is going on before it becomes apparent in the alpha band. This effect may or may not be visible in the EEG, but when it is, it does not contribute to the alpha band.

Application

The theory described in the previous section is illustrated with the EEG/fMRI data of a single subject (subject 5) of our study presented in De Munck et al. (2007a; 2008). This subject was chosen because it showed strong fluctuations in the alpha band and other EEG frequency bands, and relatively strong fluctuations in heart rate, and because fMRI/alpha band correlations were highly significant. It should be stressed that results shown in this chapter nicely illustrate the interest of HRF modeling, but the authors do not claim that all results are representative for the whole population.

As detailed in De Munck et al. (2007a), coregistered EEG-fMRI data were acquired from 16 subjects at rest with eyes closed without falling asleep, in a room that was kept in the dark. Functional images were acquired on a 1.5 T MR scanner (Magnetom Sonata, Siemens, Erlangen, Germany) using a circularly polarized head coil. For the fMRI a T2* weighted EPI sequence was used (TR = 3.000 s, echo time TE = 60 ms, 64 × 64 matrix, FOV = 211 × 211 mm, slice thickness = 3 mm (10% gap), voxel size = 3.3 × 3.3 × 3 mm^3) with 24 transversal slices covering the complete occipital, parietal, and frontal lobes. Slices were recorded from bottom to top, with a constant time-interval of 125 ms. In the protocol, 600 volumes were acquired, resulting in 1800 s of EPI recording.

A T1-weighted anatomical scan was made, consisting of 160 coronal slices of 1.5 mm thickness. fMRI data were matched onto the anatomical scan (Maes et al., 1997), motion corrected, and spatially smoothed with Gaussian kernel with standard deviation of 5 mm. Motion parameters were saved and used as regressors of noninterest in the correlation analysis (Friston et al., 1996).

Simultaneous to the fMRI recording, EEG data were acquired with an MR compatible EEG amplifier (SD MRI 64, MicroMed, Treviso, Italy) and a cap providing 64 Ag/AgCl electrodes positioned according to an extended 10/20 system. Also ECG, pulse oxygenation and respiration were recorded. EEG data were re-referenced to average reference. Gradient and cardioballistic artifacts were removed using the algorithm of Gonçalves et al. (2007).

To study EEG/fMRI correlations occipital channels were selected. Contrary to De Munck et al. (2007a; De Munck et al., 2008) slice specific spectrogram regressors were made. For that purpose a 3 s time window was shifted over the data with steps of 0.125 s, corresponding to the slice acquisition onset times. On each time window the power spectrum was computed using the FFT algorithm of Frigo and Johnson (2005). The EEG powers were averaged over different frequencies (Table 3.6.1) according to the delta, theta, alpha, beta, and gamma band and for each slice different power variations were used as regressor, dependent on slice acquisition onset time. Frequency band regressors were normalized after removing outliers.

The delta and theta bands are more or less standard, but the alpha band was adjusted according to subject's alpha peak frequency. Furthermore, the beta and gamma bands were somewhat narrowed in order to avoid overlap with the second and third harmonic of the alpha peak. It should be noted however, that the fourth harmonic of the alpha band is within our definition of gamma band. As described in detail in De Munck et al. (2008), slice time dependent regressors were also derived from the heartbeat intervals. Figure 3.6.2 presents the regressors so obtained for the first slice. One

observes that, despite the lack of overlap of the alpha and beta bands, there is a correlation between them. Also the alpha and gamma bands are correlated.

In Figures 3.6.3 and 3.6.4 the robustness of the alpha band correlation is explored by computing fMRI-alpha band correlations and HRF estimations in different ways. The "standard" way in this chapter is to use slice dependent regressors, and to take an offset, trend, parabola, six motion parameters, 6 RETROICOR regressors, and shifted heartbeat intervals as confounders (equation 8, with $M_{start} = N_{start} = -2$ and $M_{end} = N_{end} = 8$). Correlation results are shown in Figure 3.6.3, where ρ^2 (Equation 14) is truncated and overlaid over the anatomical scan. The truncation in Figure 3.6.3 is done such that the false detection rate of all tested correlations is smaller than 7×10^{-9}, or $\rho_{min}^2 = 0.32$. Truncation of statistical maps on the basis of an estimated false detection rate is invented by Benjamini and Hochberg (1995) and first applied to fMRI by Genovese et al. (2002).

When the HBI regressors are omitted from the model, it appears that the correlations get larger (Figure 3.6.3B) and it also appears that in general slightly larger brain areas exceed the 1% FDR threshold (De Munck et al., 2007b; De Munck et al., 2008). This is due to the fact that alpha power and HBI generally have a strong correlation. For that reason we always include HBI regressors in the results presented in this chapter.

When regressors are derived from EEG frequency bands one faces the choice of using the power or the RMS value. To find out whether this makes any difference the computations of Figure 3.6.3A were repeated using either the logarithm or the RMS instead of power. Although there is no obvious physiological reason to take the logarithm, we consider it as a worst case model. Figure 3.6.3C shows the results of using logarithms of alpha power. It appears that the correlation pattern is virtually identical to Figure 3.6.3A at the FDR level used. The correlations themselves are generally somewhat higher. The use of RMS hardly made a difference (results not shown).

In Figure 3.6.4, four samples of estimated HRFs are shown, derived from a left and right parietal point (corresponding to subject's hand area of the primary sensory cortex), an occipital point, and the thalamus (De Munck et al., 2007a). These samples are computed using different methods. Similar to Figure 3.6.3, they show the effect of omitting HBI regressors and taking logarithms. We also compared the use of either slice time corrected regressors "intrinsic" to the use of identical regressors for all slices and applying a slice time correction afterward on the estimated HRF. It appears from Figures 3.6.3 and 3.6.4 that both the determination of correlation patterns and the HRF estimation are quite robust, and not very sensitive to the precise implementation of the model. Largest effects are due to ignoring of HBI-regressors.

Robustness of the model appears furthermore from the normalized parameter covariance matrix (Equation 13), which is presented in Figure 3.6.5. It appears that despite

Table 3.6.1.
EEG frequency bands used in the presented study.

Band name	Frequency range [Hz]
Delta	1–4
Theta	4–8
Alpha	9–11
Beta	12–17
Gamma	35–49

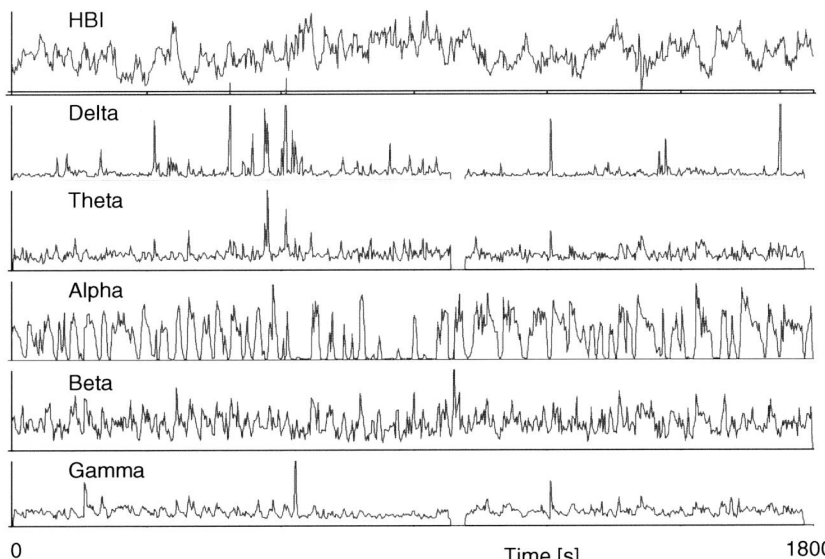

Figure 3.6.2. The upper graph shows the heartbeat interval variations during 1800 s recording time. The other graphs show the auto-scaled delta band, theta band, alpha band, beta band, and gamma band variations. Extreme outliers in the second half of the recordings in the delta, theta, and gamma band are set to zero, including a range corresponding to the size of the HRF window.

the fact that shifts applied to the alpha band profile are small with respect to the intrinsic time scale of this profile (see Figure 3.6.2), the estimated parameters are very independent. In our software (http://demunck.info/software/) this parameter covariance matrix is always computed and therefore we can report that Figure 3.6.5 is a very typical result.

A drawback of graphs like Figure 3.6.4 is that they only present the HRF of four selected points of interest, whereas in practice these curves can be derived from all points of the brain where the HRF is statistically significant. In case of the subject presented here, this would imply that 10 thousands of HRF curves would have to be visualized. To make such visualization possible, we proposed in De Munck et al. (2007a) to apply a clustering analysis (Ward, 1963) on the 10 thousand most significant points and to present the cluster averages only instead of the individual curves. It appeared that differences in HRF shapes were characterized by differences in peak time delay. For that reason, hemodynamic responses were interpolated using a modulated sine model,

$$h(t) = \begin{cases} 0 & t \leq 0 \\ At^2 e^{-\alpha t^2} \sin(\omega t - \varphi) & 0 < t \end{cases} \quad (15)$$

and this parameterization was used to determine peak time of the HRF of each cluster. When subsequently HRFs are color coded according to peak time one obtains a representation as depicted in Figure 3.6.6.

Figure 3.6.6 demonstrates that there are, at least for this subject, systematic differences in HRF peak times. The thalamus peaks first, then the parietal cortex, and finally the occipital cortex. Also within each of these parts of cortex there are systematic time delays. In De Munck et al. (2007a) two principal explanations for these effects are discussed. One explanation could be that there are systematic differences in cortical vasculature as described by Harrison et al.

(2002) in the cerebral cortex of chinchillas. Another explanation could be that in the regression Equation 8 it is implicitly assumed that the input of the impulse response time filter is equal for all points of the brain and also that the input equals the occipital alpha power. Regional differences in the alpha power modulations are ignored and therefore all such differences will result in regional differences of the estimated HRF. Therefore, an alternative explanation for the results in Figure 3.6.6 would be provided by assuming that differences in HRF are small and that Figure 3.6.6 presents a spreading pattern of alpha activity.

To obtain more insight into this matter we explored the other EEG frequency bands and correlated these EEG power variations to the BOLD. If Figure 3.6.6 would represent true systematic differences in HRF, then, the same HRF shapes would be expected when for the other frequency bands, at least at those points of the brain where the input is the same as the alpha band. Furthermore, we investigate more systematically where the noncausal parts of the HRF curves are located. True HRF curves can only be significant in the causal domain because blood volume and oxygenation simply must follow electrical activation. Significant anticausal correlation therefore points to local input that has been ignored in the modeling Equation 8.

Slice dependent band power regressors of interest were used and HBI regressors were added to the standard regressors of no interest. Figure 3.6.7 shows the results, where a common FDR threshold of 1% was applied. One observes that all correlation patterns include the occipital and parietal lobe, except the theta band. The theta band seems to correlate merely at the brain-skull interface and is therefore mostly artifactual. The alpha and beta bands show additional correlation at other parts of the brain. However, when the FDR threshold is decreased (as in Figure 3.6.2A) these extra correlations disappear. It should be noted that the beta band does not include alpha band harmonic and therefore its

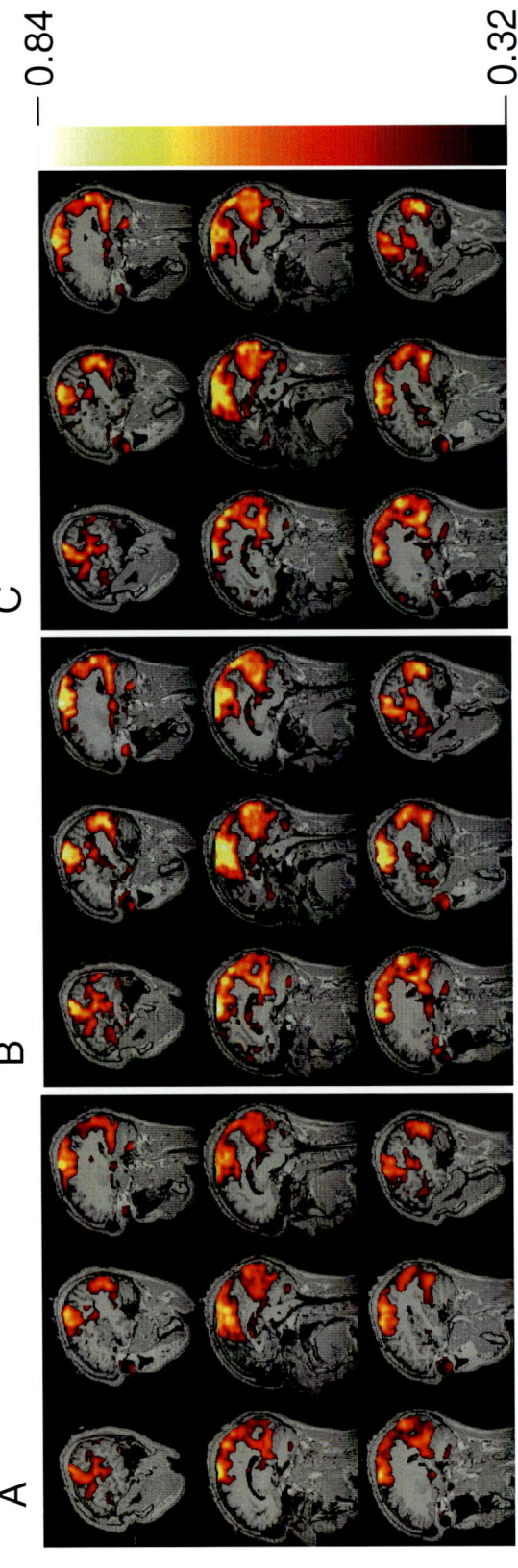

Figure 3.6.3. Three variants of fMRI-alpha band correlation (Equation 14) maps are shown. In all cases slice-specific alpha regressors were shifted from 2 (−6 s) to 7 (21 s), and in all cases motion parameters and RETROICOR regressors were used as confounders. In panel A these were used as confounders, in panel B these were omitted, and in panel C the same regressors were used as in A, except that the logarithm of the alpha power was taken rather than the alpha power itself. In all cases the maps were scaled between .32 and .84. The lower bound corresponded in three cases to a false detection rate of less than 7×10^{-9}.

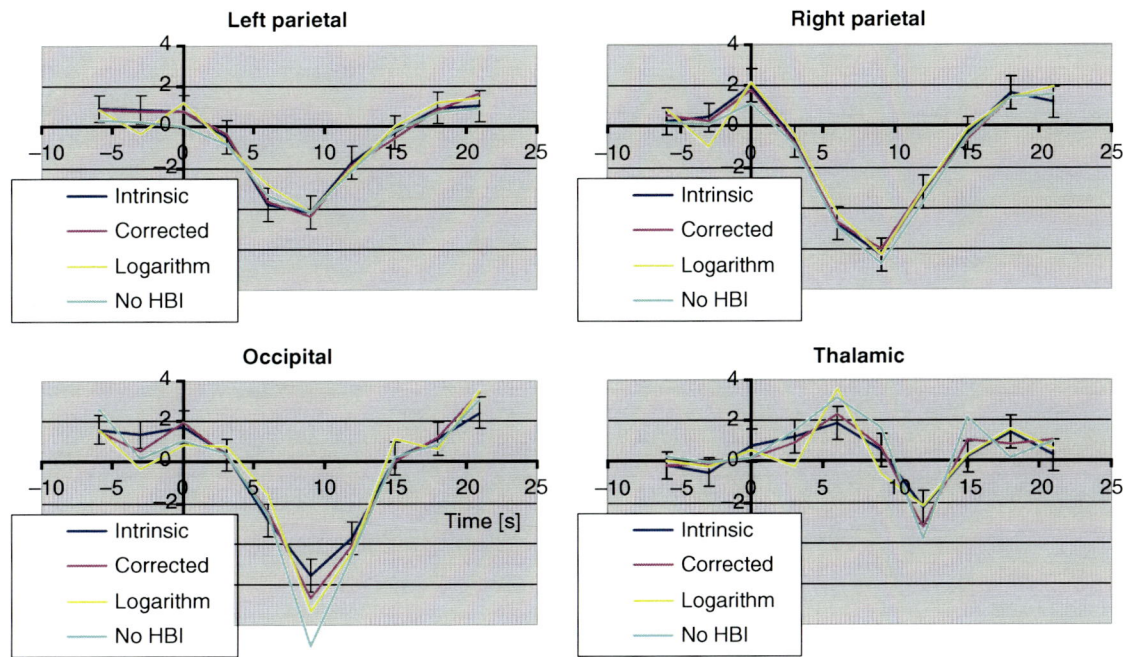

Figure 3.6.4. Four samples of estimated HRFs of the alpha power are shown (left and right parietal, occipital, and thalamic) that are estimated in four different ways each. The functions labeled "Intrinsic" use slice-dependent regressors and correspond to Figure 3.6.3A. The functions labeled "corrected" were computed using the same regressors for all slices and using an FFT-based shift correction afterward. Furthermore "No HBI" indicates that heartbeat interval regressors were omitted (as in Figure 3.6.3B), and finally "Logarithm" means that the logarithm of the alpha power was fitted (as in Figure 3.6.3C).

similarity to the alpha band correlation patterns does not have a straightforward explanation.

Although the correlation patterns are quite similar for different frequency bands, their corresponding HRFs appear to be quite different. In Figure 3.6.8 the (normalized) HRFs are presented, sampled, and averaged from four regions of interest, 1 cm diameter spheres located at the

left and right parietal cortex, the occipital lobe, and thalamus. The graphs are only shown when the HRF survives the 1% FDR threshold. For the theta band this only happens for the left parietal point.

It appears that the delta band has an HRF which is, except for the occipital point, opposite to those of the other bands. Whereas the alpha, beta, and gamma bands

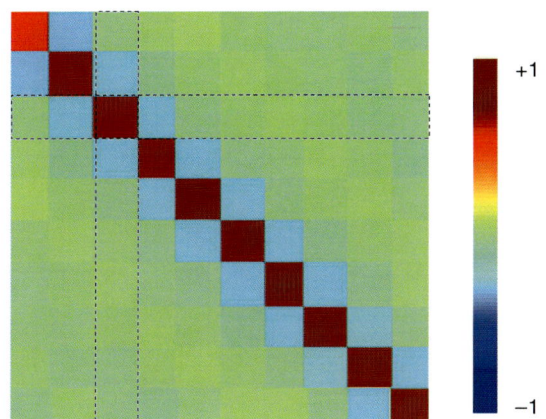

Figure 3.6.5. The auto-scaled parameter covariance matrix (Equation 13) of the analysis of Figure 3.6.3A is shown. The elements within the dashed lines give to zero-shifted parameters correlated to each of the other parameters. It appears this covariance matrix is diagonal dominant and quite stationary.

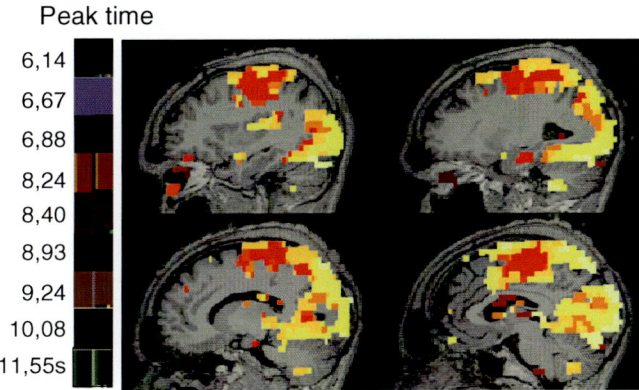

Figure 3.6.6 Cluster analysis of EEG alpha band HRF estimates. The most significant estimates (FDR$<10^{-10}$) of the HRF of the alpha band were subject to a hierarchical clustering analysis. The HRF curves were grouped in 8 clusters and cluster averages were sorted according to HRF peak time. Clusters are colour coded according to peak time (see scale at the left).

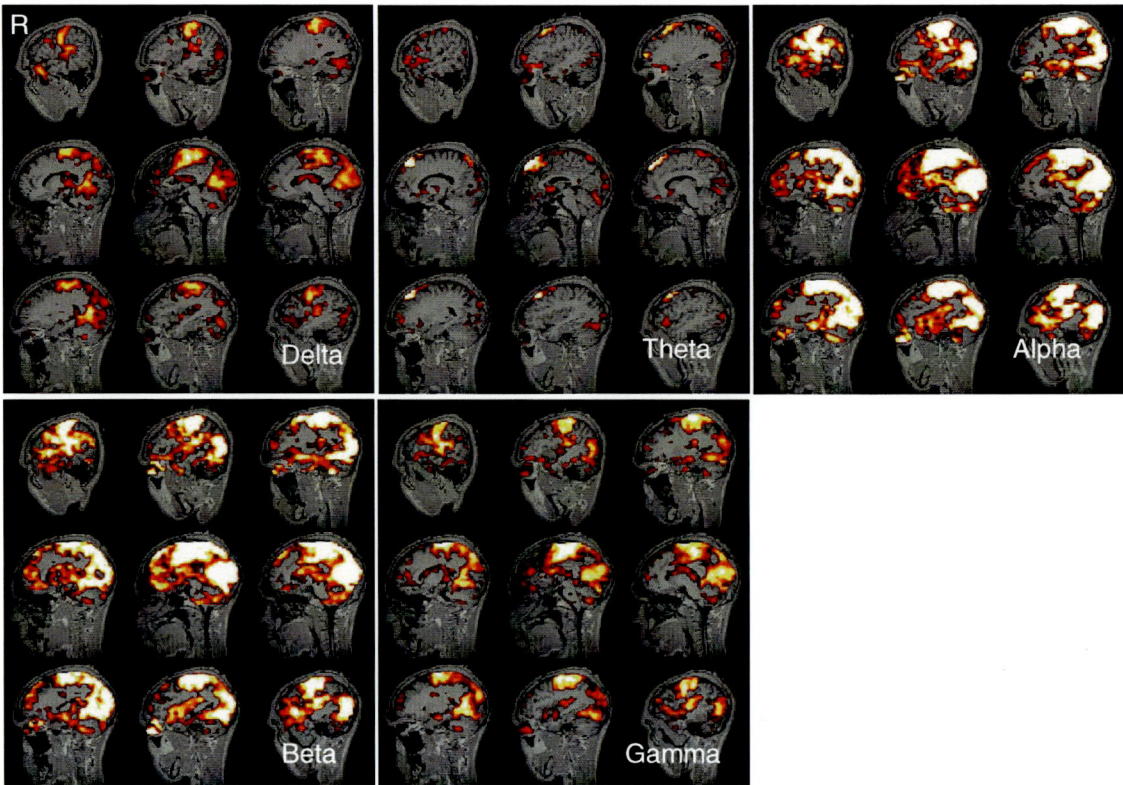

Figure 3.6.7. Correlation patterns are shown for five different analyses, where five different EEG frequency bands were used as effects of interest and the same confounders. Correlation patterns are thresholded at a false detection rate of 1%.

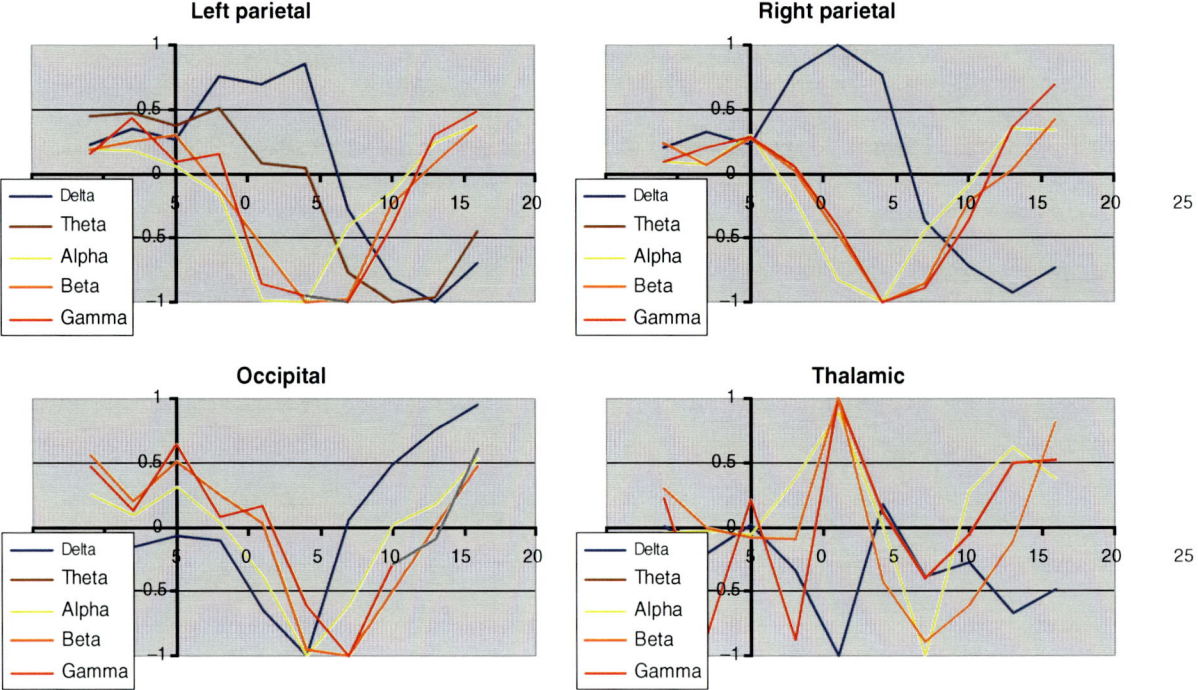

Figure 3.6.8. The estimated HRFs are presented for different correlation analysis with different shifted EEG frequency band regressors. From the four points of interest all HRFs were averaged within a distance of 5 mm from the points. Only when the significance at the selected point exceeds the 1% threshold the HRF graph is shown. For the theta band this is only the case for the left parietal point, but one also observes that the HRF shape shows an unexpected delay.

show cortical deactivation and activation at the thalamus, delta seems to activate at the parietal cortex and to deactivate at the thalamus. Furthermore, there appear to be systematic time delays in the HRFs. At the cortical points of interest, the delta band peaks first, then alpha, beta, and gamma respectively.

Anti-causal correlation was explored by using only the null and negative shifts as regressor of interest and the positive shifts as confounder (in addition to HBI and standard confounders). Only with the alpha, beta, and gamma band anti-causal correlation was found. Results are shown in Figure 3.6.9 in the form of a surface rendering of the anatomical scan, onto which the significant correlations (FDR = 1%) have been projected. Anti-causal correlation is mainly concentrated on the somatosensory cortex although for the beta band in particular there are also other cortical regions involved.

A serious concern regarding the analysis presented so far is that each frequency band is included in the model separately. Since regressors of different frequency bands are mutually correlated (see Figure 3.6.2) HRF estimates from one frequency band is contaminated with the HRF on other bands. To restrict the number of estimated parameters, we therefore performed two additional analyses, one in which the alpha was correlated to BOLD with respect to delta and another where alpha was correlated to BOLD with respect to beta and gamma. Results of alpha-delta analysis were quite similar to the analysis with alpha alone. This is illustrated in Figure 3.6.10 where the estimated HRF curves extracted from the four points of interest are plotted. Apart from a small amplitude effect at the parietal points, curves with or without delta band confounders are very similar. Also, the anti-causal correlation of the alpha band was essentially not affected. However, when using the beta and gamma regressors as confounders, the anti-causal alpha-BOLD correlation disappeared, and also the HRF estimates at the points of interest are affected (see Figure 3.6.10). In particular, the HRF curve of the occipital point is shifted to the left.

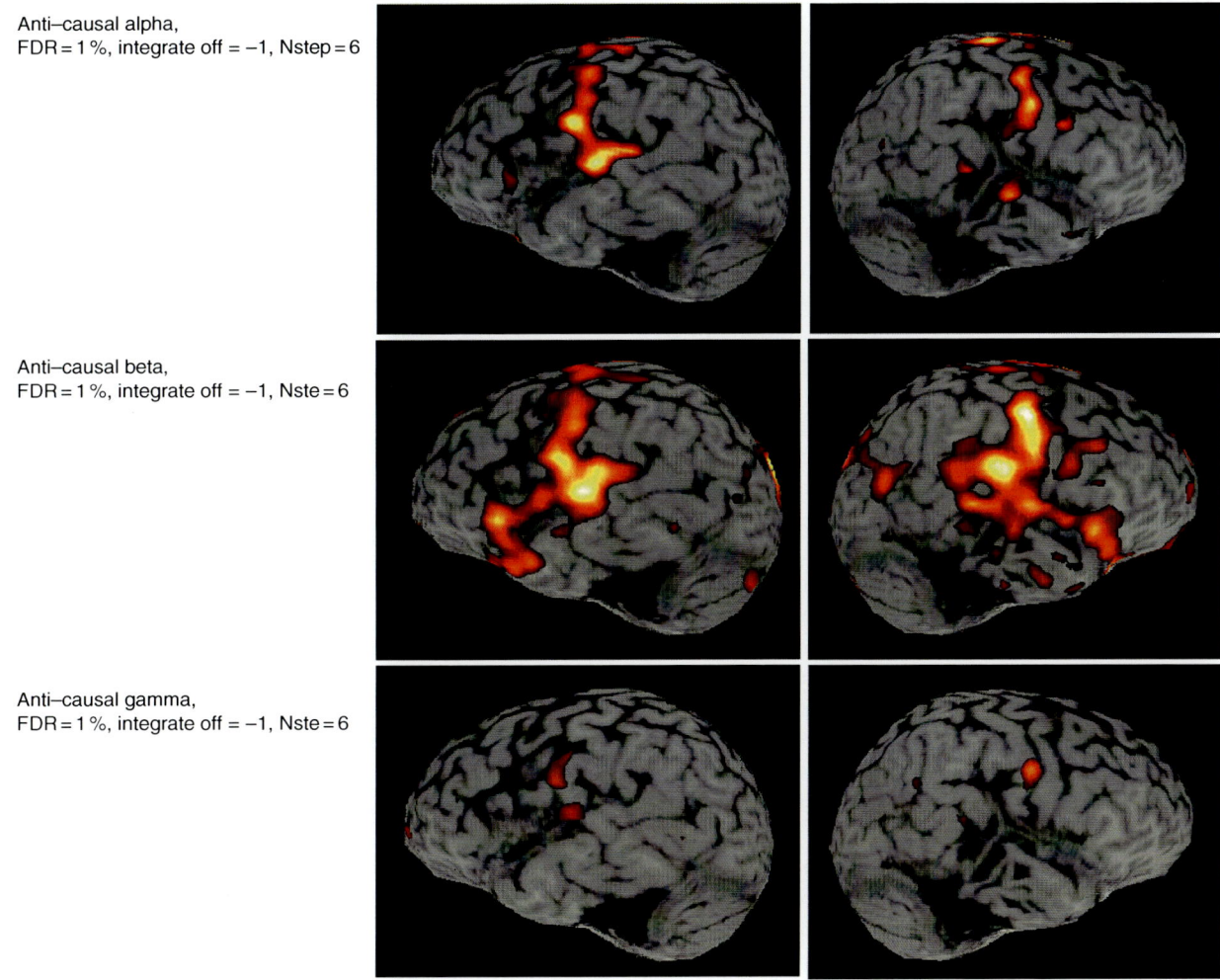

Anti–causal alpha,
FDR = 1 %, integrate off = −1, Nstep = 6

Anti–causal beta,
FDR = 1 %, integrate off = −1, Nste = 6

Anti–causal gamma,
FDR = 1 %, integrate off = −1, Nste = 6

Figure 3.6.9. Regions showing anti-causal correlations when using the alpha, beta, or gamma band regressors. For the delta and theta bands no such anti-causal correlation was found. Correlation patterns are thresholded at a false detection rate of 1%.

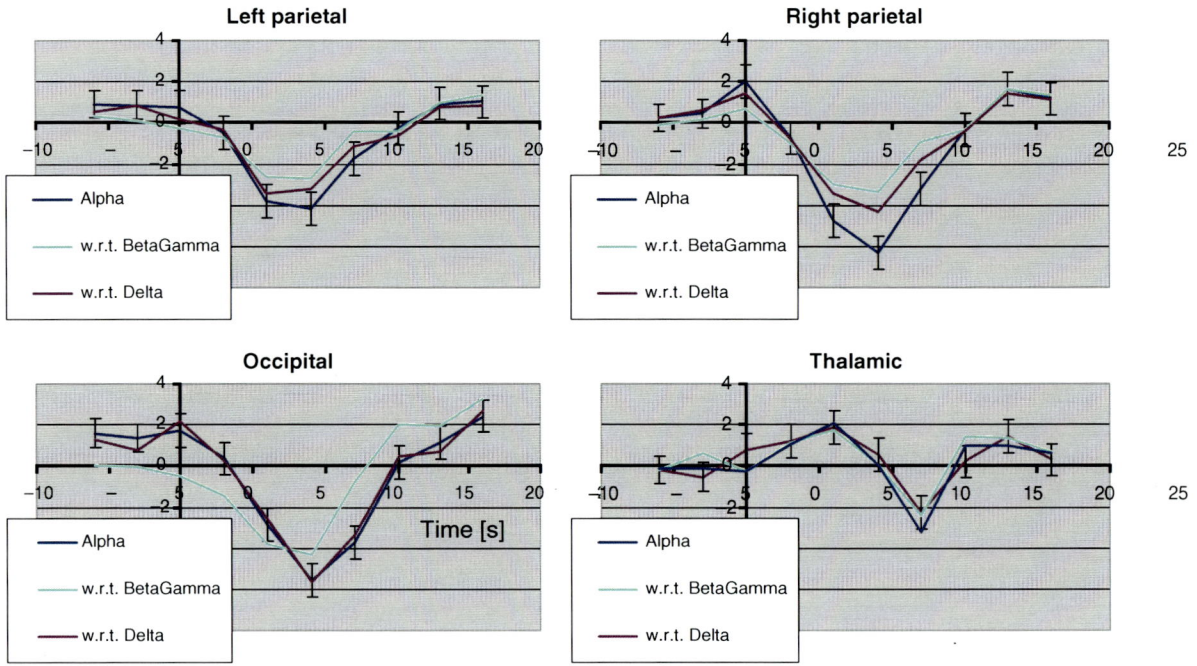

Figure 3.6.10. HRF estimates are shown for an extension of Equation 8, where either shifted delta band confounders were used, or both shifted beta and shifted gamma band confounders. One observes that inclusion of delta band confounders hardly influences results, but beta and gamma band do have an effect.

Discussion

From a study of Aguirre et al. (1998) and Handwerker et al. (2004), it is known that systematic differences in hemodynamic responses to an external stimulus exist in the human brain. However, the variations in estimated HRF found in our EEG/fMRI study of the brain's resting state cannot completely be explained by local differences in geometrical and mechanical properties of the vascular bed. In particular the finding of significant anti-causal alpha band correlation, in combination with its dependence on the inclusion of the beta and gamma band regressors, shows that the hemodynamic responses contain information about the coupling of the underlying electrical sources. For the case study presented in this chapter, this finding could imply that the occipital alpha was preceded by occipital gamma activity.

However, the latter conclusion is very preliminary because the regression model used is still far too simple. First of all, only averaged occipital leads are included. As a consequence, the spatial distribution of the EEG data over the scalp is not exploited. This problem is not easily solved (at least not from a solid theoretical model driven perspective), because for any included electrode (group), the number of free parameters increases at least with $M_{end} - M_{start}$. If multiple frequency bands are included for each electrode, then the number of parameters would increase another factor.

A second limitation of the model is that Equation 8 describes the BOLD signal as a linearly filtered version of

alpha variations. Although this approach is plausible as a first step, the physiological meaning of linearity of the filter is dependent on how the alpha variations are quantified: power or RMS values. If the filter is linear for one choice, it is non-linear in the other. Another reason to consider non-linear models is that it is not guaranteed that with linear models the heart rate and respiration effects and frequency band interaction are sufficiently removed.

A general way to include non-linear correlations in the model would be to use RMS regressors that are raised to some powers p and incorporate an unknown multiplication factor for each power. Ignoring the shifted HBI-regressors, the non-linear model would look like this:

$$\text{BOLD}_j = \sum_{p=1}^{P} \sum_{m=M_{Start}}^{M_{End}-1} h_{m,p}\left(\alpha_{j-m}\right)^p + \sum_{k=0}^{K-1} c_k \gamma_{j,k} + \eta_j \quad (16)$$

The advantage of Equation 16 is that it remains a linear regression model, where the $h_{m,p}$ are the parameters of interest. However, when all combinations of powers and time shifts are allowed, the number of parameters increases as $P \times (M_{end} - M_{start} - 1)$. To reduce the number of parameters, it might therefore be necessary to adopt a non-linear parameterization and to take the extra computational burden for granted.

A third concern with regression models like Equation 8 is that they are implicitly based on the assumption that the model

$$\sum_{m=M_{Start}}^{M_{End}-1} h_m \alpha_{j-m} + \sum_{n=N_{Start}}^{N_{End}-1} b_n \beta_{j-n} + \sum_{k=0}^{K-1} c_k \gamma_{j,k}$$

is correct, and that there are only statistical errors in the BOLD-signal. However, the EEG-band regressors result from a frequency smoothed estimate of the true EEG power spectrum and therefore also the model is contaminated with noise. Therefore a parameter estimation method that treats both kinds of noises in a balanced way (like total least squares, Golub and van Loan, 1989) needs to be developed.

REFERENCES

Aguirre GK, Zarahn E, D'Esposito M (1998) The variability of human BOLD hemodynamic responses. NeuroImage 8:360–369.

Benjamini Y, Hochberg Y (1995) Controlling the false discovery rate: a practical and powerful approach to multiple testing. J R Statist Soc B 57:289–300.

Boynton GM, Engel SA, Glover GH, Heeger DJ (1996) Linear systems analysis of functional Magnetic Resonance Imaging in Human V1. J Neurosci 16:4207–4221.

Dale AM (1999) Optimal experimental design for event related fMRI. Hum Brain Map 8:109–114.

Damoiseaux JS, Rombouts SARB, Barkhof F, Scheltens P, Stam CJ, Smith SM, Beckmann CF (2006) Consistent resting-state networks across healthy subjects. PNAS 103:13848–13853.

Debener S, Makeig S, Delorme A, Engel AK (2005) What is novel in the novelty oddball paradigm? Functional significance of the novelty P3 event-related potential as revealed by independent component analysis. Brain Res Cogn Brain Res 22:309–321.

De Munck JC, De Jongh A, Van Dijk BW (2001) The localization of spontaneous brain activity: An efficient way to analyze large data sets. IEEE Trans Biomed Eng, BME-48:1221–1228.

De Munck JC, Gonçalves SI, Huijboom L, Kuijer JPA, Pouwels PWJ, Heethaar RM, Lopes da Silva FH (2007a) The hemodynamic response of the alpha rhythm: an EEG/fMRI study. NeuroImage 35:1142–1151.

De Munck JC, Gonçalves SI, Faes Th JC, Pouwels PJW, Kuijer JPA, Heethaar RM, Lopes da Silva FH (2007b) The relation between alpha band power, heart rate and fMRI. Proceedings of fourth IEEE International Symposium on Biomedical Imaging. Arlington, Virginia.

De Munck JC, Gonçalves SI, Faes Th JC, Kuijer JPA, Pouwels PJW, Heethaar RM, Lopes da Silva FH (2008) A study of the brain's resting state based on alpha band power, heart rate and fMRI. NeuroImage 42:112–121.

Ehrhart J, Toussaint M, Simon C, Gronfier C, Luthringer R, Brandenberger G (2000) Alpha activity and cardiac correlates: three types of relationships during nocturnal sleep. Clin Neurophysiol 111:940–946.

Eichele T, Specht K, Moosmann M, Jongsma ML, Quiroga RQ, Nordby H, Hugdahl K (2005) Assessing the spatiotemporal evolution of neuronal activation with single-trial event-related potentials and functional MRI. Proc Natl Acad Sci U S A 102:17798–17803.

Fox MD, Raichle ME (2007) Spontaneous fluctuations in brain activity observed with functional magnetic resonance imaging. Nat Rev Neurosci 8:700–711.

Frigo M, Johnson, SG (2005) The design and implementation of FFTW. In: P IEEE 93:216–231.

Friston KJ, Williams S, Howard R, Frackowiak RS, Turner R (1996) Movement-related effects in fMRI time-series. Magn Reson Med 35:346–355.

Genovese CR, Lazar NA, Nichols T (2002) Thresholding of statistical maps in functional neuroimaging using the false discovery rate. NeuroImage 15:870–878.

Glover GH (1999) Deconvolution of impulse response in event related BOLD fMRI. NeuroImage 9:416–429.

Glover GH, Li TQ, Ress D (2000) Image-based method for retrospective correction of physiological motion effects in fMRI: RETROICOR, Magnetic Resonance in Medicine 44:162–167.

Goldman RI, Stern JM, Engel J, Jr., Cohen M (2002) Simultaneous EEG and fMRI of the alpha rhythm. NeuroReport 13:2487–2492.

Golub GH, Van Loan CF (1989) Matrix computations, 2nd Edition. Baltimore, MD: Johns Hopkins University Press.

Gonçalves SI, de Munck JC, Pouwels PJW, Schoonhoven R, Kuijer JPA, Maurits NM, Hoogduin JM, Van Someren EJW, Heethaar RM, Lopes da Silva FH (2006) Correlating the alpha rhythm to BOLD using simultaneous EEG/fMRI: inter-subject variability. NeuroImage 30:203–213.

Gonçalves SI, Pouwels PJW, Kuijer JPA, Heethaar RM, De Munck JC (2007) Automatic artifact removal in co-registered EEG/fMRI. Clin Neuro Physiol 118:2437–2450.

Gotman J, Benar C-G, Dubeau F (2004) Combining EEG and fMRI in epilepsy: methodological challenges and clinical results. J. Clin. Neuroph 21:229–240.

Greicius MD, Krasnow B, Reiss AL, Menon V (2003) Functional connectivity in the resting brain: A network analysis of the default mode hypothesis. PNAS 100:253–258.

Handwerker DA, Ollinger JM, D'Esposito M (2004) Variation of BOLD hemodynamic responses across subjects and brain regions and their effects on statistical analyses. NeuroImage 21:1639–1651.

Harrison RV, Harel N, Panesar J, Mount RJ (2002) Blood capillary distribution correlates with hemodynamic-based functional imaging in cerebral cortex. Cereb Cortex 12:225–233.

Hawco CS, Bagshaw AP, Lu Y, Dubeau F, Gotman J (2007) BOLD changes occur prior to epileptic spikes seen on scalp EEG. NeuroImage 35:1450–1458.

Hinrichs H, Scholz M, Tempelmann C, Woldorff MG, Dale AM, Heinze HJ (2000) Deconvolution of event-related fMRI responses in fast-rate experimental designs: tracking amplitude variations. J Cogn Neurosci 12 Suppl 2:76–89.

Ives JR, Warach S, Schmitt F, Edelman RR, Schomer DL (1993) Monitoring the patient's EEG during echo planar MRI. Electroenc Clin Neurophysiol 87:417–420.

Laufs H, Krakow K, Sterzer P, Eger E, Beyerle A, Salek-Haddadi A, Kleinschmidt A (2003a) Electroencephalographic signatures of attentional and cognitive default modes in spontaneous brain fluctuations at rest. PNAS 100:11053–11058.

Laufs H, Kleinschmidt A, Beyerle A, Eger E, Salek-Haddadi A, Preibisch C, Krakow K (2003b) EEG-correlated fMRI of human alpha activity. NeuroImage 19:1463–1476.

Lemieux L, Krakow K, Fish DR (2001) Comparison of spike-triggered functional MRI BOLD activation and EEG dipole model localization. NeuroImage 14:1097–1104.

Liston AD, De Munck JC, Hamandi K, Laufs H, Ossenblok P, Lemieux L (2006a) Analysis of EEG-fMRI of epileptiform discharges based on automated alassification of interictal epileptiform discharges. NeuroImage, 31:1015–1024.

Liston AD, Lund TE, Salek-Haddadi A, Hamandi K, Friston KJ, and Lemieux L (2006b) Modelling cardiac signal as a confound in EEG-fMRI and its application in focal epilepsy studies. NeuroImage 30:827–834.

Lopes da Silva FH, Van Rotterdam A (1982) Biophysical aspects of EEG and MEG generation. In: Electroencephalography basic principles. Clinical applications and related fields (Niedermeyer E, Lopes da Silva FH, eds), 4th Edition, pp 93–109. Munich, Vienna, Baltimore: Urban & Schwarzenberg.

Lu Y, Bagshaw AP, Grova C, Kobayashi E, Dubeau F, Gotman J (2006) Using voxel-specific hemodynamic response function in EEG-fMRI data analysis. NeuroImage 32:238–247.

Logothetis NK (2007) The ins and outs of fMRI signals. Nature Neuroscience 10:1230–1231.

Lund TE, Madsen KH, Sidaros K, Luo W-L, Nichols TE (2006) Non-white noise in fMRI: Does modelling have an impact? NeuroImage 29:54–66.

Maes F, Collignon A, Vandermeulen D, Marchal G, Suetens P (1997) Multimodality image registration by maximization of mutualinformation. IEEE T Med Imaging 16:187–198.

Mantini D, Perrucci MG, Del Gratta C, Romani GL, Corbetta M (2007) Electrophysiological signatures of resting state networks in the human brain. PNAS 104:13170–13175.

Moosmann M, Ritter P, Krastel I, Brink A, Thees S, Blankenburg F, Taskin B, Obrig H, Villringer A (2003) Correlates of alpha rhythm in functional magnetic resonance imaging and near infrared spectroscopy. NeuroImage 20:145–158.

Mosher JC, Leahy RM (1998) Recursive MUSIC: A framework for EEG and MEG source localization. IEEE Trans Biomed Eng 45:1342–1354.

Pascual-Marqui RD (1999) Review of methods for solving the EEG inverse problem. Int. J. Bioelectromagnetism 1999:75–86.

Sarvas J (1987) Basic mathematical and electromagnetic concepts of the basic biomagnetic inverse problem. Phys Med Biol 32:11–22.

Shmueli K, Van Gelderen P, De Zwart J, Horovitz SG, Fukanaga M, Jansma JM, Van Duyn JF (2007) Low frequency fluctuations in the cardiac rate as a source of variance in the resting state fMRI BOLD signal. NeuroImage 38:306–320.

Warach S, Ives JR, Schlaug G, Patel MR, Darby DG, Thanggaraj V, Edelman RR, Schomer DL (1996) EEG-triggered echoplanar functional MRI in epilepsy. Neurology 47:89–93.

Ward JH (1963) Hierarchical grouping to optimize an objective function. J Am Stat Assoc 58:236–244.

Worsley KJ, Liao CH, Aston J, Petre V, Duncan GH, Morales F, Evans AC (2002) A general statistical analysis for fMRI data. NeuroImage 15:1–15.

Windischberger C, Langenberger H, Sycha T, Tschernko EM, Fuchsjger-Mayerl G, Schmetterer L, Moser E (2002) On the origin of respiratory artifacts in BOLD-EPI of the human brain. Magn Reson Imaging 20:575–582.

Zijlmans M, Huiskamp G, Hersevoort M, Seppenwoolde JH, Van Huffelen AC, Leijten FSS (2007) EEG-fMRI in the preoperative work-up for epilepsy surgery. Brain 130:2343–2353.

3.7 Michael Wibral, Christoph Bledowski, and Georg Turi

Integration of Separately Recorded EEG/MEG and fMRI Data

Overview

This chapter presents various strategies of combining *separately* recorded EEG/MEG and fMRI data sets. To help the experimenter decide in the first place whether to use concurrent recordings of EEG and fMRI or separate recordings we try to weigh the relative merits of combined versus separate EEG/MEG and fMRI measurements and to put them in perspective with respect to various experimental goals. We also briefly describe the principle of MEG recording and its advantages as compared to EEG; these particular advantages of MEG recordings are important to consider because, at present, they are only available when data are recorded separately, due to the current incompatibility of MRI and MEG measurement equipment.

We then present various approaches to solve the underdetermined electromagnetic inverse problem by using constraints—possibly derived from separately recorded fMRI data—to arrive at a unique solution. We start by reviewing the basic algorithms like distributed linear inverse solutions, discrete dipole analysis, and source estimation using Bayesian inference. This should prepare the reader to see where and how exactly knowledge obtained from separately recorded fMRI is incorporated into these algorithms. We proceed from a minimal incorporation of fMRI data used to bias distributed linear inverse solutions to heavily constrained approaches where number, location, and orientation of dipolar sources are fixed by the use of fMRI data and source time courses are simply extracted. Mathematical formulations are presented where necessary. However, we try to motivate these mathematical constructs by a more intuitive informal formulation of the same subject matter as much as possible. Particularly for the description of beamformer source reconstruction we chose to thoroughly motivate this relatively novel approach by various thought experiments and examples,

rather than just presenting a compact mathematical treatment. What is equally important is that fMRI data can also be used for other purposes than constraining localization approaches. In fact, all uses of fMRI data as constraints in localization algorithms assume some interdependency of EEG and fMRI data; in most cases even a linear or at least monotonic dependency is assumed. This assumption is not necessarily justified (see Arthurs et al., 2004 for explicit intra individual variations in coupling) and needs to be put to the test. Here, the comparison of MEG source activity obtained from an fMRI-*independent* source reconstruction with BOLD-fMRI activity can yield extremely valuable information as demonstrated in the last section of this chapter.

Aims of Combining EEG/MEG and fMRI

A major aim motivating the integration of separately recorded EEG/MEG and fMRI data over the last decade (George et al., 1995; Liu et al., 1998; Dale et al., 2000; Mangun et al., 2000) has been the desire to overcome the limitation of poor spatial and temporal accuracy of MEG/EEG and fMRI, respectively, when these techniques are used separately. Various approaches to achieve this aim will be presented in the following sections. However, the use of electrophysiological information is not limited to enhancing the temporo-spatial accuracy of the description of neuronal processes in a certain task defined by the researcher: Information gained from electrophysiological data recorded *concurrently* with fMRI can be used instead to generate predictors to drive BOLD fMRI analysis in a variety of ways as exemplified in other chapters of this book (Laufs et al., 2003a; Laufs et al., 2003b; Debener et al., 2006; Laufs et al., 2006b; Laufs et al., 2006a; Tiége et al., 2007; Lemieux et al., 2008). On a simpler level one could just use *separately* recorded EEG information to verify that certain well-known

EEG components were indeed elicited by a novel paradigm in question, as expected, before proceeding with the respective fMRI experiment.

If one succeeds in reconstructing source activity and locations sufficiently well *without* resorting to fMRI-derived information first, then a comparison of BOLD fMRI activity and reconstructed source activity at corresponding locations can yield important insights into the relation of BOLD fMRI signal levels and electrophysiological signals. Two of the most influential studies on the issue of the dependence between electrophysiological signals—especially local field potentials—and hemodynamic signals have used data recorded invasively in anesthetized animals (Logothetis, 2002; Niessing et al., 2005). In the last section of this chapter we present studies demonstrating that similar results can possibly be obtained non-invasively using MEG beamforming and BOLD fMRI measurements recorded separately (Brookes et al., 2005). This approach has the advantage of eliminating the need for recording in an animal model and that of eliminating a potential confounding influence of anaesthetic agents on neurovascular coupling (e.g. Wibral et al., 2007 and references therein).

When to Use Concurrent EEG-fMRI and When to Use Separate Recordings

Given the availability of suitable equipment there is hardly any kind of analysis that works for separately recorded electrophysiological and fMRI data that cannot also be performed on concurrently recorded data sets, the combination of MEG and fMRI possibly being the only notable exception. This said, it is important, however, to distinguish between scenarios where concurrent recordings have a decisive advantage and those where the problems of the method, in its current state, lead to a distinctive disadvantage—such as limitations in the choice of a paradigm or a compromised data quality. To provide some guidance on these issues we will point out in this section scenarios where concurrent recordings are extremely valuable or even indispensable. In the next section we will demonstrate scenarios where it might at present still be beneficial to consider recording EEG/MEG and fMRI data separately.

Advantages of Recording EEG and fMRI Concurrently

Concurrent recordings are mandatory when the information obtained from electrophysiological measurements is necessary to drive BOLD fMRI analysis, because no other predictors for statistical analysis can be derived. Very important examples of this kind of experiments are investigations of interictal discharges in epileptic patients (e.g., Lemieux et al., 2001; Diehl et al., 2003; Salek-Haddadi et al., 2003; also see Chapter 4.2 in this book). As these discharges do not

necessarily lead to observable behavioral markers one has to resort to concurrently recorded EEG data to drive the fMRI analysis. Along similar lines there is no way around concurrent EEG fMRI recordings when generators of ongoing, stimulus independent EEG activity (like the occipital alpha activity in the wakeful resting state) are to be investigated (Laufs et al., 2003a; Laufs et al., 2003b; Moosmann et al., 2003; Gonçalves et al., 2006; Henning et al., 2006; Laufs et al., 2006b; de Munck et al., 2007; Mantini et al., 2007; Meltzer et al., 2007).

Concurrent EEG fMRI recordings also have indisputable advantages in experimental paradigms designed to investigate rapid learning processes that occur within a limited amount of time or trials.

As both EEG measurements and BOLD fMRI signals vary strongly from trial to trial, even under identical stimulation conditions and with identical behavioral results, concurrent measurements of EEG and fMRI are also very useful in searching for a possible correlation of these fluctuations at the single trial level. A common approach to the above topics has been to use single trial fluctuations in one modality—usually EEG—to search for correlated fluctuations in the other modality (Eichele et al., 2005; Debener et al., 2006; but see Mirsattari et al., 2006; Rodionov et al., 2007 for different mathematical approaches to this problem). The extraction of single-trial features of the EEG is often supported by the use of independent component analysis (ICA, Comon, 1994). Locations where BOLD fMRI activity is found to be correlated with certain features of EEG activity then possibly represent the electrical generators of the corresponding EEG feature. However, fMRI predictors derived from different EEG phenomena are often highly correlated, leading to false positives if some of these predictors are omitted from the statistical analysis. The high correlation of EEG-derived fMRI predictors with each other is due to the loss of information that usually comes with convolving the time course of the EEG signature with a hemodynamic response function (Boynton et al., 1996) for subsequent analysis using the general linear model (GLM). Hence, as many regressors—EEG features—as possible should be included simultaneously in the GLM analysis to avoid trivial false positives. Moreover, decorrelation of the predictor time courses should be performed after the convolution step and before GLM analysis. Once locations with EEG-correlated fMRI activity have been obtained, the corresponding forward model should be generated for these locations to distinguish between areas that have correlated processing at the neuronal (or metabolic) level from the actual *electrical* generators of the EEG signature under investigation.[1]

Advantages of Recording EEG/MEG and fMRI Separately

The advantages of recording EEG/MEG and fMRI data separately concern mainly the signal-to-noise-ratio (SNR) and the spatial resolution of EEG/MEG, which in turn are related to several issues that we will list shortly here and present in detail below:

1. Separate recordings allow the use of MEG, providing advantages for certain types of experiments as pointed out below. This possibility will have to be sacrificed in the case of concurrent recordings.

2. Various analysis routines that rely on independent component analysis (ICA) profit when the number of signal components does not exceed that of measurement channels. However, in concurrent recordings a considerable number of signal components will be added due to scanner related artifacts. Hence, the above requirement is much more likely to be met in the case of separately recorded data sets.

3. A related technical issue exacerbating the above problem is that some equipment that helps to record EEG from a large number of electrodes outside the scanner (such as active electrodes) is not compatible with a use inside the MR magnet.

4. Current MRI-artifact removal algorithms may introduce a certain bias or residual signal, particularly in ERP analyses, compromising signal quality.

5. Concurrent recordings a priori require the same paradigm for both measurement modalities. In contrast, separate recordings allow for separate adaptation of the paradigm to the measurement modality in order to obtain data with optimal signal-to-noise ratio (SNR).

The currents recorded by EEG and MEG differ in that EEG records mostly electric potentials generated by extracellular currents (also called "return currents"), while MEG records magnetic fields generated by both intra- and extracellular currents. Owing to the more confined nature of intracellular currents,[2] MEG measurements are in fact dominated by the intracellular currents if these current sources are closer to the respective sensor than the related extracellular return currents.

Because of these differences EEG and MEG might see different neuronal sources. Recording MEG may therefore detect sources that are not well visible in EEG and vice versa. As an example for different signals being recorded by EEG and MEG one may look at cortical oscillations in the γ-band (30–200 Hz). Here, even direct replications of EEG experiments using MEG have revealed different temporal evolution, spectral properties, or generator locations of the recorded induced gamma band activity, using illusory visual stimuli (Tallon-Baudry et al., 1996; Tallon-Baudry et al., 1997; Kaiser et al., 2004) and simple object-recognition tasks (Gruber et al., 2006; Gruber et al., 2008). The different influence of particular source configurations on EEG and MEG recordings (Tallon-Baudry and Bertrand, 1999; Tallon-Baudry et al., 1999; Gruber et al., 2008) and the fact that MEG might detect smaller source currents than EEG (Kaiser and Lutzenberger, 2005) have been proposed as possible mechanisms behind this discrepancy. An important advantage of MEG over EEG is that magnetic fields generated

by the currents (both, intra- and extracellular) are less deformed by the head tissue, which has a very low (diamagnetic) susceptibility. In contrast, electric potentials are heavily influenced by the local variations in resistivity of the various head tissues (i.e., brain, cerebrospinal fluid [CSF], dura, skull, and scalp). Hence, the forward model, or lead field matrix, L (Sarvas, 1987; Hämäläinen and Sarvas, 1989; Meijs et al., 1989; de Munck, 1992; Schlitt et al., 1995; Buchner et al., 1997; Ferguson and Stroink, 1997; Nolte, 2003; Nolte and Dassios, 2005; Schimpf, 2007), which describes the relation of source currents to sensor signals, can be more precisely approximated for the case of MEG. As will be shown below, certain source analysis methods (e.g., beamforming) depend extremely sensitively on correct assumptions about L. To date, it is unclear if common approximations of L are sufficiently accurate to allow the application of beamforming to EEG data (see discussion in Brookes et al., 2008), while the same methods have been successfully applied to MEG data in healthy controls and clinical populations (Singh et al., 2002; Ukai et al., 2002; Cheyne et al., 2003; Gaetz and Cheyne, 2003; Fawcett et al., 2004; Hall et al., 2004; Ukai et al., 2004; Brookes et al., 2005; Filbey et al., 2005; Hall et al., 2005a; Kawaguchi et al., 2005; Bardouille et al., 2006; Belardinelli et al., 2006; Cheyne et al., 2006; Oishi et al., 2006; Cheyne et al., 2007; Luo et al., 2007; Barbati et al., 2008; Muthukumaraswamy and Singh, 2008; Popescu et al., 2008; Taylor et al., 2008). In fact, source reconstruction via MEG beamforming has been sufficiently accurate to replicate results on the relationship of oscillatory brain activity and the BOLD fMRI signal that had been obtained only with invasive recordings techniques before (Brookes et al., 2005).

Separately recorded EEG/MEG data are also more easily analyzed with ICA, because no components contributed by the typical scanner artifacts or their remainders after artifact removal are present in the data. Gradient artifacts (Allen et al., 2000), cardioballistic artifacts (Allen et al., 1998; Debener et al., 2007; Debener et al., 2008) and induced voltages related to small subject movements in inhomogeneous magnetic fields increase the number of signal components. The number of artifactual components may reach a level where the results of an ICA decomposition become difficult to interpret or unreliable. This is especially true for movement-related artifacts, as their sources violate a basic assumption of the ICA mixing model (Jutten and Herault, 1991), that of a stationary mixing system. A stationary mixing system does not exist if spatially moving sources (Everson and Roberts, 1999) are present in the data. A related disadvantage of current MRI-compatible EEG systems is that they do not offer some of the recent technical advances—like active electrodes—that allow for a rapid application of a montage with a large number of electrodes. As a consequence of this practical limitation, EEG is often recorded with a suboptimal number of channels in concurrent recordings. The availability of many channels is, however, highly desirable if ICA analysis of EEG/MEG data is planned, because chances increase that the EEG ICA problem will not be underdetermined. This is because the maximum number of components that can be extracted from the data using basic ICA algorithms is smaller than or equal to the number of sensors used in the recordings (for an extension of basic ICA algorithms for the case of more sources than sensors see Amari, 1999; Inki and Hyvarinen, 2002). EEG recordings made concurrently with fMRI with as few as 32 or 64 channels can be problematic in this respect. We have discussed the importance of a large number of recording channels in the context of ICA here. A large number of recording channels and a good coverage of the head are also advantageous to the various source analysis techniques presented throughout this chapter.

Separately recorded data usually have a superior SNR, because their SNR is not degraded by residual or overcompensated scanner-related artifacts. A high SNR is especially important for experimental designs that use double differences in their analysis—e.g., (task1 - control1) - (task2 - control2)—and for analyses where weak signals like those typically observed in the high gamma frequency range are to be detected (Kaiser et al., 2008).

Another important practical merit of separate EEG/MEG and fMRI recordings, that has received little attention so far, is that they allow the researcher to optimize the paradigm independently for each recording. That is, long intertrial intervals or partial trials as they are often used in rapid event-related fMRI paradigms can be shortened or omitted in the EEG/MEG session, respectively. This may allow the researcher to collect more trials in the separate recordings of EEG/MEG data, thereby considerably improving the SNR. Alternatively, additional control conditions may be run in the same amount of time, improving the overall study design.

Neuroelectromagnetic Source Analysis

In order to overcome the limitation of poor spatial resolution of scalp-recorded EEG/MEG one wishes to localize its underlying neuroelectromagnetic source activity within the human brain. Localization of the neuroelectromagnetic sources requires the solution of two separate but related problems: the "forward problem" and the "inverse problem." The forward problem is to compute the scalp EEG/MEG signals when we know the exact location and properties of the neuroelectromagnetic sources and the properties of the surrounding head tissues. The necessary computations of the signal transduction coefficients from the sources to the sensors (i.e., the so-called leadfield L) can be performed based on simple physical principles (see e.g. Sarvas, 1987). These coefficients can be found with sufficient accuracy if detailed knowledge on the geometry and properties of the tissue compartments in the head is available. The inverse problem, on the other hand, consists in finding the locations and activation time courses of the neuronal sources given a set

of recorded sensor signals. This problem is severely ill posed, meaning that there are infinitely many source distributions within the head that can explain the scalp recorded EEG/MEG signal. We will first present a discrete formulation of both problems and then describe how different source analysis techniques try to solve the ill-posed inverse problem by placing constraints on the otherwise infinite solution space. In the next two sections we will introduce the forward and inverse problems in more detail. Throughout this presentation regular lowercase letters represent scalar variables, bold lowercase letters and bold uppercase letters represent vectors and matrices respectively. Bold italic lowercase letters are used for continuous vector fields (densities).

The Neuroelectromagnetic Forward Problem in Discrete Formulation

In MEG and EEG we measure magnetic fields and electric potentials respectively that are generated by the flow of ions in the conductive media of the head. The initial forces that make these ions move are due to biological processes in cell membranes and at synapses that make use of electrochemical gradients and active transport processes to relocate ions, i.e., to start current flows. These currents are driven by chemical forces and cannot be explained by the electromagnetic field equations alone. They are usually called the primary or impressed currents (Figure 3.7.1a).

By definition, primary currents only flow where there are chemical concentration gradients or active ion pumps, i.e., they flow across the cell membrane (e.g. Speckmann and Elger, 1993). In reaction to these impressed currents other ions will start to move in the conductive media to avoid the local accumulation of charges. That is, for the case of an excitatory synaptic potential, ions will move away from the current influx into a nerve cell along the dendrite inside the cell. Outside the cell currents will stream from all other extracellular locations in the head toward the local depletion left behind by the primary current influx. These currents are called *secondary* currents (Figure 3.7.1a). They flow—at a microscopic level—both, intracellularly and extracellularly, to and away from the ion channels at the synapse, where the primary currents were generated. These secondary currents are also called Ohmic currents, because they will lead to the generation of electric potential differences according to Ohm's law (see formula (3) in Sarvas, 1987 where the electric field is proportional to the total current minus the primary currents, meaning that it is proportional to the secondary currents). Depending on whether our measurement and reference electrodes are located intra- or extracellularly, we measure the potential differences generated by the intra- or extracellular *secondary* currents. As EEG electrodes are located extracellularly we measure the potentials generated by the extracellular *secondary* currents in the resistive media of the head tissue. In contrast, both, intra- and extracellular currents together will produce the magnetic fields measured by MEG. However, it should be kept in mind that all secondary currents simply flow because of the existence of the primary

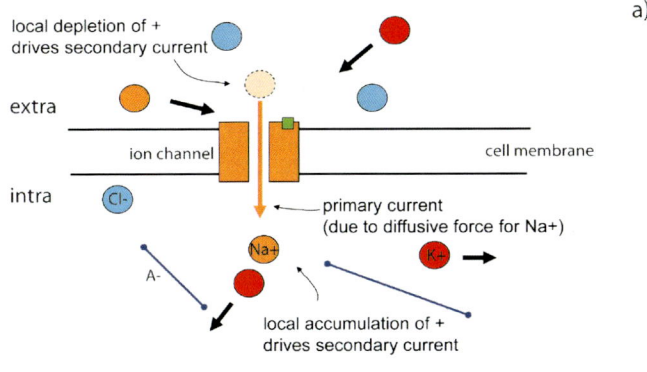

a)

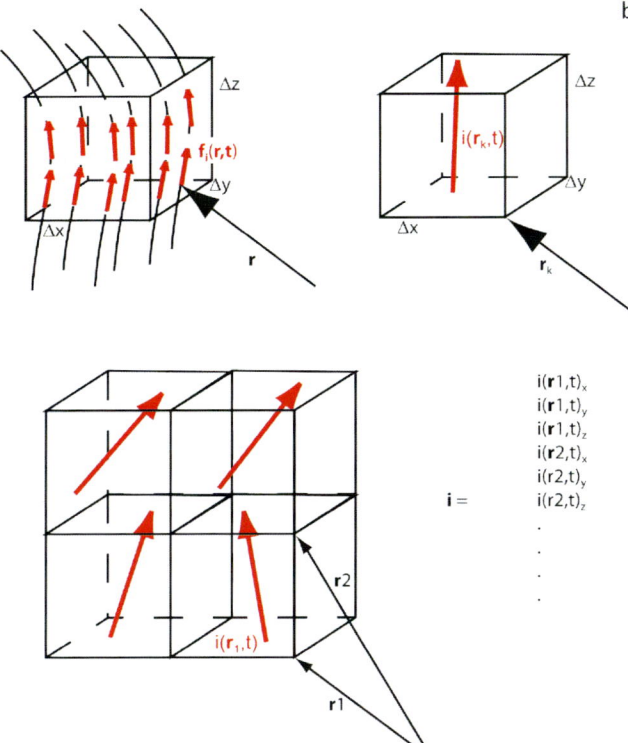

b)

$$i = \begin{matrix} i(\mathbf{r}1,t)_x \\ i(\mathbf{r}1,t)_y \\ i(\mathbf{r}1,t)_z \\ i(\mathbf{r}2,t)_x \\ i(\mathbf{r}2,t)_y \\ i(\mathbf{r}2,t)_z \\ \cdot \\ \cdot \\ \cdot \end{matrix}$$

Figure 3.7.1. (a) Distinction between primary currents and secondary currents. Primary currents are driven by chemical concentration gradients across the cell membrane (orange arrow). In this example the gradient of Na+ (orange circles) drives the primary current for the case of an excitatory postsynaptic potential. Primary currents lead to local charge imbalances that instantaneously start the secondary currents (black arrows). Positive Na+ and K+ ions (orange/red circles) are moving away from the site of current influx intracellularly and toward the site of current influx extracellularly. Blue bars/A- large indicate large, immobile, and negatively charged ions; Blue circles/Cl- indicate chloride ions. (b) Discretization of the current vector field. The continuous current vector field (top left) is integrated over small discrete volumes (voxels) of size $\Delta x \cdot \Delta y \cdot \Delta z$ as indicated in Formula 2 to yield an effective current vector $\mathbf{i}(\mathbf{r}_k)$ for a voxel at location $\mathbf{r}_k$ (top right). Information for all voxels of the headmodel is then collected in one large vector $\mathbf{i}$ of size 3N where N is the number of voxels (bottom).

currents in the case of neuroelectromagnetic activity, and that the dependence between the two is effectively linear. Hence, all generated magnetic fields and electric potentials are ultimately due to the action of primary currents, as will be shown below, and we will try to find these primary currents. The generation of secondary currents by the primary currents and the ensuing potentials and fields are mathematically described by Maxwell's equations for electromagnetic fields. Conductivities and geometrical arrangements of the tissue compartments in the human head are constant over time. This means that a given primary current will always produce the same pattern of secondary current flows and hence the same electric potentials and magnetic fields. In addition, the relatively low frequencies contained in bioelectromagnetic signals allow for the use of the quasistatic approximation of Maxwell's equations, meaning that the effects of temporal *changes* of the magnetic field on the electric field and vice versa are negligible. We thus strive to explain the measured sensor signals $\mathbf{m}$ by the instantaneous contributions of the primary currents that are seen via a constant transfer function at the sensors. This transfer function only depends on the conductivities and the geometries of the various tissue compartments in the head. To formalize the above considerations let us denote the continuous vector field of *all* currents in the head by $fi(\mathbf{r}, t)$ and write it as the sum of primary—or impressed currents $f i_{(1)}(\mathbf{r}, t)$ and the secondary or return currents $f i_{(2)}(\mathbf{r}, t)$:

$$f i(\mathbf{r}, t) = f i_{(1)}(\mathbf{r}, t) + f i_{(2)}(\mathbf{r}, t) \tag{1}$$

As we deal with macroscopic measurements that are typically several tens of millimeters away from the generating synaptic events that have themselves geometrical scales well below a millimeter we typically use a macroscopic model of these primary current sources by replacing $\mathbf{f} \mathbf{i}_{(1)}(\mathbf{r}, t)$ with the local integral $\mathbf{i}_{(1)}(\mathbf{r}_k, t)$ over a small piece of tissue at location $\mathbf{r}_k$ (Figure 3.7.1b):

$$\mathbf{i}_{(1)}(\mathbf{r}_k, t) = \int\limits_{(\mathbf{r}_k)_x}^{(\mathbf{r}_k)_x + \Delta x} \int\limits_{(\mathbf{r}_k)_y}^{(\mathbf{r}_k)_y + \Delta y} \int\limits_{(\mathbf{r}_k)_z}^{(\mathbf{r}_k)_z + \Delta z} f i_{(1)}(\mathbf{r}) d^3 r \tag{2}$$

Seen from a distance, such a current $\mathbf{i}_{(1)}(\mathbf{r}_k, t)$ at location $\mathbf{r}_k$ looks like a current sink (charges vanishing from one direction) and a source (charges emanating in the other direction) compressed into a single point. Hence, one often speaks of a current dipole.[3] This is one possible way of simplifying the description of primary currents by a source model. Other possibilities exist, however—see for example the ELECTRA source model by Grave de Peralta Menendez and colleagues, where sources and sinks of primary currents are treated separately (de Peralta Menendez et al., 2000). Henceforth, we will stick to the use of a dipolar source model, denoting the component moments of a primary current dipole $\mathbf{i}_{(1)}(\mathbf{r}_k, t)$ at location $\mathbf{r}_k$ in direction x, y, z with $\mathbf{j}(\mathbf{r}_k) = \left(\mathbf{j}(\mathbf{r}_k)_x, \mathbf{j}(\mathbf{r}_k)_y, \mathbf{j}(\mathbf{r}_k)_z\right)^T$, using the letter $\mathbf{j}$ instead of $\mathbf{i}$ to indicate that we are now dealing with current dipole moments instead of local integrals over the primary currents. The fixed electric potential or magnetic field configuration generated by a local dipole moment of unit strength at a location $\mathbf{r}_k$ pointing in direction l is typically summed up in its so called leadfield $\mathbf{L}(\mathbf{r}_k, l)$. Given sufficient information on the geometries and conductivities of tissue compartments in the head, $\mathbf{L}(\mathbf{r}_k, l)$ can be computed from physical principles, or can be at least numerically approximated (Sarvas, 1987; Hämäläinen and Sarvas, 1989; Meijs et al., 1989; de Munck, 1992; Schlitt et al., 1995; Buchner et al., 1997; Ferguson and Stroink, 1997; Nolte, 2003; Nolte and Dassios, 2005; Schimpf, 2007). We collect the information for the *primary* currents at all possible locations $\mathbf{r}_k$ in a single vector of dipole moment components:

$$j(t) = \big(j(r_1, t)_x, j(r_1, t)_y, j(r_1, t)_z, \ldots, \\ j(r_N, t)_x, j(r_N, t)_y, j(r_N, t)_z \big) T \qquad (3)$$

Note that the allowed locations $\mathbf{r}_k$ for non-zero dipole moments are now limited to tissues that can contain sources and sinks of the primary electric currents, whereas the currents in Formula 1 were distributed in all tissues. The so-called forward problem of explaining our measured sensor data $\mathbf{m}(t)$ by the currents in the brain can now be written as:

$$\mathbf{m}(t) = \mathbf{L}j(t) + \mathbf{n}(t) \qquad (4)$$

where $\mathbf{m}$ is the vector of M measured sensor signals, and $\mathbf{j}(t)$ is the vector containing 3N dipole strength components at N locations in the brain. In this formula, the leadfield $\mathbf{L}$ is a matrix whose elements $L_{k(ix)}, L_{k(iz)}, L_{k(iy)}$ describe how a dipole of unit strength at location i and with an orientation in x, y, or z direction is picked up by sensor k (Figure 3.7.2). The vector $\mathbf{n}$ describes sensor noise added by the measurement equipment.

In practice, some of the necessary information for the precise numerical approximation of $\mathbf{L}$ may be missing, and one typically resorts to approximate descriptions of the tissue compartments in the head by simpler geometrical shapes (e.g. concentric ellipsoids of homogeneous conductivity: Blimke et al., 2008; Gutiérrez and Nehorai, 2008 and references therein) that allow the computation of $\mathbf{L}$ in closed mathematical form. These simplifications usually lead to an error that may be tolerable—a four-shell ellipsoidal head model is usually thought to be sufficient for dipole fitting—or may challenge the accuracy of the obtained results—see for example the discussion of the precision of EEG-beamformer source reconstruction based on ellipsoidal head models in (Brookes et al., 2008).

The Ill-Posed Inverse Problem

The inverse problem consists in determining the dipole strengths $\mathbf{j}(t)$ from the measured data $\mathbf{m}(t)$ at each time instant t. As we use the quasistatic approximation of Maxwell's equations we now drop the explicit reference to any time dependence and only return to it where necessary. A formal approach to solve the inverse problem would be to vary the components of $\mathbf{j}$ in order to minimize the mismatch

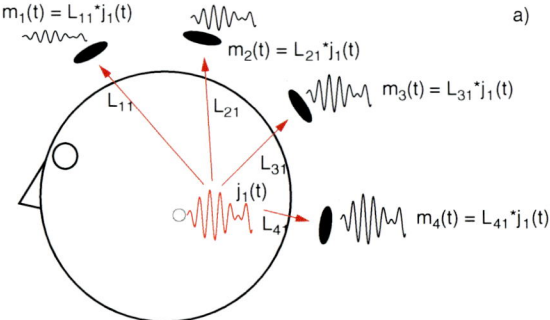

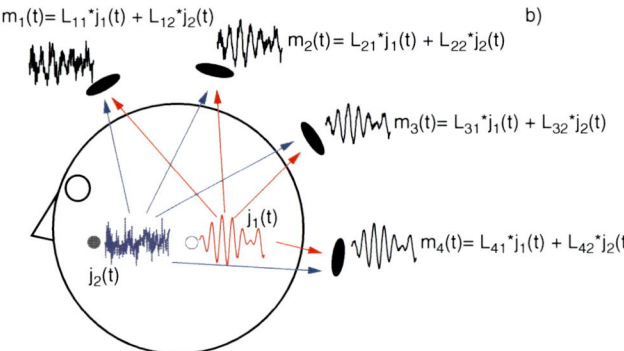

Figure 3.7.2. Relation of measured signals $m_i(t)$ and the dipole moments $j_i(t)$ of the primary currents: (a) A time dependent dipole moment $j_1(t)$ (red trace) in one of the principal directions (say $\hat{\mathbf{x}}$) is seen by the sensor 1 as a scaled version of the original signal, with a scaling coefficient L_{11}, called the leadfield coefficient for source $j_i(t)$ and sensor 1. L_{11} only depends on the geometries and conductivities of the various tissue compartments of the head. Similar relations hold for all other source orientations and all sensors. (b) In the presence of a second source $j_2(t)$ all sensors capture linear mixtures of the source signals weighted with the respective leadfield coefficients.

$\|\widetilde{\mathbf{W}}(\mathbf{L}j - \mathbf{m}^2)\|$ between the true measurements $\mathbf{m}$ and the computed measurements by the forward model given by $\mathbf{L}j$ (weighted by some matrix $\widetilde{\mathbf{W}}$) to arrive at an estimate $\hat{\mathbf{j}}$ of the true $\mathbf{j}$. This can be formally written as:

$$\hat{\mathbf{j}} = \arg \min_{\mathbf{j}} \left[(\mathbf{L}j - \mathbf{m})^t \mathbf{W}(\mathbf{L}j - \mathbf{m}) \right] \qquad (5)$$

Where the matrix $\mathbf{W} = \widetilde{\mathbf{W}}^T \widetilde{\mathbf{W}}$ represents a certain metric—a weighting—to determine the mismatch. This matrix $\mathbf{W}$ lets us decide which of the measurements in $\mathbf{m}$ we trust more than others and which we, therefore, want to see well approximated. The term $\left[(\mathbf{L}j - \mathbf{m})^T \mathbf{W}(\mathbf{L}j - \mathbf{m})\right]$ is nothing but the weighted least square error between the measurements $\mathbf{m}$ and our estimate $\mathbf{j}$ projected to the sensors via $\mathbf{L}$. The above problem is difficult to solve for several reasons:

In practice, one tries to determine the currents at many more discrete positions in the brain than there are sensors (number of locations N >> M, the number of sensors). Thus, the system of linear equations implied by (5) is necessarily underdetermined, because the matrix $\mathbf{L}$ has many more columns than rows. Therefore, the null space of **L**, i.e., the set of vectors $\{\mathbf{j}_n\}$ that satisfy $\mathbf{L}\mathbf{j} = \mathbf{0}$ is trivially different from the zero vector $\{\mathbf{0}\}$. Hence, any vector $\mathbf{j}_n$ can be added to the estimated $\mathbf{j}$ again yielding a solution $\hat{\mathbf{j}}' = \hat{\mathbf{j}} + \mathbf{j}_n$ with minimal mismatch. Interestingly enough, the above problem is rather of a *physical* than of a mathematical nature. The problem will persist, irrespective of the number of measurements sensors one uses, even if one uses as many sensors as sources in $\mathbf{j}$. This is because given a measurement $\mathbf{m}$ of electromagnetic sensor signals on a closed surface D, there is any number of current configurations with sources and sinks inside D that can produce these measurements (Helmholtz, 1853). This means, the null space of **L** stays non-trivial, even for a square **L**. These source configurations that do not produce measurable scalp signals are called *closed* field (or closed source) configurations, in contrast to those configurations that contribute to the measured signals, which are called open field configurations. It is usually assumed that measurable scalp signals are almost exclusively generated by synaptic currents at the dendrites of large pyramidal cells in the cortex. In addition, some sources with measurable signals cannot be reconstructed by *linear* methods (for a proof consult de Peralta-Menendez and Gonzalez-Andino, 1998, Appendix II). To arrive at a unique solution, one therefore tries to constrain the solution space by incorporating prior knowledge from physiology or additional mathematical assumptions. It is the choices of various additional constraints and assumptions that distinguish the source analysis techniques presented below from each other.

In the following sections we first present various source analysis techniques one by one, without explicit reference to the incorporation of fMRI data. We then explain how fMRI data can be incorporated into each of these methods. This way, source analysis methods can be directly compared and their differences can be appreciated. Later on, the various ways and underlying assumptions involved in the integration of fMRI data can be directly compared. If the reader is only interested in a particular source analysis technique, she or he may read the section explaining this particular method and then directly skip ahead to the respective section on the integration of fMRI data for that method.

Source Analysis Techniques

There are two major properties that distinguish the most popular source analysis techniques from each other. First, various source analysis techniques differ in whether they consider the scalp-recorded EEG/MEG activity to be generated by a small number of distinct dipolar sources that differ in location and/or orientation (discrete dipole source analysis; Scherg and Berg, 1991; Mosher et al., 1992) or whether they interpret the scalp-recorded signal in terms of a large number of (dipolar) sources at distributed locations within the brain (distributed linear inverse solutions; Hämäläinen and Ilmoniemi, 1984). Source analysis using Bayesian inference (Baillet and Garnero, 1997; Schmidt et al., 1999) allows

for a principled way of incorporating both source types and allows the data to decide about the most probable configuration (Trujillo-Barreto et al., 2004; Mattout et al., 2006; Friston et al., 2008). Second, source analysis techniques differ in their use of temporal information. Classical source analysis techniques like distributed linear inverse solutions and discrete dipole source analysis allow for a reconstruction of the sources at each single point in time separately but typically discard information contained in the temporal correlation of the sensor signals. This information is exploited by beamformer source reconstruction (van Veen et al., 1997; Robinson and Vrba, 1999; Sekihara et al., 2001). We will now describe each of these various approaches in detail and then review how they integrate spatial information from separately recorded fMRI data to solve the underdetermined neuroelectromagnetic inverse problem.

Distributed Linear Inverse Solutions

For the sake of an intuitive explanation, let's assume that we have some idea about what the dipole moments should be. If any such prior guess $\mathbf{j}_p$ can be made on the expected dipole moments, this could be incorporated into our estimation problem as:

$$\hat{\mathbf{j}} = \arg \min_{\mathbf{j}} \left[(\mathbf{L}\mathbf{j} - \mathbf{m})^T \mathbf{W} (\mathbf{L}\mathbf{j} - \mathbf{m}) \right] + \lambda^2 \left[(\mathbf{j} - \mathbf{j}_p)^t \mathbf{W}_P (\mathbf{j} - \mathbf{j}_p) \right] \tag{6}$$

i.e., by trying to simultaneously minimize the mismatch $(\mathbf{L}\mathbf{j} - \mathbf{m})$ between our estimate $\mathbf{j}$ and the measurements $\mathbf{m}$ on the one hand and the mismatch between our estimate $\mathbf{j}$ and the guessed prior currents $\mathbf{j}_p$ as measured by the metric $\mathbf{W}_p$ on the other hand. This problem now has a unique solution in the least square sense.[4] This solution can be obtained by standard linear algebra methods and is given by (de Peralta-Menendez and Gonzalez-Andino, 1998):

$$\hat{\mathbf{j}} = \mathbf{j}_p + \left[\mathbf{L}^t \mathbf{W} \mathbf{L} + \lambda^2 \mathbf{W}_P \right]^{-1} \mathbf{L}^t \mathbf{W} \left[\mathbf{m} - \mathbf{L}\mathbf{j}_p \right] \tag{7}$$

This formula can be read as follows: If our guess $\mathbf{j}_p$ completely explains our measurements then $\left[\mathbf{m} - \mathbf{L}\mathbf{j}_p \right] = \mathbf{0}$ and $\hat{\mathbf{j}} = \mathbf{j}_p$ is already a good estimate of the currents $\mathbf{j}$ because the measurements $\mathbf{m}$ did not yield any additional information. If $\mathbf{m}$ has additional information, then we have an error $\boldsymbol{\varepsilon} = \left[\mathbf{m} - \mathbf{L}\mathbf{j}_p \right]$ in our explanation of the measurements that should be used to update our estimate $\hat{\mathbf{j}}$. This is done by projecting the sensor-space error term $\left[\mathbf{m} - \mathbf{L}\mathbf{j}_p \right]$ by the optimal weighting $\left[\mathbf{L}^t \mathbf{W} \mathbf{L} + \lambda^2 \mathbf{W}_P \right]^{-1} \mathbf{L}^t \mathbf{W}$ into the source space $\mathbf{j}$ and adding this to our prior guess $\mathbf{j}_p$. Even when no information on $\mathbf{j}_p$ is available ($\mathbf{j}_p = \mathbf{0}$) the incorporation of the remaining second term $\lambda^2 \mathbf{j}^t \mathbf{W}_p \mathbf{j}$ in Equation 6 is enough of a constraint to yield a unique solution[5] in the least square sense given by:

$$\hat{\mathbf{j}} = \mathbf{W}_p^{-1}\mathbf{L}^t\left[\mathbf{L}\mathbf{W}_p^{-1}\mathbf{L}^t + \lambda^2\mathbf{W}^{-1}\right]^{-1}\mathbf{m} \qquad (8)$$

Various choices of a metric $\mathbf{W}_p$ result in well-known distributed source localization algorithms:

$\mathbf{W} = \mathbf{W}_p = \mathbf{I}$ corresponds to the well-known minimum norm approach. $\mathbf{W} = \mathbf{I}$ simply states that the squared error between measurements $\mathbf{m}$ and estimates $\mathbf{L}\mathbf{j}$ is minimized. $\mathbf{W}_p = \mathbf{I}$ leads to an equally weighted penalty for increasing currents independent of their depth and the corresponding values in the respective columns of $\mathbf{L}$ at their location. As deep sources usually have smaller values of $\mathbf{L}(\mathbf{r})$ they need larger values of $\mathbf{j}(\mathbf{r},t)$ to explain the data. This ultimately leads to a preference for solutions with superficial sources. To avoid this undesired bias it has been tried to choose $\mathbf{W} = \mathbf{I}$ and $(\mathbf{W}_p)_{ii} = |\mathbf{L}(\mathbf{r}_i)|$ to alleviate this problem. Here currents come with a smaller penalty for sources with smaller leadfield coefficients, allowing larger currents for deeper sources. This approach is known as weighted minimum norm (wMN). More advanced approaches exist, e.g., $\mathbf{W}_p$ can have operator form, performing discrete first order or Laplacian spatial derivation on $\mathbf{j}$. The latter case is known as low resolution electromagnetic tomography (LORETA; Pascual-Marqui et al., 1994) and chooses the smoothest of all possible solutions for LORETA can also be combined with anatomical constraints (cLORETA; Pascual-Marqui, 1999) or noise normalized (sLORETA; Pascual-Marqui, 2002). $\mathbf{W}_p$ can also be chosen as the inverse of the covariance matrix of the sources (if something about it is known or imposed as a constraint), and $\mathbf{W}$ as the inverse of the covariance matrix of the sensor noise. The latter implies that a mismatch between $\mathbf{L}\mathbf{j}$ and $\mathbf{m}$ is accepted more readily at sensors with a high noise contribution, i.e., one ascribes this mismatch to the presence of the sensor noise. This choice of $\mathbf{W}$ requires that an estimate of the sensor noise covariance is available, e.g., from a suitable baseline recording. One may also try to reconstruct a weighted *local average* of $\mathbf{j}$ that is consistent with the data (the LAURA algorithm; see de Peralta Menendez et al., 2001) by introducing off-diagonal elements in $\mathbf{W}_p$ that are motivated by the physics of signal crosstalk in tissue. In combination with the latter approach one also resorts to modeling current sources for EEG signals as separate (scalar) sources and sinks instead of using a (vectorial) local dipole model, thereby reducing the numbers of parameters to be estimated by a factor of 3 (the ELECTRA source model; see de Peralta Menendez et al., 2000). If anatomical MRI data are available, the number of dipole moments in $\mathbf{j}$ can be reduced. This is done by confining the search space to grey matter and by using a fixed dipole orientation perpendicular to the cortical sheet of grey matter at each location in the computation of $\mathbf{L}$ instead of three spatial components (representing dipoles in x, y, and z direction). This considerably reduces the number of components of $\mathbf{j}$ that have to be estimated. It is important to be aware of the fact that the use of anatomical constraints on the search space a priori excludes the detection of sources not contained in that space, e.g., sources localized in deeper structures of the brain will evidently not be found when

confining the search to *cortical* grey matter. Due to volume conduction, these deep lying sources can contribute significantly to the scalp signal, however, at least in EEG recordings. If these sources are not accounted for in the space of possible source locations their contributions to the signal will distort the rest of the solution. This will also hold for signals due to residual artifacts when recording EEG fMRI simultaneously. Both the accuracy of localization and that of the reconstructed source signal time courses may be compromised. The latter point is particularly important because distributed inverse solutions of the kind described here are not optimized to suppress contributions from other sources (in contrast to minimum variance beamforming approaches; see below). A possible solution to this problem may be to investigate several ways of incorporating anatomical constraints (i.e., models) and use Bayesian statistics to decide on the final set of constraints (Trujillo-Barreto et al., 2004).

Discrete Dipole Source Analysis

Dipole source analysis uses the constraint that only a limited and small number of dipolar sources in the brain contribute to the measured sensor signals. This assumption is in principle sufficient to guarantee that the inverse problem has a unique solution in the least square sense. By setting all components of $\mathbf{j}$ to zero except for a limited number N_s of locations one can rewrite the inverse problem as:

$$\mathbf{m} = \sum_{i=1}^{N_s} \mathbf{L}(\mathbf{r}_i,\boldsymbol{\theta}_i)\mathbf{j}_i + \mathbf{n} \qquad (9)$$

where $\mathbf{L}(\mathbf{r}_i,\boldsymbol{\theta}_i)$ is the column of $\mathbf{L}$ belonging to a dipole moment at location $\mathbf{r}_i$ with orientation $\boldsymbol{\theta}_i$ whereas $\mathbf{j}_i$ is the size of the dipole moment. Hence, 6 parameters per assumed dipole need to be found (3 location coordinates, two angles, and its strength). In the noise-free case, this inverse problem (9) is overdetermined and has a unique solution in the least square sense as long as the number of assumed sources N_s is smaller than the number of sensors divided by six (M/6). However, because of the influence of the noise $\mathbf{n}$ the number of dipoles that can actually be fitted from experimental data is usually much smaller and a maximum number of 7 has been given in (Ramírez, 2008). It should be noted that while the above equation looks like a standard linear equation, $\mathbf{L}(\mathbf{r}_i,\boldsymbol{\theta}_i)$ is a non-linear function of the parameters $\mathbf{r}_i,\boldsymbol{\theta}_i$ that we wish to estimate. Hence non-linear optimization algorithms (e.g., Nelder-Mead downhill simplex, Levenberg-Marquardt) are required for its solution. A fundamental problem of this approach is that a correct assumption on the number N_s of dipoles has to be made in the first place. As will be demonstrated below, fMRI data can be incorporated in a variety of ways to alleviate this problem.

MEG Beamforming

So far all attempts to solve the electromagnetic linear inverse problem presented here had in common that they tried to satisfy the constraints posed by the inverse problem at single points in time and tried to satisfy additional constraints that were physiologically informed and necessary to guarantee the existence of a unique solution. Therefore, these solution algorithms were targeted at and capable of reconstructing the electrical activity at a single point in time but limited in their capability of exploiting available temporal information beyond simple averaging over consecutive time points. It is quite straightforward to see that this may be a disadvantage, because sources may be active over prolonged intervals. Some points in time may be better suited to localize a certain source than others, not because its dipole moment is maximal at that point but interfering signals from other sources may be weakest. The time varying dipole moments of the source may in fact be used to disentangle their signals. This information is implicitly contained in the data covariance matrix $\mathbf{C} = \mathbf{m}\,\mathbf{m}^T$. This information can be used to construct a spatial filter, i.e., a weighted sum of sensor signals to represent the source activity. The spatial filter used here on the one hand satisfies the requirements of the linear inverse problem for a given location in the head while, at the same time, minimizing interfering signals from all other points in the head. This particular set of weights is called a beamformer. For an intuitive understanding of beamforming it is best to start with a very simple source configuration. Imagine having just one active source a in the brain at a known location $\mathbf{r}_a$ oriented in one of the principal directions (e.g., $\boldsymbol{\theta}_a = \hat{\mathbf{x}}$) with activity time course a(t) (see Figure 3.7.2a). We can now compute the corresponding column $\mathbf{L}(\mathbf{r}_a, \boldsymbol{\theta}_a)$ of the leadfield for this source location and all sensors and obtain the measured sensor signals $\mathbf{m}$:

$$\mathbf{m}(t) = \mathbf{L}(\mathbf{r}_a, \boldsymbol{\theta}_a)\mathrm{a}(t) \qquad (10)$$

One perfect reconstruction of the source activity a(t) would then be given by:

$$\mathrm{a}(t) = \frac{1}{N}\sum_{i=1}^{N}\frac{1}{L_i(\mathbf{r}_a, \boldsymbol{\theta}_a)}\,\mathrm{m}_i(t) \qquad (11)$$

where $L_i(\mathbf{r}_a, \boldsymbol{\theta}_a)$ is the coeffcient of the leadfield that describes the signal transmission from source a to sensor i. Of course, one could also simply compute a(t) from a single sensor, say the first one:

$$\mathrm{a}(t) = \frac{1}{L_1(\mathbf{r}_a, \boldsymbol{\theta}_a)}\,\mathrm{m}_1(t) \qquad (12)$$

In fact, any linear combination $\hat{\mathrm{a}}(t)$ of sensor signals $\mathrm{m}_i(t)$:

$$\hat{\mathrm{a}}(t) = \sum_{i=1}^{N} w_{ai}\mathrm{m}_i(t) \qquad (13)$$

where the coefficients w_{ai} satisfy the criterion:

$$\sum_{i=1}^{N} w_{ai}L_i(\mathbf{r}_a, \boldsymbol{\theta}_a) = 1 \quad (\text{"unity gain"}) \qquad (14)$$

leads to a perfect reconstruction $\hat{\mathrm{a}}(t)$ of a(t) in our simple example. Thus, there is no preference for any of the possible

sets of filter coefficients as long as they satisfy the *unity gain* constraint (Equation 14). This changes, however, if we consider the presence of a second source b at location $\mathbf{r}_b$, with orientation in one of the principal directions (e.g. $\boldsymbol{\theta}_b = \hat{\mathbf{y}}$) and time course b(t) (Figure 3.7.2b). Now the choice of a set of coefficients $\{w_{ai}\}$ used to reconstruct a(t) via its estimate $\hat{\mathrm{a}}(t, \{w_{ai}\})$ will strongly influence the quality of the reconstruction: We would like to weight preferentially those sensors strongly that are close to source a while weighting those close to b with small, zero, or alternating weights, such that the influence of b(t) on our estimate $\hat{\mathrm{a}}(t, \{w_{ai}\})$ becomes small. Since b is at an unknown location this is not straightforward to achieve, however. In a thought experiment we might still search all possible sets $\{w_{ai}\}$ that satisfy the *unity gain* constraint for the one set $\{\hat{w}_{ai}\}$ that minimizes the power P of our estimated signal $\hat{\mathrm{a}}(\{w_{ai}\})$:

$$\begin{aligned}\{\hat{w}_{ai}\} &= \arg\min_{\{w_{ai}\}} P(\hat{\mathrm{a}}(\{w_{ai}\})) \\ &= \arg\min_{\{w_{ai}\}} \sum_t \hat{\mathrm{a}}(\{w_{ai}\},t)\hat{\mathrm{a}}(\{w_{ai}\},t) \qquad (15)\end{aligned}$$

or, writing the signal $\hat{\mathrm{a}}(t)$ as a row vector $\hat{\mathbf{a}}$ and our set of weights $\{w_{ai}\}$ as a column vector $\mathbf{w}_a$:

$$\begin{aligned}\mathbf{w}_a &= \arg\min_{\mathbf{w}_a}\ \left(\hat{\mathbf{a}}\,\hat{\mathbf{a}}^T\right) = \arg\min_{\mathbf{w}_a}\ \left(\mathbf{w}_a^T\mathbf{m}\mathbf{m}^T\mathbf{w}_a\right) \\ &= \arg\min_{\mathbf{w}_a}\ \left(\mathbf{w}_a^T\mathbf{C}\mathbf{w}_a\right) \qquad (16)\end{aligned}$$

where $\mathbf{C}$ is the covariance matrix of the data. The idea here is that, since we know we are only choosing from sets of coefficients that would perfectly reconstruct a(t) if it were the only source (unity gain), we can be sure that our minimization will not take away any power coming from a. Hence, searching through all sets of coefficients we will finally pick the set that reconstructs the power of a with the least possible amount of interference of b. Fortunately, we do not have to search through all possible sets of weights, because a closed form solution to the above minimization problem exists:

$$\mathbf{w}_a = \mathbf{w}(\mathbf{r}_a, \boldsymbol{\theta}_a) = \mathbf{C}^{-1}\mathbf{L}(\mathbf{r}_a, \boldsymbol{\theta}_a)\left(\mathbf{L}^t(\mathbf{r}_a, \boldsymbol{\theta}_a)\mathbf{C}^{-1}\mathbf{L}(\mathbf{r}_a, \boldsymbol{\theta}_a)\right)^{-1} \qquad (17)$$

We can now scan our head model point by point ($\mathbf{r}_a$) and orientation by orientation ($\boldsymbol{\theta}_r = \hat{\mathbf{x}}, \hat{\mathbf{y}}, \hat{\mathbf{z}}$) and reconstruct the corresponding source power via the weights $\mathbf{w}(\mathbf{r}, \boldsymbol{\theta}_r)$. This source power P for one source at $\mathbf{r}$ in one principal direction $\boldsymbol{\theta}_r$ is then given by:

$$\mathrm{P}(\mathbf{r}, \boldsymbol{\theta}_r) = \mathbf{w}(\mathbf{r}, \boldsymbol{\theta}_r)^t\mathbf{C}\mathbf{w}(\mathbf{r}, \boldsymbol{\theta}_r) = \left(\mathbf{L}(\mathbf{r}, \boldsymbol{\theta}_r)^t\mathbf{C}^{-1}\mathbf{L}(\mathbf{r}, \boldsymbol{\theta}_r)\right)^{-1} \qquad (18)$$

If we are interested in an estimate of local signal power without being interested in the orientation of the sources, there exist several ways to sum up the power obtained in the principal directions as explained below. One popular choice is to take the trace of the local covariance matrix of source power in the principal directions $\boldsymbol{\theta}_r = \hat{\mathbf{x}}, \hat{\mathbf{y}}, \hat{\mathbf{z}}$ at $\mathbf{r}$:

$$P(\mathbf{r}) = trace\left(\tilde{\mathbf{L}}(\mathbf{r})^t \mathbf{C}^{-1} \tilde{\mathbf{L}}(\mathbf{r})\right)^{-1}$$
$$\text{with} \quad \tilde{\mathbf{L}}(\mathbf{r}) = [\mathbf{L}(\mathbf{r}, \hat{\mathbf{x}}), \mathbf{L}(\mathbf{r}, \hat{\mathbf{y}}), \mathbf{L}(\mathbf{r}, \hat{\mathbf{z}})] \tag{19}$$

In addition, we face the problem that an optimum source reconstruction—in the sense that we have a minimal interference from other sources—by no means guarantees that this interference is actually small. Hence, suitable normalization or subtraction procedures are necessary to obtain an interpretable signal. Usually one estimates the residual noise power, that could not be removed by the beamforming procedure from a suitable baseline or control condition. Huang and colleagues (Huang et al., 2004), for example, propose to use the following normalization:

$$P_{norm}(\mathbf{r}_i) = \frac{\left(\mathbf{L}(\mathbf{r}_i, \hat{\mathbf{x}})^T \mathbf{C}^{-1} \mathbf{L}(\mathbf{r}_i, \hat{\mathbf{x}})\right)^{-1}}{\left(\mathbf{L}(\mathbf{r}_i, \hat{\mathbf{x}})^T \boldsymbol{\Sigma}^{-1} \mathbf{L}(\mathbf{r}_i, \hat{\mathbf{x}})\right)^{-1}}$$
$$+ \frac{\left(\mathbf{L}(\mathbf{r}_i, \hat{\mathbf{y}})^T \mathbf{C}^{-1} \mathbf{L}(\mathbf{r}_i, \hat{\mathbf{y}})\right)^{-1}}{\left(\mathbf{L}(\mathbf{r}_i, \hat{\mathbf{y}})^T \boldsymbol{\Sigma}^{-1} \mathbf{L}(\mathbf{r}_i, \hat{\mathbf{y}})\right)^{-1}}$$
$$+ \frac{\left(\mathbf{L}(\mathbf{r}_i, \hat{\mathbf{z}})^T \mathbf{C}^{-1} \mathbf{L}(\mathbf{r}_i, \hat{\mathbf{z}})\right)^{-1}}{\left(\mathbf{L}(\mathbf{r}_i, \hat{\mathbf{z}})^T \boldsymbol{\Sigma}^{-1} \mathbf{L}(\mathbf{r}_i, \hat{\mathbf{z}})\right)^{-1}} \tag{20}$$

where $\boldsymbol{\Sigma}$ is the covariance matrix of the noise estimate. Various other measures of neuronal source activity and reconstructed source time course have been proposed (see Huang et al., 2004 for an excellent overview). Together with different possibilities to sum the vectorized information at each point, this leads to a variety of measures for source activities (Huang et al., 2004).

The Bayesian Approach to the Inverse Problem

The problem of constraining and conditioning the inverse problem can be also be treated using Bayesian estimation techniques (Baillet and Garnero, 1997; Schmidt et al., 1999; Friston et al., 2002; Phillips et al., 2002a). In fact, all algorithms presented in the previous sections can also be found to be limiting cases of an appropriate Bayesian formulation of the inverse problem (see for example the Scholarpedia article by Ramírez, 2008 for a review). Bayesian inference is a technique to construct a probability distribution for certain parameters of interest (the dipole moments $\mathbf{j}$ in our case), incorporating prior knowledge on these parameters in the form of a

probability distribution $p(\mathbf{j})$. For example, such prior knowledge could be derived from anatomy and consist in the fact that primary currents originate at synapses in grey matter. This prior knowledge is then combined with the knowledge obtained from the data (the sensor data $\mathbf{m}$ in our case) to obtain the most likely estimate of $\mathbf{j}$. In other words, we would like to know how likely it is that the true dipole moments were $\mathbf{j}$ under the assumption that these dipole moments produced the measurements $\mathbf{m}$ and in addition have to satisfy certain (e.g., anatomical) constraints. To give an example, it might be highly likely that a current source in the exact center of the head produced our measurements if we only look at the relation between the position of the current sources and the corresponding potential distribution as measured by $\mathbf{m}$. If we add knowledge on the anatomically plausible locations of current sources we may rule out a current source in the exact center of the head a priori and thus rather ascribe the observed potential distribution $\mathbf{m}$ to noise contributions.[7]

The above probability distribution of $\mathbf{j}$ that incorporates the prior knowledge and information from the measurements is termed the *posterior* probability distribution of $\mathbf{j}$ given the measurements $\mathbf{m}$ and the prior knowledge H: $p(\mathbf{j}|\mathbf{m}, H)$. Once we have this posterior probability for the parameter of interest, $\mathbf{j}$, we can for example choose the maximum of this distribution as a valid guess—a reconstruction—of the parameter $\mathbf{j}$. The construction of the posterior probability $p(\mathbf{j}|\mathbf{m}, H)$ relies on Bayes' Theorem, which allows us to write the posterior probability as a product of probabilities that are much easier to asses:

$$p(\mathbf{j}|\mathbf{m}, H) = \frac{p(\mathbf{m}|\mathbf{j}, H) p(\mathbf{j}|H)}{p(\mathbf{m}|H)} \tag{21}$$

Where $p(\mathbf{m}|\mathbf{j}, H)$ is the probability that a parameter $\mathbf{j}$ would produce the data $\mathbf{m}$ given the constraints H hold (likelihood), whereas $p(\mathbf{j}|H)$ is the probability (the prior, dependent on our prior knowledge incorporated in H) that the parameter of interest is indeed $\mathbf{j}$ if we would not know anything else but H, that is if we didn't measure any data. In our example this probability would be non-zero for dipole moment distributions $\mathbf{j}$ that are non-zero only in grey matter and zero for all dipole moment distributions that have significant contributions at locations outside of grey matter. The so called evidence $p(\mathbf{m}|H)$ in the denominator of Equation 21 is just a normalizing factor that guarantees that $p(\mathbf{j}|\mathbf{m}, H)$ is a probability distribution, i.e., its integral is normalized to one. Once the posterior probability is decomposed into simpler known probabilities as described above, Bayesian estimation reduces to finding either the maximum of this posterior probability (maximum a posteriori or MAP estimator) or its mean (minimal mean square error or MMSE estimator). While this sounds simple, finding the maximum of a distribution on a high dimensional parameter space or evaluating the mean of this distribution can be a highly complex task. In fact both, theoretical formulation (Wipf and Nagarajan, 2008), algorithms (like Variational Bayes or Markov Chain Monte Carlo algorithms: Daunizeau et al.,

2007; Nummenmaa et al., 2007b; Jun et al., 2008; Kiebel et al., 2008; Trujillo-Barreto et al., 2008), and the necessary computational power have only recently reached a level where the application of Bayesian techniques to the neuroelectromagnetic inverse problem is practical (Henson et al., 2007; Trujillo-Barreto et al., 2008) and available with standard software packages (e.g., spm8: www.fil.ion.ucl.ac.uk/spm/software/spm8b). However, even using the latest solution algorithms, problems with (hyper-) parameter estimation may arise, e.g., due to certain approximations made in the Variational Bayes algorithm (Nummenmaa et al., 2007b; Nummenmaa et al., 2007a). Another complication is how to explicitly incorporate the necessary prior information. New approaches are being continuously developed (Friston et al., 2008; Jun et al., 2008; Kiebel et al., 2008; Trujillo-Barreto et al., 2008), although recently a unifying formulation covering most or all of these approaches has been proposed (Wipf and Nagarajan, 2008). While the Bayesian approach may seem overly formal at this point of presentation it has considerable strength in that it is capable of incorporating and weighting competing constraints on **j**, using the data to determine their relative importance (Trujillo-Barreto et al., 2004; Mattout et al., 2006; Friston et al., 2008). In the following paragraph we will demonstrate how typical priors (e.g., spatial constraints from anatomical MRI or smoothness constraints as used in LORETA) are practically implemented in Bayesian source estimation, following the material presented in (Mattout et al., 2006).

Priors can be given in sensor space (e.g., some knowledge on sensor noise is available) and/or in source space (e.g., anatomical constraints on source locations, smoothness constraints). Hence, it makes sense to formulate the forward problem (the model in Bayesian terms) in a hierarchical model (see e.g. Friston et al., 2002; Sato et al., 2004 for an introduction to hierarchical Bayesian estimation):

$$\mathbf{m} = \mathbf{Lj} + \boldsymbol{\varepsilon}_1 \qquad (22)$$

$$\mathbf{j} = \mathbf{0} + \boldsymbol{\varepsilon}_2 \qquad (23)$$

Where the error terms of the model are separated into the errors at the sensor level (instrumentation noise) and those at the source level (modeling errors). In the absence of other knowledge it is practical to assume that the errors $\boldsymbol{\varepsilon}_1$, $\boldsymbol{\varepsilon}_2$ are multivariate Gaussian with zero mean:

prior on sensor noise $p(\varepsilon_1) = N_M(\mathbf{0}, \mathbf{C}_m) \Leftrightarrow p(\mathbf{m} - \mathbf{Lj}|\mathbf{j}, \mathbf{C}_m)$
$$= N_M(\mathbf{0}, \mathbf{C}_m) \qquad (24)$$

prior on dipole moments **j** $p(\varepsilon_2) = N_N(\mathbf{0}, \mathbf{C}_{jp}) \Leftrightarrow p(\mathbf{j}|\mathbf{C}_{jp})$
$$= N_N(\mathbf{0}, \mathbf{C}_{jp}) \qquad (25)$$

where $N_k(\mathbf{x}, \mathbf{C})$ is a k-dimensional multivariate Gaussian distribution with mean $\mathbf{x}$ and covariance matrix $\mathbf{C}$. Prior knowledge on the sources **j** can now be incorporated via $p(\mathbf{j}|\mathbf{C}_{jp})$ by specifying $\mathbf{C}_{jp}$: Smoothness constraints for example could be

implemented using non-zero off-diagonal elements, that enforce currents at neighboring locations to be correlated to some extent—dependent on their distance. Anatomical knowledge could be incorporated either by setting the diagonal elements $\left(\mathbf{C}_{jp}\right)_{ii}$ of $\mathbf{C}_{jp}$ for location i to zero (hard constraints) or by giving them a very small prior variance (soft constraints), if this location i has a low probability to contain a current source (e.g., location i lies in white matter). Several constraints can be incorporated by making $\mathbf{C}_{jp}$ a weighted linear sum of various constraint matrices:

$$\mathbf{C}_{jp} = \lambda_1 \mathbf{C}_{jp1} + \ldots + \lambda_l \mathbf{C}_{jpl} + \ldots \qquad (26)$$

Where the $\mathbf{C}_{jpl}$ describe different priors l and the hyperparameters λ_l describe the relative importance of these priors. If several priors at the sensor level must be incorporated this

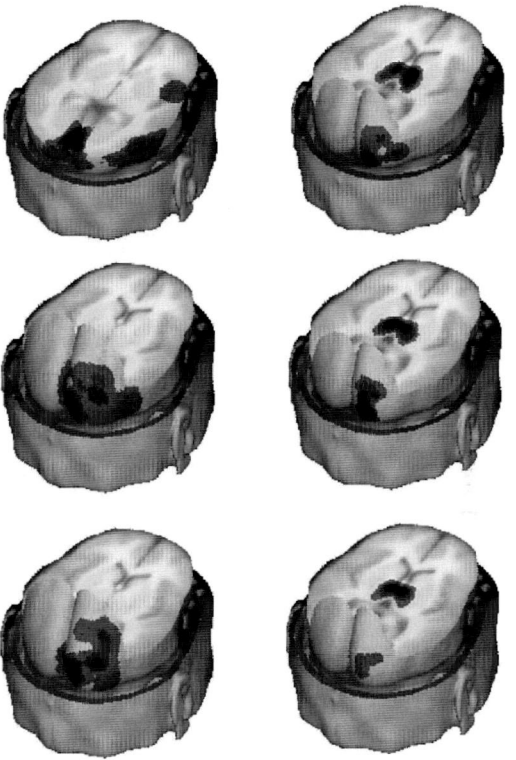

Figure 3.7.3. 3D reconstructions of the absolute values of primary current densities using Bayesian model averaging (BMA, right) and the constrained LORETA algorithm (cLORETA, left) for simulated measurements for a two-source configuration consisting of one source at the right occipital pole and one source in the thalamus. Simulated sensor arrays were: 19-channel EEG (top), 120-channel EEG (middle), 151-channel MEG (bottom). The maximum of the scale is different for each case. For cLORETA (from top to bottom): max = 0.21, 0.15, and 0.05; for BMA (from top to bottom): max = 0.41, 0.42, and 0.27. Note how cLORETA fails to recover the thalamic source, while Bayesian model averaging places sufficient weight on one of the prior models that contain a thalamic source. Figure 7 from Trujillo-Barreto NJ, Aubert-Vasquéz E, and Valdés-Sosa PA (2004) Bayesian model averaging in EEG/MEG imaging. Neuroimage 21:1300–1319. Copyright Elsevier Inc. 2004.

could be done analogously by splitting $C_m = \sum_k \mu_k C_{mk}$. The resulting posterior density of $\mathbf{j}$ then writes:

$$
\begin{aligned}
&\mathrm{p}\big(\mathbf{j}|\mathbf{m}, \{\mathbf{C}_{mk}\}, \{\mu_k\}, \{\mathbf{C}_{jpl}\}, \{\lambda_l\}\big) \\
&= \frac{\mathrm{p}(\mathbf{m}|\mathbf{j}, \{\mathbf{C}_{mk}\}, \{\mu_k\})\mathrm{p}(\mathbf{j}|\{\mathbf{C}_{jpl}\}, \{\lambda_l\})}{\mathrm{p}(\mathbf{m}|\{\mathbf{C}_{mk}\}, \{\mu_k\}, \{\mathbf{C}_{jpl}\}, \{\lambda_l\})}
\end{aligned}
\tag{27}
$$

Two minor problems arise with this approach: First, one has to deal with a hierarchical model where $\mathrm{p}(\mathbf{j}|\{\mathbf{C}_{jpl}\}, \{\lambda_l\})$ would have to be estimated by a second level of Bayesian estimation. Second, instead of just estimating the parameters $\mathbf{j}$, in addition the hyperparameters $\{\lambda_l\}, \{\mu_k\}$ have to be estimated from the data (parametrical empirical Bayes). Again we can incorporate prior knowledge on the expected values of the hyperparameters by specifying hyperpriors for these parameters. Fortunately, substitution of (25) into (24) yields a single level model (Friston et al., 2002). Hyperparameters and parameters can then be estimated recursively using an EM-algorithm (Friston et al., 2002; Phillips et al., 2002b; Phillips et al., 2002a; Phillips et al., 2005; Mattout et al., 2006) where first the Bayesian MAP estimator for $\mathbf{j}$ is computed from given some arbitrary initial values for the hyperparameters $\{\lambda_l\}, \{\mu_k\}$. For this particular estimate of $\mathbf{j}$ the values for the errors $\boldsymbol{\varepsilon}_1, \boldsymbol{\varepsilon}_2$ can be computed, and the estimate of the hyperparameters can be updated accordingly. Using the updated hyperparameters a new MAP estimate of $\mathbf{j}$ is computed and so on, until convergence. The resulting estimate then is a restricted maximum likelihood estimate of $\mathbf{j}$.

So far we have only laid out an alternative way of formulating the distributed linear inverse solution presented in one of the previous sections. This approach has the advantage that the importance of priors can be guessed from the data (Phillips et al., 2002a), instead of choosing the regularization λ ad hoc, as it was done with distributed linear inverse solutions above. Bayesian methods however unfold their true power when various competing constraints have to be incorporated in an unbiased, data driven way, or when we have to decide between various models M1, M2, ... that have the potential to explain the measured data. Such competing models could consist of one model that constrains sources to be cortical and another model that in addition searches for sources buried in the brain (Trujillo-Barreto et al., 2004). The competing models are then written as (sums of) matrices $\mathbf{C}_{jpl}$ and each model is given its own hyperparameter λ_l. Now, estimating the hyperparameters λ_l is equivalent to weighting the relative importance of the models. Using this framework it is posssible to compare and weight models that consist either of sparse activations (like discrete dipoles) or favor extended activation patches (Mattout et al., 2006; Friston et al., 2008).

We can then use Bayesian model selection (Mattout et al., 2006; Friston et al., 2008) or Bayesian model averaging (Trujillo-Barreto et al., 2004) to treat these selection problems in an unbiased manner.

Integrating Knowledge from Separately Recorded fMRI Data to Constrain the Source Analysis

The Necessity of Assumptions for the Integration of EEG and fMRI Data

Given that the neuroelectromagnetic problem is severely underdetermined one would like to include as many plausible constraints as possible in the source reconstruction process. Knowledge gained from fMRI can be easily integrated with any of the presented source localization techniques under the assumption that the BOLD fMRI signal at location $\mathbf{r}_i$ contains at least some information on the local dipole moments $\mathbf{j}(\mathbf{r}_i) = (\mathbf{j}(\mathbf{r}_i)_x, \mathbf{j}(\mathbf{r}_i)_y, \mathbf{j}(\mathbf{r}_i)_z)^T$. This assumption can take one of several forms that we list here ordered from weak to strong assumptions:

(a). "Overlapping substrates of task related activity": One assumes that the set of locations with task-related changes in the BOLD fMRI signal and the set of locations with task related local dipole moments $\Delta\mathbf{j}(\mathbf{r}_i)$ overlap:

$$
\exists \mathbf{r}_i : \quad \Delta\mathrm{BOLD}(\mathbf{r}_i) \neq 0 \quad \mathrm{AND} \quad \Delta\mathbf{j}(\mathbf{r}_i) \neq 0
\tag{28}
$$

This assumption is used (and tested) in the symmetrical Bayesian Integration of EEG and fMRI data (Trujillo-Barreto et al., 2001; Daunizeau et al., 2007).

(b). "Common substrate of task related activity": The task-related local dipole moments $\Delta\mathbf{j}(\mathbf{r}_i)$ are non-zero where the task-related BOLD fMRI signal change ($\Delta\mathrm{BOLD}$) is non-zero. However, changes in the magnitude of the task related local dipole moments $\Delta\mathbf{j}(\mathbf{r}_i)$ and in $\Delta\mathrm{BOLD}$ can in principle have a different sign. This assumption is at the heart of fMRI-constrained dipole analysis:

$$
\forall \mathbf{r}_i : \quad \Delta\mathrm{BOLD}(\mathbf{r}_i) \neq 0 \quad \Leftrightarrow \quad \Delta\mathbf{j}(\mathbf{r}_i) \neq 0
\tag{29}
$$

In fMRI-constrained dipole analysis, one would typically start assuming (29), but would check this assumption using certain validation procedures described below.

(c). "Monotonic dependency" of local dipole moments and BOLD fMRI signals: Here, the BOLD fMRI signal level is thought to depend in a monotonically increasing manner on the magnitude of the local dipole moments $\mathbf{j}(\mathbf{r}_i)$:

$$
\mathrm{BOLD}(\mathbf{r}_i) \propto f(|\mathbf{j}(\mathbf{r}_i)|) \quad f \text{ monotonically increasing}
\tag{30}
$$

This assumption is typically used in fMRI-constrained distributed linear inverse solutions.

(d). "Linearity assumption": The local BOLD fMRI signal level is thought to be strictly linearly dependent on the magnitude of the local dipole moments $\mathbf{j}(\mathbf{r}_i)$:

$$\text{BOLD}(\mathbf{r}_i, t) = |\mathbf{j}(\mathbf{r}_i, t)| \ \otimes \ \text{HRF}(\mathbf{r}_i, \tau) + c_0(\mathbf{r}_i) \quad (31)$$

Here $\otimes$ signifies the convolution operator, $\text{HRF}(\mathbf{r}_i, \tau)$ the hemodynamic response function (Boynton et al., 1996) in reaction to changing neuronal currents underlying $\mathbf{j}(\mathbf{r}_i, t)$, and $c_0(\mathbf{r}_i)$ is the offset of the local MRI signal level. All of these measures are allowed to depend on the location $\mathbf{r}_i$. The above assumption of linearity (31) is implicitly made when EEG signals are convolved with a hemodynamic response function and used as regressors for BOLD fMRI analysis and the obtained activated locations are subsequently treated as being the *electrical* generators of the scalp signal (Eichele et al., 2005; Debener et al., 2006; see also the discussion in Bledowski et al., 2007). This is because only signals conforming to this linear model have a chance to be picked up by the subsequent analysis using the general linear model (GLM). A linearity assumption is also implicit when one uses ICA to unmix concatenated EEG and fMRI data as a concatenation is only allowed when both EEG and fMRI share the same mixing matrix over trials or subjects. Hence, using the ICA decomposition over concatenated data is only correct when the linearity assumption holds (for a study that uses this approach see Calhoun et al., 2006). Note that no linearity assumption is implicit when data from both modalities are first decomposed separately and one then searches for correspondences. In this case it depends on the type of correspondence sought after which of the above assumptions (28) to (31) is explicitly used (Matsumoto et al., 2005; Eichele et al., 2008; Moosmann et al., 2008).

As pointed out by Nunez and Silberstein (Nunez and Silberstein, 2000) all of the above assumptions can be problematic. In the next sections we will describe which particular assumption is used by a particular fMRI-constrained source analysis method and whether checks of the validity of the respective assumption are possible within the framework of that source analysis method.

fMRI-Constrained Distributed Linear Inverse Solutions

If the above assumption of a monotonous dependency (30) or even that of linearity (31) holds, fMRI information can be directly used to improve the accuracy of distributed linear inverse solutions via incorporating this information into the source space metric $\mathbf{W}_p$ (see equation). This is implemented by having large penalty factors at locations, i.e., matrix elements of $\mathbf{W}_p$, where we find little BOLD fMRI activity. Hence, dipole moment estimates at these locations will lead to large undesired contributions in and will be suppressed by the minimization. A weighting matrix $\mathbf{W}_p$ that implements these principles would be given by (Babiloni et al., 2000; Babiloni et al., 2002):

$$\left(\mathbf{W}_p^{-1}\right)_{ij} = \delta_{ij}|\mathbf{L}_i|_2^{-2} f\left(\alpha_{k(i)}\right)^2 \quad (32)$$

where δ_{ij} is Kronecker's Delta and $\left(\mathbf{W}_p^{-1}\right)_{ij}$ is the ij^{th} element of the inverse of the diagonal matrix $\mathbf{W}_p$. $|\mathbf{L}_i|_2$ is the L2 norm of the vector consisting of the ith column of the leadfield $\mathbf{L}$ (corresponding to the ith dipole moment). $\alpha_{k(i)}$ describes some measure of BOLD fMRI activation at location $k(i)$[8]. Usually α is chosen to be the percentage of BOLD signal change, possibly clipped by a statistical significance mask. The function f is some suitable transformation of α. A typical choice for f is given in (Babiloni et al., 2004):

$$f\left(\alpha_{k(i)}\right) = \max\left\{1 + (K-1)\left(\frac{\alpha_{k(i)}}{\max_{k(i)}\left\{\alpha_{k(i)}\right\}}\right), K-1\right\}$$
$$(33)$$

Based on prior simulations studies Babiloni and colleagues (2003) suggest a choice of K $\approx$10. As pointed out above, the resulting metric $\mathbf{W}_p$ will punish currents in locations that were unlikely to be activated as they had little observed BOLD fMRI activity. Depending on the function f and the representation of the BOLD fMRI activity via α the influence of the fMRI based metric $\mathbf{W}_p$ can range from a subtle influence on the solution to constraining possible sources solely to the locations of significant fMRI clusters.

Note, that the incorporation of fMRI data to bias distributed inverse solutions only improves source reconstruction accuracy if the underlying assumption (30) holds. When fMRI clusters are electrically silent at the scalp level or when phase resets in ongoing electrical activity of the brain lead to detectable signals of interest (say, in an ERP analysis) at no metabolic cost, these locations may be overemphasized or eliminated from the distributed solution. As the minimum norm approach usually guarantees a unique solution with an error that is minimal in some sense, errors of this kind might prove rather difficult to detect. In contrast, fMRI-constrained dipole analysis, as presented in the next section, offers the possibility of validation steps that allow to probe the relationship between BOLD-fMRI clusters and electrical generators on a cluster-to-cluster basis. Thus, gross errors are more likely to be detected. fMRI-constrained dipole source analysis may not be applicable, however, when the true sources are spatially extended and, therefore, non-dipolar in nature.

fMRI-Constrained Dipole Source Analysis

As pointed out in the introduction to source analysis using discrete dipoles, a fundamental problem consists in choosing the right number of dipoles for the analysis. fMRI data can be used to estimate this number. In addition, further constraints can be extracted from fMRI data that might enhance the quality of the model, given that certain checks of validity are performed. Henceforth, the possible constraints derived from fMRI data will be presented sorted from weak constraints that constrain only a very limited number of degrees of freedom of our dipole model to constraints that fix all model parameters except the time course $j_i(t)$ of each dipole moment.

The weakest constraint would be to simply infer the number of dipolar sources from the number of—positively and negatively—activated fMRI clusters at a certain threshold while *fitting* all necessary six parameters per assumed dipolar source, given the number of clusters/dipoles is small enough (e.g. < 7; Ramírez, 2008). This incorporates only as little fMRI information as possible, but nevertheless relies on assumption (29) being true. Even if assumption (29) in principle holds, we encounter a practical problem with this approach: One assumes that all fMRI activations are electrically active and all electrical generators show up as fMRI activations; i.e., one assumes that fMRI activations are neither a subset nor superset of electrical generator locations. It is easy to see that in this case the "correct" choice of a statistical threshold for fMRI activations is essential for a meaningful solution. In addition, it has been shown that BOLD fMRI activations sometimes correlate well with non-stimulus-locked neuronal activations (Logothetis et al., 2001; Brookes et al., 2005; Niessing et al., 2005). Hence, when searching generators of the event-related potentials, locations of fMRI activations may very well prove to be electrically silent as far as their stimulus-locked signal content is concerned. A similar problem arises if neuronal activations from a source configuration that does not produce signals that are visible at the scalp (i.e., a closed field configuration) drive metabolic demand and produce a significant BOLD fMRI activation. In contrast, changes of the electrical activity that only reset the phase of ongoing electrical activities but do not change metabolic demand too much may well fail to elicit a sufficient BOLD fMRI response. This will lead to a true source not being considered in the model. For a more detailed discussion of these issues the reader may also refer to the treatment in (Nunez and Silberstein, 2000). These problems are particularly severe when just the number of sources and no additional information is obtained from the fMRI data.

These problems can be partially alleviated by incorporating more information from fMRI data in order to enable subsequent sanity checks (Ahlfors et al., 1999; Bledowski et al., 2004; Bledowski et al., 2006; Bledowski et al., 2007; Wibral et al., 2008; Wibral et al., 2009): If one assumes that fMRI activations are electrically active and one therefore places dipolar sources directly at these locations (rather than merely inferring their number) only their orientations and moments need to be subsequently fit. Now, electrically silent fMRI clusters have a high probability of yielding very small noise-like dipole moment time courses j(t) and can be subsequently removed from the model. This possibility may be absent if dipole locations were fitted, because in the latter case all dipoles are allowed to move during the fitting procedure and will eventually do so to pick up as much source strength/

activity as possible. Hence, there might be no chance to detect the presence of a superfluous source in the model by looking at the dipole moment time courses. Thus, fixing dipole locations takes care of the problem of electrically silent fMRI clusters, at least partially. The reciprocal problem of metabolically silent generators of electrical activations can be partially taken care of by subsequently scanning the source space with a probe source trying to explain signal variance that is not yet explained by the fMRI-constrained model. If a source location explaining a large portion of variance is found, a source is added to the model at this location. Finally, it should be checked whether dipolar sources have been positioned (and oriented) such that their leadfield coefficients (L_i) are very similar. In this case source waves will inevitably have a high degree of similarity, or "crosstalk" between the sources. If such a pair or set of sources is found, these sources should be summed and replaced by a single effective source and it should be stated that this set of sources cannot be further resolved by the analysis (Vanni et al., 2004). This guarantees that the results reported are within the limits of accuracy of this method. The above validation procedures are also schematically depicted in Figure 3.7.4. One may further assess the validity of the resulting sources by manipulating the source configuration via changes in the experimental paradigm that have known consequences at the source level (Wibral et al., 2009).

A third possibility of incorporating information from fMRI and anatomical MRI is to constrain source number and location by information derived from fMRI activations and to use the local orientation of the sheet of grey matter obtained from anatomical MRI at the locations of fMRI activations to fix the *orientation* parameters (Vanni et al., 2004). All that remains to be fitted by the (now linear) least squares procedure are the dipole moments j_i. If this approach is chosen, the additional validity checks described above (removal of silent sources, search for sources without corresponding fMRI activation, and cross-talk analysis) can and should be performed. One problem of this approach is that dipole moment time courses sensitively depend on dipole orientation. Due to the convoluted geometry of the cortical surface even relatively small displacements of the sources may lead to rather large changes in orientation. These changes in the assumed orientation will in turn lead to large errors in the reconstruction of dipole moments. Unfortunately, activated fMRI clusters may often be slightly misplaced on the cortical surface when using fMRI images obtained by normal echo planar imaging (EPI) using the T2* contrast (Ogawa et al., 1990; Ogawa et al., 1993), because the obtained fMRI images are usually distorted with respect to the anatomical MRI. Hence, utmost care has to be taken to minimize distortions in fMRI images. Possibilities for low distortion fMRI data acquisition comprise a mapping of the point spread function and subsequent image correction (Zeng and Constable, 2002; Zaitsev et al., 2004; see Wibral et al., 2009 for an application to fMRI-constrained source analysis), the use of a sequence with inherently low distortion (Liu et al., 1993;

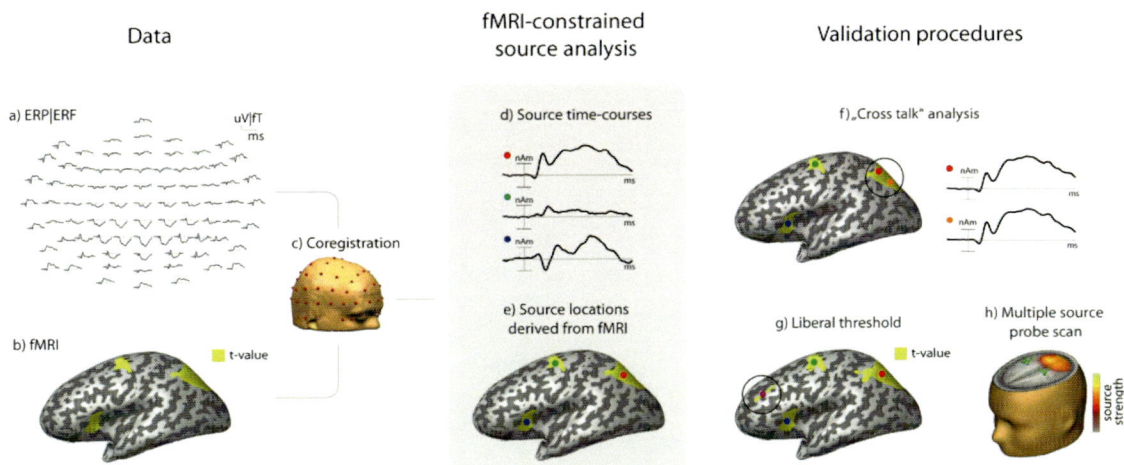

Figure 3.7.4. fMRI constrained dipole analysis with seeded source positions: In this approach, event-related potentials/fields (ERP/ERF) and fMRI data are acquired separately or simultaneously and co-registered into a common coordinate system (a–c). Neuroelectromagnetic sources are placed in candidate locations as derived from the task-related fMRI activity (e). In a fitting step, source orientations are adjusted to explain the maximum variance of the data. The source time courses then reflect localized neuroelectromagnetic activity in the cluster with millisecond resolution (d). Validation procedures: A "crosstalk" analysis excludes the possibility that the model overestimates the number of sources (f) by joining sources with near-identical time courses. Conversely, the risk of underestimating the number of sources can be addressed by lowering statistical thresholds for the fMRI data and assessing whether any additional sources make a notable contribution in explaining scalp ERP/ERF variance (g). Scanning the brain with an additional ("probe") source added to the current solution will detect locations of possible generators not included in the current model (fMRI silent electrical generators, e.g., due to phase resetting processes); these locations will be indicated by a large fraction of scalp signal variance explained by the probe source (e.g., posterior brain activity in h). If a location of this kind is found a source can be added to the model. Figure 1 from Bledowski C, Linden DEJ, Wibral M (2007) Combining electrophysiology and functional imaging: different methods for different questions, Trends Cogn Sci 11:500–502. Copyright Elsevier Inc. 2007.

Vanni et al., 2004) or optimized shimming strategies (Constable and Spencer, 1999; Glover, 1999), and careful selection of the phase encoding direction (Weiskopf et al., 2006).

Bayesian Approaches to Source Analysis Using fMRI Data as Priors

As pointed out above, prior knowledge can be incorporated within a Bayesian framework (Baillet and Garnero, 1997; Schmidt et al., 1999). For knowledge obtained from fMRI this is done in a relatively straightforward manner by specifying this information via (hyper-)priors on the hyperparameters λ_l for those constraint matrices $\mathbf{C}_{jpl}$ in Equation 27 that reflect the locations of activated fMRI clusters. The advantage of using the Bayesian approach, compared to using a classical distributed linear inverse with fMRI weighting as in Equation 32 is that the relative importance of the information from fMRI can be obtained from the data (Mattout et al., 2006; Friston et al., 2008), i.e., irrelevant information from fMRI will result in a very small hyperparameter λ_l for the respective covariance component $\mathbf{C}_{jpl}$. In this framework it is also possible to adjust the importance of prior knowledge from subject to subject (Henson et al., 2007). This approach still assumes a graded applicability of one of the assumptions 28 to 31. However, Bayesian estimation also allows to confront this problem of partial correspondence of EEG-visible and fMRI-visible neuronal activity more directly: Within a

Bayesian framework it is possible to estimate sources that are both EEG- and fMRI-visible ("common substrate") using constraints from both modalities while using only EEG data for sources that are fMRI-silent (Trujillo-Barreto et al., 2001; Daunizeau et al., 2007; Trujillo-Barreto et al., 2008). As no a priori assumption on the correspondence of EEG- and fMRI-visible generators at a certain location is made, this approach has also been called a "symmetrical" fusion of EEG and fMRI data (Trujillo-Barreto et al., 2001). When one plans to use the above symmetrical Bayesian approach to integrate EEG and fMRI data it is important to note that for separately recorded data it suffices to assume neuronal activity $a(\mathbf{r},t)$ that produces both types of measurements via two different spatiotemporal transfer functions of this neuronal activity into measurable EEG or fMRI signals, respectively. These assumptions would be incomplete for the case of *concurrently* recorded data: Here, a second set of generators $b(\mathbf{r},t)$ for the residual—scanner related—artifactual activity in the EEG trace will have to be included.

Validation by Comparison of Source Time Courses Obtained from fMRI-Constrained Source Analysis and ICA

Results of the various fMRI-constrained source analysis techniques are only reliable to the degree that the constraints used to obtain a unique solution hold. Independent validation

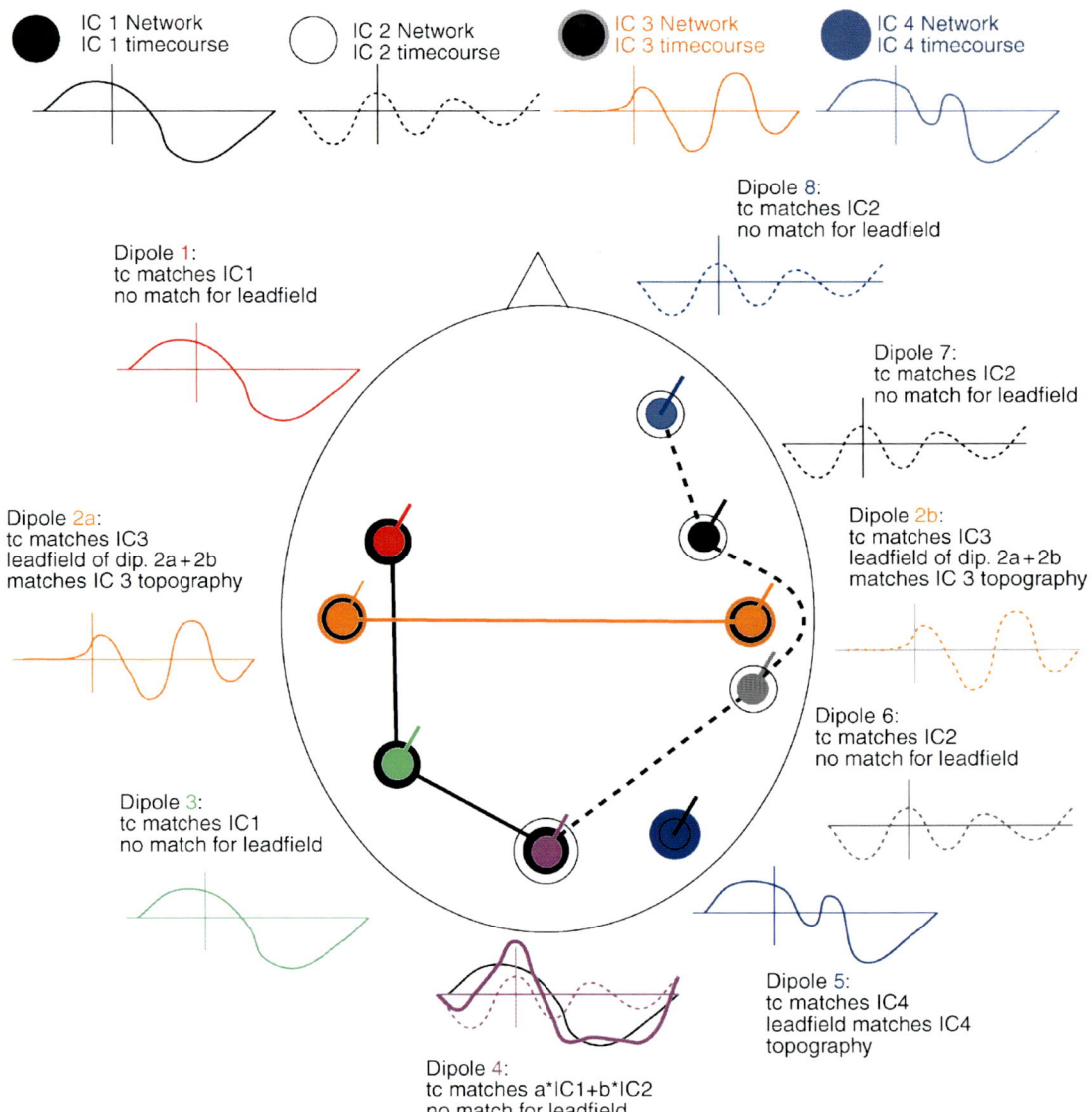

Figure 3.7.5. Schematic model of time courses (tc) and locations (circles and dipole symbols) extracted by ICA and discrete dipole source analysis, respectively. ICA separates multi-channel data into linear combinations that have maximal statistical independence, called independent components (ICs). These ICs can be generated by synchronized neurons at a single location (IC4), bilaterally symmetric (IC3) or multiple locations in the brain (ICs 1 and 2). The sets of generator locations for different ICs can partially overlap, as different neurons at the same macrosopic locations may subserve different processes. In contrast, discrete dipolar source analysis extracts the full signal at a single location. Hence, different processes may overlap in the extracted time course of a dipolar source (see dipole 4). In contrast several ICs may overlap in a certain cortical location. If an IC does not comprise generators at multiple locations both, scalp topography and time course should exactly match that of a dipolar source, thereby allowing for a cross-validation.

procedures to test the results of the source analysis can therefore enhance the reliability of the estimated results considerably. We will now present an exemplary validation step that can be applied to discrete dipolar source models and to local activation time courses from distributed models. The proposed validation is based on a statistical comparison of source time courses obtained from one of the above fMRI-informed source analysis techniques and those obtained from ICA (Figure 3.7.5). It may not be applicable to all sources of a given model, but it can establish a high degree of reliability for those sources that are successfully validated by it. A validation

is possible because the proposed procedure is based on properties of the measured data that are fully independent of fMRI-derived information. In the specific example presented in Figure 3.7.6 we compare the dipole moment time courses obtained via fMRI-constrained dipole source analyses to the independent component time courses obtained via ICA decomposition of the scalp data (Wibral et al., 2008) and search for statistically significant correlations. While there is no fundamental reason forcing all dipole moment time courses and independent component time courses to match, they have to match if a dipole moment time course

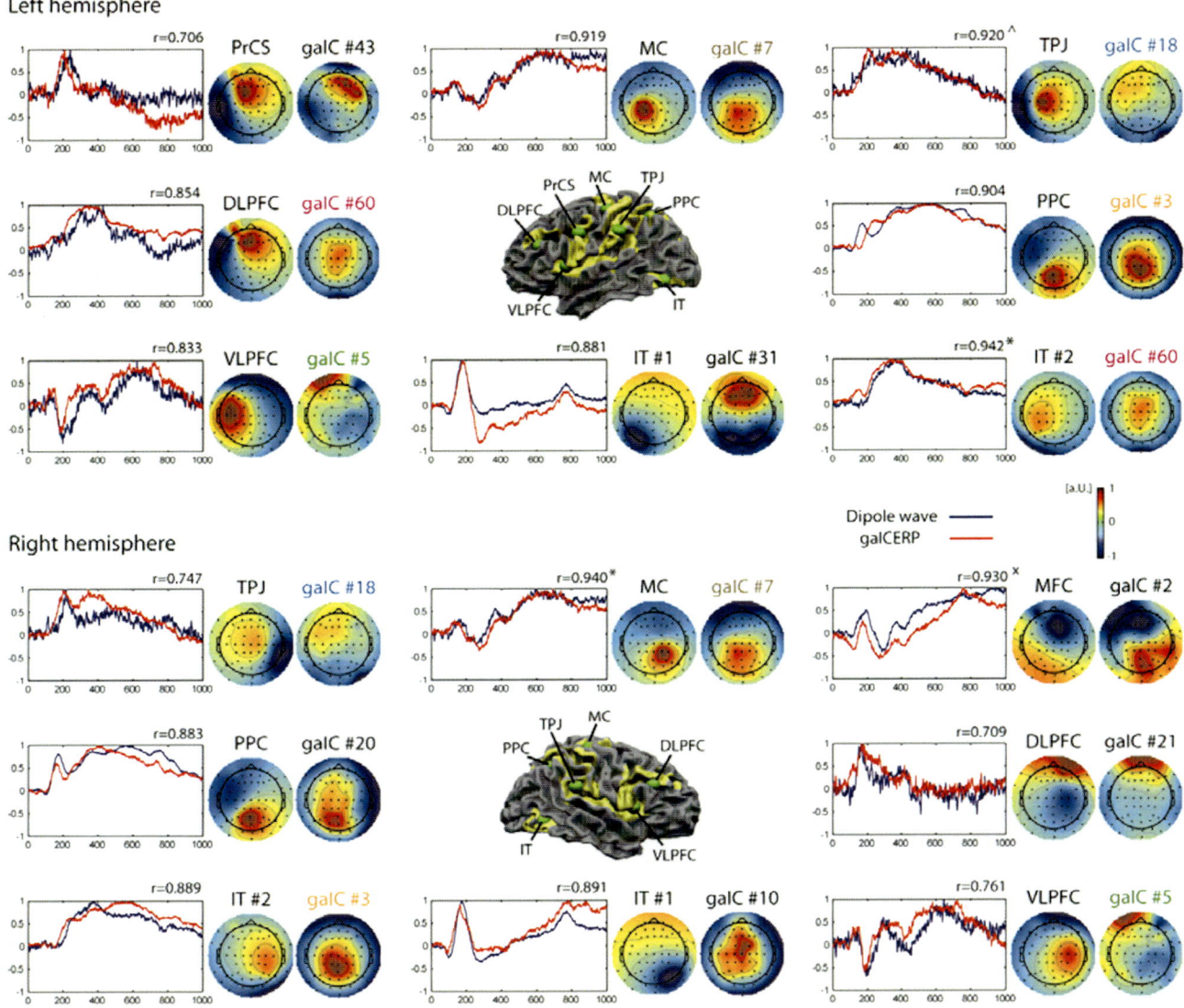

Figure 3.7.6. Results from a comparison of independent component time courses averaged over trials and subjects (gaIC) and grand average dipole moment time courses from an fMRI-constrained dipole analysis of data from a delayed match to sample visual working memory experiment. The inserts show the localization of the dipolar sources and of significant fMRI activations on a reconstruction of the grey-white matter boundary of the MNI template brain. Blue traces in time course displays are the dipole source waves, red traces are grand average IC event-related potentials. To the right of each time course display the corresponding scalp topographies are compared. Note the high degree of overlap in time courses, but not in scalp topographies perhaps pertaining to extended sets of generators for the respective independent components. Statistically significant correlations of ICs and dipole source waves and trends are indicated by $^*p < 0.05$, $^xp < 0.1$ and $^\wedge p = 0.1$. Anatomical abbreviations: DLPFC—dorsolateral prefrontal cortex, IT inferior temporal cortex, MC—motor cortex, MFC—medial frontal cortex, PPC—posterior parietal cortex, TPJ temporo-parietal junction, VLPFC—ventrolateral prefrontal cortex. Figure 1 from Wibral M, Turi G, Linden DEJ, Kaiser J, Bledowski C (2008) Decomposition of working memory related scalp ERPs: crossvalidation of fMRI-constrained source analysis and ICA, Int J Psychophysiol 67:200–211. Copyright Elsevier Inc. 2008.

representing a single and localized independent brain process has been correctly reconstructed by the fMRI-constrained source analysis. As pointed out in Figure 3.7.5, the set of dipole moment time courses with *significantly correlated* IC time courses is possibly smaller than the sets of source time courses obtained by either analysis technique alone. Interestingly enough, significantly correlated dipole moment time courses and IC time courses have indeed been found in experimental data (see Figure 6 and Wibral et al., 2008).

Comparing BOLD fMRI and Independently Localized Electrophysiological Signals

Despite numerous efforts, the mechanisms of neurovascular coupling (Magistretti et al., 1994; Pellerin and Magistretti, 1994, 1997; Magistretti and Pellerin, 1999; Magistretti and Pellerin, 2000; Zonta et al., 2003b; Zonta et al., 2003a; Cauli et al., 2004; Kasischke et al., 2004; Rancillac et al., 2006;

Pellerin et al., 2007) and the relationship between invasively (Mathiesen et al., 1998; Caesar et al., 1999; Logothetis et al., 2001) or non-invasively recorded electrophysiological signals (Arthurs and Boniface, 2002; Arthurs and Boniface, 2003; Arthurs et al., 2004; Devor et al., 2005; Niessing et al., 2005; Arthurs et al., 2007; Devor et al., 2007) and the BOLD fMRI response are still a topic of active research (also see Chapters 1.1 and 1.2 in this book). Given that there is considerable uncertainty about the degree of local coupling between EEG- and fMRI-visible neuronal activity, and that both measures do not necessarily always correlate (e.g. Liu et al., 1998; Arthurs et al., 2004; Schulz et al., 2004; Im et al., 2005), it is worthwhile considering a comparison of data from both imaging modalities to elucidate their relationship (Brookes et al., 2005), perhaps using detailed models of underlying cortical dynamics and neurovascular coupling (Riera et al., 2007). A prerequisite for this is a source analysis of electrophysiological data that, without resorting to constraints derived from fMRI data, yields reasonably accurate and reliable source localization. In the past one had to rely on results from invasive electrophysiological recordings—with their very direct means of "localizing" activity—and concurrent fMRI (Logothetis et al., 2001) or optical imaging (Devor et al.,

2005; Niessing et al., 2005) to describe the relationship of hemodynamic and electrophysiological responses. Several complications are related to these approaches. First, the very local measures of spiking or LFP activity comprise the activity of a few up to 10^3 neurons while EEG or MEG activity is thought to be due to mass action of at least 10^4 or more synchronized neurons. In addition, only a fraction of the cells that contribute to LFP activity will also contribute to measurable scalp signals (mostly the large pyramidal cells). Hence, invasive electrophysiological measures bear no simple one-to-one relationship to scalp signals like MEG or EEG, introducing an additional level of inference. Second, perhaps owing to the formidable technical challenges of this approach, the initial studies in this field were all performed in anesthetized animals, possibly compromising neurovascular coupling between neuronal activity and blood flow (see e.g. Hendrich et al., 2001; Leopold et al., 2002; Brevard et al., 2003; Wibral et al., 2007). Therefore, there is still a considerable need for analyses that allow the direct comparison of EEG and MEG signals to BOLD fMRI signals in awake human subjects. With the advent of MEG beamforming (van Veen et al., 1997; Robinson and Vrba, 1999; Sekihara et al., 2001) and newer Bayesian approaches to EEG/MEG source analysis (Baillet

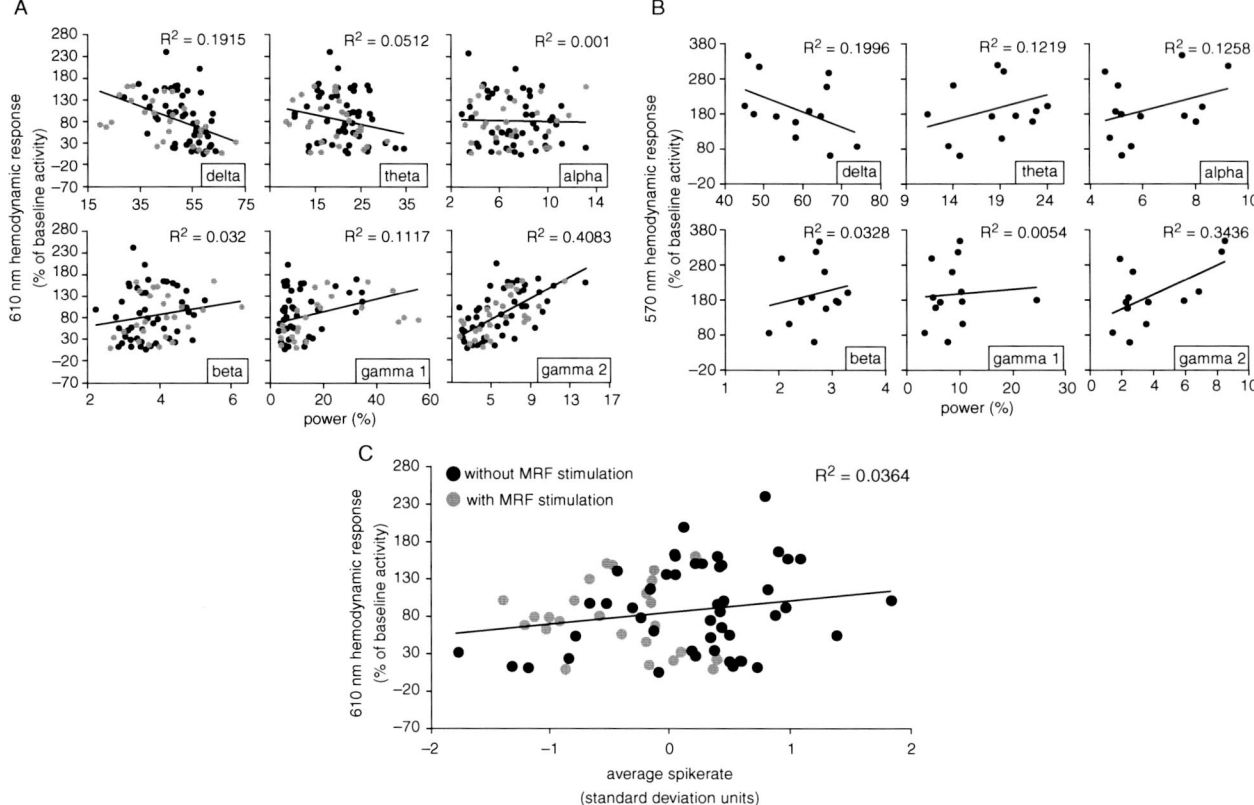

Figure 3.7.7. Correlation analysis between hemodynamic responses measured by optical imaging of intrinsic signals and local field potential (LFP) responses under constant stimulus conditions. (A and B) Scatter plots showing the relationship between hemodynamic responses obtained at 610 nm (A) and 570 nm (B) and the LFP power in different frequency bands. (C) Regression plot of hemodynamic responses at 610 nm against the spike rates averaged over all normalized multi-unit activity (MUA) channels. Figure 2 from Niessing et al. (2005) Hemodynamic signals correlate tightly with synchronized gamma oscillations. Science 309:948. Reprinted with permission from AAAS.

and Garnero, 1997; Schmidt et al., 1999; Friston et al., 2002; Trujillo-Barreto et al., 2004; Phillips et al., 2005; Friston et al., 2006; Mattout et al., 2006; Daunizeau et al., 2007; Friston et al., 2008; Kiebel et al., 2008; Trujillo-Barreto et al., 2008), localization quality has improved considerably, at least for data that have a sufficient SNR (e.g., oscillatory activities of a reasonably long duration). This gives rise to the hope that it may be possible in the future to gain insight into the relationship of non-invasive measures of electrophysiological activity and the BOLD fMRI signal by a direct comparison of reconstructed source activity and the BOLD signal. In the next paragraph we will present results that demonstrate the capability of MEG beamforming to uncover a relationship of reconstructed source signals to BOLD fMRI signals that closely matches the relationship observed with invasive electrophysiology.

Figure 3.7.7 presents results obtained from invasive electrophysiological recordings and concurrent optical imaging in the primary visual cortex of the anesthetized cat (Niessing et al., 2003; Niessing et al., 2005). Under constant stimulus conditions the hemodynamic response amplitudes, as measured by optical imaging, were negatively correlated with the

spontaneous amplitude fluctuations of local field potential (LFP) response in the delta and theta band (0.1–3 Hz and 4–8 Hz, respectively) and were positively correlated with LFP amplitudes in the beta (15–21 Hz), the low (22–48 Hz), and the high gamma band (52–90 Hz). A tight correlation of hemodynamic responses, as measured with BOLD fMRI, and LFP response amplitudes in the gamma band (40–130 Hz, peak amplitude at 73 Hz) had also previously been found for changing stimulus conditions in the visual cortex of the anesthetized macaque monkey (Logothetis et al., 2001).

A remarkably similar positive correlation between oscillatory brain activity in the higher gamma frequency range (55–70Hz), as measured with MEG beamforming, and the BOLD fMRI response was found in the visual cortex of awake human subjects as shown in Figure 3.7.8 (Brookes et al., 2005). These results compare extremely well to data obtained invasively from the macaque as pointed out by Hall and colleagues (Hall et al., 2005b; their figure 2). Interestingly enough, several potential discrepancies were observed as well. Very low frequency activity (delta waves, 0.1–4 Hz) correlated negatively with hemodynamic responses in the study of Niessing and colleagues, whereas

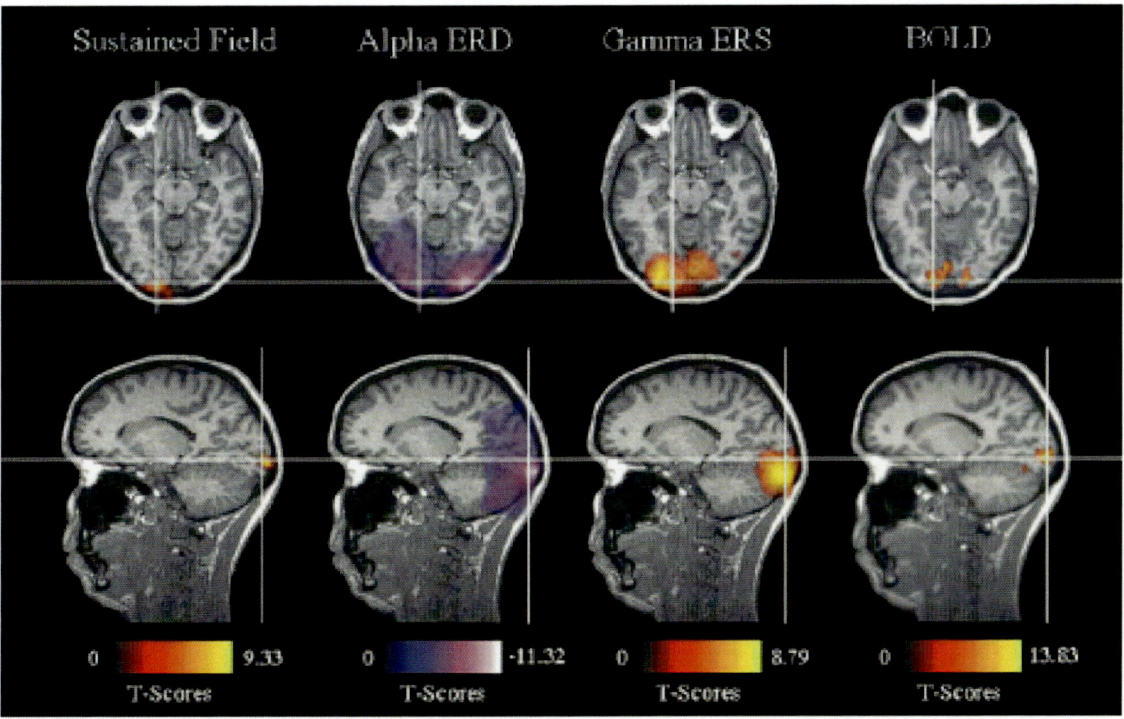

Figure 3.7.8. Comparison of beamformer general linear model source reconstructions of sustained and oscillatory neuronal activity in various frequency bands (sustained field activity, alpha band activity, gamma band activity; from left to right) in response to a visual checkerboard stimulus and the localization of BOLD fMRI activity in response to the same stimulus. In accordance with the results in (Logothetis et al., 2001; Niessing et al., 2005) gamma band activity is positively correlated with increased BOLD fMRI activity. Note the interesting positive correlation of sustained field activity and BOLD fMRI, that had not been found in the studies above before, as sustained field signals had not been recorded. This positive correlation is in line with findings of a positive correlation between slow wave ERPs and the BOLD fMRI signal (Schicke et al., 2006). Figure 1 from Brookes MJ, Gibson AM, Hall SD, Furlong PL, Barnes GR, Hillebrand A, Singh KD, Holliday IE, Francis ST, and Morris PG (2005) GLM-beamformer method demonstrates stationary field, alpha ERD and gamma ERS co-localisation with fMRI BOLD response in visual cortex. Neuroimage 26:302–308. Copyright Elsevier Inc. 2005.

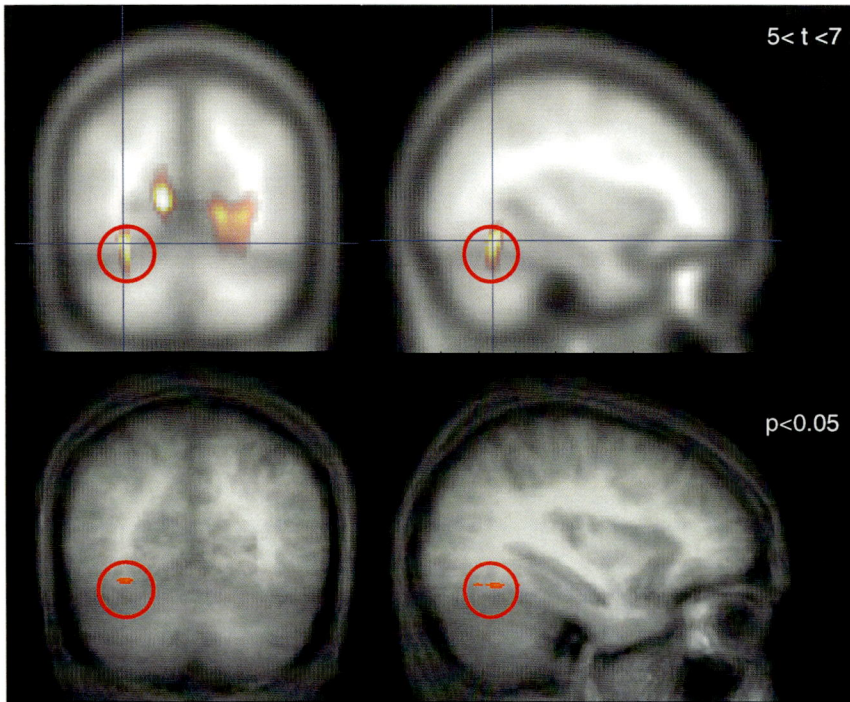

5< t <7

p<0.05

Figure 3.7.9. Face specific activity localized with MEG beamforming and BOLD fMRI. (Top) MEG beamformer localization of significant differences in power in the high gamma band (60–90Hz) in response to a stimulus correctly identified as a face compared to a stimulus correctly rejected as being a non-face stimulus. Color coded pseudo t-values run from 5 (red) to 7 (white). (Bottom) Significant BOLD fMRI activity for the same stimulus contrast ($p <$ 0.05, corrected for multiple comparisons). Talairach coordinates obtained from both localization approaches overlap and are compatible with a localization of the respective activity in the fusiform face area. (Figure courtesy of C. Tillmann; Tillmann C, Uhlhaas PJ, Kohler A, Singer W, Wibral M (2007) Using MEG and cluster randomization testing to investigate the role of oscillatory brain activty in face processing. In: Society for Neuroscience Annual Meeting. San Diego, CA.)

sustained field amplitudes in the study of Brookes and colleagues (2005) and slow ERPs in a study of Schicke and colleagues (Schicke et al., 2006) were positively correlated with BOLD fMRI responses. Alpha band activity was only weakly correlated to hemodynamic responses in the study of Niessing and colleagues (2005), whereas it was strongly negatively correlated with BOLD fMRI responses in the study of Brookes and colleagues. One reason for this apparent mismatch may be that Niessing and colleagues investigated spontaneous fluctuations of LFP power under constant stimulus conditions, whereas Brookes and colleagues used the difference between stimulation and baseline condition to establish a correlation. In order to obtain results that would be fully comparable to those obtained by Niessing and colleagues one would have to look at single trial fluctuations of the respective signals under constant stimulus conditions. This would necessitate *concurrent* recordings of electrophysiological and BOLD fMRI signals. Unfortunately, beamforming is at present only well evaluated for MEG data and a *concurrent* recording of MEG and BOLD fMRI data is not feasible to date. Two possibilities exist to resolve this problem: Attempts have been made to record MEG and MRI concurrently (Volegov et al., 2004). Perhaps more importantly, a successful evaluation of beamformer source reconstruction for *EEG* data would pave the way to combine the strengths of concurrent recordings and beamformer source reconstructions (Brookes et al., 2008).

Figure 3.7.9 shows unpublished results from our laboratory (see Tillmann et al., 2007 for a conference abstract) comparing the BOLD fMRI response that was specific to face versus non-face stimuli with results obtained using MEG beamforming of oscillatory activity in the high gamma frequency range (60–90 Hz) for the same statistical contrast (face versus non-face). These results suggest that the correspondence of BOLD fMRI responses and oscillatory activity in the high gamma range may hold beyond primary sensory cortices and for complex stimulus comparisons.

As demonstrated by the above examples the direct comparison of results from fMRI-independent source reconstructions and BOLD fMRI signals can yield important insight, with MEG beamforming being the source reconstruction technique best evaluated in this respect (Brookes et al., 2005; Hillebrand et al., 2005).

Conclusion

With the advent of concurrent EEG/fMRI recordings the researcher today is faced with the difficult question whether this new method is worth the considerable investment of time, effort and funding with regard to her or his research goals. As described elsewhere in this book, concurrent recordings of EEG/fMRI data open up exciting new possibilities like the analysis of single-trial fluctuations and joint decomposition via ICA. Concurrent recordings are mandatory in experiments where rapid learning is involved or where the predictors for the analysis of BOLD fMRI data must be obtained from electrophysiological signals. An important example for the latter scenario is the application of concurrent recordings in epilepsy research by Laufs and colleagues presented in the Chapter 4.2. We hope to have shown, however, that several traditional analyses profit from the superior signal-to-noise ratio currently offered by combining separately recorded

EEG/MEG and fMRI data sets. Both ICA and Bayesian estimation profit from the presence of fewer sources in the data, because no components or prior distributions for residual MRI related artifacts have to be incorporated in the data model. In addition, certain types of studies require the flexibility to optimize the paradigm separately for the incongruent requirements of EEG and fMRI recordings. In all these cases the researcher may consider sticking with recording EEG and fMRI separately. Ultimately, the comparison of *independently* localized MEG/EEG and BOLD fMRI activity and the identification of the shared and disparate sets of their generators may foster our understanding of BOLD fMRI activity and of brain function. It is here that the full usefulness of concurrently or separately recorded datasets of high quality from both measurement modalities may be found.

NOTES

1. BOLD fMRI clusters that emerge in this kind of correlation analysis with EEG-derived predictors are, of course, very likely to be related to the process generating the EEG phenomenon under investigation. It is a lot less certain, however, that all of the found clusters represent *electrical* generators that are really visible in the recorded scalp signals. Thus the problem here is rather one of careful interpretation of results.
2. Intracellular currents have to pass through the dendrite; the return path for extracellular currents comprises all conducting tissue in the head.
3. Although when approaching $\mathbf{r}_k$, there are differences in the fields generated by a true current dipole and $\mathbf{i}_{(1)}(\mathbf{r}_k, t)$.
4. While Equation 5 had no unique solution. In addition, $\mathbf{W}$ and $\mathbf{W}_p$ are assumed to be positive definite here. If $\mathbf{W}$ and $\mathbf{W}_p$ are not positive definite but positive semidefinite, the additional condition Null space($\mathbf{W}$) $\cap$ Null space ($\mathbf{W}_p$) = $\{\mathbf{0}\}$ is required for a unique solution.
5. However, the existence of a unique solution by no means implies that this solution is anywhere near the true $\mathbf{j}$ when $\mathbf{W}_p$ is not chosen wisely to reflect reasonable constraints derived from anatomy and/or physiology.
6. Strictly speaking, this is only true if no other source b has an activity time course that is highly correlated with a(t). This is because the above algorithm will choose coefficients $\{w_{ai}\}$ such that output power is minimized while adhering to the unity gain constraint. Some allowed sets of weights under this constraint have large negative weights for sensors close to an hypothetical source b. Now, if b(t) is highly correlated to a(t), such a particular set of weights can be used to minimize the power even further than it would be possible for uncorrelated sources, without violating the unity gain constraint. As a rule of thumb, this effect seriously affects the results of MEG beamforming once normalized correlation coefficients between two sources start to exceed 0.7.
7. Consider the influence of excessive sensor noise, for example, that often leads to sources being shifted toward the center of the head in discrete dipole source analysis.
8. The index k only covers the 3D locations in space, i.e. It runs from 1...N, whereas i runs from 1...3N, due to the

decomposition of the local vector $\mathbf{j}$ into its three components: j_x, j_y, j_z. The location vector $\mathbf{r}(k(i))$ therefore is the same for three subsequent indices i: $k(i)$ = ceiling($i/3$)

REFERENCES

Ahlfors SP, Simpson GV, Dale AM, Belliveau JW, Liu AK, Korvenoja A, Virtanen J, Huotilainen M, Tootell RB, Aronen HJ, Ilmoniemi RJ (1999) Spatiotemporal activity of a cortical network for processing visual motion revealed by MEG and fMRI. J Neurophysiol 82:2545–2555.

Allen PJ, Josephs O, Turner R (2000) A method for removing imaging artifact from continuous EEG recorded during functional MRI. Neuroimage 12:230–239.

Allen PJ, Polizzi G, Krakow K, Fish DR, Lemieux L (1998) Identification of EEG events in the MR scanner: the problem of pulse artifact and a method for its subtraction. Neuroimage 8:229–239.

Amari S (1999) Natural gradient learning for over- and under-complete bases In ICA. Neural Comput 11:1875–1883.

Arthurs OJ, Boniface S (2002) How well do we understand the neural origins of the fMRI BOLD signal? Trends Neurosci 25:27–31.

Arthurs OJ, Boniface SJ (2003) What aspect of the fMRI BOLD signal best reflects the underlying electrophysiology in human somatosensory cortex? Clin Neurophysiol 114:1203–1209.

Arthurs OJ, Johansen-Berg H, Matthews PM, Boniface SJ (2004) Attention differentially modulates the coupling of fMRI BOLD and evoked potential signal amplitudes in the human somatosensory cortex. Exp Brain Res 157:269–274.

Arthurs OJ, Donovan T, Spiegelhalter DJ, Pickard JD, Boniface SJ (2007) Intracortically distributed neurovascular coupling relationships within and between human somatosensory cortices. Cereb Cortex 17:661–668.

Babiloni F, Babiloni C, Carducci F, Gratta CD, Romani GL, Rossini PM, Cincotti F (2002) Cortical source estimate of combined high resolution EEG and fMRI data related to voluntary movements. Methods Inf Med 41:443–450.

Babiloni F, Carducci F, Cincotti F, Gratta CD, Roberti GM, Romani GL, Rossini PM, Babiloni C (2000) Integration of high resolution EEG and functional magnetic resonance in the study of human movement-related potentials. Methods Inf Med 39:179–182.

Babiloni F, Mattia D, Babiloni C, Astolfi L, Salinari S, Basilisco A, Rossini PM, Marciani MG, Cincotti F (2004) Multimodal integration of EEG, MEG and fMRI data for the solution of the neuroimage puzzle. Magn Reson Imaging 22:1471–1476.

Baillet S, Garnero L (1997) A Bayesian approach to introducing anatomo-functional priors in the EEG/MEG inverse problem. IEEE Trans Biomed Eng 44:374–385.

Barbati G, Porcaro C, Hadjipapas A, Adjamian P, Pizzella V, Romani GL, Seri S, Tecchio F, Barnes GR (2008) Functional source separation applied to induced visual gamma activity. Hum Brain Mapp 29:131–141.

Bardouille T, Picton TW, Ross B (2006) Correlates of eye blinking as determined by synthetic aperture magnetometry. Clin Neurophysiol 117:952–958.

Belardinelli P, Ciancetta L, Pizzella V, Gratta CD, Romani GL (2006) Localizing complex neural circuits with MEG data. Cogn Process 7:53–59.

Bledowski C, Linden DEJ, Wibral M (2007) Combining electrophysiology and functional imaging - different methods for different questions. Trends Cogn Sci 11:500–502.

Bledowski C, Prvulovic D, Hoechstetter K, Scherg M, Wibral M, Goebel R, Linden DEJ (2004) Localizing P300 generators in visual target and distractor processing: a combined event-related potential and functional magnetic resonance imaging study. J Neurosci 24:9353–9360.

Bledowski C, Kadosh KC, Wibral M, Rahm B, Bittner RA, Hoechstetter K, Scherg M, Maurer K, Goebel R, Linden DEJ (2006) Mental chronometry of working memory retrieval: a combined functional magnetic resonance imaging and event-related potentials approach. J Neurosci 26:821–829.

Blimke J, Myklebust J, Volkmer H, Merrill S (2008) Four-shell ellipsoidal model employing multipole expansion in ellipsoidal coordinates. Med Biol Eng Comput 46:859–869.

Boynton GM, Engel SA, Glover GH, Heeger DJ (1996) Linear systems analysis of functional magnetic resonance imaging in human V1. J Neurosci 16:4207–4221.

Brevard ME, Duong TQ, King JA, Ferris CF (2003) Changes in MRI signal intensity during hypercapnic challenge under conscious and anesthetized conditions. Magn Reson Imaging 21:995–1001.

Brookes MJ, Mullinger KJ, Stevenson CM, Morris PG, Bowtell R (2008) Simultaneous EEG source localisation and artifact rejection during concurrent fMRI by means of spatial filtering. Neuroimage 40:1090–1104.

Brookes MJ, Gibson AM, Hall SD, Furlong PL, Barnes GR, Hillebrand A, Singh KD, Holliday IE, Francis ST, Morris PG (2005) GLM-beamformer method demonstrates stationary field, alpha ERD and gamma ERS co-localisation with fMRI BOLD response in visual cortex. Neuroimage 26:302–308.

Buchner H, Knoll G, Fuchs M, Rienäcker A, Beckmann R, Wagner M, Silny J, Pesch J (1997) Inverse localization of electric dipole current sources in finite element models of the human head. Electroencephalogr Clin Neurophysiol 102:267–278.

Caesar K, Akgören N, Mathiesen C, Lauritzen M (1999) Modification of activity-dependent increases in cerebellar blood flow by extracellular potassium in anaesthetized rats. J Physiol 520 Pt 1:281–292.

Calhoun VD, Adali T, Pearlson GD, Kiehl KA (2006) Neuronal chronometry of target detection: fusion of hemodynamic and event-related potential data. Neuroimage 30:544–553.

Cauli B, Tong X-K, Rancillac A, Serluca N, Lambolez B, Rossier J, Hamel E (2004) Cortical GABA interneurons in neurovascular coupling: relays for subcortical vasoactive pathways. J Neurosci 24:8940–8949.

Cheyne D, Bakhtazad L, Gaetz W (2006) Spatiotemporal mapping of cortical activity accompanying voluntary movements using an event-related beamforming approach. Hum Brain Mapp 27:213–229.

Cheyne D, Bostan AC, Gaetz W, Pang EW (2007) Event-related beamforming: a robust method for presurgical functional mapping using MEG. Clin Neurophysiol 118:1691–1704.

Cheyne D, Gaetz W, Garnero L, Lachaux J-P, Ducorps A, Schwartz D, Varela FJ (2003) Neuromagnetic imaging of cortical oscillations accompanying tactile stimulation. Brain Res Cogn Brain Res 17:599–611.

Comon P (1994) Independent Component Analysis, a new concept? Signal Processing 36:287–314.

Constable RT, Spencer DD (1999) Composite image formation in z-shimmed functional MR imaging. Magn Reson Med 42:110–117.

Dale AM, Liu AK, Fischl BR, Buckner RL, Belliveau JW, Lewine JD, Halgren E (2000) Dynamic statistical parametric mapping: combining fMRI and MEG for high-resolution imaging of cortical activity. Neuron 26:55–67.

Daunizeau J, Grova C, Marrelec G, Mattout J, Jbabdi S, Pélégrini-Issac M, Lina J-M, Benali H (2007) Symmetrical event-related EEG/fMRI information fusion in a variational Bayesian framework. Neuroimage 36:69–87.

de Munck JC (1992) A linear discretization of the volume conductor boundary integral equation using analytically integrated elements. IEEE Trans Biomed Eng 39:986–990.

de Munck JC, Gonçalves SI, Huijboom L, Kuijer JPA, Pouwels PJW, Heethaar RM, da Silva FHL (2007) The hemodynamic response of the alpha rhythm: an EEG/fMRI study. Neuroimage 35:1142–1151.

de Peralta-Menendez RG, Gonzalez-Andino SL (1998) A critical analysis of linear inverse solutions to the neuroelectromagnetic inverse problem. IEEE Trans Biomed Eng 45:440–448.

de Peralta Menendez RG, Andino SLG, Morand S, Michel CM, Landis T (2000) Imaging the electrical activity of the brain: ELECTRA. Hum Brain Mapp 9:1–12.

de Peralta Menendez RG, Andino SG, Lantz G, Michel CM, Landis T (2001) Noninvasive localization of electromagnetic epileptic activity. I. Method descriptions and simulations. Brain Topogr 14:131–137.

Debener S, Ullsperger M, Siegel M, Engel AK (2006) Single-trial EEG-fMRI reveals the dynamics of cognitive function. Trends Cogn Sci 10:558–563.

Debener S, Mullinger KJ, Niazy RK, Bowtell RW (2008) Properties of the ballistocardiogram artefact as revealed by EEG recordings at 1.5, 3 and 7 T static magnetic field strength. Int J Psychophysiol 67:189–199.

Debener S, Strobel A, Sorger B, Peters J, Kranczioch C, Engel AK, Goebel R (2007) Improved quality of auditory event-related potentials recorded simultaneously with 3-T fMRI: removal of the ballistocardiogram artefact. Neuroimage 34:587–597.

Devor A, Ulbert I, Dunn AK, Narayanan SN, Jones SR, Andermann ML, Boas DA, Dale AM (2005) Coupling of the cortical hemodynamic response to cortical and thalamic neuronal activity. Proc Natl Acad Sci U S A 102:3822–3827.

Devor A, Tian P, Nishimura N, Teng IC, Hillman EMC, Narayanan SN, Ulbert I, Boas DA, Kleinfeld D, Dale AM (2007) Suppressed neuronal activity and concurrent arteriolar vasoconstriction may explain negative blood oxygenation level-dependent signal. J Neurosci 27:4452–4459.

Eichele T, Specht K, Moosmann M, Jongsma MLA, Quiroga RQ, Nordby H, Hugdahl K (2005) Assessing the spatiotemporal evolution of neuronal activation with single-trial event-related potentials and functional MRI. Proc Natl Acad Sci U S A 102:17798–17803.

Eichele T, Calhoun VD, Moosmann M, Specht K, Jongsma MLA, Quiroga RQ, Nordby H, Hugdahl K (2008) Unmixing concurrent EEG-fMRI with parallel independent component analysis. Int J Psychophysiol 67:222–234.

Everson R, Roberts SJ (1999) Non-stationary independent component analysis. In: Proc. Artificial Neural Networks Ninth International Conference on (Conf. Publ. No. 470), pp 503–508. Edinburgh, UK.

Fawcett IP, Barnes GR, Hillebrand A, Singh KD (2004) The temporal frequency tuning of human visual cortex investigated using synthetic aperture magnetometry. Neuroimage 21:1542–1553.

Ferguson AS, Stroink G (1997) Factors affecting the accuracy of the boundary element method in the forward problem–I: Calculating surface potentials. IEEE Trans Biomed Eng 44:1139–1155.

Filbey FM, Holroyd T, Carver F, Sunderland T, Cohen RM (2005) A magnetoencephalography spatiotemporal analysis of neural activities during feature binding. Neuroreport 16:1747–1752.

Friston K, Henson R, Phillips C, Mattout J (2006) Bayesian estimation of evoked and induced responses. Hum Brain Mapp 27:722–735.

Friston K, Penny W, Phillips C, Kiebel S, Hinton G, Ashburner J (2002) Classical and Bayesian inference in neuroimaging: theory. Neuroimage 16:465–483.

Friston K, Harrison L, Daunizeau J, Kiebel S, Phillips C, Trujillo-Barreto N, Henson R, Flandin G, Mattout J (2008) Multiple sparse priors for the M/EEG inverse problem. Neuroimage 39:1104–1120.

Gaetz WC, Cheyne DO (2003) Localization of human somatosensory cortex using spatially filtered magnetoencephalography. Neurosci Lett 340:161–164.

George JS, Aine CJ, Mosher JC, Schmidt DM, Ranken DM, Schlitt HA, Wood CC, Lewine JD, Sanders JA, Belliveau JW (1995) Mapping function in the human brain with magnetoencephalography, anatomical magnetic resonance imaging, and functional magnetic resonance imaging. J Clin Neurophysiol 12:406–431.

Glover GH (1999) 3D z-shim method for reduction of susceptibility effects in BOLD fMRI. Magn Reson Med 42:290–299.

Gonçalves SI, de Munck JC, Pouwels PJW, Schoonhoven R, Kuijer JPA, Maurits NM, Hoogduin JM, Someren EJWV, Heethaar RM, da Silva FHL (2006) Correlating the alpha rhythm to BOLD using simultaneous EEG/fMRI: inter-subject variability. Neuroimage 30:203–213.

Gruber T, Maess B, Trujillo-Barreto NJ, Muller MM (2008) Sources of synchronized induced Gamma-Band responses during a simple object recognition task: a replication study in human MEG. Brain Res 1196:74–84.

Gruber T, Trujillo-Barreto NJ, Giabbiconi CM, Valdes-Sosa PA, Muller MM (2006) Brain electrical tomography (BET) analysis of induced gamma band responses during a simple object recognition task. Neuroimage 29:888–900.

Gutiérrez D, Nehorai A (2008) Array response kernels for EEG and MEG in multilayer ellipsoidal geometry. IEEE Trans Biomed Eng 55:1103–1111.

Hall SD, Barnes GR, Hillebrand A, Furlong PL, Singh KD, Holliday IE (2004) Spatio-temporal imaging of cortical desynchronization in migraine visual aura: a magnetoencephalography case study. Headache 44:204–208.

Hall SD, Holliday IE, Hillebrand A, Furlong PL, Singh KD, Barnes GR (2005a) Distinct contrast response functions in striate and extra-striate regions of visual cortex revealed with magnetoencephalography (MEG). Clin Neurophysiol 116:1716–1722.

Hall SD, Holliday IE, Hillebrand A, Singh KD, Furlong PL, Hadjipapas A, Barnes GR (2005b) The missing link: analogous human and primate cortical gamma oscillations. Neuroimage 26:13–17.

Hämäläinen MS, Ilmoniemi RJ (1984) Interpreting measured magnetic fields of the brain: Estimates of current distributions. In: Technical Report TKK-F-A559: Helsinki University of Technology, Dept. of Technical Physics.

Hämäläinen MS, Sarvas J (1989) Realistic conductivity geometry model of the human head for interpretation of neuromagnetic data. IEEE Trans Biomed Eng 36:165–171.

Helmholtz H (1853) Über einige Gesetze der Vertheilung elektrischer ströme in körperlichen leitern mit Anwendung auf die thierisch-elektrischen Versuche. Annalen der Physik und Chemie 89:211–233 and 353–377.

Hendrich KS, Kochanek PM, Melick JA, Schiding JK, Statler KD, Williams DS, Marion DW, Ho C (2001) Cerebral perfusion during anesthesia with fentanyl, isoflurane, or pentobarbital in normal rats studied by arterial spin-labeled MRI. Magn Reson Med 46:202–206.

Henning S, Merboldt K-D, Frahm J (2006) Task- and EEG-correlated analyses of BOLD MRI responses to eyes opening and closing. Brain Res 1073–1074: 359–364.

Henson RN, Mattout J, Singh KD, Barnes GR, Hillebrand A, Friston K (2007) Population-level inferences for distributed MEG source localization under multiple constraints: application to face-evoked fields. Neuroimage 38:422–438.

Hillebrand A, Singh KD, Holliday IE, Furlong PL, Barnes GR (2005) A new approach to neuroimaging with magnetoencephalography. Hum Brain Mapp 25:199–211.

Huang MX, Shih JJ, Lee RR, Harrington DL, Thoma RJ, Weisend MP, Hanlon F, Paulson KM, Li T, Martin K, Millers GA, Canive JM (2004) Commonalities and differences among vectorized beamformers in electromagnetic source imaging. Brain Topogr 16:139–158.

Im C-H, Jung H-K, Fujimaki N (2005) fMRI-constrained MEG source imaging and consideration of fMRI invisible sources. Hum Brain Mapp 26:110–118.

Inki M, Hyvarinen A (2002) Two approaches to estimation of overcomplete independent component bases. In: Proc. International Joint Conference on Neural Networks IJCNN '02, pp 454–459.

Jun SC, George JS, Kim W, Paré-Blagoev J, Plis S, Ranken DM, Schmidt DM (2008) Bayesian brain source imaging based on combined MEG/EEG and fMRI using MCMC. Neuroimage 40:1581–1594.

Jutten C, Herault J (1991) Blind separation of sources, part I: An adaptive algorithm based on neuromimetic architecture. Signal Processing 24:1–10.

Kaiser J, Lutzenberger W (2005) Human gamma-band activity: a window to cognitive processing. Neuroreport 16:207–211.

Kaiser J, Bühler M, Lutzenberger W (2004) Magnetoencephalographic gamma-band responses to illusory triangles in humans. Neuroimage 23:551–560.

Kaiser J, Heidegger T, Wibral M, Altmann CF, Lutzenberger W (2008) Distinct Gamma-Band Components Reflect the Short-Term Memory Maintenance of Different Sound Lateralization Angles. Cereb Cortex in press.

Kasischke KA, Vishwasrao HD, Fisher PJ, Zipfel WR, Webb WW (2004) Neural activity triggers neuronal oxidative metabolism followed by astrocytic glycolysis. Science 305:99–103.

Kawaguchi S, Ukai S, Shinosaki K, Ishii R, Yamamoto M, Ogawa A, Mizuno-Matsumoto Y, Fujita N, Yoshimine T, Takeda M (2005) Information processing flow and neural activations in the dorsolateral prefrontal cortex in the Stroop task in schizophrenic patients. A spatially filtered MEG analysis with high temporal and spatial resolution. Neuropsychobiology 51:191–203.

Kiebel SJ, Daunizeau J, Phillips C, Friston KJ (2008) Variational Bayesian inversion of the equivalent current dipole model in EEG/MEG. Neuroimage 39:728–741.

Laufs H, Lengler U, Hamandi K, Kleinschmidt A, Krakow K (2006a) Linking generalized spike-and-wave discharges and resting state brain activity by using EEG/fMRI in a patient with absence seizures. Epilepsia 47:444–448.

Laufs H, Kleinschmidt A, Beyerle A, Eger E, Salek-Haddadi A, Preibisch C, Krakow K (2003a) EEG-correlated fMRI of human alpha activity. Neuroimage 19:1463–1476.

Laufs H, Krakow K, Sterzer P, Eger E, Beyerle A, Salek-Haddadi A, Kleinschmidt A (2003b) Electroencephalographic signatures of attentional and cognitive default modes in spontaneous brain activity fluctuations at rest. Proc Natl Acad Sci U S A 100:11053–11058.

Laufs H, Holt JL, Elfont R, Krams M, Paul JS, Krakow K, Kleinschmidt A (2006b) Where the BOLD signal goes when alpha EEG leaves. Neuroimage 31:1408–1418.

Lemieux L, Laufs H, Carmichael D, Paul JS, Walker MC, Duncan JS (2008) Noncanonical spike-related BOLD responses in focal epilepsy. Hum Brain Mapp 29:329–345.

Leopold DA, Plettenberg HK, Logothetis NK (2002) Visual processing in the ketamine-anesthetized monkey. Optokinetic and blood oxygenation level-dependent responses. Exp Brain Res 143:359–372.

Liu AK, Belliveau JW, Dale AM (1998) Spatiotemporal imaging of human brain activity using functional MRI constrained magnetoencephalography data: Monte Carlo simulations. Proc Natl Acad Sci U S A 95:8945–8950.

Liu G, Sobering G, Duyn J, Moonen CT (1993) A functional MRI technique combining principles of echo-shifting with a train of observations (PRESTO). Magn Reson Med 30:764–768.

Logothetis NK (2002) The neural basis of the blood-oxygen-level-dependent functional magnetic resonance imaging signal. Philos Trans R Soc Lond B Biol Sci 357:1003–1037.

Logothetis NK, Pauls J, Augath M, Trinath T, Oeltermann A (2001) Neurophysiological investigation of the basis of the fMRI signal. Nature 412:150–157.

Luo Q, Holroyd T, Jones M, Hendler T, Blair J (2007) Neural dynamics for facial threat processing as revealed by gamma band synchronization using MEG. Neuroimage 34:839–847.

Magistretti PJ, Pellerin L (1999) Astrocytes Couple Synaptic Activity to Glucose Utilization in the Brain. News Physiol Sci 14:177–182.

Magistretti PJ, Pellerin L (2000) The astrocyte-mediated coupling between synaptic activity and energy metabolism operates through volume transmission. Prog Brain Res 125:229–240.

Magistretti PJ, Sorg O, Naichen Y, Pellerin L, de Rham S, Martin JL (1994) Regulation of astrocyte energy metabolism by neurotransmitters. Ren Physiol Biochem 17:168–171.

Mangun GR, Hopfinger JB, Jha AP (2000) Integrating electrophysiology and neuroimaging in the study of brain function. Adv Neurol 84:35–49.

Mantini D, Perrucci MG, Gratta CD, Romani GL, Corbetta M (2007) Electrophysiological signatures of resting state networks in the human brain. Proc Natl Acad Sci U S A 104:13170–13175.

Mathiesen C, Caesar K, Akgören N, Lauritzen M (1998) Modification of activity-dependent increases of cerebral blood flow by excitatory synaptic activity and spikes in rat cerebellar cortex. J Physiol 512 (Pt 2):555–566.

Matsumoto A, Iidaka T, Haneda K, Okada T, Sadato N (2005) Linking semantic priming effect in functional MRI and event-related potentials. Neuroimage 24:624–634.

Mattout J, Phillips C, Penny WD, Rugg MD, Friston KJ (2006) MEG source localization under multiple constraints: an extended Bayesian framework. Neuroimage 30:753–767.

Meijs JW, Weier OW, Peters MJ, van Oosterom A (1989) On the numerical accuracy of the boundary element method. IEEE Trans Biomed Eng 36:1038–1049.

Meltzer JA, Negishi M, Mayes LC, Constable RT (2007) Individual differences in EEG theta and alpha dynamics during working memory correlate with fMRI responses across subjects. Clin Neurophysiol 118:2419–2436.

Mirsattari SM, Wang Z, Ives JR, Bihari F, Leung LS, Bartha R, Menon RS (2006) Linear aspects of transformation from inter-ictal epileptic discharges to BOLD fMRI signals in an animal model of occipital epilepsy. Neuroimage 30:1133–1148.

Moosmann M, Eichele T, Nordby H, Hugdahl K, Calhoun VD (2008) Joint independent component analysis for simultaneous EEG-fMRI: principle and simulation. Int J Psychophysiol 67:212–221.

Moosmann M, Ritter P, Krastel I, Brink A, Thees S, Blankenburg F, Taskin B, Obrig H, Villringer A (2003) Correlates of alpha rhythm in functional magnetic resonance imaging and near infrared spectroscopy. Neuroimage 20:145–158.

Mosher JC, Lewis PS, Leahy RM (1992) Multiple dipole modeling and localization from spatio-temporal MEG data. IEEE J BME 39:541–557.

Muthukumaraswamy SD, Singh KD (2008) Spatiotemporal frequency tuning of BOLD and gamma band MEG responses compared in primary visual cortex. Neuroimage 40:1552–1560.

Niessing J, Ebisch B, Schmidt KE, Niessing M, Singer W, Galuske RAW (2005) Hemodynamic signals correlate tightly with synchronized gamma oscillations. Science 309:948–951.

Niessing M, Schmidt K, Singer W, Galuske R (2003) Precise placement of multiple electrodes into functionally predefined cortical locations. J Neurosci Methods 126:195–207.

Nolte G (2003) The magnetic lead field theorem in the quasi-static approximation and its use for magnetoencephalography forward calculation in realistic volume conductors. Phys Med Biol 48:3637–3652.

Nolte G, Dassios G (2005) Analytic expansion of the EEG lead field for realistic volume conductors. Phys Med Biol 50:3807–3823.

Nummenmaa A, Auranen T, Hämäläinen MS, Jääskeläinen IP, Sams M, Vehtari A, Lampinen J (2007a) Automatic relevance determination based hierarchical Bayesian MEG inversion in practice. Neuroimage 37:876–889.

Nummenmaa A, Auranen T, Hämäläinen MS, Jääskeläinen IP, Lampinen J, Sams M, Vehtari A (2007b) Hierarchical Bayesian estimates of distributed MEG sources: theoretical aspects and comparison of variational and MCMC methods. Neuroimage 35:669–685.

Nunez PL, Silberstein RB (2000) On the relationship of synaptic activity to macroscopic measurements: does co-registration of EEG with fMRI make sense? Brain Topogr 13:79–96.

Ogawa S, Lee TM, Kay AR, Tank DW (1990) Brain magnetic resonance imaging with contrast dependent on blood oxygenation. Proc Natl Acad Sci U S A 87:9868–9872.

Ogawa S, Menon RS, Tank DW, Kim SG, Merkle H, Ellermann JM, Ugurbil K (1993) Functional brain mapping by blood oxygenation level-dependent contrast magnetic resonance imaging. A comparison of signal characteristics with a biophysical model. Biophys J 64:803–812.

Oishi M, Otsubo H, Iida K, Suyama Y, Ochi A, Weiss SK, Xiang J, Gaetz W, Cheyne D, Chuang SH, Rutka JT, Snead OC (2006) Preoperative simulation of intracerebral epileptiform discharges: synthetic aperture magnetometry virtual sensor analysis of interictal magnetoencephalography data. J Neurosurg 105:41–49.

Pascual-Marqui RD (1999) Review of methods for solving the EEG inverse problem. Int J Bioelectromagn 1:75–86.

Pascual-Marqui RD (2002) Standardized low-resolution brain electromagnetic tomography (sLORETA): technical details. Methods Find Exp Clin Pharmacol 24 Suppl D:5–12.

Pascual-Marqui RD, Michel CM, Lehmann D (1994) Low resolution electromagnetic tomography: a new method for localizing electrical activity in the brain. Int J Psychophysiol 18:49–65.

Pellerin L, Magistretti PJ (1994) Glutamate uptake into astrocytes stimulates aerobic glycolysis: a mechanism coupling neuronal activity to glucose utilization. Proc Natl Acad Sci U S A 91:10625–10629.

Pellerin L, Magistretti PJ (1997) Glutamate uptake stimulates Na+, K+-ATPase activity in astrocytes via activation of a distinct subunit highly sensitive to ouabain. J Neurochem 69:2132–2137.

Pellerin L, Bouzier-Sore A-K, Aubert A, Serres S, Merle M, Costalat R, Magistretti PJ (2007) Activity-dependent regulation of energy metabolism by astrocytes: an update. Glia 55:1251–1262.

Phillips C, Rugg MD, Fristont KJ (2002a) Systematic regularization of linear inverse solutions of the EEG source localization problem. Neuroimage 17:287–301.

Phillips C, Rugg MD, Friston KJ (2002b) Anatomically informed basis functions for EEG source localization: combining functional and anatomical constraints. Neuroimage 16:678–695.

Phillips C, Mattout J, Rugg MD, Maquet P, Friston KJ (2005) An empirical Bayesian solution to the source reconstruction problem in EEG. Neuroimage 24:997–1011.

Popescu M, Popescu E-A, Chan T, Blunt SD, Lewine JD (2008) Spatio-temporal reconstruction of bilateral auditory steady-state responses using MEG beamformers. IEEE Trans Biomed Eng 55:1092–1102.

Ramírez RR (2008) Source localization. In: Scholarpedia.

Rancillac A, Rossier J, Guille M, Tong X-K, Geoffroy H, Amatore C, Arbault S, Hamel E, Cauli B (2006) Glutamatergic Control of Microvascular Tone by Distinct GABA Neurons in the Cerebellum. J Neurosci 26:6997–7006.

Riera JJ, Jimenez JC, Wan X, Kawashima R, Ozaki T (2007) Nonlinear local electrovascular coupling. II: From data to neuronal masses. Hum Brain Mapp 28:335–354.

Robinson SE, Vrba J (1999) Functional neuroimaging by synthetic aperture magnetometry (SAM). In: Recent Advances in Biomagnetism (Yoshimoto T, Kotani M, Kuriki S, Karibe H, Nakasato N, eds), pp 302–305: Tohoku University Press, Sendai, Japan.

Rodionov R, Martino FD, Laufs H, Carmichael DW, Formisano E, Walker M, Duncan JS, Lemieux L (2007) Independent component analysis of interictal fMRI in focal epilepsy: comparison with general linear model-based EEG-correlated fMRI. Neuroimage 38:488–500.

Sarvas J (1987) Basic mathematical and electromagnetic concepts of the biomagnetic inverse problem. Phys Med Biol 32:11–22.

Sato M-a, Yoshioka T, Kajihara S, Toyama K, Goda N, Doya K, Kawato M (2004) Hierarchical Bayesian estimation for MEG inverse problem. Neuroimage 23:806–826.

Scherg M, Berg P (1991) Use of prior knowledge in brain electromagnetic source analysis. Brain Topogr 4:143–150.

Schicke T, Muckli L, Beer AL, Wibral M, Singer W, Goebel R, Rösler F, Röder B (2006) Tight covariation of BOLD signal changes and slow ERPs in the parietal cortex in a parametric spatial imagery task with haptic acquisition. Eur J Neurosci 23:1910–1918.

Schimpf PH (2007) Application of quasi-static magnetic reciprocity to finite element models of the MEG lead-field. IEEE Trans Biomed Eng 54:2082–2088.

Schlitt HA, Heller L, Aaron R, Best E, Ranken DM (1995) Evaluation of boundary element methods for the EEG forward problem: effect of linear interpolation. IEEE Trans Biomed Eng 42:52–58.

Schmidt DM, George JS, Wood CC (1999) Bayesian inference applied to the electromagnetic inverse problem. Hum Brain Mapp 7:195–212.

Schulz M, Chau W, Graham SJ, McIntosh AR, Ross B, Ishii R, Pantev C (2004) An integrative MEG-fMRI study of the primary somatosensory cortex using cross-modal correspondence analysis. Neuroimage 22:120–133.

Sekihara K, Nagarajan SS, Poeppel D, Marantz A, Miyashita Y (2001) Reconstructing spatio-temporal activities of neural sources using an MEG vector beamformer technique. IEEE Trans Biomed Eng 48:760–771.

Singh KD, Barnes GR, Hillebrand A, Forde EME, Williams AL (2002) Task-related changes in cortical synchronization are spatially coincident with the hemodynamic response. Neuroimage 16:103–114.

Speckmann EJ, Elger CE (1993) Introduction to the Neurophysiological basis of the EEG and DC Potentials. In: Electroencephalography: Basic Principles, Clinical Applications, and Related Fields (Lopes da Silva F, Niedermeyer E, eds), pp 15–26. Baltimore: Williams & Wilkins.

Tallon-Baudry C, Bertrand O (1999) Oscillatory gamma activity in humans and its role in object representation. Trends Cogn Sci 3:151–162.

Tallon-Baudry C, Bertrand O, Pernier J (1999) A ring-shaped distribution of dipoles as a source model of induced gamma-band activity. Clin Neurophysiol 110:660–665.

Tallon-Baudry C, Bertrand O, Delpuech C, Pernier J (1996) Stimulus specificity of phase-locked and non-phase-locked 40 Hz visual responses in human. J Neurosci 16:4240–4249.

Tallon-Baudry C, Bertrand O, Wienbruch C, Ross B, Pantev C (1997) Combined EEG and MEG recordings of visual 40 Hz responses to illusory triangles in human. Neuroreport 8:1103–1107.

Taylor MJ, Mills T, Smith ML, Pang EW (2008) Face processing in adolescents with and without epilepsy. Int J Psychophysiol 68:94–103.

Tiége XD, Laufs H, Boyd SG, Harkness W, Allen PJ, Clark CA, Connelly A, Cross JH (2007) EEG-fMRI in children with pharmacoresistant focal epilepsy. Epilepsia 48:385–389.

Tillmann C, Uhlhaas PJ, Kohler A, Singer W, Wibral M (2007) Using MEG and cluster randomization testing to investigate the role of oscillatory brain activty in face processing. In: Society for Neuroscience Annual Meeting. San Diego.

Trujillo-Barreto NJ, Martínez-Montes E, Valdés-Sosa PA (2001) A symmetrical Bayesian Model for fMRI and EEG/MEG

Neuroimage Fusion. International Journal of Bioelectromagnetism 3(1).

Trujillo-Barreto NJ, Aubert-Vázquez E, Valdés-Sosa PA (2004) Bayesian model averaging in EEG/MEG imaging. Neuroimage 21:1300–1319.

Trujillo-Barreto NJ, Aubert-Vázquez E, Penny WD (2008) Bayesian M/EEG source reconstruction with spatio-temporal priors. Neuroimage 39:318–335.

Ukai S, Shinosaki K, Ishii R, Ogawa A, Mizuno-Matsumoto Y, Inouye T, Hirabuki N, Yoshimine T, Robinson SE, Takeda M (2002) Parallel distributed processing neuroimaging in the Stroop task using spatially filtered magnetoencephalography analysis. Neurosci Lett 334:9–12.

Ukai S, Kawaguchi S, Ishii R, Yamamoto M, Ogawa A, Mizuno-Matsumoto Y, Robinson SE, Fujita N, Yoshimine T, Shinosaki K, Takeda M (2004) SAM(g2) analysis for detecting spike localization: a comparison with clinical symptoms and ECD analysis in an epileptic patient. Neurol Clin Neurophysiol 2004:57.

van Veen BD, van Drongelen W, Yuchtman M, Suzuki A (1997) Localization of brain electrical activity via linearly constrained minimum variance spatial filtering. IEEE Trans Biomed Eng 44:867–880.

Vanni S, Warnking J, Dojat M, Delon-Martin C, Bullier J, Segebarth C (2004) Sequence of pattern onset responses in the human visual areas: an fMRI constrained VEP source analysis. Neuroimage 21:801–817.

Volegov P, Matlachov AN, Espy MA, George JS, Kraus RH (2004) Simultaneous magnetoencephalography and SQUID detected nuclear MR in microtesla magnetic fields. Magn Reson Med 52:467–470.

Weiskopf N, Hutton C, Josephs O, Deichmann R (2006) Optimal EPI parameters for reduction of susceptibility-induced BOLD sensitivity losses: a whole-brain analysis at 3 T and 1.5 T. Neuroimage 33:493–504.

Wibral M, Turi G, Linden DEJ, Kaiser J, Bledowski C (2008) Decomposition of working memory-related scalp ERPs: cross-validation of fMRI-constrained source analysis and ICA. Int J Psychophysiol 67:200–211.

Wibral M, Bledowski C, Kohler A, Singer W, Muckli L (2009) The timing of feedback to early visual cortex in the perception of long-range apparent motion. Cerebral Cortex: in press.

Wibral M, Muckli L, Melnikovic K, Scheller B, Alink A, Singer W, Munk MH (2007) Time-dependent effects of hyperoxia on the BOLD fMRI signal in primate visual cortex and LGN. Neuroimage 35:1044–1063.

Wipf D, Nagarajan S (2008) A unified Bayesian framework for MEG/EEG source imaging. Neuroimage.

Zaitsev M, Hennig J, Speck O (2004) Point spread function mapping with parallel imaging techniques and high acceleration factors: fast, robust, and flexible method for echo-planar imaging distortion correction. Magn Reson Med 52:1156–1166.

Zeng H, Constable RT (2002) Image distortion correction in EPI: comparison of field mapping with point spread function mapping. Magn Reson Med 48:137–146.

Zonta M, Sebelin A, Gobbo S, Fellin T, Pozzan T, Carmignoto G (2003a) Glutamate-mediated cytosolic calcium oscillations regulate a pulsatile prostaglandin release from cultured rat astrocytes. J Physiol 553:407–414.

Zonta M, Angulo MC, Gobbo S, Rosengarten B, Hossmann K-A, Pozzan T, Carmignoto G (2003b) Neuron-to-astrocyte signaling is central to the dynamic control of brain microcirculation. Nat Neurosci 6:43–50.

3.8 Stefan J. Kiebel, Marta I. Garrido, and Karl J. Friston

Analyzing Effective Connectivity with EEG and MEG

Introduction

A key goal in M/EEG methods research is to identify models that describe the mapping from the underlying neuronal system to the observed M/EEG response. These models should incorporate known or assumed constraints (David and Friston, 2003; Sotero et al., 2007). By using biophysically and neuronally informed forward models we can use the M/EEG to make explicit statements about the underlying biophysical and neuronal parameters (David et al., 2006). This approach, informed by biophysics and neurobiology, is not only critical to link M/EEG models (and any inferences made) to existing knowledge about neuronal mechanisms, but will also be a cornerstone for future models of multimodal data (Kiebel and Friston, 2004; Riera et al., 2007; Sotero and Trujillo-Barreto, 2008).

One important class of constraints is the assumption that M/EEG data can be explained as the output of a few interconnected brain sources. To employ and make inference about these temporal effective-connectivity parameters, one has to deal with another important physical constraint: In M/EEG, brain sources express themselves in many sensors instantaneously. To estimate temporal parameters like effective connectivity one has to either *(1)* remove this spatial mixing by estimating the time courses of the underlying brain sources (Chen et al., 2008; Gross et al., 2001; Kujala et al., 2007), or *(2)* specify a full spatiotemporal model that explains M/EEG data in the sensors (Daunizeau et al., 2006; Friston et al., 2008; Jun et al., 2005). In this chapter, we will describe a model of the second kind, a full spatiotemporal model, which can be used to infer about effective connectivity among a few interconnected brain sources. In the following, we will motivate this model, dynamic causal modeling (DCM), by observing that there have been three important developments in M/EEG analysis in recent years.

The first development is that standard computers are now powerful enough to perform sophisticated analyses in a routine fashion (David et al., 2006). This and many other analyses would have been impractical ten years ago, even for low-density EEG measurements. Second, the way methods researchers describe their M/EEG models has changed dramatically in the last decade. Recent descriptions tend to specify the critical assumptions underlying the model, followed by the inversion technique. This is useful because models for M/EEG can be complex; specifying the model explicitly also makes a statement about how one believes data were generated. This makes model development more effective and transparent, because fully specified models can be compared to other models.

The third substantial advance is the advent of Empirical or hierarchical Bayesian approaches to M/EEG model inversion. Bayesian approaches are important, because they allow for the introduction of constraints that ensure robust parameter estimation, for example (Auranen et al., 2007; Nummenmaa et al., 2007; Penny et al., 2007; Zumer et al., 2007). This is vital once the model is complex enough to generate ambiguities (conditional dependencies) among groups of parameters. One could avoid these correlations among parameter estimates by avoiding complex models. However, this would preclude further research into the mechanisms behind the M/EEG. An empirical Bayesian formulation allows the data to resolve these ambiguities and uncertainties. The traditional argument against the use of Bayesian methods is that the priors introduce "artificial" or "biased" information not solicited by the data. Essentially, the claim is that the priors enforce solutions that are desired by the researcher. This argument can be discounted for three reasons: *(1)* In Empirical Bayesian procedures the weight afforded by the priors is determined by the data, not the analyst. *(2)* Bayesian analysis provides the posterior distribution, which encodes uncertainty about the parameters, after observing the data. If the posterior is similar to the prior, then the data do not contain sufficient information to enable qualitative inference. This can be tested explicitly using the model evidence (see below); the fact that a parameter cannot be resolved is informative in itself. *(3)* Usually, Bayesian analysis explores a selection of models, followed by model comparison (Garrido et al., 2007a). For example, one can invert a model[1] derived from one's favorite cognitive neuroscience theory, along with other alternative models. The best model can then be found by comparing model evidences using standard decision criteria (Penny et al., 2004).

In summary, we argue that the combination of these developments allows for models that are sophisticated enough to capture the full richness of the data. The Bayesian approach is central to this new class of models; without it, it is not possible to constrain complex models or deal with inherent correlations among parameter estimates. Bayesian model comparison represents the important tool of selecting the best among competing models, which is central to the scientific process.

Dynamic causal modeling (DCM) provides a generative spatiotemporal model for M/EEG responses. The idea central to DCM is that M/EEG data are the response of a dynamic input-output system to experimental inputs. It is assumed that the sensory inputs are processed by a network of discrete but interacting neuronal sources. For each source, we use a neural mass model, which describes responses of neuronal subpopulations. Each population has its own (intrinsic) dynamics governed by the neural mass equations, but also receives extrinsic input, either directly as sensory input or from other sources. The whole set of sources and their interactions are fully specified by a set of first-order differential equations that are formally related to other neural mass models used in computational models of M/EEG (Breakspear et al., 2006; Rodrigues et al., 2006; Sotero et al., 2007; Marreiros et al., 2008; Sotero et al., 2007). We assume that the depolarization of pyramidal cell populations gives rise to observed M/EEG data; one specifies how these depolarizations are expressed in the sensors through a conventional leadfield. The full, spatiotemporal model takes the form of a non-linear state-space model with hidden states modeling (unobserved) neuronal dynamics, while the observation (leadfield) equation is instantaneous and linear in the states. In other words, the model consists of a temporal and spatial part with temporal (e.g., connectivity between two sources) and spatial parameters (e.g., leadfield parameters like equivalent current dipole [ECD] locations). In the next section, we describe the DCM equations and demonstrate how the ensuing model is inverted using Bayesian techniques. We illustrate inference and the usefulness of this approach using evoked responses from a multisubject EEG data set (Garrido et al., 2007b; Garrido et al., 2007a). We conclude with a discussion about current DCM algorithms and point to some promising future developments.

Dynamic Causal Modeling: Theory

Intuitively, the DCM scheme regards an experiment as a designed perturbation of neuronal dynamics that are promulgated and distributed throughout a system of coupled anatomical sources to produce region-specific responses. This system is modeled using a dynamic input-state-output system with multiple inputs and outputs. Responses are evoked by deterministic inputs that correspond to experimental manipulations (i.e., presentation of stimuli). Experimental factors (i.e., stimulus attributes or context) can also change the parameters or causal architecture of the system producing these responses. The state variables cover both the neuronal activities and other neurophysiological or biophysical variables needed to form the outputs. Outputs are those components of neuronal responses that can be detected by MEG/EEG sensors. In our model, these components are depolarizations of a "neural mass" of pyramidal cells. DCM starts with a reasonably realistic neuronal model of interacting cortical regions. This model is then supplemented with a spatial forward model of how neuronal activity is transformed into measured responses, here, M/EEG scalp-averaged responses. This enables the parameters of the neuronal model (e.g., effective connectivity) to be estimated from observed data. For M/EEG data, this spatial model is a forward model of electromagnetic measurements that accounts for volume conduction effects (Mosher et al., 1999).

Hierarchical MEG/EEG Neural Mass Model

DCMs for M/EEG adopt a neural mass model (David and Friston, 2003) to explain source activity in terms of the ensemble dynamics of interacting inhibitory and excitatory subpopulations of neurons, based on the model of Jansen and Rit (1995). This model emulates the activity of a source using three neural subpopulations, each assigned to one of three cortical layers; an excitatory subpopulation in the granular layer, an inhibitory subpopulation in the supragranular layer and a population of deep pyramidal cells in the infragranular layer. The excitatory pyramidal cells receive excitatory and inhibitory input from local interneurons (via intrinsic connections, confined to the cortical sheet), and send excitatory outputs to remote cortical sources via extrinsic connections. See also Grimbert and Faugeras (2006) for a bifurcation analysis of this model.

In David et al. (2005) we developed a hierarchical cortical model to study the influence of forward, backward, and lateral connections on evoked responses. This model embodies directed extrinsic connections among a number of sources, each based on the Jansen model (Jansen and Rit, 1995), using the connectivity rules described in (Felleman and Van Essen, 1991). Using these rules, it is straightforward to construct any hierarchical cortico-cortical network model of cortical sources. Under simplifying assumptions, directed connections can be classified as: *(1)* Bottom-up or forward connections that originate in the infragranular layers and terminate in the granular layer. *(2)* Top–down or backward connections that connect infragranular to agranular layers. *(3)* Lateral connections that originate in infragranular layers and target all layers. These long-range or extrinsic cortico-cortical connections are excitatory and are mediated through the axonal processes of pyramidal cells. For simplicity, we do not consider thalamic connections, but model thalamic afferents as a function encoding subcortical input (see below).

The Jansen and Rit model emulates the MEG/EEG activity of a cortical source using three neuronal subpopulations. A population of excitatory pyramidal (output) cells receives inputs from inhibitory and excitatory populations of inter-neurons, via intrinsic connections. Within this model, exci-tatory interneurons can be regarded as spiny stellate cells found predominantly in layer 4 and in receipt of forward connections. Excitatory pyramidal cells and inhibitory inter-neurons occupy agranular layers and receive both intrinsic and extrinsic backward and lateral inputs. The ensuing DCM is specified in terms of its state-equations and an observer or output equation

$$
\begin{aligned}
x &= f(x, u, \theta) \\
h &= g(x, \theta)
\end{aligned}
\tag{1}
$$

where x is the neuronal states of cortical sources, u is exogenous inputs, and h is the system's response. θ is quantities that parameterize the state and observer equations (see also below under "Prior assumptions"). The state-equations are ordinary first-order differential equations and are derived from the behavior of the three neu-ronal subpopulations, which operate as linear damped oscillators. The integration of the differential equations pertaining to each subpopulation can be expressed as a convolution of the exogenous input to produce the response (David and Friston, 2003). This convolution transforms the average density of presynaptic inputs into an average postsynaptic membrane potential, where the convolution kernel is given by

$$
p(t)_e =
\begin{cases}
\dfrac{H_e}{\tau_e} t \exp(-t/\tau_e) & t \geq 0 \\
0 & t < 0
\end{cases}
\tag{2}
$$

Here, the subscript "e" stands for "excitatory". Similarly sub-script "i" is used for inhibitory synapses. H controls the maximum postsynaptic potential, and τ represents a lumped rate constant. An operator S transforms the potential of each subpopulation into firing rate, which is the exogenous input to other subpopulations. This operator is assumed to be an instantaneous sigmoid nonlinearity of the form

$$
S(x) = \frac{1}{1 + \exp(-\rho_1(x - \rho_2))} - \frac{1}{1 + \exp(\rho_1 \rho_2)}
\tag{3}
$$

where the free parameters ρ_1 and ρ_2 determine its slope and translation. Interactions, among the subpopulations, depend on internal coupling constants, $\gamma_{1,2,3,4}$, which con-trol the strength of intrinsic connections and reflect the total number of synapses expressed by each subpopulation (see Figure 3.8.1). The integration of this model, to form predicted responses, rests on formulating these two opera-tors (Equations 2 and 3) in terms of a set of differential

equations as described in David and Friston (2003). These equations, for all sources, can be integrated using the matrix exponential of the systems Jacobian as described in the appendices of David et al. (2006). Critically, the integration scheme allows for conduction delays on the connections, which are free parameters of the model. A DCM, at the network level, obtains by coupling sources with extrinsic forward, backward, and lateral connections as described above.

Event-Related Input and Event-Related Response-Specific Effects

To model event-related responses, the network receives inputs from the environment via input connections. These connections are exactly the same as forward connections and deliver inputs u to the spiny stellate cells in layer 4 of specified sources. In the present context, inputs u model afferent activity relayed by subcortical structures and are modeled with two components: The first is a gamma density function (truncated to peristimulus time). This models an event-related burst of input that is delayed with respect to stimulus onset and dispersed by subcortical synapses and axonal conduction. Being a density function, this component integrates to one over peristimulus time. The second compo-nent is a discrete cosine set modeling systematic fluctuations in input, as a function of peristimulus time. In our imple-mentation, peristimulus time is treated as a state variable, allowing the input to be computed explicitly during integra-tion. Critically, the event-related input is exactly the same for all ERPs. The effects of experimental factors are mediated through event-related response (ERR)-specific changes in connection strengths. See Figure 3.8.1 for a summary of the resulting differential equations.

We can model differential responses to different stimuli in two ways. The first is when the effects of experimental factors are mediated through changes in extrinsic connection strengths (David et al., 2006). For example, this extrinsic mechanism can be used to explain ERP (event-related poten-tial) differences by modulating forward (bottom-up) or back-ward (top-down) coupling. The second mechanism involves changing the intrinsic architecture; of the sort mediating local adaptation. Changes in connectivity are expressed as differences in intrinsic, forward, backward, or lateral con-nections that confer a selective sensitivity on each source, in terms of its response to others. The experimental or sti-mulus-specific effects are modeled by coupling gains

$$
\begin{aligned}
A_{ijk}^F &= A_{ij}^F B_{ijk} \\
A_{ijk}^B &= A_{ij}^B B_{ijk} \\
A_{ijk}^L &= A_{ij}^L B_{ijk}
\end{aligned}
\tag{4}
$$

Here, A_{ij} encodes the strength of a connection to the ith source from the jth and B_{ijk} encodes its gain for the kth ERP. The superscripts (F, B, or L) indicate the type of connection, i.e., forward, backward, or lateral (see also Figure 3.8.1). By

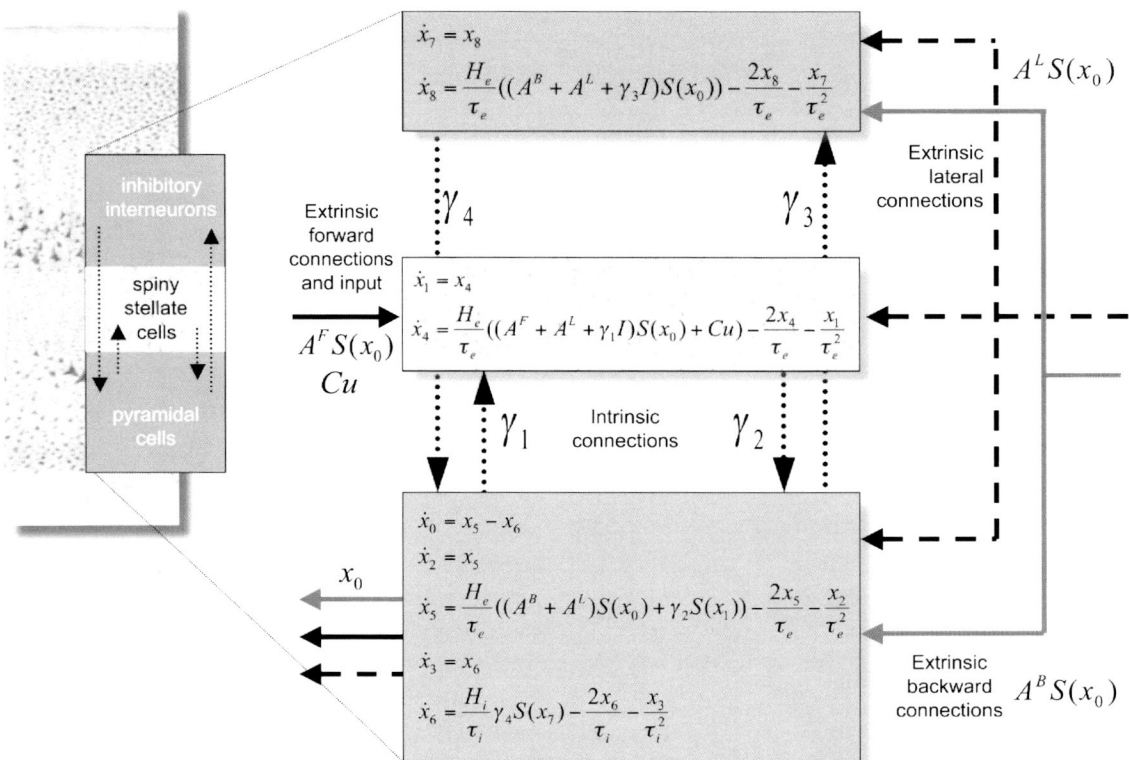

Figure 3.8.1. Neuronal state-equations. A source consists of three neuronal subpopulations, which are connected by four intrinsic connections with weights $\gamma_{1,2,3,4}$. Mean firing rates (Equation 3) from other sources arrive via forward A^F, backward A^B, and lateral A^L connections. Similarly, exogenous input Cu enters receiving sources. The output of each subpopulation is its transmembrane potential (Equation 2). From Olivier et al. (2006) with permission.

convention, we set the gain of the first ERP to unity, so that the gains of subsequent ERPs are relative to the first. The reason we model extrinsic modulations in terms of gain (a multiplicative factor), as opposed to additive effects, is that by construction, connections should always be positive. This is assured; provided both the connection and its gain are positive. In this context, a (positive) gain of less than one represents a decrease in connection strength.

Note that if we considered the gains as elements of a gain matrix, the intrinsic gain would occupy the leading diagonal. Intrinsic modulation can explain important features of typical evoked responses, which are difficult to model with a modulation of extrinsic connections (Kiebel et al., 2007). We model the modulation of intrinsic connectivity by a gain on the amplitude H_e of the synaptic kernel (Equation 2). A gain greater than one effectively increases the maximum response that can be elicited from a source. For the ith source:

$$H_{ek}^{(i)} = H_e^{(i)} B_{iik} \qquad (5)$$

The Spatial Forward Model

The dendritic signal of the pyramidal subpopulation of the ith source $x_0^{(i)}$ is detected remotely on the scalp surface in M/

EEG. The relationship between scalp data h and source activity is assumed to be linear and instantaneous

$$h = g(x, \theta) = L(\theta^L)x_0 \qquad (6)$$

where L is a leadfield matrix (i.e., spatial forward model), which accounts for passive conduction of the electromagnetic field (Mosher et al., 1999). Here, we assume that the spatial expression of each source is caused by one equivalent current dipole (ECD). Of course, one can use different source models, e.g., extended patches on the cortical surface (Daunizeau et al. 2009). The head model for the dipoles is based on four concentric spheres, each with homogeneous and isotropic conductivity. The four spheres approximate the brain, skull, cerebrospinal fluid, and scalp. The parameters of the model are the radii and conductivities for each layer. Here, we use as radii 71, 72, 79, and 85 mm, with conductivities 0.33, 1.0, 0.0042, and 0.33 s/m respectively. The potential at the sensors requires an evaluation of an infinite series, which can be approximated using fast algorithms (Mosher et al., 1999; Zhang, 1995). The leadfield of each ECD is then a function of three location and three orientation or moment parameters $\theta^L = \{\theta^{pos}, \theta^{mom}\}$. For the ECD forward model, we used a Matlab (Mathworks) routine that is freely available as part of the FieldTrip package (http://fieldtrip.fcdonders.nl/), under the GNU general public license.

Data Reduction

For computational expediency, we generally reduce the dimensionality of the sensor data: in previous versions of DCM (David et al., 2006; Kiebel et al., 2006), we projected the data onto the principal eigenvectors of the sample covariance matrix of the data. This retained the maximum amount of information in the reduced data. However, this projection is not informed about which data can be explained by the model. Effectively, this projection spans data that cannot be generated by the model. In more recent versions of our software, we use the principal components of the prior covariance of the data, which are a function of, and only of, the model:

The prior covariance of the signal in sensor space C^h follows from Equation 6

$$
\begin{aligned}
C^h &= \left\langle hh^T \right\rangle_{p(\theta)} = \left\langle Lx_0 x_0^T L^T \right\rangle_{p(\theta)} \\
&= \left\langle \sum_{ij} \Delta\theta_i \frac{\partial L}{\partial \theta_i} C^x \frac{\partial L}{\partial \theta_j}^T \Delta\theta_j \right\rangle_{p(\theta)} = \sum_{ij} C_{ij}^L \frac{\partial L}{\partial \theta_i} C^x \frac{\partial L}{\partial \theta_j}^T \\
C_{ij}^L &= \left\langle \Delta\theta_i \Delta\theta_j \right\rangle_{p(\theta)} \\
C^x &= \left\langle x_0 x_0^T \right\rangle_{p(\theta)} \\
\Delta\theta_i &= \theta_i - \mu_i
\end{aligned}
\tag{7}
$$

where C^x and C^L correspond to the prior covariances of the pyramidal cell depolarization and the leadfield parameters respectively. For simplicity, we assume that $C^x = 1$ and compute the principal components of C^h from Equation 7. We then retain a specified number of components or spatial modes. This procedure furnishes a subspace which spans signals that can be explained by the model. Note that generally this projection results in different data subspaces for models that differ in the number and (prior) placement of the sources. To facilitate model comparison, we used the same projection in all model inversions. This is because the model evidence pertains to the data explained by the model.

The Observation or Likelihood Model

In summary, our DCM comprises a state-equation that is based on neurobiological heuristics and an observer equation based on an electromagnetic forward model. By integrating the state-equation and passing the ensuing states through the observer equation, we generate a predicted measurement. This corresponds to a generalized convolution of the inputs to generate a response $h(\theta)$ (Equation 6). This generalized convolution gives an observation model for the vectorized data y and the associated likelihood

$$
\begin{aligned}
y &= vec(h(\theta) + X\theta^X) + \varepsilon \\
p(y/\theta, \lambda) &= N(vec(h(\theta) + X\theta^X), diag(\lambda) \otimes V)
\end{aligned}
\tag{8}
$$

Measurement noise, ε is assumed to be zero-mean Gaussian and independent over channels, i.e., $Cov(vec(\varepsilon)) = diag(\lambda) \otimes V$, where λ is an unknown vector of channel-specific variances. V represents the error's temporal autocorrelation matrix, which we assume is the identity matrix. This is tenable because we downsample the data to about 8 ms. Low-frequency noise or drift components are modeled by X, which is a block diagonal matrix with a low-order discrete cosine set for each evoked response and channel. The order of this set can be determined by Bayesian model selection (see below). This model is fitted to data by tuning the free parameters θ to minimize the discrepancy between predicted and observed MEG/EEG time-series under model complexity constraints (more formally, the parameters minimize the variational free energy; see below). In addition to minimizing prediction error, the parameters are constrained by a prior specification of the range they are likely to lie in (Friston et al., 2003). These constraints, which take the form of a prior density $p(\theta)$, are combined with the likelihood, $p(y|\theta)$, to form a posterior density $p(\theta|y) \propto p(y|\theta)p(\theta)$ according to Bayes' rule. It is this posterior or conditional density we want to estimate. Gaussian assumptions about the errors in Equation 8 enable us to compute the likelihood from the prediction error. The only outstanding quantities we require are the priors, which are described next.

Model Priors

The connectivity architecture is constant over peristimulus time and defines the dynamic behavior of the DCM. We have to specify prior assumptions about the connectivity parameters to estimate their posterior distributions. Priors have a dramatic impact on the landscape of the objective function to be optimized: precise prior distributions ensure that the objective function has a global minimum that can be attained robustly. Under Gaussian assumptions, the prior distribution $p(\theta_i)$ of the ith parameter is defined by its mean and variance. The mean corresponds to the prior expectation. The variance reflects the amount of prior information about the parameter. A tight distribution (small variance) corresponds to precise prior knowledge. The parameters of the state-equation can be divided into six subsets: *(1)* extrinsic connection parameters, which specify the coupling strengths among sources; *(2)* intrinsic connection parameters, which reflect our knowledge about canonical micro-circuitry within a source; *(3)* conduction delays; *(4)* synaptic and sigmoid parameters controlling the dynamics within a source; *(5)* input parameters, which control the subcortical delay and dispersion of event-related responses; and, importantly, *(6)* intrinsic and extrinsic gain parameters. Table 3.8.1 list the priors for these parameters; see also David et al. (2006) for details. Note that we fixed the values of intrinsic coupling parameters as described in Jansen and Rit (1995). Interlaminar conduction delays are usually fixed at 2 ms and interregional delays have a prior expectation of 16 ms.

Table 3.8.1.
Prior densities of parameters (for connections to the *i*-th source from the *j*-th, in the *k*-th evoked response)

Extrinsic coupling parameters

$$
\begin{aligned}
A_{ijk}^{F} &= A_{ij}^{F} B_{ijk} & A_{ij}^{F} &= 32 \exp(\theta_{ij}^{F}) & \theta_{ij}^{F} &\sim N(0, \tfrac{1}{2}) \\
A_{ijk}^{B} &= A_{ij}^{B} B_{ijk} & A_{ij}^{B} &= 16 \exp(\theta_{ij}^{B}) & \theta_{ij}^{B} &\sim N(0, \tfrac{1}{2}) \\
A_{ijk}^{L} &= A_{ij}^{L} B_{ijk} & A_{ij}^{L} &= 4 \exp(\theta_{ij}^{L}) & \theta_{ij}^{L} &\sim N(0, \tfrac{1}{2}) \\
 & & B_{ijk} &= \exp(\theta_{ijk}^{B}) & \theta_{ij}^{B} &\sim N(0, \tfrac{1}{2}) \\
 & & C_{i} &= \exp(\theta_{i}^{C}) & \theta_{i}^{C} &\sim N(0, \tfrac{1}{2})
\end{aligned}
$$

Intrinsic coupling parameters
Conduction delays (ms)

$\gamma_1 = 128 \quad \gamma_2 = \tfrac{4}{5}\gamma_1 \quad \gamma_3 = \tfrac{1}{4}\gamma_1 \quad \gamma_4 = \tfrac{1}{4}\gamma_1$

$\Delta_{ii} = 2 \quad \Delta_{ij} = 16 \exp(\theta_{ij}^{\Delta}) \quad \theta_{ij}^{\Delta} \sim N(0, \tfrac{1}{16})$

Synaptic parameters (ms)

$T_e^{(i)} = 8 \exp(\theta_i^{T}) \quad \theta_i^{T} \sim N(0, \tfrac{1}{8})$

$H_{e,k}^{(i)} = B_{iik} H_e^{(i)} \quad H_e^{(i)} = 4 \exp(\theta_i^{H}) \quad \theta_i^{H} \sim N(0, \tfrac{1}{8})$

$T_i = 16 \qquad H_i = 32$

Sigmoid parameters

$\rho_1^{(i)} = \tfrac{2}{3} \exp(\theta_i^{\rho_1}) \quad \theta_i^{\rho_1} \sim N(0, \tfrac{1}{8})$

$\rho_2^{(i)} = \tfrac{1}{3} \exp(\theta_i^{\rho_2}) \quad \theta_i^{\rho_2} \sim N(0, \tfrac{1}{8})$

Input parameters (sec)

$$
\begin{aligned}
u(t) &= b(t, \eta_1, \eta_2) + \Sigma \theta_i^{c} \cos(2\pi(i-1)t) & \theta_i^{c} &\sim N(0, 1) \\
\eta_1 &= \exp(\theta_1^{\eta}) & \theta_1^{\eta} &\sim N(0, \tfrac{1}{16}) \\
\eta_2 &= 16 \exp(\theta_2^{\eta}) & \theta_2^{\eta} &\sim N(0, \tfrac{1}{16})
\end{aligned}
$$

Spatial (ECD) parameters (mm)

$\theta_i^{pos} \sim N(L_i^{pos}, 32 I_3)$

$\theta_i^{mom} \sim N(0, 8 I_3)$

Inference and Model Comparison

For a given DCM, say model m, parameter estimation corresponds to approximating the moments of the posterior distribution given by Bayes' rule

$$
p(\theta|y, m) = \frac{p(y|\theta, m) p(\theta, m)}{p(y|m)} \tag{9}
$$

The estimation procedure employed in DCM is described in (Friston et al., 2003). The posterior moments (mean η and covariance Σ) are updated iteratively using Variational Bayes under a fixed-form Laplace (i.e., Gaussian) approximation to the conditional density $q(\theta) = N(\eta, \Sigma)$. This can be regarded as an expectation-maximization (EM) algorithm that employs a local linear approximation of Equation 8 about the current conditional expectation. The E-step conforms to a Fisher-scoring scheme (Fahrmeir and Tutz, 1994) that performs a descent on the variational free energy $F(q, \lambda, m)$ with respect to the conditional moments. In the M-Step, the error variances λ are updated in exactly the same way. The estimation scheme can be summarized as follows:

Repeat until convergence

$$
\begin{aligned}
E - Step \quad q &\leftarrow \min_q F(q, \lambda, m) \\
M - Step \quad \lambda &\leftarrow \min_\lambda F(q, \lambda, m)
\end{aligned}
$$

$$
\begin{aligned}
F(q, \lambda, m) &= \langle \ln q(\theta) - \ln p(y|\theta, \lambda, m) - \ln p(\theta|m) \rangle_q \\
&= D(q \| p(\theta|y, \lambda, m)) - \ln p(y|\lambda, m)
\end{aligned} \tag{10}
$$

Note that the free energy is simply a function of the log-likelihood and the log-prior for a particular DCM and $q(\theta)$. The expression $\langle \cdot \rangle_q$ denotes the expectation under the density q. $q(\theta)$ is the approximation to the posterior density $p(\theta|y, \lambda, m)$ we require. The E-step updates the moments of $q(\theta)$ (these are the variational parameters η and Σ) by minimizing the variational free energy. The free energy is the Kullback-Leibler divergence (denoted by $D(\cdot\|\cdot)$), between the real and approximate conditional density minus the log-likelihood. This means that the conditional moments or variational parameters maximize the marginal log-likelihood, while minimizing the discrepancy between the true and approximate conditional density. Because the divergence does not depend on the covariance parameters, minimizing the free energy in the M-step is equivalent to finding the maximum likelihood estimates of the covariance parameters. This scheme is identical to that employed by DCM for functional magnetic resonance imaging (Friston et al., 2003). Source code for this routine can be found in the Statistical Parametric Mapping software package (see "Software note" below), in the function "spm_nlsi_N.m."

Bayesian inference proceeds using the conditional or posterior density estimated by iterating Equation 10. Usually this involves specifying a parameter or compound of parameters as a contrast, $c^T \eta$. Inferences about this contrast are made using its conditional covariance, $c^T \Sigma c$. For example, one can compute the probability that any contrast is greater than zero or some meaningful threshold, given the data. This inference is conditioned on the particular model specified. In other words, given the data and model, inference is based on the probability that a particular contrast is bigger than a specified threshold. In some situations one may want to compare different models. This entails Bayesian model comparison.

Different models are compared using their evidence (Penny et al., 2004). The model evidence is

$$p(y|m) = \int p(y|\theta, m)p(\theta|m)d\theta \qquad (11)$$

Note that the model evidence is simply the normalization constant in Equation 9. The evidence can be decomposed into two components: an accuracy term, which quantifies the data fit, and a complexity term, which penalizes models with a large number of parameters. Therefore, the evidence embodies the two conflicting requirements of a good model, that it explains the data and is as simple as possible. In the following, we approximate the model evidence for model m, under a normal approximation (Friston et al., 2003), by

$$\ln\ p(y|m) \approx \ln p(y|\lambda, m) \qquad (12)$$

This is the maximum value of the objective function attained by EM (see the **M**-Step in Equation 10). The most likely model is the one with the largest log-evidence. This enables Bayesian model selection. Model comparison rests on the likelihood ratio B_{ij} (i.e., Bayes Factor) of the evidence or relative log-evidence for two models. For models i and j

$$\ln\ B_{ij} = \ln p(y|m = i) - \ln p(y|m = j) \qquad (13)$$

Conventionally, strong evidence in favor of one model requires the difference in log-evidence to be three or more (Penny et al., 2004). This threshold criterion plays a similar role as a p-value of 0.05 = 1/20 in classical statistics (used to reject the null hypothesis in favour of the alternative model). A difference in log-evidence of greater than three (i.e., a Bayes factor more than $\exp(3) \sim 20$) indicates that the data provide strong evidence in favor of one model over the other. This is a standard way to assess the differences in log-evidence quantitatively.

Illustrative Examples

Mismatch Negativity

In this section, we illustrate the use of DCM for evoked responses by analyzing EEG data acquired under a mismatch negativity (MMN) paradigm. Critically, DCM allows us to test hypotheses about the changes in connectivity between sources. In this example study, we will test a specific hypothesis (see below) about the MMN generation and compare various models over a group of subjects. The results shown here are a part of a series of papers that consider the MMN and its underlying mechanisms in detail (Garrido et al., 2007b; Garrido et al., 2007a).

Novel sounds, or oddballs, embedded in a stream of repeated sounds, or standards, produce a distinct response that can be recorded non-invasively with MEG and EEG. The MMN is the negative component of the waveform obtained by subtracting the event-related response to a standard from the response to an odd-ball, or deviant. This response to sudden changes in the acoustic environment peaks at about 100–200 ms from change onset (Sams et al., 1985) and exhibits an enhanced negativity that is distributed over fronto-temporal areas, with prominence in frontal regions.

The MMN is believed to be an index of automatic change detection reflecting a pre-attentive sensory memory mechanism (Tiitinen et al., 1994). There have been several compelling mechanistic accounts of how the MMN might arise. The most common interpretation is that the MMN can be regarded as a marker for error detection, caused by a break in a learned regularity, or familiar auditory context. The early work by Näätänen and Winkler suggested that the MMN results from a comparison between the auditory input and a memory trace of previous sounds. In agreement with this theory, others (Näätänen and Winkler, 1999; Sussman et al., 1999; Winkler et al., 1996) have postulated that the MMN would reflect online modifications of the auditory system, or updates of the perceptual model, during incorporation of a newly encountered stimulus into the model—the *model-adjustment hypothesis*. Hence, the MMN would be a specific response to stimulus change and not to stimulus alone. This hypothesis has been supported by Escera et al. (2003), who provided evidence that the prefrontal cortex is involved in a top-down modulation of a deviance detection system in the temporal cortex. In the light of the Näätänen model, it has been claimed that the MMN is caused by two underlying functional processes, a sensory memory mechanism related to temporal generators and an automatic attention-switching process related to the frontal generators (Giard et al., 1990). Accordingly, it has been shown that the temporal and frontal MMN sources have distinct behaviors over time (Rinne et al., 2000) and that these sources interact with each other (Jemel et al., 2002). Thus the MMN could be generated by a temporofrontal network (Doeller et al., 2003; Opitz et al., 2002), as revealed by M/EEG and fMRI studies. This work has linked the early component (in the range of about 100–140 ms) to a sensorial, or noncomparator account of the MMN, elaborated in the temporal cortex, and a later component (in the range of about 140–200 ms) to a cognitive part of the MMN, involving the frontal cortex (Maess et al., 2007).

Using DCM, we modeled the MMN generators with a fronto-temporal network comprising bilateral sources over the primary and secondary auditory and frontal cortex. Following the model-adjustment hypothesis, we assume that the early and late component of the MMN can be explained by an interaction of temporal and frontal sources or network nodes. The MMN itself is defined as the difference between the responses to the oddball and the standard stimuli. Here, we modeled both evoked responses and explained the MMN, i.e., differences in the two ERPs, by a modulation of DCM parameters. There are two kinds of parameters that seem appropriate to induce the difference between oddballs and standards: *(1)* modulation of extrinsic connectivity between sources, and *(2)* modulation of intrinsic parameters in each source. Modulation of intrinsic parameters would correspond to a mechanism that is more akin to an *adaptation* hypothesis, i.e., the MMN is generated by local adaptation of populations. This is the hypothesis considered by Jaaskelainen et al. (2004) who report evidence that the MMN is explained by differential adaptation of two pairs of bilateral temporal sources. In a recent paper, we have compared models derived from both hypotheses: *(1)* the model-adjustment hypothesis and *(2)* the adaptation hypothesis (Garrido et al., under review). Here, we will constrain ourselves to demonstrate inference based on DCMs derived from the model-adjustment hypothesis only, which involves a fronto-temporal network. Note that we recently used a so-called roving paradigm to further disambiguate between model-adjustment and the adaptation hypothesis (Garrido et al., 2008).

Experimental Design

We studied a group of 13 healthy volunteers aged 24–35 (5 female). Each subject gave signed informed consent before the study, which proceeded under local ethical committee guidelines. Subjects sat on a comfortable chair in front of a desk in a dimly illuminated room. Electroencephalographic activity was measured during an auditory "oddball" paradigm, in which subjects heard of "standard" (1000 Hz) and "deviant" tones (2000 Hz), occurring 80% (480 trials) and 20% (120 trials) of the time, respectively, in a pseudo-random sequence. The stimuli were presented binaurally via headphones for 15 min every 2 s. The duration of each tone was 70 ms with 5 ms rise and fall times. The subjects were instructed not to move, to keep their eyes closed and to count the deviant tones.

EEG was recorded with a Biosemi system with 128 scalp electrodes. Data were recorded at a sampling rate of 512Hz. Vertical and horizontal eye movements were monitored using EOG (electro-oculograms) electrodes. The data were epoched offline, with a peristimulus window of − 100 to 400 ms, downsampled to 200 Hz, band-pass filtered between 0.5 and 40 Hz and re-referenced to the average of the right and left ear lobes. Trials in which the absolute amplitude of the signal exceeded 100 µV were excluded. Two subjects were eliminated from further analysis due to excessive trials containing artifacts. In the remaining subjects, an average 18% of trials were excluded.

Specification of Dynamic Causal Model

In this section, we specify three plausible models defined under a given architecture and dynamics. The network architecture was motivated by recent electrophysiological and neuroimaging studies looking at the sources underlying the MMN (Doeller et al., 2003; Opitz et al., 2002). We assumed five sources, modeled as equivalent current dipoles (ECDs), over left and right primary auditory cortices (A1), left and right superior temporal gyrus (STG), and right inferior frontal gyrus (IFG), see Figure 3.8.2. Our mechanistic model attempts to explain the generation of each individual response, i.e., responses to standards and deviants. Therefore, left and right primary auditory cortex (A1) were chosen as cortical input stations for processing the auditory information. Opitz et al. (2002) identified sources for the differential response, with fMRI and EEG measures, in both left and right superior temporal gyrus (STG), and right inferior frontal gyrus (IFG). Here we employ the coordinates reported by Opitz et al. (2002) (for left and right STG and right IFG) and Rademacher et al. (2001) (for left and right A1) as prior source location means, with a prior variance of 32 mm. We converted these coordinates, given in the literature in Talairach space, to MNI space using the algorithm described in http://imaging.mrc-cbu.cam.ac.uk/imaging/ MniTalairach. The moment parameters had prior mean of 0 and a variance of 8 in each direction. We have used these parameters as priors to estimate, for each individual subject, the posterior locations and moments of the ECDs (Table 3.8.2). Using these sources and prior knowledge about the functional anatomy we constructed the following DCM: An extrinsic input entered bilaterally to A1, which were connected to their ipsilateral STG. Right STG was connected with the right IFG. Interhemispheric (lateral) connections were placed between left and right STG. All connections were reciprocal (i.e., connected with forward and backward connections or with bilateral connections). Given this connectivity graph, specified in terms of its nodes and connections, we tested three models. These models differed in the connections that could show putative learning-related changes, i. e., differences between listening to standard or deviant tones. Models F, **B,** and **FB** allowed changes in forward, backward, and both forward and backward connections, respectively (see Figure 3.8.2). All three models were compared against a baseline or null model. The null model had the same architecture described above but precluded any coupling changes between standard and deviant trials.

Table 3.8.2.
Prior coordinates for the locations of the equivalent current dipoles in Montreal Neurology Institute (MNI) space [mm].

left primary auditory cortex (**lA1**)	−42,−22, 7
right primary auditory cortex (**rA1**)	46, −14, 8
left superior temporal gyrus (**lSTG**)	−61, −32, 8
right superior temporal gyrus (**rSTG**)	59, −25, 8
right inferior frontal gyrus (**rIFG**)	46, 20, 8

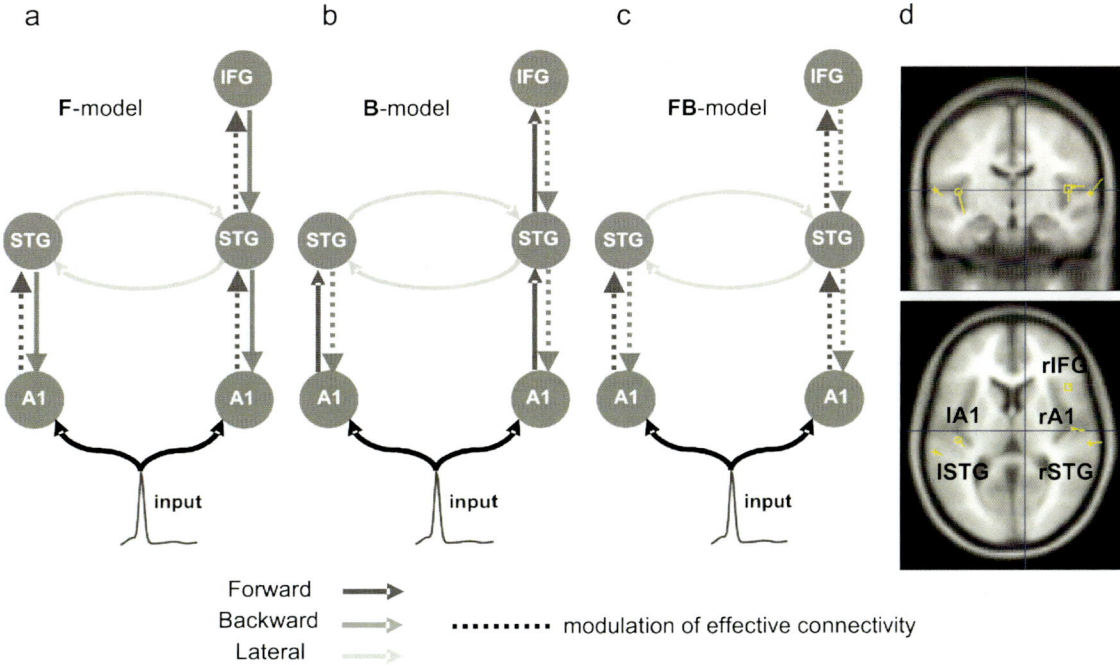

Forward ⟶
Backward ⟶ ·········· modulation of effective connectivity
Lateral ⟶

Figure 3.8.2. Model specification. The sources comprising the network are connected with forward (dark grey), backward (grey), or lateral (light grey) connections as shown. **A1**: primary auditory cortex, **STG**: superior temporal gyrus, **IFG**: inferior temporal gyrus. Three different models were tested within the same architecture (**a–c**), allowing for learning-related changes in forward **F**, backward **B**, and forward and backward **FB** connections, respectively. The broken lines indicate the connections we allowed to change. (**d**): Sources of activity, modeled as dipoles (estimated posterior moments and locations), are superimposed in an MRI of a standard brain in MNI space. From Garrido et al. (2007) with permission.

Results

The difference between the ERPs evoked by the standard and deviant tones revealed a standard MMN. This negativity was present from 90 to 190 ms and had a broad spatial pattern, encompassing electrodes previously associated with auditory and frontal areas. Four different DCMs, forward only (**F**-model), backward only (**B**-model), forward and backward (**FB**-model), and the null model were inverted for each subject. Figure 3.8.3 illustrates the model comparison based on the increase in log-evidence over the null model, for all subjects. Figure 3.8.3a shows the log-evidence for the three models, relative to the null model, for each subject, revealing that the three models were significantly better than the null in all subjects. The diamond attributed to each subject identifies the best model on the basis of the highest log-evidence. The **FB**-model was significantly better in 7 out of 11 subjects. The **F**-model was better in four subjects but only significantly so in three (for one of these subjects [subject 6], model comparison revealed only weak evidence in favor of the **F**-model over the **FB**-model, though still very strong evidence over the B-model). In all but one subject, the **F** and **FB**-models were better than the B-model. Figure 3.8.3b shows the log-evidences for the three models at the group level. The log-evidence for the group is the sum of the log-evidences from all subjects, because of the independent measures over subjects. Both **F** and **FB** are clearly more likely than **B** and, over subjects, there is very strong evidence in favor of model **FB** over model **F**. Figure 3.8.4a shows, for the best model **FB**, the predicted responses at each node of the network for each trial type (i.e., standard or deviant) for a single subject (subject 9). For each connection in the network, the plot shows the coupling gains and the conditional probability that the gains are different from one. For example, a coupling change of 2.04 from **lA1** to **lSTG** means that the effective connectivity increased 104% for rare events relative to frequent events. The response, in measurement space, of the three principal spatial modes is shown on the right (Figure 3.8.4b). This figure shows a remarkable agreement between predicted (solid) and observed (dotted) responses. Figure 3.8.5 summarizes the conditional densities of the coupling parameters for the F-model (Figure 3.8.5a) and **FB**-model (Figure 3.8.5b). For each connection in the network, the plot shows the coupling gains and the conditional probability that the gains are different from one, pooled over subjects. For the F-model the effective connectivity has increased in all connections with a conditional probability of almost 100%. For the **FB**-model the effective connectivity has changed in all forward and backward connections with a probability of almost 100%. Equivalently, and in accord with theoretical predictions, all extrinsic connections (i.e., influences) were modulated for rare events as compared to frequent events.

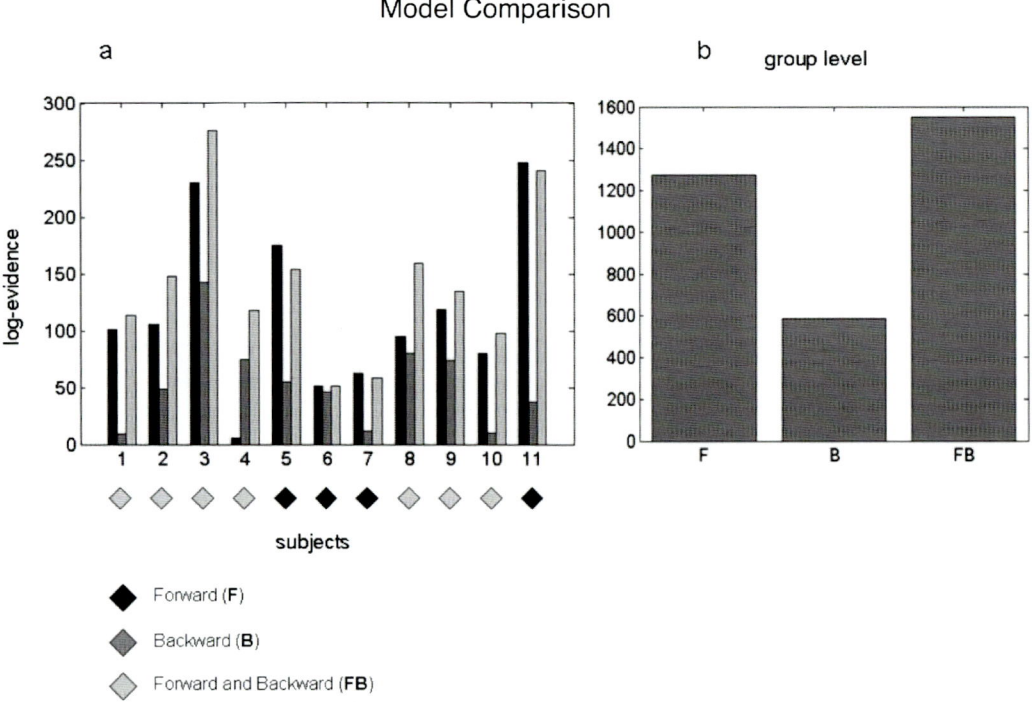

Figure 3.8.3. Bayesian model selection among DCMs for the three models, **F, B,** and **FB,** expressed relative to a DCM in which no connections were allowed to change (null model). The graphs show the free energy approximation to the log-evidence. **a:** Log-evidence for models **F, B,** and **FB** for each subject (relative to the null model). The diamond attributed to each subject identifies the best model on the basis of the subject's highest log-evidence. **b:** Log-evidence at the group level, i.e., pooled over subjects, for the three models. From Garrido et al. (2007) with permission.

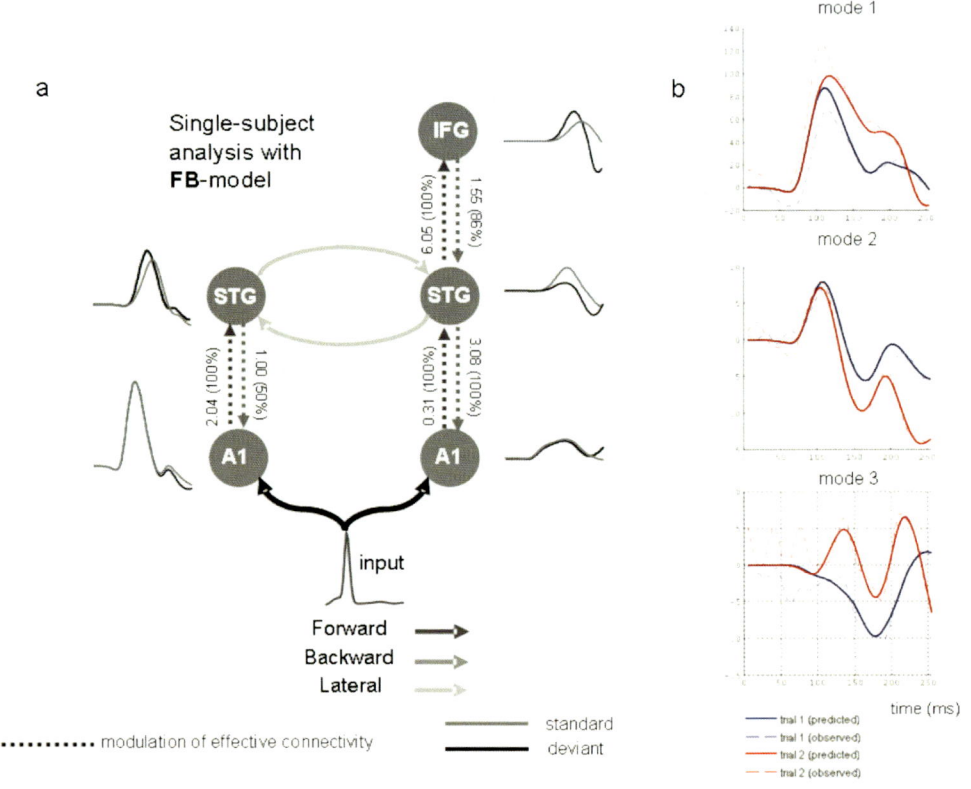

Figure 3.8.4. DCM results for a single subject [subject 9] (**FB** model). **a:** Reconstructed responses for each source and changes in coupling during oddball processing relative to standards. The numbers next to each connection are the gain modulation in connection strength and the posterior probability that the modulation is different from one. The mismatch response is expressed in nearly every source. **b:** Predicted (solid) and observed (broken) responses in measurement space, which result from a projection of the scalp data onto their first three spatial modes. From Garrido et al. (2007) with permission.

Group-analysis

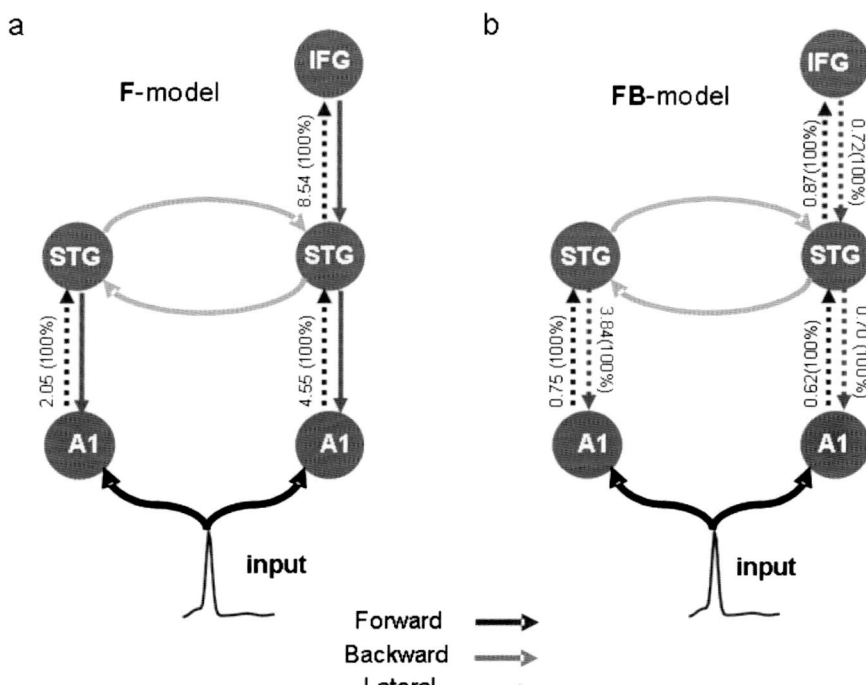

Figure 3.8.5. Coupling gains and their posterior probability estimated over subjects for each connection in the network for models **F** (**a**) and **FB** (**b**). There are widespread learning-related changes in all connections, expressed as modulations of coupling for deviants relative to standards. From Garrido et al. (2007) with permission.

Evidence for Feedback Loops

Early and Late Components in the Evoked Response

The mismatch negativity is just one example of many known M/EEG phenomena. In general, event-related potentials (ERPs) or fields (ERFs) are one of the mainstays of non-invasive neuroscience. Typically, the response evoked by a stimulus evolves in a systematic way showing a series of waves or components. Many of these components are elicited so reliably that they are studied in their own right. These include very early sensory-evoked potentials, observed within a few milliseconds, early cortical responses such as the N1 and P2 components and later components expressed several hundred milliseconds afterward. Broadly speaking, ERP components can be divided into early and late. Early or short-latency stimulus-dependent (exogenous) components reflect the integrity of primary afferent pathways. Late stimulus-independent (endogenous) components entail long-latency (more than 100 ms) responses that are thought to reflect cognitive processes (Gaillard, 1988). Early components have been associated with exogenous bottom-up stimulus-bound effects, whereas late components have been ascribed to endogenous dynamics involving top-down influences. Indeed, the amplitude and latency of early (e.g., P1 and N1) and late (e.g., N2pc) components have been used as explicit indices of bottom-up top-down processing

respectively (Schiff et al., 2006). In this section we briefly summarize results that demonstrate that late components are mediated by recurrent interactions among remote cortical regions; specifically we show that late components rest on backward extrinsic cortico-cortical connections that enable recurrent or reentrant dynamics.

Results

To investigate this, we used the multisubject data (EEG) described above but only analyzed the responses to the odd-ball stimuli. Note that the detailed analysis can be found in (Garrido et al., 2007a). The network architecture was the same as employed above, i.e., five sources with left and right primary auditory cortices (A1), left and right superior temporal gyrus (STG), and right inferior frontal gyrus (IFG). See Table 3.8.2 for their prior locations. We tested two models: model **FB** had reciprocal, i.e., forward and backward connections, and model **F** lacked backward connections, having forward connections only. In other words, model **FB** resembles recurrent dynamics, or parallel bottom-up and top-down processing, whereas model **F** emulates simple bottom-up mechanism. Note that these **F** and **FB** models are different from those above in the MMN analysis, because here we model a single response, whereas the models above pertain to two evoked responses.

To test the hypothesis that backward connections mediate late components selectively, we evaluated the model-evidence $L_i = p(y(\tau)|m_i) \approx \exp(F_i)$ for models m_1 and m_0, with and

A

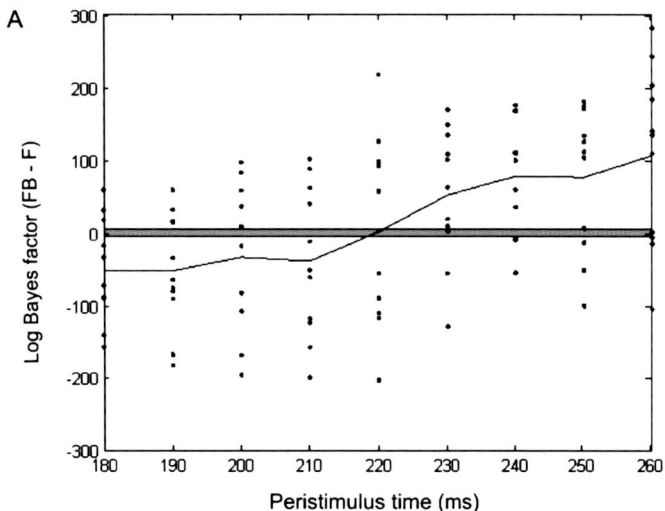

B

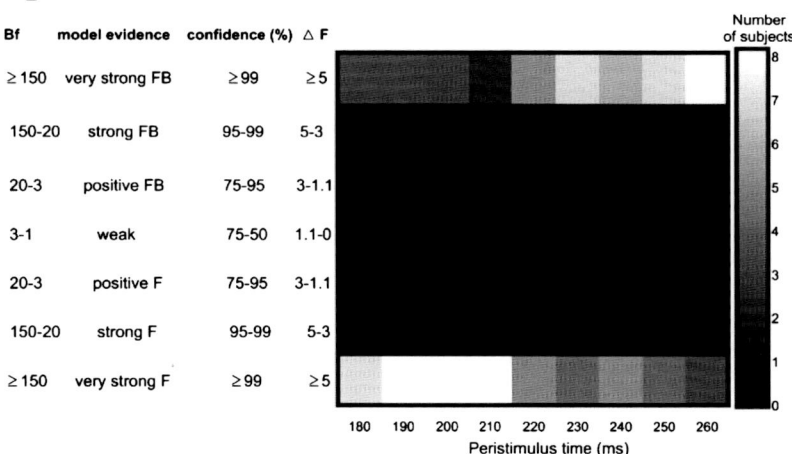

Figure 3.8.6. Bayesian model comparison across subjects. **(a)** Comparison of the model with backward connections (**FB**) against the model without (**F**), across all subjects over the peristimulus interval 180 to 260 ms. The dots correspond to differences in log-evidence for 11 subjects over time. The solid line shows the average log-evidence differences over subjects. The points outside the gray zone imply very strong inference (≥99% confidence that one model is more likely), i.e., model **FB** supervenes over **F** for positive points and the converse for negative points. **(b)** Histogram showing the number of subjects in each of seven levels of inference on models with and without backward connections across the peristimulus interval 180 to 260 ms. From Garrido et al. (2007a) with permission.

without backward connections as a function of peristimulus time τ; **FB** and **F** respectively. This involved inverting the model using data, from stimulus onset to a variable poststimulus time, ranging from 120ms to 400ms, in 10 ms steps. A difference in log-evidence of about three is usually taken as strong evidence for one model over the other (i.e., the likelihood of one model is about twenty times the other). We compared the evidence, or marginal likelihood (Penny et al., 2004) of the two models as a function of increasing peristimulus time windows for both the grand average ERP across subjects and for each subject individually (Figure 3.8.6). Both analyses revealed the same result. The longer evoked responses evolve, the more likely backward connections appear. For the group data this is evident in Figure 3.8.6a, which shows that the model with backward connections (**FB**) supervenes over the model without (**F**). This is particularly clear later in peristimulus time (220 ms poststimulus or later). For the majority of subjects (8 out of 11), the forward model supervenes over the model with backward connections, when explaining the data in the first half of peristimulus time (Figure 3.8.6b). Conversely, in the second half, for most subjects (8 out of 11), the model with backward connections (**FB**) supervenes over the model

without. This means that forward connections are sufficient to explain ERP generation in early periods, but backward connections become essential in later periods. This effect occurs after 220 ms and is more evident for longer latencies. In short, backward connections are not necessary to explain early data and only incur a complexity penalty, without increasing accuracy. This does not mean backward connections are "switched off"; it simply means their effects are not manifest until later in peristimulus time, by which time activity has returned from higher levels. At this point, backward connections become necessary to explain the data. This can be seen quantitatively in a plot of the log-evidence over time and qualitatively, in terms of the number of subjects supporting each models, at larger peristimulus time (Figure 3.8.6a, b respectively).

Discussion

Dynamic causal modeling (DCM) for M/EEG entails the inversion of informed spatiotemporal models of observed responses. The idea is to model condition-specific responses over channels and peristimulus time with the same model, where the differences among conditions are explained by changes in only a few key parameters. The face and predictive validity of DCM have been established, which makes it a potentially useful tool for group studies (David et al., 2006; Garrido et al., 2007b; Kiebel et al., 2006). In principle, the same approach can be applied to the analysis of single trials, where one would use a parametric modulation of parameters to model the effects of trial-to-trial changes in an experimental variable (e.g., reaction time or forgotten vs. remembered).

One can also view DCM for evoked responses as a source reconstruction device using biophysically informed temporal constraints. This is because DCM has two components; a neural-mass model of the interactions among a small number of dipole sources and a classical electromagnetic forward model that links these sources to extracranial measurements. Inverting the DCM implicitly optimizes the location and moments of the dipole sources. This is in contrast to traditional equivalent current dipole fitting approaches, where dipoles are fitted sequentially to the data; using user-selected periods and/or channels of the data. Classical approaches have to proceed in this way, because there is usually too much spatial and temporal dependency among the sources to identify the parameters precisely. With our approach, we place temporal constraints on the model that are consistent with the way that signals are generated biophysically. As we have shown, these allow simultaneous fitting of multiple dipoles to the data.

We used the equivalent current dipole (ECD) model because it is analytic, fast to compute, and a quasi-standard when reconstructing evoked responses. However, the ECD model is just one candidate for spatial forward models. Given the leadfield, one can use any spatial model in the observation equation (Equation 6). A further example would be some linear distributed approach (Baillet et al., 2001; Daunizeau et al., 2006; Phillips et al., 2005), where a "patch" of dipoles, confined to the cortical surface, would act as the spatial expression of one area (Daunizeau et al., 2009). With DCM, one could also use different forward models for different areas (hybrid models). For example, one could employ the ECD model for early responses while using a distributed forward model for higher areas.

We anticipate that Bayesian model comparison will become a ubiquitous tool in M/EEG. This is because further development of M/EEG models and their fusion with other imaging modalities requires more complex models embodying useful constraints. The appropriateness of such models for any given data cannot necessarily be intuited, but can be assessed formally using Bayesian model comparison. The key is to compute the model evidence $p(y/m)$ (Equation 11), for using a variational approach (see above) or as described in Sato et al. (2004), or by employing sampling approaches like the Monte Carlo Markov Chain (MCMC) techniques (Auranen et al., 2007; Jun et al., 2005; Jun et al., 2008). In principle, one can compare models based on different concepts or, indeed, inversion schemes, for a given data set y. For example, one can easily compare different types of source reconstruction (ECD vs. source imaging) with

DCM. This cannot be done with classical, non-Bayesian approaches, for which model comparisons are only feasible under certain constraints ("nested models"); precluding comparisons among qualitatively different models. Although other approximations to the model evidence exist, e.g., the Akaike Information Criterion, they are not generally useful with informative priors (Beal, 2003).

SOFTWARE NOTE

All procedures described in this chapter have been implemented as Matlab (MathWorks) code. The source code is freely available in the DCM and neural model toolboxes of the Statistical Parametric Mapping package (SPM8) under http://www.fil.ion.ucl.ac.uk/spm/.

ACKNOWLEDGMENTS

This work was supported by the Wellcome Trust and the Portuguese Foundation for Science and Technology.

NOTE

1. Model "inversion" is a technical term and stands for "fitting the model," i.e., computing the posterior distributions of the model parameters.

REFERENCES

Auranen T, Nummenmaa A, Hamalainen MS, Jaaskelainen IP, Lampinen J, Vehtari A, Sams M (2007) Bayesian inverse analysis of neuromagnetic data using cortically constrained multiple dipoles. Hum Brain Mapp 28:979–994.

Baillet S, Mosher JC, Leahy RM (2001) Electromagnetic brain mapping. IEEE Signal Proc Mag 18:14–30.

Beal, MJ (2003) Variational algorithms for approximate Bayesian inference. London: University College London (Thesis/Dissertation).

Breakspear M, Roberts JA, Terry JR, Rodrigues S, Mahant N, Robinson PA (2006) A unifying explanation of primary generalized seizures through nonlinear brain modeling and bifurcation analysis. Cereb Cortex 16:1296–1313.

Chen CC, Kiebel SJ, Friston KJ (2008) Dynamic causal modelling of induced responses. Neuroimage 41:1293–1312.

Daunizeau J, Mattout J, Clonda D, Goulard B, Benali H, Lina JM (2006) Bayesian spatio-temporal approach for EEG source reconstruction: conciliating ECD and distributed models. IEEE Trans Biomed Eng 53:503–516.

Daunizeau J, Kiebel SJ, Friston KJ (Aug 2009) Dynamic causal modelling of distributed electromagnetic responses. Neuroimage. 15;47(2):590–601.

David O, Friston KJ (2003) A neural mass model for MEG/EEG: coupling and neuronal dynamics. Neuroimage 20: 1743–1755.

David O, Harrison L, Friston KJ (2005) Modelling event-related responses in the brain. Neuroimage 25:756–770.

David O, Kiebel SJ, Harrison LM, Mattout J, Kilner JM, Friston KJ (2006) Dynamic causal modeling of evoked responses in EEG and MEG. Neuroimage 30:1255–1272.

Doeller CF, Opitz B, Mecklinger A, Krick C, Reith W, Schroger E (2003) Prefrontal cortex involvement in preattentive auditory deviance detection: neuroimaging and electrophysiological evidence. Neuroimage 20:1270–1282.

Escera C, Yago E, Corral MJ, Corbera S, Nunez MI (2003) Attention capture by auditory significant stimuli: semantic analysis follows attention switching. Eur J Neurosci 18:2408–2412.

Fahrmeir L, Tutz G (1994) Multivariate statistical modelling based on generalized linear models. New York: Springer-Verlag.

Felleman DJ, Van Essen DC (1991) Distributed hierarchical processing in the primate cerebral cortex. Cereb Cortex 1:1–47.

Friston K, Harrison L, Daunizeau J, Kiebel S, Phillips C, Trujillo-Barreto N, Henson R, Flandin G, Mattout J (2008) Multiple sparse priors for the M/EEG inverse problem. Neuroimage 39:1104–1120.

Friston KJ, Harrison L, Penny W (2003) Dynamic causal modelling. Neuroimage 19:1273–1302. Gaillard AW (1988) Problems and paradigms in ERP research. Biol Psychol 26:91–109.

Garrido MI, Kilner JM, Kiebel SJ, Friston KJ (2007a) Evoked brain responses are generated by feedback loops. Proc Natl Acad Sci U S A 104:20961–20966.

Garrido MI, Kilner JM, Kiebel SJ, Stephan KE, Friston KJ (2007b) Dynamic causal modelling of evoked potentials: a reproducibility study. Neuroimage 36:571–580.

Garrido MI, Friston KJ, Kiebel SJ, Stephan KE, Baldeweg T, Kilner JM (2008) The functional anatomy of the MMN: A DCM study of the roving paradigm. Neuroimage 42:936–944.

Giard MH, Perrin F, Pernier J, Bouchet P (1990) Brain generators implicated in the processing of auditory stimulus deviance: a topographic event-related potential study. Psychophysiology 27:627–640.

Grimbert F, Faugeras O (2006) Bifurcation analysis of Jansen's neural mass model. Neural Comput 18:3052–3068.

Gross J, Kujala J, Hamalainen M, Timmermann L, Schnitzler A, Salmelin R (2001) Dynamic imaging of coherent sources: studying neural interactions in the human brain. Proc Natl Acad Sci U S A 98:694–699.

Jaaskelainen IP, Ahveninen J, Bonmassar G, Dale AM, Ilmoniemi RJ, Levanen S, Lin FH, May P, Melcher J, Stufflebeam S, Tiitinen H, Belliveau JW (2004) Human posterior auditory cortex gates novel sounds to consciousness. Proc Natl Acad Sci U S A 101:6809–6814.

Jansen BH, Rit VG (1995) Electroencephalogram and visual evoked potential generation in a mathematical model of coupled cortical columns. Biol Cybern 73:357–366.

Jemel B, Achenbach C, Muller BW, Ropcke B, Oades RD (2002) Mismatch negativity results from bilateral asymmetric dipole sources in the frontal and temporal lobes. Brain Topogr 15:13–27.

Jun SC, George JS, Pare-Blagoev J, Plis SM, Ranken DM, Schmidt DM, Wood CC (2005) Spatiotemporal Bayesian inference dipole analysis for MEG neuroimaging data. Neuroimage 28:84–98.

Jun SC, George JS, Kim W, Pare-Blagoev J, Plis S, Ranken DM, Schmidt DM (2008) Bayesian brain source imaging based on combined MEG/EEG and fMRI using MCMC. Neuroimage 40:1581–1594.

Kiebel SJ, Friston KJ (2004) Statistical parametric mapping for event-related potentials. I: Generic considerations. Neuroimage 22:492–502.

Kiebel SJ, David O, Friston KJ (2006) Dynamic causal modelling of evoked responses in EEG/MEG with lead field parameterization. Neuroimage 30:1273–1284.

Kiebel SJ, Garrido MI, Friston KJ (2007) Dynamic causal modelling of evoked responses: the role of intrinsic connections. Neuroimage 36:332–345.

Kujala J, Pammer K, Cornelissen P, Roebroeck A, Formisano E, Salmelin R (2007) Phase coupling in a cerebro-cerebellar network at 8-13 Hz during reading. Cereb Cortex 17:1476–1485.

Maess B, Jacobsen T, Schroger E, Friederici AD (2007) Localizing pre-attentive auditory memory-based comparison: magnetic mismatch negativity to pitch change. Neuroimage 37:561–571.

Marreiros AC, Daunizeau J, Kiebel SJ, Friston KJ (2008) Population dynamics: variance and the sigmoid activation function. Neuroimage 42:147–157.

Mosher JC, Leahy RM, Lewis PS (1999) EEG and MEG: forward solutions for inverse methods. IEEE Trans Biomed Eng 46:245–259.

Näätänen R, Winkler I (1999) The concept of auditory stimulus representation in cognitive neuroscience. Psychol Bull 125:826–859.

Nummenmaa A, Auranen T, Hamalainen MS, Jaaskelainen IP, Lampinen J, Sams M, Vehtari A (2007) Hierarchical Bayesian estimates of distributed MEG sources: theoretical aspects and comparison of variational and MCMC methods. Neuroimage 35:669–685.

Opitz B, Rinne T, Mecklinger A, von Cramon DY, Schroger E (2002) Differential contribution of frontal and temporal cortices to auditory change detection: fMRI and ERP results. Neuroimage 15:167–174.

Penny WD, Stephan KE, Mechelli A, Friston KJ (2004) Comparing dynamic causal models. Neuroimage 22:1157–1172.

Penny WD, Kilner J, Blankenburg F (2007) Robust Bayesian general linear models. Neuroimage 36:661–671.

Phillips C, Mattout J, Rugg MD, Maquet P, Friston KJ (2005) An empirical Bayesian solution to the source reconstruction problem in EEG. Neuroimage 24:997–1011.

Rademacher J, Morosan P, Schormann T, Schleicher A, Werner C, Freund HJ, Zilles K (2001) Probabilistic mapping and volume measurement of human primary auditory cortex. Neuroimage 13:669–683.

Riera JJ, Jimenez JC, Wan X, Kawashima R, Ozaki T (2007) Nonlinear local electrovascular coupling. II: From data to neuronal masses. Hum Brain Mapp 28:335–354.

Rinne T, Alho K, Ilmoniemi RJ, Virtanen J, Näätänen R (2000) Separate time behaviors of the temporal and frontal mismatch negativity sources. Neuroimage 12:14–19.

Rodrigues S, Terry JR, Breakspear M (2006) On the genesis of spike-wave oscillations in a mean-field model of human thalamic and corticothalamic dynamics. Phys Lett A 355:352–357.

Sams M, Paavilainen P, Alho K, Näätänen R (1985) Auditory frequency discrimination and event-related potentials. Electroencephalogr Clin Neurophysiol 62:437–448.

Sato MA, Yoshioka T, Kajihara S, Toyama K, Goda N, Doya K, Kawato M (2004) Hierarchical Bayesian estimation for MEG inverse problem. Neuroimage 23:806–826.

Schiff S, Mapelli D, Vallesi A, Orsato R, Gatta A, Umilta C, Amodio P (2006) Top-down and bottom-up processes in the extrastriate cortex of cirrhotic patients: an ERP study. Clin Neurophysiol 117:1728–1736.

Sotero RC, Trujillo-Barreto NJ (2008) Biophysical model for integrating neuronal activity, EEG, fMRI and metabolism. Neuroimage 39:290–309.

Sotero RC, Trujillo-Barreto NJ, Iturria-Medina Y, Carbonell F, Jimenez JC (2007) Realistically coupled neural mass models can generate EEG rhythms. Neural Comput 19:478–512.

Sussman E, Winkler I, Ritter W, Alho K, Näätänen R (1999) Temporal integration of auditory stimulus deviance as reflected by the mismatch negativity. Neurosci Lett 264:161–164.

Tiitinen H, May P, Reinikainen K, Näätänen R (1994) Attentive novelty detection in humans is governed by pre-attentive sensory memory. Nature 372:90–92.

Winkler I, Karmos G, Näätänen R (1996) Adaptive modeling of the unattended acoustic environment reflected in the mismatch negativity event-related potential. Brain Res 742:239–252.

Zhang Z (1995) A fast method to compute surface potentials generated by dipoles within multilayer anisotropic spheres. Phys Med Biol 40:335–349.

Zumer JM, Attias HT, Sekihara K, Nagarajan SS (2007) A probabilistic algorithm integrating source localization and noise suppression for MEG and EEG data. Neuroimage 37:102–115.

3.9 Klaas Enno Stephan and Karl J. Friston

Analyzing Functional and Effective Connectivity with fMRI

Introduction

Functional neuroimaging techniques, e.g., positron emission tomography (PET) and functional magnetic resonance imaging (fMRI), and neurophysiological methods, e.g., electroencephalography (EEG) and magnetoencephalograpy (MEG), are used widely in cognitive and clinical neuroscience. A common aim is to understand brain function along two dimensions: functional specialization and functional integration (Friston, 2002a). *Functional specialization* assumes that distinct brain regions are specialized for certain aspects of information processing but allows for the possibility that this specialization is anatomically segregated across multiple regions. Most current functional neuroimaging experiments have adopted this view and interpret the areas that are activated by a certain task component as the elements of a distributed system. However, this characterization does not address how the locally specialized areas are bound together by context-dependent interactions among these areas, i.e., the *functional integration* within the system. This integration can be quantified in two ways, functional connectivity and effective connectivity (Friston, 1994; Horwitz et al., 1999; Stephan, 2004). While functional connectivity describes statistical dependencies between remote neuronal data, effective connectivity rests on a mechanistic model of how these data were caused. This article reviews established techniques for characterizing functional integration on the basis of fMRI data.

Functional Connectivity

Functional connectivity is operationally defined as the presence of statistical dependencies between two sets of neurophysiological data. If one assumes that these data conform to Gaussian assumptions, one only needs to investigate second-order dependencies, i.e., covariances or correlations. For non-Gaussian processes, higher-order dependencies need to be taken into account. This can be done, for example, with independent component analysis (ICA). Since this technique is described in detail elsewhere in this book (see Chapters 3.1, 3.2, 3.3, and 3.4 in this book), the present chapter concentrates on functional connectivity expressed in terms of second-order dependencies and thus deals with temporal covariances between time-series of different brain regions. In fMRI, such time series are available for each volume element (voxel) of the brain. For example, given two voxels with time-series x and y, their functional connectivity corresponds to the Pearson correlation coefficient r of the two time-series

$$r_{xy} = \frac{\mathrm{cov}_{xy}}{s_x \cdot s_y} \tag{1}$$

where s_x, s_y are the standard deviations and cov_{xy} is the covariance of the two time-series. Note that functional connectivity suffers from the general problem of interpreting correlations: Are the two time-series correlated because *(1) x* influences *y, (2) y* influences *x, (3)* both influence each other, or *(4)* both are influenced by a third variable? Disambiguating these possibilities requires a model of the causal influences (i. e., effective connectivity, as described below).

The above definition of functional connectivity can be applied practically in different ways. For example, for fMRI data one can compute functional connectivity maps with reference to a particular seed region (e.g., Bokde et al., 2001) or, alternatively, use a variety of multivariate techniques that find sets of voxels whose time-series represent distinct (orthogonal or independent) components of the covariance structure of the data. Because of their central role in analyses of functional connectivity, the following section summarizes approaches that are based on eigenimage decomposition of spatiotemporal data.

Eigendecomposition of Spatiotemporal Imaging Data

Given a matrix A, a vector x is called the *eigenvector* of A if there is a scalar *eigenvalue* λ such that

$$Ax = \lambda x \qquad (2)$$

In other words, eigenvectors are those vectors that are only scaled by A; their direction remains unchanged. Eigenvectors thus represent the principal axes of the linear function encoded by A.

Let us now consider an fMRI data set of m scans obtained for n voxels that is represented by a mean-corrected $m \times n$ matrix Y. The temporal covariance matrix of this data set is given by YY^T and the spatial covariance matrix is given by Y^TY (where ^{T} denotes the transpose operator). The challenge is to characterize those patterns in time and space, respectively, that contribute most to the covariance structure of the data. Focusing on temporal covariance for a moment, one could perform a *principal components analysis* (PCA) that re-expresses the data Y in terms of a new orthonormal basis set U comprising the eigenvectors of the temporal covariance matrix YY^T:

$$Y^* = UY \qquad (3)$$

Here, Y^* is the data after projection onto the space defined by U. In this space, the axes account for extreme and orthogonal components of the temporal covariance structure.

A more general and powerful procedure for eigendecomposition of spatiotemporal data is *singular value decomposition* (SVD). SVD decomposes the spatiotemporal data matrix Y into three matrices:

$$SVD(Y) = USV^T \qquad (4)$$

This is a so-called *eigendecomposition* because the column vectors of U and V represent the eigenvectors of the temporal and spatial covariance matrices, respectively. Each spatial eigenvector (i.e., each column of the $n \times n$ matrix V) contains one value per voxel, therefore it can be displayed as an image and is also called an *eigenimage* (or *spatial mode*). The first eigenimage is the spatial pattern that accounts for the greatest amount of the covariance structure of the data. The second eigenimage is orthogonal to the first and explains the greatest amount of the remaining covariance, and so on. The amount of covariance explained by each eigenimage is given by the *singular values* (the square root of the eigenvalues) contained by the $m \times n$ matrix S. Note that the eigenvalues of the temporal and spatial covariance matrices are identical and, given a data matrix Y with rank r, S has r singular values, which occupy the leading diagonal in decreasing order:

$$S = \begin{bmatrix} s_1 & 0 & 0 \\ 0 & \ddots & 0 \\ 0 & 0 & s_r \\ 0 & 0 & 0 \end{bmatrix} \qquad (5)$$

Finally, the temporal eigenvectors, or *eigenvariates*, contained by the columns of the $m \times n$ matrix U, reflect the degree to which an eigenimage is expressed over time and can help to interpret the function of the distributed neural system defined by the associated eigenimage (by comparing the temporal evolution of the eigenvariate to the temporal sequence of task conditions (for an example, see Friston and Büchel, 2004).

Eigenimage analysis based on SVD has been elaborated in several ways. Notable among these is canonical variate analysis (CVA) that uses a generalized eigenvector solution to maximize the variance that can be explained by some explanatory variables relative to variance that cannot. CVA can be considered as an extension of eigenimage analysis that refers explicitly to some explanatory variables and allows for statistical inference (Friston et al., 1995; Worsley et al., 1997). A technique closely related to SVD is partial least squares (PLS), which has been applied in the context of neuroimaging using behavioral data or time series from a reference voxel as explanatory variables (McIntosh and Lobaugh, 2004).

As explained above, analyses of functional connectivity only refer to statistical dependencies among measured data and do not incorporate any knowledge or assumptions about the structure and mechanisms of the neural system of interest. This is appropriate if the system of interest is largely unknown and needs to be approached in an exploratory fashion. The results from functional connectivity analyses can then be used to generate hypotheses about the system. However, given a specific mechanistic hypothesis how system function results from system structure, models of effective connectivity are more appropriate and powerful.

Effective Connectivity

The term *effective connectivity* has been defined by various authors in convergent ways. A general definition is that effective connectivity describes the causal influences that neurons or neuronal populations exert over one another (Friston, 1994). More specifically, other authors have proposed that "effective connectivity should be understood as the experiment- and time-dependent, simplest possible circuit diagram that would replicate the observed timing relationships between the recorded neurons" (Aertsen and Preißl, 1991). Both definitions emphasize that determining effective connectivity requires a causal model of the interactions between the elements of the neural system of interest. Before we describe specific implementations of particular models of effective connectivity, we briefly describe a general mathematical form for dynamic systems (see Stephan, 2004). For this purpose, we choose deterministic differential equations with time-invariant parameters as a mathematical framework. Note that these are not the only possible mathematical representation of systems; in fact, many alternatives exist, e.g., state space models or iterative maps. The underlying concept, however, is quite universal: a *system* is defined by a set of elements with n time-variant properties that interact with each other. Each time-variant property x_i ($1 \leq i \leq n$) is called a *state variable*, and the n-vector $x(t)$ of all state variables in the system is called the *state vector* (or simply *state*) of the system at time t:

$$x(t) = \begin{bmatrix} x_1(t) \\ \vdots \\ x_n(t) \end{bmatrix} \qquad (6)$$

Taking an ensemble of interacting neurons as an example, the system elements would correspond to the individual neurons, each of which is represented by one or several state variables. These state variables could refer to various neurophysiological properties, e.g., postsynaptic potentials, status of ion channels, etc. Critically, the state variables interact with each other, i.e., the evolution (temporal derivative) of each state variable depends on the current value of other state variables. For example, the postsynaptic membrane potential depends on which and how many ion channels are open; vice versa, the probability of voltage-dependent ion channels opening depends on the membrane potential. Such mutual functional dependencies between the state variables of the system can be expressed quite naturally by a set of ordinary differential equations that operate on the state vector:

$$\frac{dx}{dt} = \begin{bmatrix} f_1(x_1, \ldots, x_n) \\ \vdots \\ f_n(x_1, \ldots, x_n) \end{bmatrix} = F(x) \qquad (7)$$

However, this description is not yet sufficient. First of all, the specific form of the dependencies f_i needs to be specified, i.e., the nature of the causal relations between state variables. This requires a set of parameters θ, which determine the form and strength of influences between state variables. In neural systems, these parameters usually include time constants and synaptic strengths of the connections between the system elements. The Boolean nature of θ, i.e., the pattern of absent and present connections, and the mathematical form of the dependencies f_i represent the *structure* of the system. And second, in the case of nonautonomous systems (i.e., systems that exchange matter, energy, or information with their environment) we need to consider the inputs into the system, e.g., sensory information entering the brain. We represent the set of all m known inputs by the m-vector function $u(t)$. Extending Equation 7 accordingly leads to a general state equation for nonautonomous deterministic systems

$$\frac{dx}{dt} = F(x, u, \theta) \qquad (8)$$

A model whose form follows this general state equation provides a causal description of how system dynamics results from

system structure, because it describes *(1)* when and where external inputs enter the system and *(2)* how the state changes induced by these inputs evolve in time depending on the system's structure. Given a particular temporal sequence of inputs $u(t)$ and an initial state $x(0)$, one obtains a complete description of how the dynamics of the system (i.e., the trajectory of its state vector x in time) results from its structure by integration of Equation 8:

$$x(\tau) = x(0) + \int_0^\tau F(x, u, \theta)dt \qquad (9)$$

Equation 8 therefore provides a general form for models of effective connectivity in neural systems. It should be noted that the framework outlined here is concerned with dynamic systems in continuous time and thus uses differential equations. The same basic ideas, however, can also be applied to dynamic systems in discrete time (using difference equations), as well as to "static" systems, where the system is at equilibrium at each point of observation. The latter perspective, which is useful for regression-like equations, is used by classic system models for functional neuroimaging data, e.g., psycho-physiological interactions (PPI; Friston et al., 1997), structural equation modeling (SEM; McIntosh et al., 1994; Büchel and Friston, 1997) and multivariate/vector autoregressive models (MAR/VAR; Harrison et al., 2003; Goebel et al., 2003). These will be discussed in the following sections, followed by the description of a more recent framework, i.e., dynamic causal modeling (DCM; Friston et al., 2003).

Before we proceed to these specific implementations of models of effective connectivity, it is worth pointing out that we have made two main assumptions in this section to simplify the exposition to the general state equation. First, it is assumed that all processes in the system are deterministic and occur instantaneously. Whether or not this assumption is valid depends on the particular system of interest. If necessary, random components (noise) and delays could be accounted for by using stochastic differential equations and delay differential equations, respectively. An example of the latter is found in DCM for event-related potentials (see David et al., 2006, and Chapter 3.8 in this book). Second, we assume that we know the inputs that enter the system. This is a tenable assumption in neuroimaging because the inputs are experimentally controlled variables, e.g., changes in stimuli or instructions. It may also be helpful to point out that using time-invariant dependencies f_i and parameters θ is not a restriction. Although the mathematical form of f_i per se is static, the use of time-varying inputs u allows for dynamic changes in what components of f_i are "activated." For example, input functions that can only take values of one or zero and that are multiplied with the different terms of a polynomial function can be used to induce time-dependent changes from non-linear to linear behavior (e.g., by "switching off" all higher order terms in the polynomial) or vice versa. Also, there is no principled distinction between states and time-varying parameters. Therefore, estimating time-varying parameters can be treated as a state estimation problem.

Before we start describing any specific model of effective connectivity, it is worthwhile pointing out that, in general, the choice of a particular modeling approach can be motivated by two distinct goals: prediction or inference. If one is only concerned about prediction (e.g., of how a subject will perform on future tasks or to which of several groups a particular subject belongs to), then it does not matter much whether the model rests on a plausibly mechanistic formulation of how the data were caused, what the estimates of individual model parameters are, and how they could be interpreted in neurobiological terms. All that matters is whether the model as a whole has good prediction accuracy, regardless of whether it is biologically realistic are not. In contrast, if one is interested in inference about the biological mechanisms that generated the observed data, it is critical that the formulation of the generative model reflect a specific hypothesis about those mechanisms and that model inversion yield well-defined estimates for individual parameters with a clear biological interpretation. This latter goal is pursued by all current models of effective connectivity: given a simple generative model of how the data are assumed to have been caused, they enable one to obtain probabilistic inference about mechanisms that are represented by individual model parameters (or the combination of multiple model parameters). The parameters of interest are typically those that encode the strength of connections between specific brain regions and how these connections change as a function of experimental manipulations (like task demands, attention, learning, or drugs).

Psycho-physiological Interactions (PPI)

Psycho-physiological interaction (PPI) analysis is among the simplest models available to assess functional interactions in neuroimaging data (see Friston et al., 1997, for details). Given a chosen reference time-series y_0 (obtained from a reference voxel or region), PPI computes wholebrain connectivity maps of this reference voxel with all other voxels y_i in the brain according to the regression-like equation

$$y_i = ay_0 + b(y_0 \times u) + cu + X\beta + e \qquad (10)$$

Here, a is the strength of the endogenous (context-independent) connectivity between y_0 and y_i. The bilinear term $y_0 \times u$ represents the interaction between physiological activity y_0 and a psychological variable u, which can be construed as a contextual input into the system, modulating the connectivity between y_0 and y_i ($\times$ represents the Hadamard product, i.e., element-by element multiplication). The third term describes the strength c by which the input u determines activity in y_i directly, independent of y_0. Finally, β represents parameters for effects of no

interest X (e.g., confounds), and e is a zero-mean Gaussian error term.

Notwithstanding the fact that this is a nondynamic model, Equation 10 contains the basic components of system descriptions as outlined above (cf. Equation 8), and there is some similarity between its form and that of the state equation of DCM (Equation 14, see below). However, since only pair-wise interactions are considered (i.e., separately between the reference voxel and all other brain voxels), this model is quite limited in its capacity to represent neural systems. This has also been highlighted in the initial description of PPIs (Friston et al., 1997). Although PPIs are not a proper system model, they have a useful role in exploring the functional interactions of a chosen region across the whole brain and have been applied to fMRI data with considerable success (e. g., Macaluso et al., 2000; Stephan et al., 2003). This exploratory nature bears some similarity to analyses of functional connectivity. Unlike analyses of functional connectivity, however, PPIs model the contextual modulation of connectivity, and this modulation has a directional character, i.e., testing for a PPI from y_0 to y_i is not identical to testing for a PPI from y_i to y_0. This is because regressing $y_0 \times u$ on y_i is not equivalent to regressing $y_i \times u$ on y_0.

Structural Equation Modeling (SEM)

SEM has been an established statistical technique in the social sciences for several decades, but was only introduced to neuroimaging in the early 1990s by McIntosh and Gonzalez-Lima (1991). It is a multivariate, hypothesis-driven technique that is based on a structural model that represents the hypothesis about the causal relations between several variables (see McIntosh and Gonzalez-Lima, 1994; Büchel and Friston, 1997; Bullmore et al., 2000; Penny et al., 2004a, for methodological details). In the context of fMRI, these variables are the measured BOLD (blood oxygen level dependent) time-series $y_1...y_n$ of n brain regions, and the hypothetical causal relations are based on anatomically plausible connections between the regions.[1] The strength of each connection $y_i \rightarrow y_j$ is specified by a so-called "path coefficient" which, by analogy to a partial regression coefficient, indicates how the variance of y_j depends on the variance of y_i if all other influences on y_j are held constant.

The statistical model of SEM as it is typically used for neuroimaging data,[2] can be summarized by the equation

$$y = Ay + u \qquad (11)$$

where y is a $n \times s$ matrix of n area-specific time series with s scans each, A is a $n \times n$ matrix of path coefficients (with zeros for nonexistent connections), and u is a $n \times s$ matrix of zero-mean Gaussian error terms, which are driving the modeled system ("innovations," see Equation 11). Parameter estimation usually employs maximum likelihood procedures, minimizing the difference between the observed and the modeled covariance matrix Σ of the areas (Bollen, 1989). For any given set of parameters, Σ can be computed by transforming Equation 11:

$$
\begin{aligned}
y &= (I - A)^{-1}u \\
\Sigma &= yy^T \\
&= (I - A)^{-1}uu^T(I - A)^{-1^T}
\end{aligned}
\tag{12}
$$

where I is the identity matrix and T denotes the transpose operator. The first line of Equation 12 can be understood as a generative model of how regional activity results from the system's connectional structure: the measured time-series y are obtained by applying a function of the inter-regional connectivity matrix, i.e., $(I - A)^{-1}$, to the Gaussian innovations u.

In the special case of fMRI, the path coefficients of a SEM (i.e., the parameters in A) describe the effective connectivity of the system across the entire experimental session. What one would often prefer to know, however, is how the coupling between certain regions changes as a function of experimentally controlled context, e.g., differences in coupling between two different tasks. Two alternative approaches exist for endowing connections in an SEM with such context-dependency (for details, see Penny et al., 2004a). The first approach exploits the fact that SEM does not account for temporal order: if all regional time-series were permuted in the same fashion, the estimated parameters would not change. In case of blocked designs, this makes it possible to proceed as if one were dealing with PET data, i.e., to partition the time series into condition-specific subseries and fit separate SEMs to them. These SEMs can then be compared statistically to test for condition-specific differences in effective connectivity (for examples, see Büchel et al., 1999; Honey et al., 2002). An alternative approach is to augment the model with bilinear terms (c.f. Equation 10), which represent the modulation of a given connection by experimentally controlled variables (e.g., Büchel and Friston 1997; Rowe et al., 2002). In this case, only a single SEM is fitted to the entire time-series.

One limitation of SEM is that one is restricted to using structural models of relatively low complexity with regard to the number of connections that are being tested. This is partially because the model is fitted to replicate the observed covariance matrix; therefore, only a limited number of data points are available, leaving not enough degrees of freedom for testing complex models with many parameters (Penny et al., 2004a). Furthermore, complex models with reciprocal connections and loops may be nonidentifiable (see Bollen, 1989, for details). For such cases, heuristics have been suggested that use multiple fitting steps in which different parameters are held constant while changing others (see McIntosh et al., 1994, for an example). It should be mentioned, however, that in practice, all models of effective connectivity have limitations concerning the complexity of the models that can be tested. While SEM has statistical limitations with regard to the number of connections that can be included in the model, other models like DCM exhibit computational limitations, e.g., with regard to the total number of data points (product of the number of regions and of the number of scans) to which a model can be fitted.

Multivariate and Vector Autoregressive Models (MAR, VAR)

In contrast to SEM, autoregressive models explicitly address the temporal aspect of causality in time-series. They take into account the causal dependence of the present on the past: each data point of a regional time-series is explained as a linear combination of past data points from the same region. Models that extend this approach to n brain regions have been termed multivariate or vector autoregressive models (MAR, VAR); these terms can be used interchangeably.

MAR models explain the n-vector of regional signals at time t (y_t) as a linear combination of p past data vectors whose contributions are weighted by the parameter matrices A_i:

$$
y_t = \sum_{i=1}^{p} y_{t-i}A_i + u_t
\tag{13}
$$

MAR models thus represent directed influences among a set of regions whose causal interactions are inferred via their mutual predictability from past time points. Although MAR has been an established statistical technique in time series analysis for many decades, specific implementations for neuroimaging were suggested only relatively recently. Harrison et al. (2003) suggested a MAR implementation that allowed for the inclusion of bilinear variables representing modulatory effects of contextual variables on connections and used a Bayesian parameter estimation scheme specifically developed for MAR models (Penny and Roberts, 2002). This Bayesian scheme also determined the optimal model order, i.e., the number of past time points (p in Equation 13) to be considered by the model. A complementary MAR approach, based on the idea of "Granger causality" (Granger, 1969), was proposed by Goebel et al. (2003). In this framework, given two time-series y_1 and y_2, y_1 is considered to be caused by y_2 if its dynamics can be predicted better using past values from y_1 and y_2 as opposed to using past values of y_1 alone.

Dynamic Causal Modeling (DCM)

An important limitation of the models of effective connectivity described above is that they operate at the level of the measured signals. This is a serious problem because the causal architecture of the system that we would like to identify is expressed at the level of neuronal dynamics, which is not directly observed using non-invasive techniques like fMRI.[3] In the case of fMRI data, for example, PPI, SEM, and MAR are fitted to the measured time-series that result from a hemodynamic convolution of the underlying neural activity. Since these classical models do not include the forward model linking neuronal activity to the measured hemodynamic data, analyses of inter-regional connectivity performed at the level of hemodynamic responses can be problematic. For example, different brain regions can exhibit marked differences in neurovascular coupling, and these differences, expressed in terms of different response latencies and waveforms, may lead to false inference about connectivity. It has recently been demonstrated that this is not just a theoretical concern but is practically relevant: David et al. (2008) performed simultaneous fMRI measurements and intracortical recordings in the brains of epileptic rats, demonstrating that the source of the epileptic discharges could only be identified if the model of effective connectivity explicitly accounted for the hemodynamic convolution. Specifically, they showed that a dynamic causal model enabled the correct identification of the epileptic source, whereas a MAR model based on the concept of Granger causality did not.

It follows that in order to enable inferences about connectivity between neural units we need models that combine two things: *(1)* a parsimonious but neurobiologically plausible model of neural population dynamics, and *(2)* a biophysically plausible forward model that describes the transformation from neural activity to the measured signal. Such models make it possible to fit jointly the parameters of the neural and of the forward model and provide a

mechanistic explanation for the observed time series. In principle, any of the models described above could be combined with a modality-specific forward model, and indeed, MAR models have previously been combined with linear forward models to explain EEG data (Yamashita et al., 2004). So far, however, DCM is the only approach where the marriage between models of neural dynamics and biophysical forward models is a mandatory component (see Figures 3.9.1 and 3.9.2).

Since its original inception for fMRI (Friston et al., 2003), a variety of DCM implementations have been introduced for additional data modalities, including event-related potentials (David et al., 2006) and induced responses as measured by EEG/MEG (Chen et al., 2008), as well as frequency spectra measured by local field potential recordings or EEG (Moran et al., 2008; Moran et al., 2009). These models, all formulated under the same theoretical framework, have enjoyed considerable success in the practical analysis of neuroimaging data, resulting in more than 70 published studies to date (with more than 50 studies on DCM for fMRI). In this chapter, we focus on DCM for fMRI as originally described by Friston et al. (2003) and on some recent non-linear extensions of this model (Stephan et al., 2008).

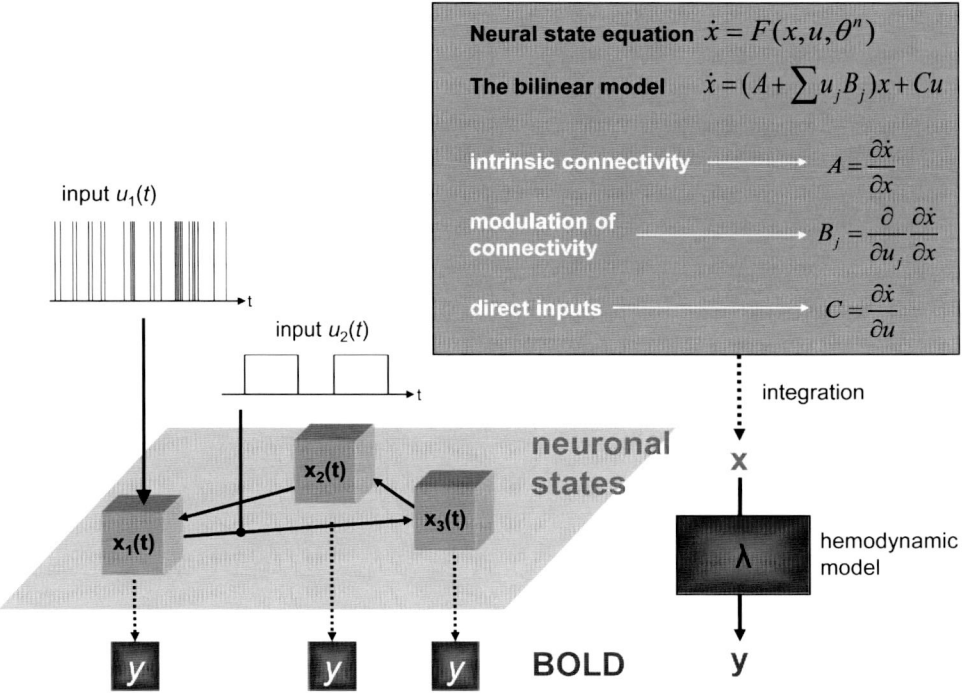

Figure 3.9.1. Schematic summary of the conceptual basis of DCM. The dynamics in a system of interacting neuronal populations (left lower panel), which are not directly observable by fMRI, is modeled using a bilinear state equation (right upper panel). Integrating the state equation gives predicted neural dynamics (*z*) that enter a model of the hemodynamic response (λ) to give predicted BOLD responses (*y*) (right lower panel). The parameters at both neural and hemodynamic levels are adjusted such that the differences between predicted and measured BOLD series are minimized. Critically, the neural dynamics are determined by experimental manipulations. These enter the model in the form of external inputs (left upper panel). Driving inputs (u_1; e.g., sensory stimuli) elicit local responses directly that are propagated through the system according to the intrinsic connections. The strengths of these connections can be changed by modulatory inputs (u_2; e.g., changes in cognitive set, attention, or learning). In this figure, the structure of the system and the scaling of the inputs are arbitrary. (This figure was reproduced, with permission, from Figure 1 in Stephan et al. (2005)).

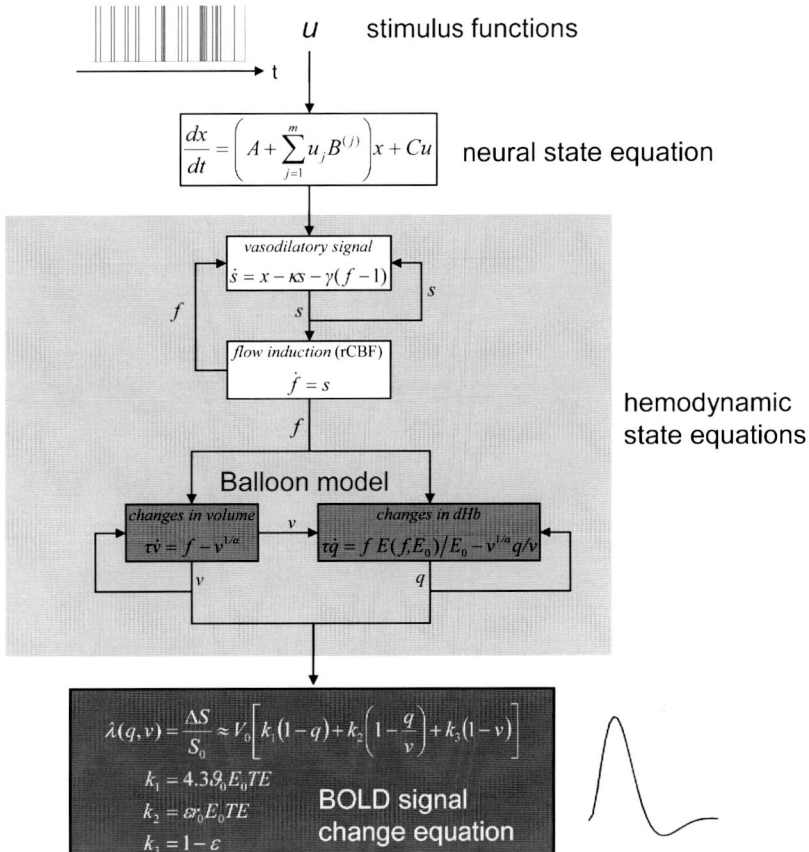

Figure 3.9.2. Schematic summary of the neural state equation and the hemodynamic forward model in DCM. Experimentally controlled input functions u evoke neural responses x, modeled by a bilinear differential state equation, which trigger a hemodynamic cascade, modeled by 4 state equations with 5 parameters. These hemodynamic parameters comprise the rate constant of the vasodilatory signal decay (κ), the rate constant for autoregulatory feedback by blood flow (γ), transit time (τ), Grubb's vessel stiffness exponent (α), and capillary resting net oxygen extraction (ρ). The so-called balloon model consists of the two equations describing the dynamics of blood volume (v) and deoxyhemoglobin content (q) (light grey boxes). Integrating the state equations for a given set of inputs and parameters produces predicted time-series for v and q, which enter a BOLD signal equation λ (dark grey box) to give a predicted BOLD response. (Reproduced, with permission, from Figure 1 in Stephan et al. 2007a.)

DCM for fMRI uses a simple model of neural dynamics in a system of n interacting brain regions (see Figure 3.9.1 for a schematic summary). In its classical form, Friston et al. (2003), it models the change of a neural state vector x in time, with each region in the system being represented by a single state variable, using the following bilinear differential equation:

$$\frac{dx}{dt} = F(x, u, \theta^n)$$
$$= \left(A + \sum_{j=1}^{m} u_j B^{(j)}\right) x + Cu \tag{14}$$

Note that this neural state equation follows the general form for deterministic system models introduced by Equation 8: the modeled state changes are a function of the current system state, the inputs u and some parameters $\theta^{(n)}$ that define the nature of the interactions among brain regions at a neuronal level. The neural state variables represent a summary index of neural population dynamics in the respective regions. The neural dynamics are driven by experimentally controlled external inputs that can enter the model in two different ways: they can elicit responses through direct influences on specific regions (e.g., evoked responses in early sensory cortices; the C matrix) or they can modulate the coupling among regions (e.g., during learning or attention; the B matrices). Note that Equation 14 does not account for

conduction delays in either inputs or inter-regional influences. This is not necessary because, due to the large regional variability in hemodynamic response latencies, fMRI data do not posses enough temporal information to enable estimation of inter-regional axonal conduction delays, which are typically in the order of 10–20 ms (note that the differential latencies of the hemodynamic response are accommodated by region-specific biophysical parameters in the hemodynamic model described below). This was verified by Friston et al. (2003), who showed in simulations that DCM parameter estimates were not affected by introducing artificial delays of up to ±1 second. In contrast, conduction delays are an important part of DCM for event-related potentials (David et al., 2006).

Given the bilinear state equation (Equation 14), the neural parameters $\theta^{(n)} = \{A, B, C\}$ can be expressed as partial derivatives of F:

$$A = \frac{\partial F}{\partial x}\bigg|_{u=0}$$
$$B^{(j)} = \frac{\partial^2 F}{\partial x \partial u_j} \tag{15}$$
$$C = \frac{\partial F}{\partial u}\bigg|_{x=0}$$

As can be seen from these equations, the matrix A represents the endogenous (fixed or context-independent) connectivity among the regions in the absence of input, the matrices $B^{(j)}$ encode the change in connectivity induced by the jth input u_j, and C embodies the strength of direct (driving) inputs on neuronal activity. In most instances, the parameters of primary interest are the modulatory ones (i.e., the matrices $B^{(j)}$) since they encode how experimentally controlled manipulations change the connection strengths in the system.

DCM for fMRI combines this model of neural dynamics with an experimentally validated hemodynamic model that describes the transformation of neuronal activity into a BOLD response. This so-called balloon model was initially formulated by Buxton et al. (1998) and later extended and refined by Friston et al. (2000) and Stephan et al. (2007a). Briefly, it consists of a set of differential equations that describe the relations between different hemodynamic state variables, using a set of parameters $\theta^{(h)}$. More specifically, changes in neural activity elicit a vasodilatory signal that leads to increases in blood flow and subsequently to changes in blood volume and deoxyhemoglobin content. The predicted BOLD signal is a non-linear function of blood volume and deoxyhemoglobin content. This hemodynamic model is summarized by Figure 3.9.2 and described in detail by Stephan et al. (2007a).

The combined neural and hemodynamic parameter set $\theta = \left\{ \theta^{(n)}, \theta^{(h)} \right\}$ is estimated from the measured BOLD data, using a fully Bayesian approach with empirical priors

for the hemodynamic parameters and conservative zero-mean shrinkage priors for the coupling parameters.[4] Details of the parameter estimation scheme, which rests on a fixed-form variational Bayesian algorithm, using a Laplace (i.e., Gaussian) approximation to the true posterior, can be found in Friston (2002b) and Friston et al. (2007).

Once the parameters of a DCM have been estimated from measured BOLD data, the posterior distributions of the parameter estimates can be used to test hypotheses about connection strengths. Due to the Laplace approximation, the posterior distributions are defined by their maximum a posteriori (MAP) estimate and their posterior covariance. Usually, the hypotheses to be tested concern context-dependent changes in coupling (i.e. the matrices $B^{(j)}$ in Equation 14). An example, originally reported by Stephan et al. (2005), where DCM was applied to fMRI data from a single subject is given by Figure 3.9.3. Here, the hypothesis was tested that in the ventral stream of the visual system the strength of right-to-left interhemispheric connections would increase during a letter decision task, but only when the word stimuli were presented in the left visual field and were thus initially received by the right hemisphere, necessitating transfer of stimulus information to the specialized left hemisphere. This hypothesis was tested by constructing a four-area model of ventral stream areas, comprising the lingual and fusiform gyri in both hemispheres (Figure 3.9.3A), and comparing the

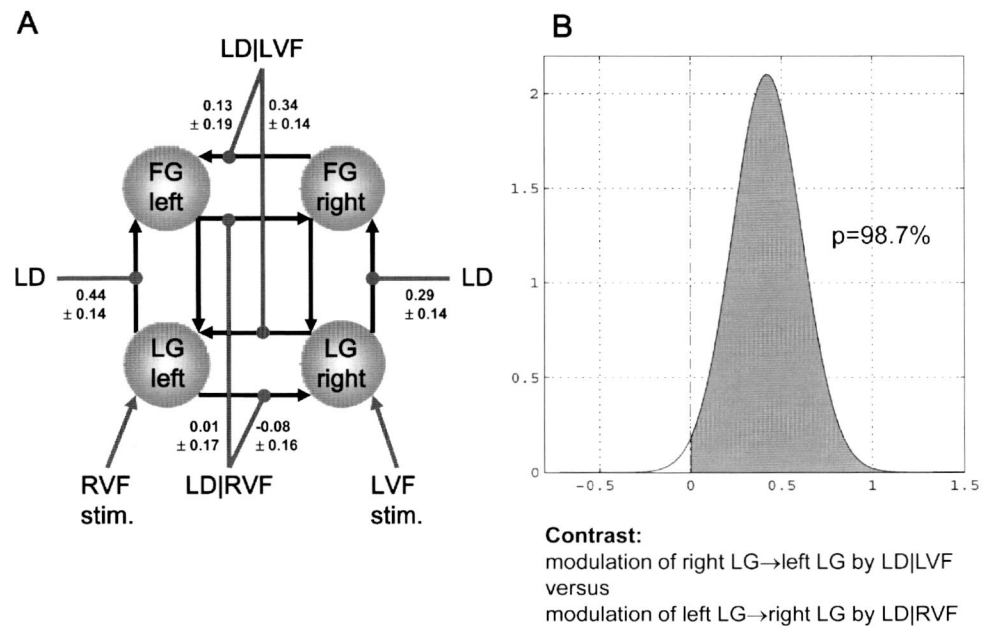

Figure 3.9.3. This figure shows an example of a single subject DCM that was used to study asymmetries in interhemispheric connections during a letter decision task. LG = lingual gyrus, FG = fusiform gyrus, LD = letter decisions, LD|VF = letter decisions conditional on the visual field of stimulus presentation. A. The values denote the maximum a posteriori (MAP) estimates of the parameters (± square root of the posterior variances; units: 1/s = Hz). For clarity, only the parameters of interest, i.e., the modulatory parameters of inter- and intrahemispheric connections, are shown. B. Asymmetry of callosal connections with regard to contextual modulation. The plots show the probability (98.7%) that the modulation of the right LG → left LG connection is stronger than the modulation of the left LG → right LG connection. (Adapted, with permission, from Figures 5 and 6 in Stephan et al. (2005)).

modulatory influences of task, conditional on the visual field of stimulus presentation, for interhemispheric connections in both directions. This comparison, based on the MAP estimates and the posterior covariances of the modulatory parameters, indicated that for this particular subject and for the connections between left and right lingual gyrus the hypothesized asymmetry in interhemispheric transfer existed with a probability of 98.7% (Figure 3.9.3B). Other examples of single-subject analyses can be found in Mechelli et al. (2003), Penny et al. (2004b), and Stephan et al. (2008).

For statistical inference at the group level, various options exist. One commonly used approach, corresponding to a random effects analysis, is to enter the conditional estimates of interest into a classical second-level analysis, e.g., a t-test on the MAP estimates of a particular parameter across subjects. For examples, see Bitan et al. (2005), Noppeney et al. (2006), Smith et al. (2006) or Stephan et al. (2007b). An alternative approach is to use Bayesian statistics at the group level as well. This can be done by computing, for a given parameter, one joint posterior density across all subjects, treating the posterior of one subject as the prior for the next (see Garrido et al., 2007). This approach can be more sensitive; its disadvantage, however, is that it corresponds to a fixed effects analysis and thus does not allow for inference beyond the particular group studied.

Bayesian Model Selection (BMS)

Model comparison and selection is central to the scientific process, in that it allows one to evaluate different hypotheses about the way data are caused (Pitt and Myung, 2002). Nearly all scientific reporting rests on some form of model comparison, which represents a probabilistic statement about the belief in one hypothesis relative to some other(s), given some observations. In other words: Given some observed data, which of several alternative models is optimal? The decision cannot be made solely by comparing the relative fit of competing models. One also needs to account for differences in complexity; i.e., the number of free parameters and the degree of their interdependency. This is important because as model complexity increases, fit increases monotonically, but at some point the model will start fitting noise that is specific to the particular data (i.e., "over-fitting") and thus becomes less generalizable across multiple realizations of the same underlying generative process. Therefore, the question "What is the optimal model?" can be reformulated as "What is the model that represents the best balance between fit and complexity?" This is the model that maximizes the model evidence:[5]

$$p(y|m) = \int p(y|\theta, m)p(\theta|m)d\theta \qquad (16)$$

Here, the numbers of free parameters (as well as the functional form of the generative model that determines their interdependencies) are subsumed by the integration. Unfortunately, this integral cannot usually be solved analytically; therefore an approximation to the model evidence is

used. This is usually a free energy bound on the log evidence (Friston et al., 2007):

$$F = \log p(y|m) - KL[q(\theta), p(\theta|y, m)] \qquad (17)$$

Because of its relation to variational calculus and free energy in statistical physics, this free energy bound F is often referred to as the "negative free energy" or "variational free energy" (Friston et al., 2007; MacKay, 2003; Neal and Hinton, 1998). Here, KL denotes the Kullback-Leibler divergence between the approximating posterior density $q(\theta)$ and the true posterior $p(\theta|y,m)$ (Friston et al., 2007). After convergence of the estimation scheme, the KL term is minimized and $F \approx \ln p(y|m)$. Rewriting Equation 17 as

$$F = \log p(y|\theta, m)_q - KL(q(\theta), p(\theta)) \qquad (18)$$

adds a useful perspective. The two terms in Equation 18 can be understood as encoding the two opposing requirements of a good model: that it explains the data and is as simple as possible (i.e., uses minimal number of parameters that deviate minimally from their priors). A derivation of Equations 17 and 18 can be found in Stephan et al. (2007a).

To quantify the relative goodness of two models m_i and m_j, the differences in their log-evidences can be transformed into a *Bayes factor* (BF):

$$BF_{ij} = \frac{p(y|m_i)}{p(y|m_j)} \approx \exp(F_i - F_j) \qquad (19)$$

The group Bayes factor (GBF) for any given model m_i, relative to m_j, is equivalent to the product of the subject-specific Bayes factors for a given model comparison

$$GBF_{ij} = \exp\left(\sum_k F_i - F_j\right) = \prod_K B_{ij}^K \qquad (20)$$

where k indexes subjects (Stephan et al., 2007b). It rests on the assumption that model evidences are independent across subjects; this is tenable if the subjects are independent samples from the population. Furthermore, given a flat prior on the model, the product of model evidences is equivalent to multiplying the posterior probabilities of all models.

The GBF suffers from two major problems. First, it corresponds to a fixed-effects analysis, making it vulnerable to the existence of outlier subjects. An alternative, random-effects procedure consists in evaluating the log-evidences across subjects as the basis for a classical log-likelihood ratio statistic, testing the null hypothesis that no single model is better (in terms of their log-evidence) than any other (Stephan et al., 2009). Effectively, this tests for differences between models that are consistent and large in relation to differences within models over subjects. The most general implementation would be a repeated measures ANOVA, where the log-evidences for the different models represent the repeated measure within a given subject. At its simplest, the comparison of just two models over subjects involves a simple paired t-test on the log-evidences (or a one-sample t-test on the log-evidence differences). Of course, it would also be possible to use nonparametric inference. However, log-evidences tend to be fairly well behaved, and the residuals of a simple ANOVA model usually suggest that parametric assumptions are not violated.

A second problem is that the GBF does not represent a formal evaluation of the density on model space itself and rests on a slightly odd generative model for group data: the *GBF* encodes the relative probability that the data were generated by one model relative to another, assuming the data were generated by the same model for all subjects. What we really want, however, is the density from which models are sampled to generate subject-specific data. In other words, we seek the conditional estimates of the model probabilities that generate indicator variables prescribing the model for the *i*th subject. We have recently developed a hierarchical model that provides such estimates of model probabilities using a variational Bayesian approach (Stephan et al., 2009). This model allows one to compute the expected probability that the *k*th model will be selected for any randomly selected subject as well as the "exceedance probability" that a given model m_1 has a higher probability of having generated the observed data across the group than any other model considered (Stephan et al., 2009).

BMS plays a central role for DCM. It has been used extensively by previous fMRI studies to select the most likely model amongst a set of alternatives before making inferences about particular parameters at the group level (e. g., Acs and Greenlee, 2008; Allen et al., 2008; den Ouden et al., 2009; Garrido et al., 2007; Garrido et al., 2008; Grol et al., 2007; Heim et al., 2008; Kumar et al., 2007; Smith et al., 2006; Stephan et al., 2007b; Summerfield and Koechlin, 2008). An alternative use of model selection is to decide about the nature of particular mechanisms without the need for any further inference about particular parameters. For example, BMS has been used to compare DCMs with non-linear versus linear BOLD equations in the hemodynamic forward model (Stephan et al., 2007a; Stephan et al., 2009). A particularly interesting approach is to go beyond the comparison of specific models and assess the importance of changes along a specific dimension of model space. This type of inference, which could be seen as a Bayesian analogue of testing for "main effects" in classical ANOVA, is made possible by the hierarchical Bayesian model described above (Stephan et al., 2009) and rests on comparing two (or more) partitions of model space. These partitions would typically reflect those components of model structure that one seeks inference about, e.g., whether a specific connection should be included in the model or not, whether a particular connection is modulated by one experimental condition or another, or whether certain effects are linear or non-linear. The advantage of this method is that arbitrarily large sets of models can be considered together, allowing one to integrate out uncertainty over any aspect of model structure other than the component of interest.

Non-linear DCM for fMRI

Since its first description by Friston et al. (2003), DCM for fMRI has been extended in several ways. Kiebel et al. (2007) have augmented the observation equation by taking into account the slice-specific sampling times in multi-slice MRI acquisitions. This enables DCM to be applied to fMRI data from any data acquisition scheme, overcoming restrictions of the original DCM formulation in this regard. Another recent extension was to represent each region in the model by two state variables and distinguish between population activity of excitatory and inhibitory neurons (Marreiros et al., 2008).

In this chapter, we focus on what we consider to be a particularly important extension of DCM for fMRI, namely the inclusion of non-linear modulatory effects. This extension, described in a recent paper by Stephan et al. (2008), was motivated by two limitations of the original bilinear neuronal state equation in DCM. First, the neuronal origin of the modulatory influence is not specified. Second, the bilinear framework may not be the most appropriate choice for modeling fast changes in effective connectivity, which are mediated by non-linear effects at the level of single neurons. These mechanisms are instances of "short-term synaptic plasticity" (STP), an umbrella term for a range of processes that alter synaptic strengths with time constants in the range of milliseconds to minutes; e.g., NMDA-controlled phosphorylation of AMPA receptors, synaptic depression/facilitation, or "early LTP." All these processes are driven by the history of prior synaptic activity and are thus non-linear (Zucker and Regehr, 2002).

A particularly interesting mechanism, which relies on STP, is "neuronal gain control." Neuronal gain, i.e., the response of a given neuron N_1 to presynaptic input from a second neuron N_2, depends on the history of inputs that N_1 receives from other neurons, e.g., a third neuron N_3. Such a non-linear modulation or "gating" of the $N_2 \rightarrow N_1$ connection by N_3 has been shown to have the same mathematical form across a large number of experiments (for review, see Salinas and Sejnowski, 2001): the change in the gain of N_1 results from a multiplicative interaction among the synaptic inputs from N_2 and N_3, i.e., a second-order non-linear effect. Biophysically, neuronal gain control can arise through various mechanisms that mediate interactions among synaptic inputs, occurring close in time but not necessarily in the same dendritic compartment (see Stephan et al., 2008, for a discussion of these mechanisms).

Critically, the bilinear framework precludes a representation, at the neuronal level, of the mechanisms described above. As stated in the original DCM paper (Friston et al., 2003), in order to model processes like neuronal gain control and synaptic plasticity properly, one needs "to go beyond bilinear approximations to allow for interactions among the states. This is important when trying to model modulatory or nonlinear connections such as those mediated by backward afferents that terminate predominantly in the supragranular layers and possibly on NMDA receptors."

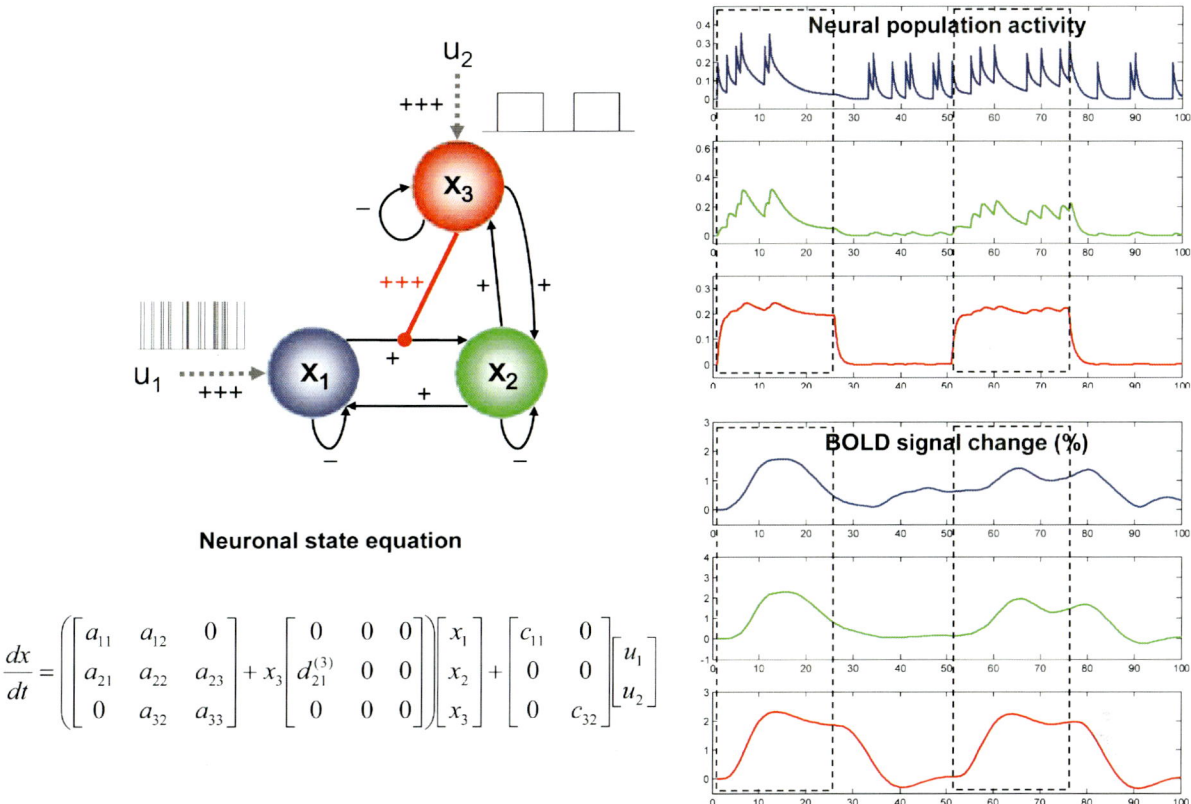

Figure 3.9.4. An example of the neuronal and hemodynamic dynamics that can be accounted for by non-linear DCMs. The right panel shows synthetic neuronal and BOLD time-series that were generated using the non-linear DCM shown on the left. In this model, neuronal population activity x_1 (blue) is driven by irregularly spaced random events (delta-functions). Activity in x_2 (green) is driven through a connection from x_1; critically, the strength of this connection depends on activity in a third population, x_3 (red), which receives a connection from x_2 but also receives a direct input from a box-car input. The effect of non-linear modulation can be seen easily: responses of x_2 to x_1 become negligible when x_3 activity is low. Conversely, x_2 responds vigorously to x_1 inputs when the $x_1 \rightarrow x_2$ connection is gated by x_3 activity. Strengths of connections are indicated by symbols (-: negative; +: weakly positive; +++: strongly positive). (Reproduced, with permission, from Figure 2 in Stephan et al. (2008)).

Therefore, to enable a realistic representation of how neuronal populations modulate the gains of other populations, one needs to model non-linear interactions among the n states of a given DCM. For this purpose, one can use a two-dimensional Taylor series, which is of second order in the states (Stephan et al., 2008):

$$f(x, u) = \frac{dx}{dt}$$
$$\approx f(0, 0) + \frac{\partial f}{\partial x} x + \frac{\partial f}{\partial u} u + \frac{\partial^2 f}{\partial x \partial u} xu + \frac{\partial^2 f}{\partial x^2} \frac{x^2}{2} \quad (21)$$

Setting $D^{(j)} = \frac{1}{2} \frac{\partial^2 f}{\partial x_j^2}\big|_{u=0}$ $(1 \le j \le n)$ makes Equation 21 equivalent to:

$$f(x, u) = \frac{dx}{dt} = \left(A + \sum_{i=1}^{m} u_i B^{(i)} + \sum_{j=1}^{n} x_j D^{(j)} \right) x + Cu$$
$$(22)$$

Here, the $D^{(j)}$ matrices encode which of the n regions gate which connections in the system. Specifically, any non-zero entry $D_{kl}^{(j)}$ indicates that responses of region k to inputs from region l depend on activity in region j. Figure 3.9.4 shows a simple example, with synthetic data generated by a non-linear DCM. This illustrates the sort of dynamics, both at the neuronal and hemodynamic level, that this sort of model exhibits.

The non-linear extension enhances the kind of dynamics that DCM can capture and enables the user to implement additional types of models. Beyond modeling how connection strengths are modulated by external inputs, one can now model how connection strengths are gated by the activity of one or several neuronal populations. This ability is critical for various applications, e.g., for marrying reinforcement learning models with DCM (c.f., Stephan, 2004), but also for mechanistic accounts of the effects of attention. Stephan et al. (2008) applied non-linear DCM to a single-subject data set from a blocked fMRI study of attention to visual motion (Büchel and Friston, 1997). They inverted and compared four different models, each of which embodied a different explanation for the empirical finding that V5 responses increased during attention to motion,

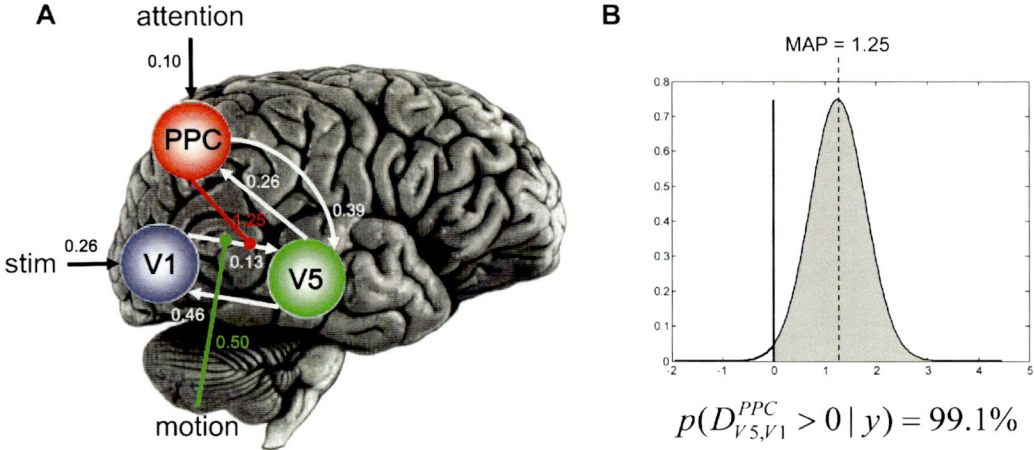

Figure 3.9.5. Application of non-linear DCM to single-subject fMRI data from an attention to motion paradigm by Büchel and Friston (1997). A. Maximum a posteriori estimates of all parameters. PPC = posterior parietal cortex. B. Posterior density of the estimate for the non-linear modulation parameter for the V1→V5 connection. Given the mean and variance of this posterior density, we have 99.1% confidence that the true parameter value is larger than zero or, in other words, that there is an increase in gain of V5 responses to V1 inputs that is mediated by PPC activity. (Reproduced, with permission, from Figure 7 in Stephan et al. (2008))T.

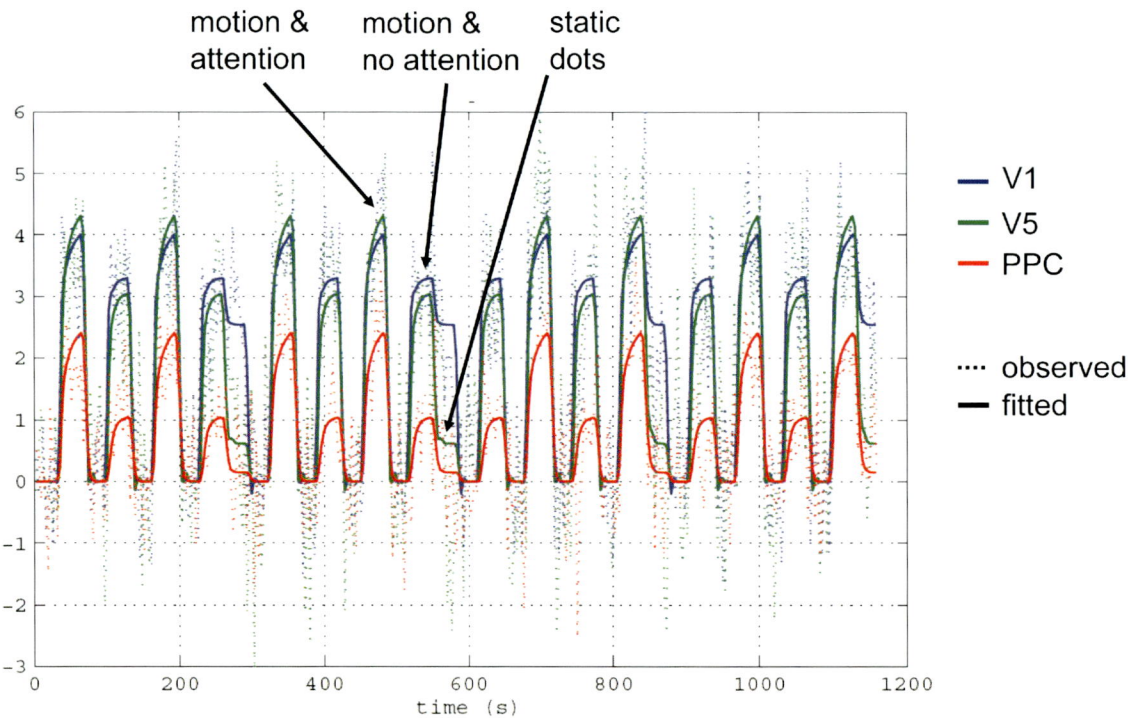

Figure 3.9.6. Fit of the non-linear model to the attention to motion data in Figure 3.9.5. Dotted lines represent the observed data, solid lines the responses predicted by the non-linear DCM. The increase in the gain of V5 responses to V1 inputs during attention is clearly visible. Reproduced, with permission, from Figure 8 in Stephan et al. (2008).

compared to unattended motion. The most likely model was one in which the gain of the V1→V5 connection depended on the activity in the posterior parietal cortex (PPC), a region on which attention was modeled to exert a direct effect (this could result, for example, from inputs

from the brainstem). Analysis of the posterior density of the modulatory parameter in this model indicated that non-linear gating of the V1→V5 connection by attention could be inferred with 99.1% confidence (see Figure 3.9.5). Figure 3.9.6 shows the observed and fitted time-series of all

Figure 3.9.7. Application of non-linear DCM to single-subject fMRI data from a binocular rivalry paradigm. A. The structure of the non-linear DCM fitted to the binocular rivalry data, along with the maximum a posteriori estimates of all parameters. The intrinsic connections between FFA and PPA are negative in both directions; i.e., FFA and PPA mutually inhibited each other. This may be seen as an expression, at the neurophysiological level, of the perceptual competition between the face and house stimuli. This competitive interaction between FFA and PPA is modulated nonlinearly by activity in the middle frontal gyrus (MFG), which showed higher activity during rivalry vs. nonrivalry conditions. B. Our confidence about the presence of this non-linear modulation is very high (99.9%), for both connections. Reproduced, with permission, from Figure 9 in Stephan et al. (2008).

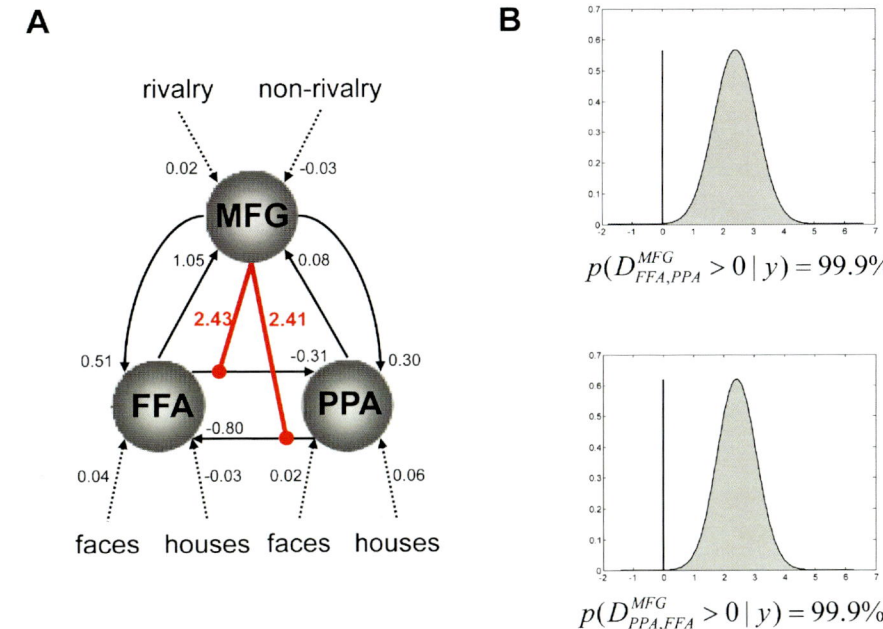

$$p(D_{FFA,PPA}^{MFG} > 0 \mid y) = 99.9\%$$

$$p(D_{PPA,FFA}^{MFG} > 0 \mid y) = 99.9\%$$

areas and highlights the attentional gating effect on V5 activity, such that V5 activity was higher when subjects attended the moving stimuli.

As a second example for the practical utility of non-linear DCMs, we show the results from a single-subject analysis of fMRI data set acquired during an event-related binocular rivalry paradigm (Stephan et al., 2008). Binocular rivalry arises when two different stimuli are projected separately to the two eyes; the subject then experiences a single percept at a time, and this percept fluctuates between the two competing stimuli with a time constant in the order of a few seconds. While there is no clear consensus about the mechanisms that underlie this phenomenon, it has been suggested that binocular rivalry *(1)* depends on nonlinear mechanisms and *(2)* may arise from modulation of connections among neuronal representations of the competing stimuli by feedback connections from higher areas (see Blake and Logothetis, 2002).

The fMRI data were acquired during a factorial paradigm in which face and house stimuli were presented either during binocular rivalry or during a matched nonrivalry (i.e., replay) condition. For the subject studied here, the conventional SPM analysis showed a rivalry × percept interaction in both the right fusiform face area (FFA) and the right parahippocampal place area (PPA): in FFA, the face vs. house contrast was higher during nonrivalry than during rivalry; conversely, in PPA the house vs. face contrast was higher during nonrivalry than during rivalry (both p < 0.05, small-volume corrected).[6] Additionally, testing for a main effect of rivalry, we replicated previous findings (Lumer et al., 1998) that the right middle frontal gyrus (MFG) showed higher activity during rivalry than during nonrivalry conditions.

These SPM results motivated a non-linear DCM in which the connections between FFA and PPA were modulated by the activity in the MFG. The structure of the resulting DCM (along with the MAP estimates for all parameters) is shown in Figure 3.9.7. First, the fixed (endogenous) connection strengths between FFA and PPA were negative in both directions, i.e., FFA and PPA exerted a mutual negative influence on each other, when the system was not perturbed by inputs (i.e., during fixation); this could be regarded as a "tonic" or "baseline" reciprocal inhibition. More importantly, however, was that during the presentation of visual stimuli this competitive interaction between FFA and PPA was modulated by activity in the middle frontal gyrus (MFG), which showed higher activity during rivalry vs. nonrivalry conditions. As shown in Figure 3.9.7, our confidence about the presence of this non-linear modulation was very high (99.9%) for both connections.

According to this model, activity levels in the MFG determine the magnitude of the face vs. house activity differences in FFA and PPA by controlling the influence that face-elicited activations and house-elicited deactivations of FFA have on PPA (and vice versa). For example, the positive non-linear modulation of the FFA→PPA connection by MFG activity (see Figure 3.9.7) means that during face-perception under rivalry conditions (which elicit positive activity in the FFA and MFG, respectively) there is a positive influence of FFA on PPA, overriding the "baseline" inhibition. This means that during binocular rivalry FFA and PPA become more tightly coupled, which destroys their stimulus selectivity: their activity becomes similar, regardless of whether a face or a house is being perceived. In contrast, deactivation of MFG during nonrivalry conditions decreases the influence that FFA has on PPA during house perception; therefore responses in

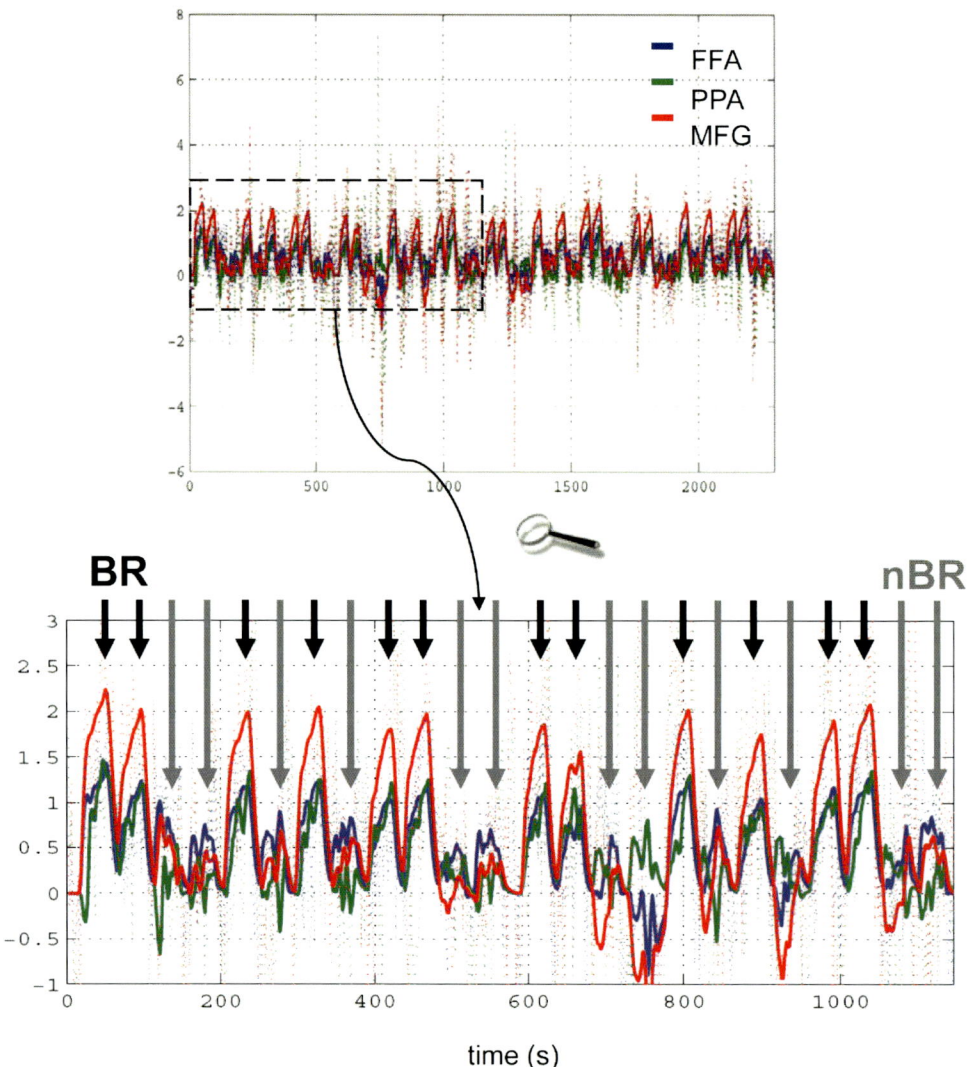

Figure 3.9.8. Fit of the non-linear model in Figure 3.9.7 to the binocular rivalry data. Dotted lines represent the observed data, solid lines the responses predicted by the non-linear DCM. The upper panel shows the entire time-series. The lower panel zooms in on the first half of the data (dotted box). One can see that the functional coupling between FFA (blue) and PPA (green) depends on the activity level in MFG (red): when MFG activity is high during binocular rivalry blocks (BR; short black arrows), FFA and PPA are strongly coupled and their responses are difficult to disambiguate. In contrast, when MFG activity is low, during nonrivalry blocks (nBR; long grey arrows), FFA and PPA are less coupled, and their activities evolve more independently. (Reproduced, with permission, from Figure 10 in Stephan et al. (2008)).

FFA and PPA become less coupled and their relative selectivity for face and house percepts is restored. This dynamic coupling and uncoupling, leading to less selectivity of FFA and PPA during rivalry and higher selectivity during nonrivalry, is clearly visible in the fitted responses shown by Figure 3.9.8. Here, the short black arrows indicate blocks with binocular rivalry (when FFA and PPA show similar time courses) and the long grey arrows denote nonrivalry blocks (when FFA and PPA activities evolve more independently). These nonlinear changes in effective connectivity, which are controlled by the activity level in MFG, provide a nice explanation for the rivalry × percept interaction in FFA and PPA that were identified by the SPM analysis.

Future Applications and Extensions of DCM

Since its inception in 2003 (Friston et al., 2003), DCM has already had a major impact on the analyses of fMRI data; this is reflected by more than 40 published studies so far. We expect that several application domains for DCM will prove to be particularly exciting and fruitful in the near future.

The first domain is the integration of the neurophysiological and computational aspects of learning and decision making. This requires that predictions from computational models (such as Rescorla-Wagner or temporal difference learning models) are integrated into DCMs. A first demonstration of this approach was recently published by den Ouden et al. (2009).

The second domain concerns the development of DCMs with clinical utility, for example as diagnostic tools. Although DCM has already been applied to clinical populations (e.g., Grefkes et al., 2008; Sonty et al., 2007), the critical challenge for the future will be to develop DCMs whose parameter estimates have sufficient sensitivity and specificity to delineate subgroups of patients that are characterized by different pathophysiological mechanisms. For example, our own work focuses on schizophrenia, trying to establish DCMs that can represent, in conjunction with pharmacological challenges and learning paradigms, specific abnormalities in the regulation of NMDA-dependent synaptic plasticity by neuromodulatory transmitters like dopamine or actylcholine (Stephan et al., 2006).

Third, as described above, the concept of DCM is very generic and can be applied to any imaging modality for which a forward model can be specified. This means that it should be possible, in principle, to employ DCM for joint analysis of brain activity data that were simultaneously acquired using different techniques, as in simultaneous recordings of fMRI and EEG, for example. In this case of multimodal fusion, a single model of neuronal processes would have to be linked to data in the different modalities by separate forward models, i.e., a hemodynamic model to explain the observed fMRI measurements and an electromagnetic forward model to explain the observed scalp potentials. The challenge will then be to invert this extended model as a whole, obtaining the posterior estimates of the neuronal parameters that are informed by both fMRI and EEG measurements. While this idea is very elegant and promising, there are several problems that need to be resolved before this approach can be implemented in practice; see David (2007) and Daunizeau et al. (2009) for further discussion of this issue.

ACKNOWLEDGMENTS

This work was funded by the Wellcome Trust (KJF) and the University Research Priority Program "Foundations of Human Social Behaviour" at the University of Zurich (KES).

NOTES

1. Note that in all models of effective connectivity, connections do not necessarily have to be direct, i.e., monosynaptic, connections (see McIntosh and Gonzalez-Lima, 1994).
2. When applied to questions in the social sciences, SEM is typically used to infer relations between unobserved or "latent" variables. In this case, Equation 11 needs to be combined with a model linking latent variables to observations.
3. A similar situation is seen with EEG data, where there is a big difference between signals measured at each electrode and the underlying neuronal activity: changes in neural activity in different brain regions lead to changes in electric potentials that superimpose linearly. The scalp electrodes therefore record a mixture, with unknown weightings, of potentials generated by a number of different sources.
4. A shrinkage prior in DCM is characterized by a mean of zero and high precision (small variance). Consequently, the posterior estimates are "shrunk" toward the prior expectation of zero unless the data contain strong evidence to the contrary. This means that the posterior expectation of parameter estimates in DCMs that are fitted to pure noise is zero.
5. Model comparison based on the evidence is appropriate if all models have identical a priori probabilities. If this is the case, the model evidence $p(y|m)$ is identical to the posterior probability of the model, $p(m|y)$.
6. This SPM result is in contradiction to the findings by Tong et al. (1998) who, using a similar paradigm, reported that activity in FFA and PPA did not differ between rivalry and nonrivalry conditions. This discrepancy might arise due to various reasons. For example, Tong et al. (1998) used a separate localizer scan whereas our design embedded the localizer contrast into a fully factorial design (c.f., Friston et al., 2006).

REFERENCES

Acs F, Greenlee MW (2008). Connectivity modulation of early visual processing areas during covert and overt tracking tasks. NeuroImage 41:380–388.

Aertsen A, Preißl H (1991) Dynamics of activity and connectivity in physiological neuronal networks. In: Non linear dynamics and neuronal networks (Schuster HG, ed), pp 281–302. New York: VCH Publishers.

Allen P, Mechelli A, Stephan KE, Day F, Dalton J, Williams S, McGuire PK (2008) Frontotemporal interactions during overt verbal initiation and suppression. J Cogn Neurosci 20:1656–1669.

Bitan T, Booth JR, Choy J, Burman DD, Gitelman DR, Mesulam MM (2005) Shifts of effective connectivity within a language network during rhyming and spelling. J Neurosci 25:5397–5403.

Blake R, Logothetis NK (2002) Visual competition. Nat Rev Neurosci 3:13–21.

Bokde AL, Tagamets MA, Friedman RB, Horwitz B (2001) Functional interactions of the inferior frontal cortex during the processing of words and word-like stimuli. Neuron 30:609–617.

Bollen KA (1989) Structural equations with latent variables. New York: John Wiley.

Büchel C, Friston KJ (1997) Modulation of connectivity in visual pathways by attention: Cortical interactions evaluated with structural equation modelling and fMRI. Cereb Cortex 7:768–778.

Büchel C, Coull JT, Friston KJ (1999) The predictive value of changes in effective connectivity for human learning. Science 283:1538–1541.

Bullmore ET, Horwitz B, Honey G, Brammer M, Williams S, Sharma T (2000) How good is good enough in path analysis of fMRI data? NeuroImage 11:289–301.

Buxton RB, Wong EC, Frank LR (1998) Dynamics of blood flow and oxygenation changes during brain activation: the balloon model. Magn Reson Med 39:855–864.

Chen CC, Kiebel SJ, Friston KJ (2008) Dynamic causal modelling of induced responses. NeuroImage 41:1293–1312.

Daunizeau J, Laufs H, Friston KJ (2009) EEG-fMRI information fusion: biophysics and data analysis. In: EEG-fMRI: physiology, technique, and applications (Mulert C, Lemieux L, eds), in press. Heidelberg: Springer.

David O (2007) Dynamic causal models and autopoietic systems. Biol Res 40:487–502.

David O, Kiebel SJ, Harrison LM, Mattout J, Kilner JM, Friston KJ (2006) Dynamic causal modeling of evoked responses in EEG and MEG. NeuroImage 30:1255–1272.

David O, Guillemain I, Saillet S, Reyt S, Deransart C, Segebarth C, Depaulis A (2008) Identifying neural drivers with functional MRI: an electrophysiological validation. PLoS Biol 6:2683–2697.

den Ouden HEM, Friston KJ, Daw ND, McIntosh AR, Stephan KE (2009) A dual role for prediction error in associative learning. Cereb Cortex 19:1175–1185.

Friston KJ (1994) Functional and effective connectivity in neuroimaging: a synthesis. Hum Brain Mapp 2:56–78.

Friston KJ (2002a) Beyond phrenology: what can neuroimaging tell us about distributed circuitry? Annu Rev Neurosci 25:221–250.

Friston KJ (2002b) Bayesian estimation of dynamical systems: an application to fMRI. NeuroImage 16:513–530.

Friston KJ, Büchel C (2004) Functional connectivity: eigenimages and multivariate analyses. In: Human brain function, 2nd edition (Frackowiack R et al., ed), pp 999–1018. New York: Elsevier.

Friston KJ, Frith CD, Frackowiak RS, Turner R (1995) Characterizing dynamic brain responses with fMRI: a multivariate approach. NeuroImage 2:166–172.

Friston KJ, Büchel C, Fink GR, Morris J, Rolls E, Dolan RJ (1997) Psychophysiological and modulatory interactions in neuroimaging. NeuroImage 6:218–229.

Friston KJ, Mechelli A, Turner R, Price CJ (2000) Nonlinear responses in fMRI: the Balloon model, Volterra kernels, and other hemodynamics. NeuroImage 12:466–477.

Friston KJ, Harrison L, Penny W (2003) Dynamic causal modelling. NeuroImage 19:1273–1302.

Friston KJ, Rotshtein P, Geng JJ, Sterzer P, Henson RN (2006) A critique of functional localisers. NeuroImage 30:1077–1087.

Friston KJ, Mattout J, Trujillo-Barreto N, Ashburner A, Penny WD (2007) Variational free energy and the Laplace approximation. NeuroImage 34:220–234.

Garrido MI, Kilner JM, Kiebel SJ, Stephan KE, Friston KJ (2007) Dynamic causal modelling of evoked potentials: a reproducibility study. NeuroImage 36:571–580.

Garrido MI, Friston KJ, Kiebel SJ, Stephan KE, Baldeweg T, Kilner JM (2008) The functional anatomy of the MMN: A DCM study of the roving paradigm. NeuroImage 42:936–944.

Goebel R, Roebroeck A, Kim DS, Formisano E (2003) Investigating directed cortical interactions in time-resolved fMRI data using vector autoregressive modeling and Granger causality mapping. Magn Res Imag 21:1251–1261.

Granger CWJ (1969) Investigating causal relations by econometric models and cross-spectral methods. Econometrica 37:424–438.

Grefkes C, Nowak DA, Eickhoff SB, Dafotakis M, Küst J, Karbe H, Fink GR (2008) Cortical connectivity after subcortical stroke assessed with functional magnetic resonance imaging. Ann Neurol 63:236–246.

Grol MJ, Majdandzic J, Stephan KE, Verhagen L, Dijkerman C, Bekkering H, Verstraten FAJ, Toni I (2007) Parieto-frontal connectivity during visually-guided grasping. J Neurosci 27:11877–11887.

Harrison LM, Penny W, Friston KJ (2003) Multivariate autoregressive modeling of fMRI time series. NeuroImage 19:1477–1491.

Heim S, Eickhoff SB, Ischebeck AK, Friederici AD, Stephan KE, Amunts K (2008) Dissociating the roles of the left BA 44 and inferior temporal gyrus during visual word processing using dynamic causal modelling. Hum Brain Mapp 30:392–402.

Honey GD, Fu CHY, Kim J, Brammer MJ, Croudace TJ, Suckling J, Pich EM, Williams SCR, Bullmore ET (2002) Effects of verbal working memory load on corticocortical connectivity modeled by path analysis of functional magnetic resonance imaging data. NeuroImage 17:573–582.

Horwitz B, Tagamets MA, McIntosh AR (1999) Neural modeling, functional brain imaging, and cognition. Trends Cogn Sci 3:91–98.

Kiebel SJ, Klöppel S, Weiskopf N, Friston KJ (2007) Dynamic causal modeling: a generative model of slice timing in fMRI. NeuroImage 34:1487–1496.

Kumar S, Stephan KE, Warren JD, Friston KJ, Griffiths TD (2007) Hierarchical processing of auditory objects in humans. PLoS Comput Biol 3:e100.

Lumer ED, Friston KJ, Rees G (1998) Neural correlates of perceptual rivalry in the human brain. Science 280:1930–1934.

Macaluso E, Frith CD, Driver J (2000) Modulation of human visual cortex by crossmodal spatial attention. Science 289:1206–1208.

MacKay DJC (2003) Information theory, inference, and learning algorithms. Cambridge: Cambridge University Press.

McIntosh AR, Gonzalez-Lima F (1991) Metabolic activation of the rat visual system by patterned light and footshock. Brain Res 547:295–302

McIntosh AR, Gonzalez-Lima F (1994) Structural equation modeling and its application to network analysis in functional brain imaging. Hum Brain Mapp 2:2–22.

McIntosh AR, Lobaugh NJ (2004) Partial least squares analysis of neuroimaging data: applications and advances. NeuroImage 23 (Suppl 1):S250–S263.

McIntosh AR, Grady CL, Ungerleider LG, Haxby JV, Rapoport SI, Horwitz B (1994) Network analysis of cortical visual pathways mapped with PET. J Neurosci 14:655–666.

Marreiros AC, Kiebel SJ, Friston KJ (2008) Dynamic causal modelling for fMRI: a two-state model. NeuroImage 39:269–278.

Mechelli A, Price CJ, Noppeney U, Friston KJ (2003) A dynamic causal modeling study on category effects: bottom-up or top-down mediation? J Cogn Neurosci 15:925–934.

Moran RJ, Stephan KE, Kiebel SJ, Rombach N, O'Connor WT, Murphy KJ, Reilly RB, Friston KJ (2008) Bayesian estimation of synaptic physiology from the spectral responses of neural masses. NeuroImage 42:272–284.

Moran RJ, Stephan KE, Seidenbecher T, Pape HC, Dolan RJ, Friston KJ (2009) Dynamic causal models of steady-state responses. NeuroImage 44:796–811.

Neal RM, Hinton GE (1998) A view of the EM algorithm that justifies incremental sparse and other variants. In: Learning in graphical models (Jordan MI, ed). Dordrecht: Kluwer Academic Publishers, pp 355–368.

Noppeney U, Price CJ, Penny WD, Friston KJ (2006) Two distinct neural mechanisms for category-selective responses. Cereb Cortex 16:437–445.

Penny WD, Roberts SJ (2002) Bayesian multivariate autoregressive models with structured priors. IEE Proc Vis Imag Sign Proc 149:33–41.

Penny WD, Stephan KE, Mechelli A, Friston KJ (2004a) Comparing dynamic causal models. NeuroImage 22:1157–1172.

Penny WD, Stephan KE, Mechelli A, Friston KJ (2004b) Modelling functional integration: a comparison of structural equation and dynamic causal models. NeuroImage 23 (Suppl 1):S264–274.

Pitt MA, Myung IJ (2002) When a good fit can be bad. Trends Cogn Sci 6:421–425.

Rowe JB, Stephan KE, Friston KJ, Frackowiak RJS, Lees A, Passingham RE (2002) Attention to action in Parkinson's disease: impaired effective connectivity among frontal cortical regions. Brain 125:276–289.

Salinas E, Sejnowski TJ (2001) Gain modulation in the central nervous system: where behavior, neurophysiology, and computation meet. Neuroscientist 7:430–440.

Smith APR, Stephan KE, Rugg MD, Dolan RJ (2006) Task and content modulate amygdala-hippocampal connectivity in emotional retrieval. Neuron 49:631–638.

Sonty SP, Mesulam MM, Weintraub S, Johnson NA, Parrish TB, Gitelman DR (2007) Altered effective connectivity within the language network in primary progressive aphasia. J Neurosci 27:1334–1345.

Stephan KE (2004) On the role of general system theory for functional neuroimaging. J Anat 205:443–470.

Stephan KE, Marshall JC, Friston KJ, Rowe JB, Ritzl A, Zilles K, Fink GR (2003) Lateralized cognitive processes and lateralized task control in the human brain. Science 301:384–386.

Stephan KE, Penny WD, Marshall JC, Fink GR, Friston KJ (2005) Investigating the functional role of callosal connections with dynamic causal models. Ann N Y Acad Sci 1064:16–36.

Stephan KE, Baldeweg T, Friston KJ (2006) Synaptic plasticity and dysconnection in schizophrenia. Biol Psychiatry 59:929–939.

Stephan KE, Weiskopf N, Drysdale PM, Robinson PA, Friston KJ (2007a) Comparing hemodynamic models with DCM. NeuroImage 38:387–401.

Stephan KE, Marshall JC, Penny WD, Friston KJ, Fink GR (2007b) Inter-hemispheric integration of visual processing during task-driven lateralization. J Neurosci 27:3512–3522.

Stephan KE, Kasper L, Harrison LM, Daunizeau J, den Ouden HEM, Breakspear M, Friston KJ (2008) Nonlinear dynamic causal models for fMRI. NeuroImage 42:649–662.

Stephan KE, Penny WD, Daunizeau J, Moran RJ, Friston KJ (2009) Bayesian model selection for group studies. NeuroImage 46:1004–1017.

Summerfield C, Koechlin E (2008) A neural representation of prior information during perceptual inference. Neuron 59:336–347.

Tong F, Nakayama K, Vaughan JT, Kanwisher N (1998) Binocular rivalry and visual awareness in human extrastriate cortex. Neuron 21:753–759.

Worsley KJ, Poline JB, Friston KJ, Evans AC (1997) Characterizing the response of PET and fMRI data using multivariate linear models. NeuroImage 6:305–319.

Yamashita O, Galka A, Ozaki T, Biscay R, Valdes-Sosa P (2004) Recursive penalized least squares solution for dynamical inverse problems of EEG generation. Hum Brain Mapp 21:221–235.

Zucker RS, Regehr WG (2002) Short-term synaptic plasticity. Annu Rev Physiol 64:355–405.

Part 4

Applications

4.1 Markus Siegel and Tobias H. Donner

Linking Band-Limited Cortical Activity to fMRI and Behavior

Introduction

Since the discovery of the electroencephalographam (EEG), it has been possible to measure neural mass activity with millisecond temporal resolution (Nunez and Srinivasan, 2006). Nowadays, neural population signals can be recorded at various spatial scales, using microelectrodes (measuring the local field potential, LFP), subdural surface electrodes (electrocorticography, ECoG), extracranial scalp electrodes (EEG), or magnetic field sensors (magnetoencephalography, MEG). Spectral analysis uncovers components of such population signals, which are "induced" by, but not necessarily "phase-locked" to, external events, such as stimulus onsets or motor responses (Pfurtscheller and Lopes da Silva, 1999; Tallon-Baudry and Bertrand, 1999).

Spectral analysis has primarily been used to characterize oscillatory patterns in the ongoing EEG (Dietsch, 1932; Grass and Gibbs, 1938). By contrast, studies of stimulus- and task-related EEG responses have long been dominated by the event-related potential (ERP) technique (Luck, 2005). This technique is based on averaging signal waveforms in the time domain across repeats of an external event, thereby isolating neural response components *phase-locked* to the event of interest. These response components are typically transient, lasting a few hundred milliseconds from the event. The rationale is to isolate the "signal" of interest from the "noise." However, neural responses to external stimulus and task events also reflect more sustained components.

We argue that, because the spectral analysis approach also captures sustained, non-phase-locked signal components, it is ideally suited for relating stimulus- and task-related neural mass activity to perception and cognition. First, many perceptual and cognitive processes (e.g., attention, short-term memory, and decision-making) unfold over time scales longer than the event-related potential. Second, these processes are not directly driven by external events, but emerge from recurrent network interactions within the brain. Such processes are thus likely to manifest themselves in the non-phase-locked neural response components. Third, investigating neural activity in the frequency domain may provide critical insights into the *mechanisms* underlying cognitive processes: Different mechanisms are often accompanied by different patterns of oscillatory neural activity (Buzsaki and Draguhn, 2004; Sejnowski and Paulsen, 2006; Steriade, 2000; Wang, 2003). For these reasons, we have recently witnessed an increasing use of spectral analysis in LFP studies in animals and in EEG and MEG studies in humans. This trend has led to an encouraging degree of convergence between these different levels of observation.

For the same reasons, we argue that spectral analysis is the prime approach for relating electrophysiological mass activity to the blood oxygenation level dependent (BOLD) contrast signal (Ogawa et al., 1990), the current mainstay of functional magnetic resonance imaging (fMRI). fMRI has proven to be an extraordinarily useful tool for identifying the large-scale cortical networks engaged in a variety of higher brain functions, including such seemingly elusive ones as attention, awareness, and decision-making (Corbetta and Shulman, 2002; Haynes and Rees, 2006; Heekeren et al., 2008; Kanwisher and Wojciulik, 2000; Kastner and Ungerleider, 2000). Cognitive neuroscience could make a major step forward if we knew how to link electrophysiological and fMRI signals measured during perception and cognition.

In this chapter, we will first address the question of how electrophysiological population signals are linked to sensory and cognitive processing. We review a wide range of studies all suggesting that such links are typically frequency-specific. We will refer to these links as the "spectral fingerprints" of the functional processes in a given brain region. We highlight that different classes of processes (and maybe even different classes of brain regions) seem to have remarkably different spectral fingerprints, a fact that is often overlooked. For example, stimulus-driven activity in sensory cortices generally seems to have a simple spectral fingerprint, the network mechanisms of which are becoming increasingly clear. By contrast, the spectral fingerprints of *intrinsic*, cognitive processes (such as "top-down" attention or switches between different perceptual states) in the same sensory regions appear to be more complex, and their underlying mechanisms are as yet elusive. We speculate that the reason for this discrepancy is that the latter kind of processes involve stronger recurrent network interactions between distant brain areas and/or neuromodulation[1] of cortical processing by ascending brainstem systems.

Second, we will discuss how the electrophysiological population signals relate to the fMRI signal. Many previous discussions of the relationship between invasive electrophysiology and the fMRI signal (e.g., Heeger and Ress, 2002; Lauritzen, 2005; Logothetis, 2008; Logothetis and Wandell, 2004) have focused on the question which aspect of neuronal activity (spiking vs. synaptic) drives the fMRI signal. We will not address this question here. Instead, we ask whether we can identify simple, general rules that govern the relationship between electrophysiological population activity and the fMRI signal at a macroscopic level. Based on the evidence reviewed below, a simple answer to this question appears to be "no." The relationship between these signals seems to depend on the specific *functional process* and, perhaps, even the *brain area* under study. While, again, a relatively simple relationship is beginning to emerge for stimulus-driven responses in sensory cortex, this relationship appears more complex, and as yet elusive, for higher cognitive processes. Thus, we propose that a fruitful approach toward integrating electrophysiology and fMRI may be an indirect one, that is, via the processes under study. We conclude with a list of open questions, answers to which might fundamentally advance our understanding of the issues addressed here.

A Brief Primer on Band-Limited Neural Activity

Electrophysiological Population Signals

Current electrophysiological techniques provide measures of neuronal population activity across a broad range of spatial scales. Intracortical microelectrode-recordings allow for directly measuring the spike output (action potentials) of individual (single-unit activity or SUA) or multiple (multi-unit activity or MUA) neurons. While spike signals are mostly confined to signal components above 500 Hz, the low-frequency signal (approx. <250 Hz) recorded from intracortical microelectrodes constitutes the local field potential (LFP), which reflects summed dendro-somatic currents surrounding the electrode tip (approx. <1 mm) (Juergens et al., 1999; Logothetis and Wandell, 2004; Mitzdorf, 1987). The LFP averages over several hundreds of neurons, and its amplitude

is thus thought to reflect predominantly *synchronized* synaptic events and other slow nonsynaptic potentials (e.g., spike afterpotentials). The electromagnetic fields corresponding to these synchronized dendritic currents can also be recorded from outside of the cortex. The ECoG measures these fields with sub- or epidurally placed electrodes, often referred to as intracranial EEG (Lachaux et al., 2003). At the most macroscopic level, scalp EEG and MEG measure the corresponding electric/magnetic fields using scalp electrodes (Nunez and Srinivasan, 2006) or magnetic field sensors (Hamalainen et al., 1993). While the intracortical LFP depends on the laminar placement of the electrode tip, the ECoG, EEG, or MEG do not provide such laminar specificity. The ECoG, EEG, or MEG mainly reflect the electromagnetic fields generated by the large dendrites of pyramidal neurons, which are arranged in parallel to one another and which are oriented perpendicular to the cortical surface.

"Frequency Bands" and Neural Oscillations

These electrophysiological signals comprise activity over a broad frequency range. Their power roughly follows a power-law decay ($1/frequency^n$) (Bedard et al., 2006; Buzsaki and Draguhn, 2004; Freeman et al., 2000). Thus, at higher frequencies, modulations of the spectral power are typically small in absolute magnitude and, without normalization, often masked by strong low-frequency components. Therefore, it is useful to calculate electrophysiological responses as power changes relative to a "baseline" (e.g., prestimulus interval) spectrum for visualizing the effects of a particular experimental manipulation, and for comparing them across different frequency ranges. Figure 4.1.1 illustrates this for MEG responses to a visual grating stimulus.

The different frequency ranges of these electrophysiological measures are commonly referred to as "bands," whose definition typically follows clinical EEG conventions: "delta" ($\sim$ 2–4 Hz), "theta" ($\sim$ 4–8 Hz), "alpha" ($\sim$ 8–12 Hz), "beta" ($\sim$ 12–30 Hz), and "gamma" ($\sim$ 30–80 Hz). This taxonomy is derived from the logarithmically scaled peaks of spectral power that are often superimposed onto the overall power decay, and it appeals to the notion of distinct oscillators producing these spectral peaks. There are considerable inconsistencies in the exact definition of frequency bands across studies. Therefore, we will state the exact frequency ranges along with the band names used by the authors in our literature review below.

In this chapter, we will use the descriptive term "band-limited" activity to refer to neural activity in specific frequency ranges. The often-used term "oscillatory" activity implies that the measured signal is generated by a single oscillator, or by a system of coupled oscillators. Indeed, (see below, "Why do different frequency bands exhibit different functional properties?"), experimental evidence suggests that the brain contains specific neural mechanisms (cellular and circuit-based) that produce oscillatory behavior in neural networks. Nevertheless, the presence of band-limited modulations in the measured

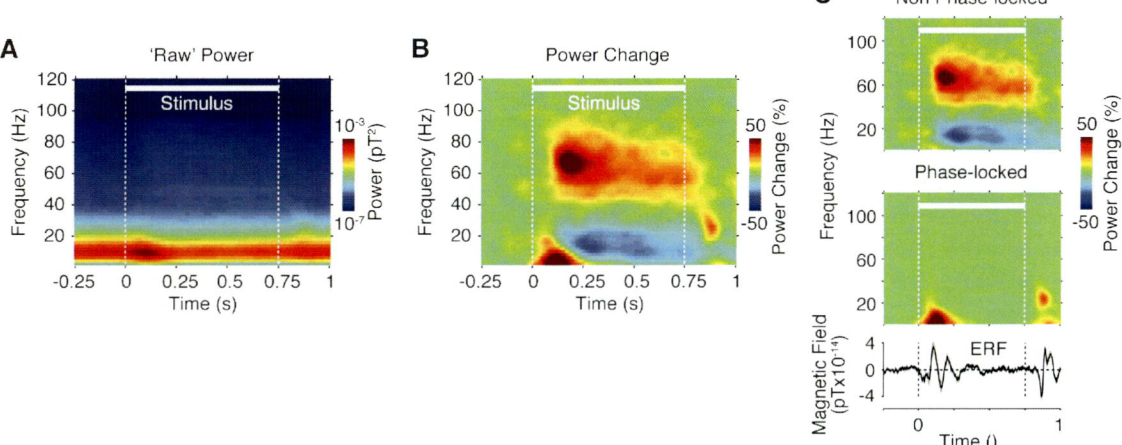

Figure 4.1.1. Illustration of the spectral analysis of human MEG responses (one occipital sensor) to a full-contrast drifting sine-wave grating presented for 750 ms. (**A**) Time-frequency representation of the *raw* MEG power, which exhibits the typical power law decay toward higher frequencies ($1/frequency^n$), masking the responses at high frequencies. (**B**) *Normalized* MEG response (percent power change relative to prestimulus baseline). By compensating for the power decay, this normalization reveals the high-frequency component of the stimulus response. (**C**) Dissociation of the response components phase-locked and non-phase-locked to stimulus onset. The stimulus-locked components correspond to the time-domain average of the MEG-signal that is displayed in the lower panel along with its time-frequency representation. The time-domain average only captures the transient phase-locked responses to stimulus on- and offset below 30 Hz. By contrast, the non-phase-locked components (upper panel) capture the prominent sustained responses induced by the stimulus: A power reduction in the 10–30 Hz range and a power enhancement in the 40–90 Hz range. The non-phase-locked response was isolated by subtracting the time-domain average from each trial before transforming the data into the frequency domain.

signals does not necessarily imply the presence of an underlying neural oscillation, for several reasons. First, population activity in a given frequency band may simply reflect the summation of relatively transient, nonperiodic signals with a specific spectral signature. For example, band-limited LFP power may reflect the summation of slow spike afterpotentials with dominant power in a specific frequency range (Buzsaki and Kandel, 1998). Second, apparently "band-limited" activity may also result from the superposition of broadband signals with band-limited effects specific to neighboring frequency ranges. For example, limb movements are typically associated with a high-frequency enhancement (50–200 Hz) and a low-frequency suppression (10–50 Hz) of the ECoG recorded over motor cortex (Crone et al., 1998a; Crone et al., 1998b; Miller et al., 2007). The high-frequency enhancement has commonly been interpreted as an induced gamma-band oscillation. However, principle component analysis (PCA) of movement-related ECoG activity revealed that the high-frequency enhancement in fact reflects a broadband (i.e., non-oscillatory) increase of $1/frequency^n$ activity, superimposed onto a movement-related decrease of low-frequency oscillations in the 10–50 Hz band (Miller et al., 2009). Analogous analyses will help to distinguish between oscillatory and non-oscillatory signals associated with other processes.

Phase-locked Versus Non-Phase-Locked Responses

Modulations of population signals correlated with external events can be classified according to the phase relationship

between these events and neural activity (see Figure 4.1.1) (Pfurtscheller and Lopes da Silva, 1999; Tallon-Baudry and Bertrand, 1999). For example, the onset of a sensory stimulus leads to transient amplitude changes of neural activity that show a constant phase-relationship to stimulus onset across several repeats. However, sensory stimulation and cognitive tasks also induce sustained neural responses, which are not phase-locked to external events. Because of their variable phase-relation to external events, time-domain averaging removes these response components. Thus, they are not reflected in the ERP. By contrast, spectral analysis allows for investigating non-phase-locked responses: First, the signal is transformed to the frequency- or time-frequency-domain on a single-trial basis. Then, the resulting complex spectrum is squared, which extracts the signal's power (i.e., variance) at a particular frequency, and discards its phase (Figure 4.1.1A). Eventually, power can be averaged across trials and normalized by a baseline-spectrum to account for the power decay toward high frequencies (Figure 4.1.1B).

For several reasons, the frequency domain is ideally suited for analyzing responses of electrophysiological population signals: First, cognitive processes often evolve over extended time periods (e.g., attention, short-term memory, decision-processes) and are thus often better reflected in sustained non-phase-locked response components than in transient phase-locked responses. Second, such cognitive processes are often not directly driven by external events (such as stimulus presentation). The corresponding neural responses are thus often not precisely aligned to external events and again better captured by sustained non-phase-locked responses. The analysis of ongoing activity unrelated to external events presents a special, and the most extreme, case for which, again, spectral analysis is ideally suited, but the ERP approach is, by definition, impossible.[2] We will here focus on task-related activity and thus not discuss studies of ongoing activity (reviewed by Laufs, 2008). Third, cognitive processes commonly display characteristic "spectral fingerprints" that presumably reflect the specific neural mechanisms and networks involved (see below, "Linking band-limited neural activity to behavior"). These fingerprints can be directly visualized in the frequency domain, which thus may provide a window into the neural mechanisms underlying the cognitive process under study.

When interpreting responses in the frequency domain, one needs to keep in mind that these reflect neural activity, which is both phase-locked and non-phase-locked to external events. Signals with sharp transients contain energy across a wide range of frequencies. Thus, ERPs are often reflected by transient broadband responses in the time-frequency domain, with significant power in the high frequency range, in the absence of a high-frequency oscillation. In other words, simply detecting significant power in any frequency band of the spectrum (e.g., "gamma") does not imply that the signal contains a neuronal oscillation in that frequency range. Furthermore, one needs to be cautious about electromagnetic activity from non-neuronal sources such as muscles that may be picked up by extracortical EEG/MEG sensors. For example, Yuval-Greenberg et al. (2008) demonstrated that the transient enhancement of spontaneous microsaccades, typically occurring around 200 ms after the onset of visual stimuli, causes a transient broadband increase of high-frequency power in the scalp EEG that is likely generated by ocular muscles. Fortunately, such artifacts have distinct spectral and temporal profiles that allow for dissociating them from the more sustained stimulus driven gamma-band responses (see Figures 4.1.1–4.1.3 and 4.1.5) (Fries et al., 2008a). This highlights the advantage of sustained stimulation protocols (stimulus durations of several seconds) as commonly used in single-unit physiology and fMRI. Furthermore, source-reconstruction or localization techniques and high-resolution eye-movement recordings will help rule out such artifacts.

Possible Functional Roles of Neuronal Phase Coherence

The band-limited power of population signals like LFP, EEG, or MEG primarily reflects neural activity that is locally synchronized across the spatial integration scale of the respective signal. More long-range synchronization of neural populations, e.g., between different brain regions, can be assessed by computing the phase consistency ("coherence") between pairs of simultaneously recorded signals (see also below, "Different windows into interactions between brain areas").

Dynamic adjustments of neuronal coherence may provide flexible mechanisms for regulating neuronal communication (Engel et al., 2001; Fries, 2005; Salinas and Sejnowski, 2001). First, synchronization of *presynaptic* spikes may enhance their functional impact on postsynaptic processing stages, and thus the effective connectivity between pre- and postsynaptic stages (König et al., 1996; Salinas and Sejnowski, 2001; Usrey and Reid, 1999). Theoretical (König et al., 1996; Salinas and Sejnowski, 2000; Shelley et al., 2002; Tiesinga et al., 2004) and experimental (Alonso et al., 1996; Azouz and Gray, 2000; Azouz and Gray, 2003; Bruno and Sakmann, 2006; Usrey et al., 1998) evidence suggests that cortical neurons act as "coincidence detectors": Presynaptic spikes that arrive synchronously on a millisecond time scale are more effective in driving a postsynaptic response than nonsynchronized inputs. In fact, neurons may be particularly sensitive to such synchronized synaptic input in regimens of high-conductance (Shelley et al., 2002) or balanced excitation and inhibition (Salinas and Sejnowski, 2000; Salinas and Sejnowski, 2001). Second, the phase alignment between *pre- and postsynaptic* processing stages in the cortex may also dynamically regulate their effective connectivity (Buzsaki and Draguhn, 2004; Fries, 2005; Womelsdorf et al., 2007): Subthreshold membrane potential oscillations induce rhythmic changes in neural excitability, and presynaptic spikes that are aligned to the excitable phase of such postsynaptic oscillations are more likely to drive spiking activity at the postsynaptic stage. In light of these biophysical considerations, it is of great interest to investigate whether the cortex in fact dynamically adjusts the local or long-range coherence of neural oscillations for regulating information flow, for example during selective attention or decision-making.

Phase coherence may not only regulate neural communication, but also play an important role for neural coding of information. Evidence suggests that the phase of neural oscillations may provide scaffolding for information coding by the spikes of individual neurons (Kayser et al., 2009; Lee H et al., 2005; Montemurro et al., 2008; Siegel et al., 2009). For example, while monkeys remembered complex visual objects over a brief delay, spikes were synchronized to prominent theta-band (4–8 Hz) oscillations of the LFP in extrastriate visual area V4 (Lee H et al., 2005), i.e., spikes preferentially occurred at a specific theta-phase. Notably, not all spikes were equally informative about memory content, but those at the preferred theta-phase of spiking conveyed most information about the remembered objects. In monkey prefrontal cortex, spikes conveyed most information about two objects simultaneously held in short-term memory at specific phases of the mid-frequency (20–50 Hz, beta and gamma) LFP (Siegel et al., 2009). Notably, the most informative phases differed between the two remembered objects. Finally, stimulus-driven spiking activity in sensory cortices also conveys more information when its timing relative to slow (<8 Hz) LFP fluctuations is taken into account (Kayser et al., 2009; Montemurro et al., 2008). In sum, the information conveyed by individual cortical neurons seems to depend critically on their spike timing, relative to coherent activity of the surrounding neural population. It is an exciting question for future research to which extent, and in which systems, the brain utilizes such a "phase-dependent coding" scheme.

Source Reconstruction of Band-Limited EEG/MEG Activity

A major challenge for understanding the functional role of band-limited population activity and relating it to fMRI responses is the comparison of results across species and spatial scales. At the sensor-level, EEG and MEG signals reflect a coarse summation of cortical activity and thus provide only limited information about the exact cortical regions involved. Reconstruction of cortical source-level activity from the sensor-level data is a critical step in relating EEG/MEG to intracortical electrophysiological or fMRI signals. Recent methodological advances yielded tools that are particularly well suited to estimate source-level activity from EEG or MEG data in the frequency domain. Specifically, adaptive linear spatial filtering techniques based on the "beamforming" approach allow for estimating the power and coherence of cortical population activity across the brain (Gross et al., 2001; Liljestrom et al., 2005; Van Veen et al., 1997). The spatial resolution of these techniques depends on the number of MEG/EEG sensors, the signal-to-noise ratio of the recorded signals, and the number of underlying cortical sources. Estimates of the spatial resolution are on the order of a few centimeters, or below for currently available recording techniques (Gross et al., 2003).

Linking Band-Limited Neural Activity to Behavior

In this section, we will review studies relating band-limited cortical population activity to specific sensory and cognitive processes, focusing on visual tasks and the primate brain. Rather than providing a comprehensive review, we will try to identify general principles underlying the spectral fingerprints of specific functional processes. To this end, we will contrast stimulus-driven signals in sensory cortex with intrinsically generated activity produced by recurrent cortical interactions and ascending neuromodulators during higher-level cognitive processing. This distinction is certainly an oversimplification, but it constitutes a very useful heuristic for sorting recent results.

Stimulus-Driven Activity in Visual Cortex

Several studies have identified the frequency ranges of cortical mass activity that exhibit, first, selectivity for visual features (such as contour orientation or motion direction),

and second, dependence on feature strength (such as luminance contrast or motion coherence).[3] These studies suggest that neural gamma-band activity reflects visual features.

Neural population responses in early visual cortex induced by visual stimuli exhibit a characteristic spectral signature. Activity is enhanced in a broad gamma band from about 30 Hz to well above 100 Hz and suppressed below 30 Hz (e.g., in the alpha and beta band, 8–30 Hz; see Figures 4.1.1, 4.1.2, 4.1.3, and 4.1.5). In particular the stimulus-driven gamma-band enhancement is consistently measured in early visual areas ranging from LFPs in cats (Brosch et al., 1995; Eckhorn et al., 1988; Gray et al., 1989; Gray and Singer, 1989; Kayser and König, 2004; Siegel and König, 2003) and monkeys (Belitski et al., 2008; Berens et al., 2008; Frien and Eckhorn, 2000; Frien et al., 2000; Henrie and Shapley, 2005; Liu and Newsome, 2006; Logothetis et al., 2001) to human EEG or MEG (Donner et al., 2007; Fries et al., 2008a; Gruber et al., 1999; Hall et al., 2005; Hoogenboom et al., 2005; Siegel et al., 2007; Siegel et al., 2008; Van Der Werf et al., 2008; Wyart and Tallon-Baudry, 2008). By comparison, in invasive recordings the low-frequency suppression is found less consistently than in non-invasive recordings. Microelectrode recordings suggest that the gamma-band response reflects synchronized oscillations of local neuronal ensembles. The strength of synchronization between neurons correlates with the similarity of their receptive fields and tuning properties (Brosch et al., 1995; Eckhorn et al., 1988; Frien and Eckhorn, 2000; Frien et al., 2000; Gray et al., 1989; Gray and Singer, 1989; Nir et al., 2007; Siegel and König, 2003). Hence, the amplitude of the local gamma-band LFP is tuned for specific sensory features and its tuning preference corresponds to the averaged selectivity of the neural population contributing to the gamma-band LFP. In primary visual cortex, the gamma-band LFP is selective for stimulus orientation (Berens et al., 2008a; Frien et al., 2000; Gray and Singer, 1989; Kayser and König, 2004; Siegel and König, 2003), spatial and temporal frequency (Kayser and König, 2004), and ocular dominance (Berens et al., 2008a). In monkey area MT, the gamma-band LFP is selective for motion direction and speed (Liu and Newsome, 2006). This selectivity is typically confined to a frequency range from about 50 to 100 Hz. In addition to the gamma band, several studies reported a second, weaker feature-selective frequency range from about 8 to 25 Hz. (Berens et al., 2008a; Kayser and König, 2004; Liu and Newsome, 2006; Siegel and König, 2003).

Comparison of LFP-selectivity across different kinds of visual features provides insight into the spatial integration properties of the LFP. Liu and Newsome (2006) observed that LFP responses to moving stimuli in area MT were selective for speed at higher frequencies (> 80 Hz) than for direction (> 40 Hz). Neurons with the same speed preference cluster in small groups of 500 μm diameter, whereas neuronal clusters ("columns") of the same direction preference span up to 2000 μm perpendicular to the cortical surface. The

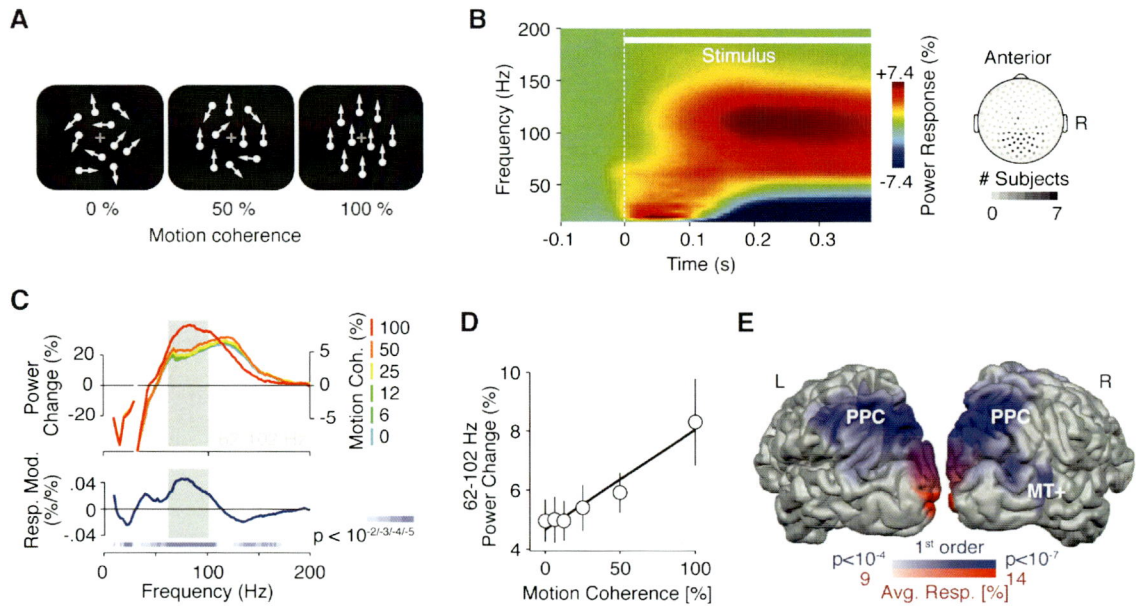

Figure 4.1.2. Modulation of band-limited MEG-activity by visual motion strength. Subjects viewed dynamic random dot patterns of different levels of motion strength. (**A**) "Motion coherence" (fraction of coherently moving dots) determines the strength of the visual motion signal. (**B**) Time-frequency response (percent power change relative to prestimulus baseline) across 30 MEG–sensors (indicated on the scalp projection). Stimuli induced a sustained broadband power enhancement in the gamma band (50–150 Hz) and a suppression below 50 Hz. Note the higher and broader gamma response as compared to moving gratings (Figure 4.1.1B). (**C**) Top panel: Spectral distribution of responses (100–500 ms past stimulus onset) for each level of motion coherence. Responses are scaled separately for frequencies below and above 30 Hz. Lower panel: Linear modulation of the response by motion coherence (percent response per percent motion coherence). The gray band (62–102 Hz) marks the strongest modulation. (**D**) 62–102 Hz responses as a function of motion coherence, evaluated with a linear fit. (**E**) Cortical distribution of the average 62–102 Hz response across all levels of motion coherence (red overlay) and of its linear modulation by visual motion strength (blue overlay). While the strongest average response was located around the calcarine, the linear modulation was maximally expressed in posterior parietal cortex (PPC) and the human motion-sensitive area MT+. (Reprinted and modified with permission from Siegel et al. (2007).)

authors concluded that lower LFP frequencies reflect neuronal activity integrated across a broader spatial scale, explaining the loss of speed information, but the persistence of direction information. This is consistent with findings from monkey V1, where ocular dominance is organized on a broader spatial scale than orientation tuning: The LFP reflects ocular dominance at frequencies above 30 Hz, but preferred orientations only at above 80 Hz (Berens et al., 2008a). These findings suggest that the high-frequency LFP (>80 Hz) reflects more local activity as compared to the more widespread activity reflected at gamma frequencies from about 30 to 80 Hz.

The EEG and MEG do not provide sufficient spatial resolution to delineate feature selectivity *within* a given cortical region (e.g., orientation columns in V1 or direction columns in MT). Thus, electrophysiological studies in humans have focused on how population responses are modulated by the *strength* of sensory features. Consistent with the above data on feature-selectivity, these demonstrate enhanced gamma-band activity with increasing strength of visual features. Combining human MEG and source-reconstruction, Hall et al. (2005) found robust visual responses in the gamma band (30–70 Hz), localized around the calcarine sulcus (i.e., area V1), and increasing

monotonically with stimulus contrast, consistent with LFPs in monkey V1 (Henrie and Shapley, 2005; Logothetis et al., 2001). These findings accord well with a human MEG study that characterized the modulation of neural activity by strength of visual motion (Figure 4.1.2) (Siegel et al., 2007). The strongest increase of neural activity with strength of motion occurred in the gamma band (60 to 100 Hz). Lower frequencies (10–30 Hz) showed a slightly weaker opposite relationship. The strongest *mean* gamma-band response was located in area V1, but the *modulation* of the response by motion strength prevailed in motion-sensitive areas in extrastriate cortex, such as area MT+ and the intraparietal sulcus (Figure 4.1.2). Thus gamma-band activity is specifically modulated in the cortical systems processing a specific visual feature.

In sum, a highly consistent picture emerges: In early visual areas, visual stimuli enhance population activity in the gamma band (30–150 Hz) and suppress population activity in the alpha and beta bands (8–30 Hz). The stimulus-driven gamma-band activity is tuned for specific sensory features and increases monotonically with feature intensity. The neural mechanisms underlying this spectral fingerprint of stimulus driven activity are becoming increasingly clear (see also "Types of Neural Networks" below). The low-frequency suppression may reflect the disruption of widespread ongoing activity involving reverberation in cortico-thalamic loops (Pfurtscheller and Lopes da Silva, 1999; Steriade 2000). By contrast, local gamma-band activity involves fast recurrent interactions between excitation and inhibition within local, activated cortical networks (Bartos et al., 2007; Cardin et al., 2009; Hasenstaub et al., 2005; Sohal et al., 2009). This mechanistic understanding of the spectral fingerprint of stimulus-driven activity stands in contrast to the comparatively poor understanding of the spectral fingerprints of more intrinsic functional processes that we will discuss in the following sections.

Perception-Related Activity in Visual Cortex

We will now discuss modulations of neural activity in visual cortex that are correlated with perception rather than with changes of the sensory input. We focus on two prime examples of such perception-related activity: First, activity correlated with spontaneous fluctuations of conscious perception, and second, the modulation of neuronal responses by selective attention. The spectral fingerprints of these processes are more complex than the stimulus-driven responses discussed above.

Perceptual phenomena, which evoke fluctuating perceptual experience in the face of constant sensory stimuli, provide ideal tools for isolating patterns of neural activity that are specifically associated with conscious visual perception (Kim and Blake, 2005). For example, during prolonged viewing of bistable stimuli (such as the "vase-face" illusion), our perception switches spontaneously between two distinctly different states (Blake and Logothetis, 2002). Similarly, stimuli near the psychophysical detection threshold are sometimes seen and sometimes not (Green and Swets, 1966). A number of electrophysiological studies in monkeys and humans have used such psychophysical tools to establish links between band-limited cortical population activity and perception. Monkey LFP studies suggest that gamma-band (about 50–100 Hz) responses in extrastriate visual cortical areas (such as MT and V4) correlate with conscious perceptual reports; this holds for both bistable and near-threshold stimuli (Liu and Newsome, 2006; Wilke et al., 2006). Thus, the gamma-band LFP is not only stimulus-selective, but also seems to reflect subjects' conscious perception of these stimuli.

But two further observations suggest that the picture is more complex than the one for stimulus-driven activity. First, in V1, modulations of the low frequency (<30 Hz) activity exhibit a *positive* correlation with visual awareness during bistable perceptual suppression phenomena (Gail et al., 2004; Wilke et al., 2006). This contrasts sharply with the typical stimulus-induced suppression of low-frequency activity; it might reflect feedback from extrastriate areas (Gail et al., 2004; Wilke et al., 2006). Second, in extrastriate areas, the low frequency LFP was negatively correlated with visual motion perception in a fine discrimination task (Liu and Newsome, 2006), but positively correlated with the perceptual suppression of a salient visual target (Wilke et al., 2006). Such differences between visual phenomena might provide hints to the specific mechanisms mediating the fluctuations of perception under the different conditions. Further studies are required to gain more insights into the significance of such perception-related LFP modulations.

Another important step in this field of research will be the regular use of protocols designed for isolating conscious perception from attention (Huk et al., 2001; Koch and Tsuchiya, 2007; Lamme, 2003), which have often been conflated. A recent MEG study provides an excellent example for such a successful dissociation (Wyart and Tallon-Baudry, 2008), suggesting that spatial attention and conscious perception have distinct spectral fingerprints within the gamma band (Figure 4.1.3). MEG activity in the range from 54 to 64 Hz was larger over visual cortex when subjects detected a faint visual target stimulus than when they did not, irrespective of the locus of attention. By contrast, the spatially specific effect of an endogenous cue (directing subjects' attention to the left or right visual hemifield) was expressed in a higher frequency range (76–90 Hz). Interestingly, these two dissociated, and relatively narrow band effects of detection and cue were superimposed onto the typical broadband, stimulus-driven gamma-band response from about 50 to above 100 Hz, suggesting distinct underlying mechanisms. The detection-related modulation in the 54–64 Hz range predicted subjects' "target present" reports even on "target absent" trials (that is, when their perceptual reports were inaccurate). This further suggests that this modulation did not simply reflect attention. Since, the authors focused their analyses on the gamma band (30–150 Hz), it is unknown whether the lower frequency activity also correlated with subjects' perceptual reports, in a similar way as in monkey V1 (see above).

Neuronal responses in visual cortex to constant sensory input can also be affected by instructing subjects to shift attention from one location or stimulus feature to another (Desimone and Duncan, 1995). Several monkey LFP studies and human EEG/MEG studies have characterized the spectral signature of the "top-down" modulation of neural activity in visual cortex by selective attention. During stimulus processing, spatially selective and feature-based attention enhance gamma-band activity (30–100 Hz) in the human MEG and EEG (Gruber et al., 1999; Muller and Keil, 2004; Siegel et al., 2008; Wyart and Tallon-Baudry, 2008) and macaque area V4 (Bichot et al., 2005; Fries et al., 2001; Fries et al., 2008; Taylor et al., 2005). By contrast, before presentation of a visual stimulus, spatial attention induces a widespread suppression of alpha-band activity across visual cortex, demonstrated again in both human EEG/MEG (Siegel et al., 2008; Thut et al., 2006; Worden et al., 2000; Wyart and Tallon-Baudry, 2008) and macaque area V4 (Fries et al., 2001; Fries et al., 2008b). Before and during stimulus presentation, the strength of these attentional modulations predicts the accuracy (Siegel et al., 2008; Taylor et al., 2005) and speed (Thut et al., 2006;

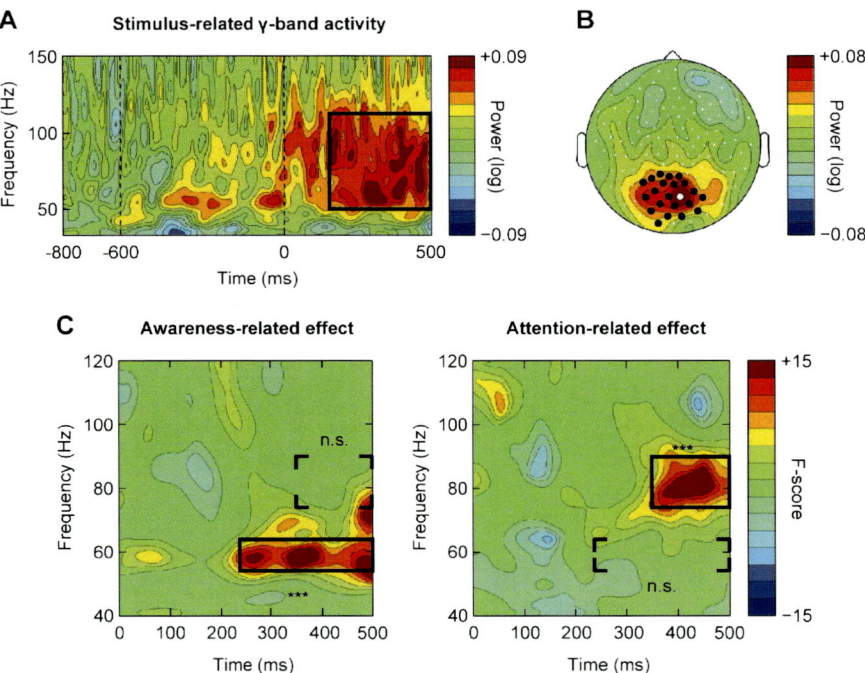

Figure 4.1.3. Dissociated spectral fingerprints of spatial attention and visual contrast detection. (**A**) Time-frequency representation of the high-frequency MEG response (in log power) of one occipital MEG sensor to low contrast gratings near psychophysical detection threshold. Following a central cue to the left or right, a grating was presented for 0.4 s in either the left or right hemifield, or no stimulus was presented at all. The first vertical line indicates cue onset, stimulus onset is at 0 ms. Subjects reported the presence/absence of the target stimulus after a variable delay. The faint grating stimuli induced an MEG response in the high gamma (50–110 Hz) range. Note the similarity to the gamma-band responses shown in Figure 4.1.1B. (**B**) Scalp topography of the high gamma-band response (50–110 Hz, 50–110 ms after stimulus onset, black box in A), averaged across left and right hemifield stimuli. Gamma-band responses were expressed over posterior sensors overlying visual and parietal cortex. The sensors marked with the peak response in black constitute the ROI for averaging responses in C. (**C**) Effects of target detection ("awareness-related") and of spatial cue ("attention-related") on the high-frequency MEG-response (statistical F-maps; ***p < 0.001 corrected: n.s., nonsignificant effect). (Reprinted with permission from Wyart and Tallon-Baudry (2008).)

Womelsdorf et al., 2006) of behavioral reports. Thus, rather than being constant or stimulus-independent, the spectral fingerprint of selective attention in visual cortex seems to depend strongly on the presence of a visual input. This suggests that band-limited activity in these regions reflects the result of a complex interaction between "bottom-up" and "top-down" signals.

The spectral fingerprint may also differ substantially between different processing stages within visual cortex (Siegel et al., 2008). By means of MEG source-reconstruction, Siegel et al. (2008) were able to separate attentional modulations in visual cortical areas V1/V2 and MT+. Area MT+ showed attentional effects in accordance with the findings from sensor-level EEG/MEG and monkey V4 studies discussed above: Prestimulus activity was strongly suppressed in the alpha (5–15 Hz) and beta (15–35 Hz) band, while attention enhanced broadband gamma-band activity (35–100 Hz) during stimulation. By contrast, in V1/V2 attention selectively *enhanced* activity in the beta band (15–35 Hz) during stimulation and, surprisingly, *suppressed* high gamma-band activity (60–100 Hz) before stimulus onset. Thus, the spectral fingerprint of attentional modulation does not only

depend on the presence of sensory input, but may also vary qualitatively between cortical processing stages. Further studies are needed to compare attentional modulations between processing stages, and to characterize their interaction with bottom-up signals. Further, a closer integration of findings between monkey and human studies is needed, which can be accomplished by the use of common experimental protocols and source-reconstruction of non-invasively recorded data.

Integrative Processes in Frontal and Parietal Association Cortex

We now turn to processes at the interface between perception and action: The control of attentional selection and the flexible mapping of perceptual representations onto voluntary actions (sensorimotor integration and decision-making). These processes are related at a functional level, and they seem to engage an overlapping network of regions in prefrontal and posterior parietal association cortex (Corbetta and Shulman, 2002; Desimone and Duncan, 1995; Gold and Shadlen, 2007; Kastner and Ungerleider, 2000; Miller and Cohen, 2001; Schall, 2001). In particular, a large number of neuroimaging studies have implicated two cortical association regions in the control of attention: the intraparietal sulcus in posterior parietal cortex, and the frontal eye fields in prefrontal cortex (Corbetta and Shulman, 2002; Donner et al., 2000; Kastner and Ungerleider, 2000; Moore et al., 2003; Serences and Yantis, 2006). Several recent studies have demonstrated that attention modulates band-limited activity within these regions, as well as their long-range coherence. However, the spectral profile of these effects differed markedly between studies. It remains to be clarified by future studies whether these discrepancies reflect differences in behavioral tasks, analysis methods, or the cortical regions under study.

In the macaque lateral intraparietal area (LIP), attention enhances population activity in the beta and low gamma band (25–45 Hz), while boosting coherence between areas MT and LIP in a broad alpha and beta frequency range (10–35 Hz) (Saalmann et al., 2007). This dissociation between effects of attention on local processing and on inter-regional coherence is consistent with the MEG results from Siegel et al. (2008) discussed above (see "Perception-related activity in visual cortex"). In this study, attention enhanced gamma-band coherence (35–100 Hz) and suppressed alpha- and beta-band coherence (5–35 Hz) between the intraparietal sulcus, frontal eye fields, and MT+ independent of visual input. This stimulus independent spectral profile stands in sharp contrast to strongly stimulus dependent modulation of local band-limited activity in MT+ and the intraparietal sulcus. Further, these modulations of inter-regional coherence contrast with an attentional suppression of beta-band (15–35 Hz) activity in the frontal eye fields. The latter results underline the regional specificity of attentional modulation in cortex.

The spectral fingerprints of attention also vary between different *modes* of attentional control. Buschman et al. (2007) compared the spectral profile of frontal-parietal coherence in macaques between visual search guided by "top-down" information (a target held in working memory) and attention guided by "bottom-up" stimulus saliency. In general, attention broadly enhanced coherence from about 15 to 70 Hz, but coherence was higher in the beta range (22–34 Hz) for "top-down" attention and higher in the low gamma range (35–55 Hz) for "bottom-up" attention. Thus, different modes of attentional control entail different modes of frontal-parietal communication, with distinct spectral fingerprints. These differences might reflect different directions of information flow (i.e., frontal to parietal in "top-down" mode and vice versa in "bottom-up" mode) or different neuronal subpopulations engaged in the two modes.

Large-scale electrophysiological recordings have also characterized the neural basis of sensorimotor integration and decision-making. These processes seem to involve frontal-parietal activity in lower and intermediate (alpha and beta) frequency ranges (Brovelli et al., 2004; Buschman and Miller, 2007; Donner et al., 2007; Gross et al., 2004; Pesaran et al., 2008; Rubino et al., 2006). This line of evidence is well illustrated by a study (Pesaran et al., 2008) correlating

neural activity between posterior parietal and dorsal premotor cortex while monkeys planned of a series of reach movements (Figure 4.1.4). In the condition of interest ("free search"), the animals were free to choose the sequence of movements. In the control condition ("instructed search"), a stimulus array instructed a particular sequence of movements. Coherence between spikes in premotor cortex and LFPs in the parietal reach region, and vice versa, increased transiently after the onset of the stimulus array (i.e., in the period of the trial in which monkeys formed their decision about the sequence of reaches). This effect occurred in the low frequency range (peaking at around 15 Hz) and was stronger during "free" than "instructed" search. Thus, decision-making seems to activate long-range coupling between the nodes of a large-scale frontal-parietal network. Further, the latency difference between the responses of each area (about 30 ms), as well as the spike-LFP coherence in both directions, further suggested that premotor cortex was influencing parietal cortex and the decision process in a feedback fashion.

Further support for the relevance of beta-band activity in decision-making comes from human MEG studies of different visual detection processes (Donner et al., 2007; Gross

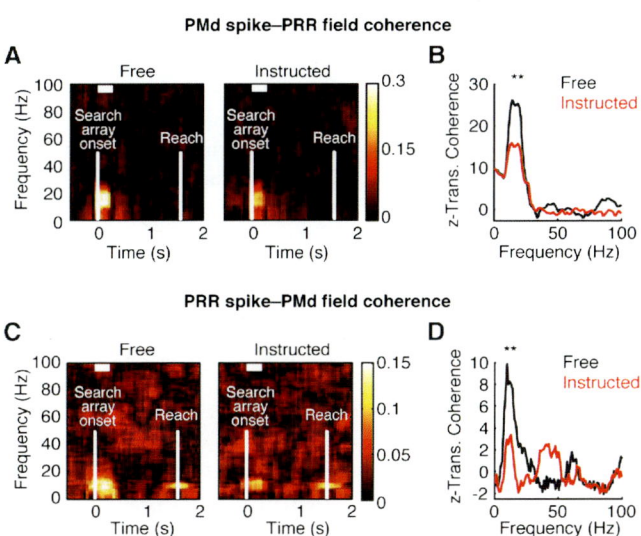

Figure 4.1.4. Frontal-parietal coherence around 15 Hz reflects decision-making during motor planning. (**A**) Time-frequency representation of coherence between spikes in the dorsal premotor area (PMd) and the LFP in the parietal reach region (PRR) during free (left panel) and instructed (right panel) search. See main text for details of the task. Neuronal activity is aligned to search array onset. The second vertical bar marks the average time of the first reach. The horizontal bar at the top shows the analysis window for panel B. (**B**) Spectra of z-transformed coherence between PMd spikes and the PRR LFP directly after search array onset. (**C**) and (**D**) display the same analyses as panels (A) and (B) but for spikes in PRR and the LFP in PMd. (******; p < 0.05). (Reprinted by permission from Pesaran B, Nelson MJ, Andersen RA (2008) Free choice activates a decision circuit between frontal and parietal cortex. Nature 453:406–409. Copyright Macmillan Publishers Ltd. (2008).)

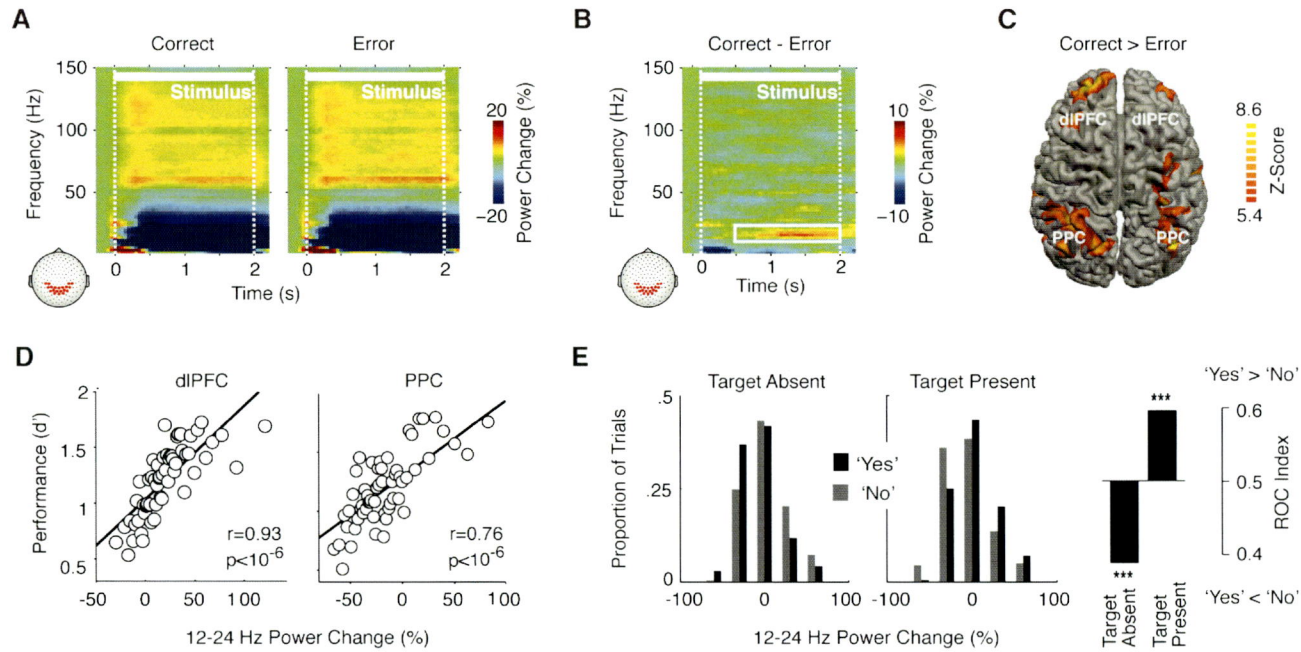

Figure 4.1.5. Frontal-parietal 12–24 Hz activity predicts correct perceptual decisions. (**A**) Time-frequency representations of MEG responses (percent power change relative to baseline) to moving random dot patterns (average across 20 sensors marked in red). Stimuli were presented for 2 s while subjects judged the presence of a weak coherent motion target signal embedded in dynamic noise. They indicated their "yes/no" decision by button press after a variable delay (0.5–1 s). The steady-state response at 60 Hz was phase-locked and driven by the large fraction of "noise" dots flickering at that frequency. The moving dot patterns induced a sustained enhancement of MEG power in the high gamma range (50–150 Hz) and suppression in the low frequency range (8–50 Hz) before both correct and incorrect decisions. (**B**) Difference between correct and incorrect decisions. 12–24 Hz (beta) range activity (white box) was enhanced before correct decisions, specifically during stimulus viewing; this effect was superimposed onto the more broadband stimulus-induced suppression. (**C**) Cortical distribution of performance-predictive 12–24 Hz activity during stimulus viewing, based on beamforming (statistical Z-map). (**D**) Trial-to-trial fluctuations of 12–24 Hz activity during stimulus viewing in dlPFC and PPC were tightly correlated with detection performance (d'). Trials are binned by response magnitude (200 trials per bin). (**E**) Left. Single-trial 12–24 Hz response distributions for the dlPFC of an example subject, sorted according to perceptual report and target absent/present conditions. Right. ROC-indices quantifying the overlap between response distributions. An index of 0.5 indicates perfect overlap, larger than 0.5 indicate "yes" > "no," and smaller than 0.5 indicate "yes" < "no" (***p < 0.001, permutation test). (Reprinted and modified with permission from Donner et al. (2007).)

et al., 2004). During a motion detection task, trial-to-trial fluctuations of MEG activity in the 12–24 Hz range predicted correct perceptual choices of the subjects (Figure 4.1.5). This predictive activity was expressed in a widespread cortical network comprising frontal, parietal, and visual cortex. It did not just reflect slow fluctuations of subjects' arousal state, but was specifically expressed during the stimulus interval. Similarly, during the "attentional blink" phenomenon, 13–18 Hz MEG activity in frontal, parietal, and visual cortex, as well as their coherence, predicted successful target detection (Gross et al., 2004).

Importantly, the 12–24 Hz activity predicted the accuracy of subjects' "yes/no" detection decisions, irrespective of their content ("yes/no"): On target-present trials, the activity tended to be higher before "yes" than before "no" choices (i.e., "hits" > "misses"), whereas, on motion-absent trials, it showed the opposite relation to the "yes/no" choice (i.e. "correct rejects" > "misses"). Thus, the 12–24 Hz activity does not reflect a cortical *representation* (of the target or of an abstract decision variable), but the *mechanism* transforming

this representation into a motor plan (deCharms and Zador, 2000).

What might be this mechanism? In many cases, perceptual decision-making involves the accumulation of "sensory evidence" over time, which in turn seems to be mediated by persistent neuronal activity (Gold and Shadlen, 2007). As originally suggested by Hebb (1949), persistent neural activity in cortex might be established by reverberant activity within local and long-range networks. Reverberant activity can be reflected in oscillations as measured by neural population signals (Wang, 2001). Indeed, several studies explicitly probing the neural correlates of short-term memory in frontal, parietal, and visual cortex found these to be specifically expressed in similar beta frequency ranges (Tallon-Baudry et al., 2001; Tallon-Baudry et al., 1998; Tallon-Baudry et al., 2004).

To sum up, the most consistent spectral fingerprints of population activity are observed for stimulus-driven activity in sensory cortex. Sensory stimulation generally induces stimulus-specific increases of gamma-band power and (less specific) decreases in low-frequency power. Similar principles seem to apply to movement-selective activity in motor cortex (Crone et al., 1998a; Crone et al., 1998b; Miller et al., 2007; Rickert et al., 2005; Spinks et al., 2008). By contrast the spectral fingerprints of higher cognitive processes (such as attention or decision-making) appear more complex. We suggest that one reason for this discrepancy might be that the latter processes involve strong recurrent interactions, within and between distant cortical networks, and various neuromodulators interacting with these cortical processes. In addition, the spectral fingerprints might also differ systematically between sensory cortex on the one hand and association cortices on the other hand, perhaps reflecting distinct network properties. In light of present evidence these ideas remain largely speculative, but we can address the more general question of what can be inferred from neural population activity in the different frequency bands.

Why Do Frequency Bands Exhibit Specific Functional Properties?

Several previous accounts of cortical frequency bands have mapped coarsely defined psychological concepts (e.g. "cognitive binding") onto specific frequency bands (such as the "gamma-band"). This approach bears some similarity to the "neo-phrenological" approach in functional neuroimaging, which aims at labeling each region of the cerebral cortex with a specific cognitive process (Friston, 2002; Nichols and Newsome, 1999). We think that it will be more fruitful to approach the question at a basic neurophysiological level (i.e., the properties of individual neurons and neuronal circuits). Do the spectral fingerprints of functional processes provide hints toward the specific neural computations underlying these processes?

Spatial Scales of Measurements and Neural Networks

To understand the significance of LFP or EEG signals in particular frequency bands, we need to consider how these signals emerge from the activity of individual neurons and their interactions. In particular, what is the relationship between signals measured at different spatial scales?

The phase-coherence of simultaneously recorded LFPs decreases with cortical distance, and coherence declines faster for higher as for lower frequencies (Frien and Eckhorn, 2000; Leopold et al., 2003). Further, feature selectivity of the LFP is confined to higher frequencies for sensory features that are represented in more local cortical clusters (Berens et al., 2008a; Liu and Newsome, 2006). These results could either reflect broader spatial scales of neural interaction at lower frequencies (i.e., an *active* process) or simply the biophysical principles governing *passive* signal propagation in the cortex. In other words, the effect could simply be caused by a stronger attenuation of high-frequency signals in the cortex, which would result in the LFP reflecting activity over a broader spatial scale at lower frequencies. Measurements of the frequency dependent cortical impedance argue against the latter explanation (Logothetis et al., 2007). Over the relevant frequency range, the impedance-spectrum along the cortical surface is largely flat within each cortical layer. This implies that the LFP propagates equally well across different spectral components, which, in turn, suggests that the frequency dependent decay of LFP coherence and feature selectivity indeed reflect more local synchronization at higher frequencies compared to more widespread synchrony at lower frequencies.

This relation between spatial scale and frequency is also supported by theoretical studies. It has been suggested that, for spatially more separate neural ensembles, longer conduction delays may constrain oscillatory interactions to lower frequencies (König and Schillen, 1991; Kopell et al., 2000), consistent with several invasive animal studies and non-invasive studies in humans: Long-range, inter-regional synchronization is typically expressed at frequencies below 40 Hz (Brovelli et al., 2004; Gross et al., 2004; Pesaran et al., 2008; Roelfsema et al., 1997; Saalmann et al., 2007; Sarnthein et al., 1998). However, some studies found also synchronization between distant brain areas well above 40 Hz (Buschman and Miller, 2007; Engel et al., 1991; Siegel et al., 2008).

Considering the spatial scale (or spatial resolution) of measured signals is also particularly important for the interpretation of the MEG and EEG. Despite the application of advanced source-reconstruction techniques, the spatial resolution of EEG/MEG is likely one order of magnitude coarser than the resolution of the LFP. Thus, changes in the spatial structure of synchronized population activity can lead to different effects for LFP signals on the one hand and EEG/MEG signals on the other hand. Suppose a visual stimulus reduces frequency specific synchronization on a broader spatial scale of a few millimeters along the cortical surface, but has little effect on synchrony on a more local scale of less than one millimeter. Then, the power of the LFP will show little decrease. By contrast, the coarser spatial resolution of the non-invasive recordings will lead to a more prominent power reduction for EEG/MEG signals. Such an effect could explain an apparent discrepancy between LFP and MEG/EEG studies of visual stimulus responses: For the EEG or MEG visual stimulation induce a strong suppression of low-frequency activity over wide, posterior brain regions (Donner et al., 2007; Hoogenboom et al., 2005; Siegel et al., 2007; Siegel et al., 2008; Tallon-Baudry et al., 1998), whereas this suppression is typically weaker, or even absent, for the LFP (Belitski et al., 2008; Berens et al., 2008a; Henrie and Shapley, 2005; Lee H et al., 2005; Liu and Newsome, 2006; Siegel and König, 2003).

Types of Neural Networks

It becomes increasingly clear that the spectral profile of neural population activity is critically determined by biophysical properties on the cellular and network level. An intensely investigated example is the mechanism underlying the cortical spindle activity (8–14 Hz) observed during slow-wave sleep (Destexhe and Sejnowski, 2003; Llinas and Steriade, 2006). Detailed in vivo and in vitro studies at the cellular and network level, combined with numerous modeling studies, underline the importance of intrinsic cellular properties of thalamic neurons for the generation of these rhythms. Thalamocortical (TC) relay cells and thalamic reticular (RE) neurons are equipped with voltage-dependent conductances that support intrinsically oscillating firing patterns. However, the spindle-activity observed in vivo does not only depend on these intrinsic cellular properties. Instead, such activity results from the interactions between these thalamic cell types as well as between thalamic and cortical neurons within large-scale cortico-thalamic loops (reviewed in Destexhe and Sejnowski, 2003).

Local, synchronized gamma-band activity in the cortex provides another prime example: Inhibitory interneurons play a key role for this type of activity. Networks of synaptically and electrically (gap-junctions) coupled interneurons engage in rhythmic gamma-band activity (Bartos et al., 2007; Whittington et al., 1995). Throughout the cortex, inhibitory neurons interact with excitatory cells in local excitatory-inhibitory loops, in which they entrain and synchronize excitatory cells in a rhythmic fashion. Within each oscillatory cycle, excitatory neurons spike with a sufficient decline of network inhibition during the depolarizing phase of the LFP. This triggers the firing of inhibitory neurons, which, in turn, shuts down excitatory neurons in a synchronized fashion until inhibition decays and the next cycle begins. Strong evidence for this mechanism has been obtained from the rodent hippocampus (Csicsvari et al., 2003) and the prefrontal cortex of anesthetized ferrets (Hasenstaub et al., 2005). Furthermore, two recent studies provided direct causal evidence for this mechanism by optogenetic manipulation of fast-spiking interneurons (Cardin et al., 2009; Sohal et al., 2009). The peak frequency and bandwidth of these local gamma-band processes seem critically determined by the cellular properties of the participating neurons (Bartos et al., 2007). It remains open to which extent this also holds for other types of neural oscillations.

Gieselmann and Thiele (2008) provided indirect evidence that gamma-band activity of the LFP indeed reflects the underlying inhibitory activity. The authors recorded spiking activity and LFPs in V1 of behaving monkeys presented with visual gratings of variable size. Gratings extending beyond the summation area of receptive fields inhibited spiking activity (presumably due to lateral inhibition), while the LFP gamma-band activity increased monotonically for all grating sizes. Thus, rather than reflecting only excitatory drive, the gamma-band LFP seems to reflect the oscillatory interaction between local excitation and inhibition. The fact that band-limited population activity reflects excitatory-inhibitory interactions, and active processing within specific functional networks, rather than mere average levels of excitation seems particularly important if one aims to link band-limited cortical population activity to the fMRI signal.

Linking Band-Limited Neural Activity to fMRI

We will now discuss attempts to uncover the relationship between band-limited neural activity (as measured by the LFP, EEG, or MEG) on the one hand and the BOLD fMRI signal on the other hand. We will adopt a descriptive perspective, searching for simple rules that may govern this relationship at the macroscopic level. In principle, we might be able to identify such rules despite our present lack of a detailed understanding of each of the signals' generation from the activity of individual neurons and neuronal circuits. As in the previous section, we will contrast stimulus-driven responses with neural activity reflecting higher-order cognitive processes. The relationship between band-limited activity and fMRI seems relatively simple and reasonably well understood for the former, but more complex, and as yet elusive, for the latter.

Simultaneous Versus Nonsimultaneous Measurements

Electrophysiological and fMRI recordings can be integrated based on either simultaneous or nonsimultaneous measurements. Nonsimultaneous recordings are technically less intricate, provide optimal signal quality in both recording modalities, and allow for optimizing the experimental design within each modality. By contrast, simultaneous recordings ensure that the data in both modalities have been obtained under exactly identical conditions and are particularly well suited for studies of dynamic changes, such as learning.

One general important issue in this context is that different sources of variance can drive correlations between the signals measured with both modalities: variance across different experimental conditions and variance across time or trials within conditions. Nonsimultaneously recorded signals can only be linked based on the covariance controlled by experimental conditions (e.g., stimulus contrast, cognitive task, or behavioral report). Simultaneously recorded signals, however, can also be linked based on the covariance of their trial-to-trial fluctuations, which are not controlled by the experimenter. Such intrinsic, stimulus-independent fluctuations are a pervasive feature of neural activity (Ermentrout et al., 2008; Faisal et al., 2008; Fox and Raichle, 2007; Leopold et al., 2003). One might obtain different correlations between electrophysiology and fMRI, depending on the source of variance (experimental conditions vs. trial-to-trial) used for the analysis. This has immediate consequences for the question of whether one should perform simultaneous or nonsimultaneous recordings: The nonsimultaneous approach seems sufficient for identifying the relationship between stimulus-driven responses in the different modalities; the same holds for cognitive processes well controlled by the task at hand. By contrast, the simultaneous approach is preferable for determining the relationship between intrinsic signal fluctuations, whether measured in the "resting state" or in the presence of a stimulus or task.

For the EEG, it is also important to consider that correlations with local fMRI signals do not necessarily identify electrophysiological activity from that same region. For example, several studies have identified a correlation between widespread alpha-band EEG activity on the human scalp and simultaneously recorded fMRI signals in the thalamus. Does this imply that the scalp-EEG alpha-band activity directly reflects the electrical fields generated by a thalamic source? Certainly not. Rather, this correlation is likely to be caused by a modulation of *cortical sources* of alpha-band EEG activity by thalamic input (Feige et al., 2005; Goldman et al., 2002; Mantini et al., 2007; Moosmann et al., 2003; Steriade, 2000). Such indirect correlations can be exploited for investigating which brain structures modulate band-limited population activity in other cortical areas. However, if one aims at identifying correlations driven by identical structures for the EEG and fMRI signal, source-reconstruction techniques (see above) should be used to project the EEG data into a common source-space where they can be more directly correlated with the fMRI data.

Different Windows into Interactions Between Brain Areas

Analyses of "functional connectivity" (i.e., correlations between remote fMRI time-series) are a common motif in fMRI research (Friston, 2002). In particular, studies of coherent resting-state fluctuations across large-scale cortical and subcortical networks are increasing in popularity (Fox and Raichle, 2007). It is by no means straightforward to establish a direct correspondence between the phase coherence of electrophysiological signals at a fine temporal scale and the temporal correlations of sluggish fMRI signals. The fMRI signal is likely to be blind to the phase coherence between cortical responses, at least in intermediate- and high-frequency (beta and gamma) ranges. Instead, experimental evidence suggests that correlations between the *amplitude envelopes* of band-limited cortical responses may be the source of the correlations between distant fMRI time-series (Leopold et al., 2003; Nir et al., 2008). However, it is important to note that the phase coherence and the correlation between the amplitude envelopes of two signals are independent of one another. For example, the amplitude envelopes (i.e., power) of the gamma-band responses of two regions can covary strongly, despite their phases' being randomly distributed.

The reverse can be true as well. Slow covariations between amplitude envelopes are typically as slow as the resting-state fluctuations of the fMRI signal, in that they have a 1/f spectrum with dominant frequencies at 0.1 Hz and below (Fox and Raichle, 2007). Such slow covariations may not play a direct role in neural coding. It has been speculated that they reflect common input from neuromodulatory projections ascending from the brainstem (Leopold et al., 2003). If so, such slow intrinsic signal fluctuations may generally have strong links to cognition and behavioral performance across a large variety of tasks (see below, "Questions for future research").

There is also ample evidence that correlations between remote fMRI time series at faster time scales reflect perception, attention, and behavioral performance (Freeman et al., 2008; Friston, 2002; Haynes et al., 2005b; Haynes et al., 2005c). These results strongly suggest that the fMRI signal provides a meaningful measure of the interaction between neuronal populations in cortex. Again, these correlations likely reflect amplitude correlations of band-limited activity, on a faster time scale than during resting state, but measurements to test this hypothesis have not yet been done.

Stimulus-Driven Responses in Sensory Cortex

Electrophysiological and fMRI measurements in primary visual cortex suggest a tight covariation between modulations of the BOLD signal and of gamma-band LFP and MEG activity correlated with stimulus strength. Logothetis et al. (2001) simultaneously recorded BOLD fMRI, spikes, and LFPs in monkey V1. Consistent with other reports (Henrie and Shapley, 2005), they found strong and sustained LFP responses to visual stimulation in the gamma band that peaked around 70 Hz and increased approximately linearly with stimulus contrast. These LFP responses were well correlated with modulations of the BOLD signal that showed a similar linear increase with stimulus contrast. A tight coupling between contrast-dependent modulation of the BOLD signal and gamma-band activity is also supported for human V1 by means of nonsimultaneous non-invasive recordings. A similar linear increase with stimulus contrast is found for the BOLD response (Boynton et al., 1999) and gamma-band activity (30–70 Hz) reconstructed from MEG (Hall et al., 2005) (see also "Linking band-limited neural activity to behavior," above).

A similarly tight relationship between the BOLD signal and gamma-band activity seems to hold for human area MT+ for modulations of visual motion strength. Rees et al. (2000) found a linear increase of the BOLD signal in human area MT+ with motion strength. Siegel et al. (2007) demonstrated a similar linear increase of MEG activity in the gamma band (60–100 Hz) in area MT+ and several other motion responsive regions along the dorsal visual pathway (Figure 4.1.2). Further, albeit weaker and less consistently, low-frequency activity (10–30 Hz) decreased with increasing motion strength.

These findings are consistent with a series of LFP recordings in the auditory cortex of epileptic patients. These exploited "inter-subject correlation"[5] to establish indirect links between the LFP and fMRI activity in normal subjects. Mukamel et al. (2005) recorded LFPs and found a *positive* correlation of LFP power in the gamma band (40–130 Hz), and a *negative* correlation of LFP power in the alpha band (5–15 Hz), each with fMRI in auditory cortex. Intermediate bands showed little effect. Nir et al. (2007) further established that this observation also holds for spontaneous activity and that occasional dissociations between SUA and the fMRI response tended to be accompanied by reductions of the correlation between the spiking activity of individual neurons and the gamma-band LFP. In other words, whenever, single neurons activate coherently with the surrounding network, their spiking activity is closely coupled to the fMRI signal; whenever they deviate from the mean of their neighborhood, their spiking activity is a poor predictor of the fMRI signal.

Perception-Related Activity in Visual Cortex

Binocular rivalry has been a major source of apparent discrepancies between electrophysiology in fMRI. In binocular rivalry, a bistable visual illusion, two dissimilar patterns presented to the two eyes cannot be fused, and are consequently perceived in alternation (Blake and Logothetis, 2002). fMRI studies of rivalry consistently found strong response modulations correlated with perception in early visual cortex including V1, and even in the LGN (Haynes et al., 2005a; Lee SH et al., 2005; Lee et al., 2007; Meng et al., 2005; Polonsky et al., 2000; Tong and Engel, 2001; Wunderlich et al., 2005). By contrast, single-unit recordings in awake, behaving monkeys found little modulation in V1 with perception (Blake and Logothetis, 2002; Leopold and Logothetis, 1996). Similarly, the LFP recordings in monkey V1 during binocular rivalry and a related perceptual suppression phenomenon reported little modulation of the gamma-band LFP with visual awareness. However, as discussed above, these studies observed strong perception-related LFP modulations in the low frequency range (< 30 Hz) correlated with perception (Gail et al., 2004; Maier et al., 2008; Wilke et al., 2006), prompting the hypothesis that these may have been the source of the fMRI responses measured in human V1 during binocular rivalry.

Maier et al. (2008) addressed this issue by comparing electrophysiological responses with the fMRI signal in macaque V1, measured within the same animals and experimental protocol. When a salient visual target was *physically* removed from the screen, responses decreased for all three measures of neural activity, and in particular for a broad frequency range of the LFP, including the gamma band (30–100 Hz). However, when the target was rendered *subjectively* invisible by means of "generalized flash suppression" (a bistable visual illusion analogous to binocular rivalry), these signals diverged: There was a strong reduction of the fMRI response with perceptual suppression, little modulation of the high frequency LFP and MUA spiking activity, and an intermediate reduction of the low frequency LFP. In other words, virtually identical decreases of the fMRI response during physical removal and subjective disappearance conditions were accompanied by distinctly different spectral fingerprints: The low-frequency suppression was paralleled by an enhancement in an intermediate frequency range (30–40 Hz), and a suppression in the high gamma frequency range (60–80 Hz). The dissociation between the spectral modulations correlated with fMRI responses during physical removal and perceptual suppression demonstrates the context-dependent relationship between these two measures of neural population activity.

A human fMRI study of "motion-induced blindness"[6] (Donner et al., 2008) indicates that the topography of response modulations correlated with perceptual suppression provides clues to the underlying mechanisms, in a similar fashion as the corresponding spectral fingerprints. Also during motion-induced blindness, the fMRI response in V1 modulated strongly with perceptual suppression. However, this modulation was not confined to the cortical representation of the small target stimulus, but expressed throughout the entire visual field representation in V1. Such a "global" modulation can hardly be a specific correlate of the localized target suppression. When this global component was removed from the fMRI signals measured in the retinotopic target subregions of areas V1 through V4, the residual target-specific responses tracked the illusory target suppression strongly only in V4 and showed no modulation in V1. These residual target-specific responses may reflect local modulations of spiking activity and/or the gamma-band LFP (Liu and Newsome, 2006; Logothetis and Wandell, 2004; Nir et al., 2007). By contrast, the "global" response component might reflect widespread modulations of the low frequency LFP, perhaps driven by subcortical inputs. Future studies should characterize the topography of the low-frequency electrophysiological signal components correlated with perceptual suppression. A more general implication may be that, for the fMRI signal, it is the spatial (rather than temporal) pattern that may be used for inferring underlying mechanisms: Stimulus representations are expressed in the spatial fine structure (Donner et al., 2008; Haynes and Rees, 2006), whereas neuromodulatory processes acting on these representations are expressed in the global modulations (Donner et al., 2008; Jack et al., 2006).

Studies of attentional modulation of neural responses in visual cortex are another source of apparent discrepancies between electrophysiology in fMRI. First, spatial attention seems to have little effect on firing rates in monkey V1 (Desimone and Duncan, 1995; Luck et al., 1997; but see Chen et al., 2008; Herrero et al., 2008; Roelfsema et al., 1998), but strong effect on the fMRI signal in human V1 (Brefczynski and DeYoe, 1999; Kastner et al., 1999; Ress et al., 2000; Somers et al., 1999). Second, in the absence of sensory stimulation, attention has only modest effect on baseline firing rates in early visual cortex (V1, V2) (Luck et al., 1997), but again a big effect on the fMRI signal (Kastner et al., 1999; Ress et al., 2000). In principle, these discrepancies could merely be due to the different species, stimuli, and behavioral protocols (e.g. near-threshold vs. suprathreshold stimuli), or they may reflect true differences between the different signals. For example, the effects of attention on the fMRI signal could reflect relatively small modulations of synaptic activity, which are coherent across large populations of neurons, and therefore have a strong impact on population signals, but are weakly reflected by single-unit activity. Alternatively, these dissociations might reflect a primary modulation of the *temporal structure* of neuronal population activity, which, in turn, might have a particularly strong effect on the fMRI response.

Although there were several differences in terms of behavioral protocols, studies of band-limited population activity are beginning to shed new light on these issues. These studies demonstrated profound attentional modulation of band-limited population activity in the human brain (Doesburg et al., 2008; Fan et al., 2007; Fries et al., 2001; Gruber et al., 1999; Siegel et al., 2008; Taylor et al., 2005; Thut et al., 2006; Worden et al., 2000; Wyart and Tallon-Baudry, 2008). One MEG study (Siegel et al., 2008) compared attentional baseline and stimulus-related effects and characterized modulations in V1 and MT+ at the cortical source-level (see also above, "Linking band-limited neural activity to behavior: perception-related activity in visual cortex"). In accordance with fMRI (Kastner et al., 1999; Sapir et al., 2005) attention modulated population activity in both regions during the baseline and stimulus intervals in a spatially selective fashion. However, the spectral fingerprints of these effects differed strongly between V1 and MT+, and even more surprisingly, between the baseline and stimulation intervals, within each area. Invasive recordings in monkey area V4 also displayed an (albeit weaker) analogous difference in attention effects between baseline and stimulation intervals (Fries et al., 2008b).

In conclusion, attentional effects in visual cortex perhaps do not exhibit a stereotype relation between the BOLD signal and electrophysiological population activity in a single frequency band. However, it remains difficult to assess to which extent the difference between regions found by means of MEG can also be observed on the LFP level. For example, it remains open to which extent extracranially recorded effects are affected by interactions of center-surround type attentional modulations (Silver et al., 2007) with the comparatively low spatial resolution of EEG/MEG (see also above "Spatial Scales of Measurements and Neural Networks").

Integrative Processes in Frontal and Parietal Association Cortex

Numerous fMRI studies have probed the involvement of prefrontal and posterior parietal association cortex in selective attention, sensorimotor integration, and decision-making (Corbetta and Shulman, 2002; Desimone and Duncan, 1995; Gold and Shadlen, 2007; Heekeren et al., 2008; Kanwisher and Wojciulik, 2000; Kastner and Ungerleider, 2000; Miller and Cohen, 2001; Schall, 2001). How closely are the fMRI correlates of these processes related to their electrophysiological correlates discussed in the previous section? Unfortunately, only few electrophysiological studies have used experimental protocols directly comparable to the fMRI studies. Also, few studies have applied source reconstruction techniques to estimate activity specifically in prefrontal and parietal cortex. Both limitations hamper a close comparison between the different measurement modalities.

Studies of saccade planning suggest a simple relationship between measurement modalities in parietal association cortex that is largely consistent with the picture emerging for stimulus-driven responses in sensory cortex. Several fMRI studies have demonstrated retinotopically specific fMRI activity in the posterior parietal cortex when human subjects remembered the position of a visual target for a delayed saccade (Hagler and Sereno, 2006; Kastner et al., 2007; Schluppeck et al., 2005; Sereno et al., 2001; Swisher et al., 2007). Converging evidence from monkey and human electrophysiology suggests that such fMRI activity is closely linked to band-limited population activity in the gamma band. Pesaran et al. (2002) demonstrated saccade direction-selective gamma-band activity in monkey area LIP during a delay before saccade execution. Van der Werf et al. (2008) found analogous saccade direction-selective gamma-band activity in the human intraparietal sulcus.

However, the situation appears more complex for studies of attention and decision processes in the same or neighboring cortical networks. There appears to be a *positive* correlation between electrophysiological activity in the low-beta frequency range (about 12–24 Hz) and fMRI activity in posterior parietal and prefrontal cortex during visual detection tasks. Successful target detection is typically associated with increased fMRI activity in prefrontal and posterior parietal cortex; this is true for motion detection in noise (Shulman et al., 2001), change detection (Beck et al., 2001), flicker detection (Carmel et al., 2006), and target letter detection (Kranczioch et al., 2005; Marois et al., 2004). Recent MEG studies found detection-related enhancements of low beta-band (12–24 Hz) activity in corresponding frontal-parietal regions (Donner et al., 2007; Gross et al., 2004; Linkenkaer-Hansen et al., 2004), suggesting that such performance-related lower frequency activity in frontal-parietal networks correlates positively with the fMRI response in these regions of association cortex, different from the stimulus-induced suppression of low frequency activity in visual cortex. This again suggests that the link between fMRI and electrophysiology may differ substantially between functional processes and cortical regions.

The above studies also illustrate the point that spectral fingerprints of different functional processes may superimpose in a complex fashion, with unknown consequences for the fMRI signal. In particular the performance-related beta activity during motion detection was superimposed onto a more broadband (about 8–50 Hz) stimulus-induced low-frequency suppression (Figure 4.1.5); these two signal components were independent of one another in their trial-to-trial fluctuations and spatial topography (Donner et al., 2007). Both, the stimulus-induced low-frequency *suppression* in visual and parietal cortex and the detection-related beta-band *enhancement* in parietal and prefrontal cortex presumably correlate with increased fMRI responses in different (partially overlapping) cortical regions. Again, this suggests a process- and perhaps area-dependence of the link between fMRI and electrophysiological mass activity.

Questions for Future Research

In the final part of this chapter, we will put forward three questions for future research, the answers to which will be particularly important for understanding the relationship between band-limited neural population activity and both, behavior and the fMRI signal.

What is the Link Between Intracortical and Extracranial Electrophysiology?

Despite the convergence between LFP and EEG/MEG studies that we have highlighted in this chapter, it is still an open question how exactly intracortical LFPs relate to extracranial EEG/MEG signals. For example, which effect does the spatial correlation-structure of neural activity have on invasively and non-invasively recorded signals? The coarser spatial resolution of the latter suggests that they are more sensitive to long-range correlations of neural activity while the LFP primarily reflects synchronized activity on a local spatial scale. Thus, depending on the signal type, the spatial correlation profile of neural activity and its modulation by stimuli or cognitive processes may have profoundly different effects. Similar open questions are to which extent the laminar profile of activity affects different population signals or which role the individual anatomical geometry (gyri, sulci) plays for the relationship between these signals. Quantitative measurements addressing these questions are largely missing (but see Juergens et al., 1999; Mitzdorf, 1987). Addressing them seems crucial for integrating results across different signal scales, and for making inferences between these different levels of observation. Simultaneous LFP and EEG/MEG recordings seem particularly promising for directly elucidating these questions. Furthermore, sub- or epidural surface electrodes (ECoG) constitute an intermediate scale, which might provide a valuable link between intracortical and extracranial signals. Such "intracranial EEG" recordings for research purposes are becoming more frequent, both in human patients (Engel et al., 2005; Lachaux et al., 2003) as

well as in nonhuman primates (Bressler et al., 1993; Tallon-Baudry et al., 2004; Taylor et al., 2005).

How Does Neural Mass Activity Relate to Local Circuit Dynamics?

Attempts to link fMRI and electrophysiological population signals will fall short if these signals are understood as simply reflecting average "activation" levels of cortical regions with different temporal resolution. Both signals are generated by complex interactions between various specialized cell-types within local neuronal circuits (e.g., Heeger and Ress, 2002; Lauritzen, 2005; Logothetis, 2008; Logothetis and Wandell, 2004). We are beginning to understand the principles underlying the processing in such micro-circuits (Douglas and Martin, 2004). It is clear that inhibitory neurons play an integral part in shaping basic tuning properties of individual cortical neurons (Carandini et al., 1997; Heeger et al., 1996; Shapley et al., 2003) as well as generating local network oscillations, e.g., in the gamma band (Bartos et al., 2007). In addition, inhibition might also play a crucial role in high-level cognitive processes such as selective attention (Mitchell et al., 2007). Yet, relatively little is known about how specific cognitive processes affect local network dynamics and how these in turn transfer into modulations of neuronal mass signals as measured with electrophysiology and fMRI. Again, integrated experimental approaches using comparable behavioral protocols and combinations of electrophysiological and functional imaging techniques are required to address these questions. Furthermore, cell-type and layer-specific recordings, as well as genetically targeted manipulations of specific cell classes seem promising techniques to further our understanding of local cortical circuit dynamics and their relation to neural mass signals.

How Does Neuromodulation Shape the Spectral Fingerprints of Cortical Processes?

Several nuclei in the basal forebrain and brainstem send massive, and relatively diffuse neuromodulatory (adrenergic, cholinerig, etc.) projections to wide regions of the cortex. These neuromodulators seem to play an important role in shaping band-limited cortical population activity (Munk et al., 1996; Rodriguez et al., 2004; Steriade, 2000). These ascending systems have traditionally been thought of as merely regulating slow fluctuations of coarse behavioral states, such as vigilance and arousal (Steriade, 2000). However, growing theoretical and empirical evidence suggests that neuromodulators play more specific computational roles in selective attention, short-term memory, and decision-making (Aston-Jones and Cohen, 2005; Hasselmo, 1995; Herrero et al., 2008; Usher et al., 1999; Wang et al., 2007; Yu and Dayan, 2005). Taken together, these lines of evidence suggest that neuromodulators may be an essential factor determining the spectral fingerprints of these cognitive processes.

Direct studies of neuromodulator effects on cortical population activity in awake, behaving animals will provide deeper insights into this issue. Such studies could use either local (Herrero et al., 2008) or systemic (Bentley et al., 2003; Coull et al., 1999; Coull et al., 2001; Minzenberg et al., 2008) pharmacological manipulations, or simultaneous measurements of activities in subcortical neuromodulatory centers and in their cortical recipients (Minzenberg et al., 2008). The latter is one area of research for which simultaneous EEG and fMRI recordings might prove to be extremely useful. Simultaneously monitoring subcortical neuromodulatory centers, such as the noradrenergic locus coeruleus with fMRI and widespread band-limited activity patterns in the cortex with EEG during the performance of cognitive tasks could provide deep insights into how the spectral fingerprints of cognitive processes are shaped by subcortical centers.

Conclusion

We have addressed the relationship of band-limited electrophysiological mass activity to behavior on the one hand, and to the BOLD fMRI signal on the other hand. Electrophysiological mass activity generally reflects several different *components* of neuronal activity, which are generated by distinct neural mechanisms and expressed in different frequency ranges. The relative strengths of these components thus determine what we have called the specific *spectral fingerprint* of a perceptual or cognitive process (and perhaps even of a given brain area involved in this process). We have highlighted a striking discrepancy between the spectral fingerprint of stimulus-driven responses in sensory cortices and the fingerprints of intrinsic processes (such as top-down attention or switches between perceptual states) within the same cortical areas. We speculate that this dissociation reflects recurrent interactions between distant cortical areas and/or neuromodulation of cortical activity patterns by ascending systems, which are both thought to play an important role in such processes. If this idea turns out to be correct, we may be able to exploit the spectral fingerprints of functional processes for inferring about the detailed mechanisms underlying these processes.

The fMRI signal, likewise, reflects several different components of neuronal activity. Since the sluggish fMRI signal does not have the temporal fine structure of electrophysiological signals, we cannot use its frequency spectrum to disentangle these different components. However, we may use the scale (local vs. global) of spatial patterns to make inferences about the underlying mechanisms: Neuronal representations are likely to be expressed in the local structure of neural population responses, whereas neuromodulatory processes may be expressed in more global response modulations. Importantly, the multi-component nature of electrophysiological activity and the fMRI signal explains why there does not seem to be a simple, stationary transformation between the two. This important point has often been overlooked in recent discussions. Instead, we suggest that there may exist a *cohort* of such transformations, one for each class of functional processes and perhaps brain areas. The close coupling between gamma-band activity and the fMRI signal for stimulus-driven responses of sensory cortical regions provides a well established example, the mechanisms of which we are beginning to understand. In this case, identifying the spectral fingerprints of the functional processes would also help define the relation between electrophysiological activity and the fMRI signal. Even if such cohorts of transformations do not exist, characterizing the neural basis of a process under study with both electrophysiology and fMRI will provide more insights than each of these measurements alone.

ACKNOWLEDGMENTS

We thank Timothy J. Buschman, Ilan Dinstein, Luke Hallum, David J. Heeger, Jörg F. Hipp, Christopher Honey, Rafael Malach, Yuval Nir, Jefferson Roy, Nava Rubin, and Robert Shapley for comments. This work has been supported by research grants from the German Academy of Science Leopoldina (THD: BMBF-LPD 9901/8-136), the National Institutes of Health (THD: R01-EY16752 to David J. Heeger, MS: R01-NS035145 to Earl K. Miller), and the National Science Foundation/CELEST (MS: CGC-187353NGA to Earl K. Miller).

NOTES

1. The term *neuromodulation* refers to the fact that these respective neurotransmitters (such as norepinephrine or acetylcholine) bind on postsynaptic receptors, which are not directly coupled to ion channels, but instead exert their effects on cortical neurons via second messenger cascades (Hasselmo, 1995).
2. In fact, this is the case, from which the spectral analysis approach to EEG has originally emerged (Mitra and Bokil, 2007).
3. We will not discuss the hypothesis that synchronized population activity serves as a *relational* code that represents which elementary features belong to the same sensory object ("binding by synchrony"). Evidence has been provided in support of (Castelo-Branco et al., 2000; Eckhorn et al., 1988; Gray et al., 1989; Kreiter and Singer, 1996) as well as against (Lamme and Spekreijse, 1998; Palanca and DeAngelis, 2005; Thiele and Stoner, 2003) this specific hypothesis, and it has been intensely debated elsewhere (Riesenhuber and Poggio, 1999; Shadlen and Movshon, 1999; Singer, 1999).
4. When two target objects (e.g., letters) are presented in close temporal succession during rapid serial presentation, subjects frequently miss the second, suggesting that attention (i.e., the mind's eye) "blinks" after detection of the first.
5. "Inter-subject correlation" refers to the phenomenon that, while subjects watch engaging movies, neural population responses tend to become highly correlated across subjects, for multiple areas of the cortical hierarchy (Hasson et al., 2004).
6. Motion-induced blindness is a bistable perceptual suppression phenomenon analogous to binocular rivalry and generalized

flash suppression, in which a salient target stimulus disappears spontaneously from conscious perception when surrounded by a moving flow field, only to reappear several seconds later (Bonneh et al., 2001).

⁝⁝⁝ REFERENCES

Alonso JM, Usrey WM, Reid RC (1996) Precisely correlated firing in cells of the lateral geniculate nucleus. Nature 383:815–819.

Aston-Jones G, Cohen JD (2005) An integrative theory of locus coeruleus-norepinephrine function: adaptive gain and optimal performance. Annu Rev Neurosci 28:403–450.

Azouz R, Gray CM (2000) Dynamic spike threshold reveals a mechanism for synaptic coincidence detection in cortical neurons in vivo. Proc Natl Acad Sci U S A 97:8110–8115.

Azouz R, Gray CM (2003) Adaptive coincidence detection and dynamic gain control in visual cortical neurons in vivo. Neuron 37:513–523.

Bartos M, Vida I, Jonas P (2007) Synaptic mechanisms of synchronized gamma oscillations in inhibitory interneuron networks. Nat Rev Neurosci 8:45–56.

Beck DM, Rees G, Frith CD, Lavie N (2001) Neural correlates of change detection and change blindness. Nat Neurosci 4:645–650.

Bedard C, Kroger H, Destexhe A (2006) Does the 1/f frequency scaling of brain signals reflect self-organized critical states? Phys Rev Lett 97:118–102.

Belitski A, Gretton A, Magri C, Murayama Y, Montemurro MA, Logothetis NK, Panzeri S (2008) Low-frequency local field potentials and spikes in primary visual cortex convey independent visual information. J Neurosci 28:5696–5709.

Bentley P, Vuilleumier P, Thiel CM, Driver J, Dolan RJ (2003) Effects of attention and emotion on repetition priming and their modulation by cholinergic enhancement. J Neurophysiol 90:1171–1181.

Berens P, Keliris GA, Ecker AS, Logothetis NK, Tolias AS (2008a) Comparing the feature selectivity of the gamma-band of the local field potential and the underlying spiking activity in primate visual cortex. Front Syst Neurosci 2:2.

Berens P, Keliris GA, Ecker AS, Logothetis NK, Tolias AS (2008b) Feature selectivity of the gamma-band of the local field potential in primate primary visual cortex. Front Neurosci 2:199–207.

Bichot NP, Rossi AF, Desimone R (2005) Parallel and serial neural mechanisms for visual search in macaque area V4. Science 308:529–534.

Blake R, Logothetis NK (2002) Visual competition. Nat Rev Neurosci 3:13–21.

Bonneh YS, Cooperman A, Sagi D (2001) Motion-induced blindness in normal observers. Nature 411:798–801.

Boynton GM, Demb JB, Glover GH, Heeger DJ (1999) Neuronal basis of contrast discrimination. Vision Res 39:257–269.

Brefczynski JA, DeYoe EA (1999) A physiological correlate of the "spotlight" of visual attention. Nat Neurosci 2:370–374.

Bressler SL, Coppola R, Nakamura R (1993) Episodic multiregional cortical coherence at multiple frequencies during visual task performance. Nature 366:153–156.

Brosch M, Bauer R, Eckhorn R (1995) Synchronous high-frequency oscillations in cat area 18. Eur J Neurosci 7:86–95.

Brovelli A, Ding M, Ledberg A, Chen Y, Nakamura R, Bressler SL (2004) Beta oscillations in a large-scale sensorimotor cortical network: directional influences revealed by Granger causality. Proc Natl Acad Sci U S A 101:9849–9854.

Bruno RM, Sakmann B (2006) Cortex is driven by weak but synchronously active thalamocortical synapses. Science 312:1622–1627.

Buschman TJ, Miller EK (2007) Top-down versus bottom-up control of attention in the prefrontal and posterior parietal cortices. Science 315:1860–1862.

Buzsaki G, Draguhn A (2004) Neuronal oscillations in cortical networks. Science 304:1926–1929.

Buzsaki G, Kandel A (1998) Somadendritic backpropagation of action potentials in cortical pyramidal cells of the awake rat. J Neurophysiol 79:1587–1591.

Carandini M, Heeger DJ, Movshon JA (1997) Linearity and normalization in simple cells of the macaque primary visual cortex. J Neurosci 17:8621–8644.

Cardin JA, Carlen M, Meletis K, Knoblich U, Zhang F, Deisseroth K, Tsai LH, Moore CI (2009) Driving fast-spiking cells induces gamma rhythm and controls sensory responses. Nature 459:663–667.

Carmel D, Lavie N, Rees G (2006) Conscious awareness of flicker in humans involves frontal and parietal cortex. Curr Biol 16:907–911.

Castelo-Branco M, Goebel R, Neuenschwander S, Singer W (2000) Neural synchrony correlates with surface segregation rules. Nature 405:685–689.

Chen Y, Martinez-Conde S, Macknik SL, Bereshpolova Y, Swadlow HA, Alonso JM (2008) Task difficulty modulates the activity of specific neuronal populations in primary visual cortex. Nat Neurosci 11:974–982.

Corbetta M, Shulman GL (2002) Control of goal-directed and stimulus-driven attention in the brain. Nat Rev Neurosci 3:201–215.

Coull JT, Buchel C, Friston KJ, Frith CD (1999) Noradrenergically mediated plasticity in a human attentional neuronal network. Neuroimage 10:705–715.

Coull JT, Nobre AC, Frith CD (2001) The noradrenergic alpha2 agonist clonidine modulates behavioural and neuroanatomical correlates of human attentional orienting and alerting. Cereb Cortex 11:73–84.

Crone NE, Miglioretti DL, Gordon B, Lesser RP (1998a) Functional mapping of human sensorimotor cortex with electrocorticographic spectral analysis. II: Event-related synchronization in the gamma band. Brain 121 (Pt 12):2301–2315.

Crone, NE, Miglioretti DL, Gordon B, Sieracki JM, Wilson MT, Uematsu S, Lesser RP (1998b) Functional mapping of human sensorimotor cortex with electrocorticographic spectral analysis. I: Alpha and beta event-related desynchronization. Brain 121 (Pt 12):2271–2299.

Csicsvari J, Jamieson B, Wise KD, Buzsaki G (2003) Mechanisms of gamma oscillations in the hippocampus of the behaving rat. Neuron 37:311–322.

deCharms RC, Zador A (2000) Neural representation and the cortical code. Annu Rev Neurosci 23:613–647.

Desimone R, Duncan J (1995) Neural mechanisms of selective visual attention. Annu Rev Neurosci 18:193–222.

Destexhe A, Sejnowski TJ (2003) Interactions between membrane conductances underlying thalamocortical slow-wave oscillations. Physiol Rev 83:1401–1453.

Dietsch G (1932) Fourier-analyse von Elektroenkephalogrammen des Menschen. Pflger's Arch Ges Physiol 230:106–112.

Doesburg SM, Roggeveen AB, Kitajo K, Ward LM (2008) Large-scale gamma-band phase synchronization and selective attention. Cereb Cortex 18:386–396.

Donner TH, Kettermann A, Diesch E, Ostendorf F, Villringer A, Brandt SA (2000) Involvement of the human frontal eye field and multiple parietal areas in covert visual selection during conjunction search. Eur J Neurosci 12:3407–3414.

Donner TH, Siegel M, Oostenveld R, Fries P, Bauer M, Engel AK (2007) Population activity in the human dorsal pathway predicts the accuracy of visual motion detection. J Neurophysiol 98:345–359.

Donner TH, Sagi D, Bonneh YS, Heeger DJ (2008) Opposite neural signatures of motion-induced blindness in human dorsal and ventral visual cortex. J Neurosci 28:10298–10310.

Douglas RJ, Martin KA (2004) Neuronal circuits of the neocortex. Annu Rev Neurosci 27:419–451.

Eckhorn R, Bauer R, Jordan W, Brosch M, Kruse W, Munk M, Reitboeck HJ (1988) Coherent oscillations: a mechanism of feature linking in the visual cortex? Multiple electrode and correlation analyses in the cat. Biol Cybern 60:121–130.

Engel AK, Kreiter AK, Konig P, Singer W (1991) Synchronization of oscillatory neuronal responses between striate and extrastriate visual cortical areas of the cat. Proc Natl Acad Sci U S A 88:6048–6052.

Engel AK, Fries P, Singer W (2001) Dynamic predictions: oscillations and synchrony in top-down processing. Nat Rev Neurosci 2:704–716.

Engel AK, Moll CK, Fried I, Ojemann GA (2005) Invasive recordings from the human brain: clinical insights and beyond. Nat Rev Neurosci 6:35–47.

Ermentrout GB, Galan RF, Urban NN (2008) Reliability, synchrony, and noise. Trends Neurosci 31:428–434.

Faisal AA, Selen LP, Wolpert DM (2008) Noise in the nervous system. Nat Rev Neurosci 9:292–303.

Fan J, Byrne J, Worden MS, Guise KG, McCandliss BD, Fossella J, Posner MI (2007) The relation of brain oscillations to attentional networks. J Neurosci 27:6197–6206.

Feige B, Scheffler K, Esposito F, Di Salle F, Hennig J, Seifritz E (2005) Cortical and subcortical correlates of electroencephalographic alpha rhythm modulation. J Neurophysiol 93:2864–2872.

Fox MD, Raichle ME (2007) Spontaneous fluctuations in brain activity observed with functional magnetic resonance imaging. Nat Rev Neurosci 8:700–711.

Freeman J, Donner TH, Heeger DJ (2008) Interactions Between Human Inferotemporal and Early Visual Areas Reflect Feature Integration. Soc Neurosci Abstr 34:316.8.

Freeman WJ, Rogers LJ, Holmes MD, Silbergeld DL (2000) Spatial spectral analysis of human electrocorticograms including the alpha and gamma bands. J Neurosci Methods 95:111–121.

Frien A. Eckhorn R (2000) Functional coupling shows stronger stimulus dependency for fast oscillations than for low-frequency components in striate cortex of awake monkey. Eur J Neurosci 12:1466–1478.

Frien A, Eckhorn R, Bauer R, Woelbern T, Gabriel A (2000) Fast oscillations display sharper orientation tuning than slower components of the same recordings in striate cortex of the awake monkey. Eur J Neurosci 12:1453–1465.

Fries P (2005) A mechanism for cognitive dynamics: neuronal communication through neuronal coherence. Trends Cogn Sci 9:474–480.

Fries P, Reynolds JH, Rorie AE, Desimone R (2001) Modulation of oscillatory neuronal synchronization by selective visual attention. Science 291:1560–1563.

Fries P, Scheeringa R, Oostenveld R (2008a) Finding gamma. Neuron 58:303–305.

Fries P, Womelsdorf T, Oostenveld R, Desimone R (2008b) The effects of visual stimulation and selective visual attention on rhythmic neuronal synchronization in macaque area V4. J Neurosci 28:4823–4835.

Friston, K (2002) Beyond phrenology: what can neuroimaging tell us about distributed circuitry? Annu Rev Neurosci 25:221–250.

Gail A, Brinksmeyer HJ, Eckhorn R (2004) Perception-related modulations of local field potential power and coherence in primary visual cortex of awake monkey during binocular rivalry. Cereb Cortex 14:300–313.

Gieselmann MA, Thiele A (2008) Comparison of spatial integration and surround suppression characteristics in spiking activity and the local field potential in macaque V1. Eur J Neurosci 28:447–459.

Gold JI, Shadlen MN (2007) The neural basis of decision making. Annu Rev Neurosci 30:535–574.

Goldman RI, Stern JM, Engel J, Jr., Cohen MS (2002) Simultaneous EEG and fMRI of the alpha rhythm. Neuroreport 13:2487–2492.

Grass AM, Gibbs FA (1938) A Fourier transform of the electroencephalogram. J Neurophysiol 1:521–526.

Gray CM, Singer W (1989) Stimulus-specific neuronal oscillations in orientation columns of cat visual cortex. Proc Natl Acad Sci U S A 86:1698–1702.

Gray CM, König P, Engel AK, Singer W (1989) Oscillatory responses in cat visual cortex exhibit inter-columnar synchronization which reflects global stimulus properties. Nature 338:334–337.

Green DM, Swets JA (1966) Signal detection theory and psychophysics. New York: Wiley.

Gross J, Kujala J, Hamalainen M, Timmermann L, Schnitzler A, Salmelin R (2001) Dynamic imaging of coherent sources: Studying neural interactions in the human brain. Proc Natl Acad Sci U S A 98:694–699.

Gross J, Timmermann L, Kujala J, Salmelin R, Schnitzler A (2003) Properties of MEG tomographic maps obtained with spatial filtering. Neuroimage 19:1329–1336.

Gross J, Schmitz F, Schnitzler I, Kessler K, Shapiro K, Hommel B, Schnitzler A (2004) Modulation of long-range neural synchrony reflects temporal limitations of visual attention in humans. Proc Natl Acad Sci U S A 101:13050–13055.

Gruber T, Muller MM, Keil A, Elbert T (1999) Selective visual-spatial attention alters induced gamma band responses in the human EEG. Clin Neurophysiol 110:2074–2085.

Hagler DJ, Jr., Sereno MI (2006) Spatial maps in frontal and prefrontal cortex. Neuroimage 29:567–577.

Hall SD, Holliday IE, Hillebrand A, Singh KD, Furlong PL, Hadjipapas A, Barnes GR (2005) The missing link: analogous human and primate cortical gamma oscillations. Neuroimage 26:13–17.

Hamalainen M, Hari R, Ilmoniemi R., Knuutila J, Lounasmaa OV (1993) Magnetoencephalography: theory, instrumentation, and applications to noninvasive studies of the working human brain. Rev Mod Phys 65:413–497.

Hasenstaub A, Shu Y, Haider B, Kraushaar U, Duque A, McCormick DA (2005) Inhibitory postsynaptic potentials carry synchronized frequency information in active cortical networks. Neuron 47:423–435.

Hasselmo ME (1995) Neuromodulation and cortical function: modeling the physiological basis of behavior. Behav Brain Res 67:1–27.

Hasson U, Nir Y, Levy I, Fuhrmann G, Malach R (2004) Intersubject synchronization of cortical activity during natural vision. Science 303:1634–1640.

Haynes JD, Rees G (2006) Decoding mental states from brain activity in humans. Nat Rev Neurosci 7:523–534.

Haynes JD, Deichmann R, Rees G (2005a) Eye-specific effects of binocular rivalry in the human lateral geniculate nucleus. Nature 438:496–499.

Haynes JD, Driver J, Rees G (2005b) Visibility reflects dynamic changes of effective connectivity between V1 and fusiform cortex. Neuron 46:811–821.

Haynes JD, Tregellas J, Rees G (2005c) Attentional integration between anatomically distinct stimulus representations in early visual cortex. Proc Natl Acad Sci U S A 102:14925–14930.

Hebb DO (1949) The organization of behavior: a neuropsychological theory. New York: Wiley.

Heeger DJ, Ress D (2002) What does fMRI tell us about neuronal activity? Nat Rev Neurosci 3:142–151.

Heeger DJ, Simoncelli EP, Movshon JA (1996) Computational models of cortical visual processing. Proc Natl Acad Sci U S A 93:623–627.

Heekeren HR, Marrett S, Ungerleider LG (2008) The neural systems that mediate human perceptual decision making. Nat Rev Neurosci 9:467–479.

Henrie JA, Shapley R (2005) LFP power spectra in V1 cortex: the graded effect of stimulus contrast. J Neurophysiol 94:479–490.

Herrero JL, Roberts MJ, Delicato LS, Gieselmann MA, Dayan P, Thiele A (2008) Acetylcholine contributes through muscarinic receptors to attentional modulation in V1. Nature 454:1110–1114.

Hoogenboom N, Schoffelen JM, Oostenveld R, Parkes LM, Fries P (2005) Localizing human visual gamma-band activity in frequency, time, and space. Neuroimage 29:764–773.

Huk AC, Ress D, Heeger DJ (2001) Neuronal basis of the motion aftereffect reconsidered. Neuron 32:161–172.

Jack AI, Shulman GL, Snyder AZ, McAvoy M, Corbetta M (2006) Separate modulations of human V1 associated with spatial attention and task structure. Neuron 51:135–147.

Juergens E, Guettler A, Eckhorn R (1999) Visual stimulation elicits locked and induced gamma oscillations in monkey intracortical- and EEG-potentials, but not in human EEG. Exp Brain Res 129:247–259.

Kanwisher N, Wojciulik E (2000) Visual attention: insights from brain imaging. Nat Rev Neurosci 1:91–100.

Kastner S, Ungerleider LG (2000) Mechanisms of visual attention in the human cortex. Annu Rev Neurosci 23:315–341.

Kastner S, Pinsk MA, De Weerd P, Desimone R, Ungerleider LG (1999) Increased activity in human visual cortex during directed attention in the absence of visual stimulation. Neuron 22:751–761.

Kastner S, DeSimone K, Konen CS, Szczepanski SM, Weiner KS, Schneider KA (2007) Topographic maps in human frontal cortex revealed in memory-guided saccade and spatial working-memory tasks. J Neurophysiol 97:3494–3507.

Kayser C, König P (2004) Stimulus locking and feature selectivity prevail in complementary frequency ranges of V1 local field potentials. Eur J Neurosci 19:485–489.

Kayser C, Montemurro MA, Logothetis NK, Panzeri S (2009) Spike-phase coding boosts and stabilizes information carried by spatial and temporal spike patterns. Neuron 61:597–608.

Kim CY, Blake R (2005) Psychophysical magic: rendering the visible "invisible." Trends Cogn Sci 9:381–388.

Koch C, Tsuchiya N (2007) Attention and consciousness: two distinct brain processes. Trends Cogn Sci 11:16–22.

König P, Schillen TB (1991) Stimulus-Dependent assembly formation of oscillatory responses. I: Synchronization. Neural Computation 3:155–166.

König P, Engel AK, Singer W (1996) Integrator or coincidence detector? The role of the cortical neuron revisited. Trends Neurosci 19:130–137.

Kopell N, Ermentrout GB, Whittington MA, Traub RD (2000) Gamma rhythms and beta rhythms have different synchronization properties. Proc Natl Acad Sci U S A 97:1867–1872.

Kranczioch C, Debener S, Schwarzbach J, Goebel R, Engel AK (2005) Neural correlates of conscious perception in the attentional blink. Neuroimage 24:704–714.

Kreiter AK, Singer W (1996) Stimulus-dependent synchronization of neuronal responses in the visual cortex of the awake macaque monkey. J Neurosci 16:2381–2396.

Lachaux JP, Rudrauf D, Kahane P (2003) Intracranial EEG and human brain mapping. J Physiol Paris 97:613–628.

Lamme VA (2003) Why visual attention and awareness are different. Trends Cogn Sci 7:12–18.

Lamme VA, Spekreijse H (1998) Neuronal synchrony does not represent texture segregation. Nature 396:362–366.

Laufs H (2008) Endogenous brain oscillations and related networks detected by surface EEG-combined fMRI. Hum Brain Mapp 29:762–769.

Lauritzen, M (2005) Reading vascular changes in brain imaging: is dendritic calcium the key? Nat Rev Neurosci 6:77–85.

Lee H, Simpson GV, Logothetis NK, Rainer G (2005) Phase locking of single neuron activity to theta oscillations during working memory in monkey extrastriate visual cortex. Neuron 45:147–156.

Lee SH, Blake R, Heeger DJ (2005) Traveling waves of activity in primary visual cortex during binocular rivalry. Nat Neurosci 8:22–23.

Lee SH, Blake R, Heeger DJ (2007) Hierarchy of cortical responses underlying binocular rivalry. Nat Neurosci 10:1048–1054.

Leopold DA, Logothetis NK (1996) Activity changes in early visual cortex reflect monkeys percepts during binocular rivalry. Nature 379:549–553.

Leopold DA, Murayama Y, Logothetis NK (2003) Very slow activity fluctuations in monkey visual cortex: implications for functional brain imaging. Cereb Cortex 13:422–433.

Liljestrom M, Kujala J, Jensen O, Salmelin R (2005) Neuromagnetic localization of rhythmic activity in the human brain: a comparison of three methods. NeuroImage 25:734.

Linkenkaer-Hansen K, Nikulin VV, Palva S, Ilmoniemi RJ, Palva JM (2004) Prestimulus oscillations enhance psychophysical performance in humans. J Neurosci 24:10186–10190.

Liu J, Newsome WT (2006) Local field potential in cortical area MT: stimulus tuning and behavioral correlations. J Neurosci 26:7779–7790.

Llinas RR, Steriade M (2006) Bursting of thalamic neurons and states of vigilance. J Neurophysiol 95:3297–3308.

Logothetis NK (2008) What we can do and what we cannot do with fMRI. Nature 453:869–878.

Logothetis NK, Wandell BA (2004) Interpreting the BOLD signal. Annu Rev Physiol 66:735–769.

Logothetis NK, Pauls J, Augath M, Trinath T, Oeltermann A (2001) Neurophysiological investigation of the basis of the fMRI signal. Nature 412:150–157.

Logothetis NK, Kayser C, Oeltermann A (2007) In vivo measurement of cortical impedance spectrum in monkeys: implications for signal propagation. Neuron 55:809–823.

Luck SJ (2005) An introduction to the event-related potential technique. Cambridge, MA: MIT Press.

Luck SJ, Chelazzi L, Hillyard SA, Desimone R (1997) Neural mechanisms of spatial selective attention in areas V1, V2, and V4 of macaque visual cortex. J Neurophysiol 77:24–42.

Maier A, Wilke M, Aura C, Zhu C, Ye FQ, Leopold DA (2008) Divergence of fMRI and neural signals in V1 during perceptual suppression in the awake monkey. Nat Neurosci 11:1193–1200.

Mantini D, Perrucci MG, Del Gratta C, Romani GL, Corbetta M (2007) Electrophysiological signatures of resting state networks in the human brain. Proc Natl Acad Sci U S A 104:13170–13175.

Marois R, Yi DJ, Chun MM (2004) The neural fate of consciously perceived and missed events in the attentional blink. Neuron 41:465–472.

Meng M, Remus DA, Tong F (2005) Filling-in of visual phantoms in the human brain. Nat Neurosci 8:1248–1254.

Miller EK, Cohen JD (2001) An integrative theory of prefrontal cortex function. Annu Rev Neurosci 24:167–202.

Miller KJ, Leuthardt EC, Schalk G, Rao RP, Anderson NR, Moran DW, Miller JW, Ojemann JG (2007) Spectral changes in cortical surface potentials during motor movement. J Neurosci 27:2424–2432.

Miller KJ, Zanos S, Fetz EE, den Nijs M, Ojemann JG (2009) Decoupling the cortical power spectrum reveals real-time representation of individual finger movements in humans. J Neurosci 29:3132–3137.

Minzenberg MJ, Watrous AJ, Yoon JH, Ursu S, Carter CS (2008) Modafinil shifts human locus coeruleus to low-tonic, high-phasic activity during functional MRI. Science 322:1700–1702.

Mitchell JF, Sundberg KA, Reynolds JH (2007) Differential attention-dependent response modulation across cell classes in macaque visual area V4. Neuron 55:131–141.

Mitra P, Bokil H (2007) Observed brain dynamics. New York: Oxford University Press.

Mitzdorf U (1987) Properties of the evoked potential generators: current source-density analysis of visually evoked potentials in the cat cortex. Int J Neurosci 33:33–59.

Montemurro MA, Rasch MJ, Murayama Y, Logothetis NK, Panzeri S (2008) Phase-of-firing coding of natural visual stimuli in primary visual cortex. Curr Biol 18:375–380.

Moore T, Armstrong KM, Fallah M (2003) Visuomotor origins of covert spatial attention. Neuron 40:671–683.

Moosmann M, Ritter P, Krastel I, Brink A, Thees S, Blankenburg F, Taskin B, Obrig H, Villringer A (2003) Correlates of alpha rhythm in functional magnetic resonance imaging and near infrared spectroscopy. Neuroimage 20:145–158.

Mukamel R, Gelbard H, Arieli A, Hasson U, Fried I, Malach R (2005) Coupling between neuronal firing, field potentials, and FMRI in human auditory cortex. Science 309:951–954.

Muller MM, Keil A (2004) Neuronal synchronization and selective color processing in the human brain. J Cogn Neurosci 16:503–522.

Munk MH, Roelfsema PR, Konig P, Engel AK, Singer W (1996) Role of reticular activation in the modulation of intracortical synchronization. Science 272:271–274.

Nichols MJ, Newsome WT (1999) The neurobiology of cognition. Nature 402:C35–38.

Nir Y, Fisch L, Mukamel R, Gelbard-Sagiv H, Arieli A, Fried I, Malach R (2007) Coupling between neuronal firing rate, gamma LFP, and BOLD fMRI is related to interneuronal correlations. Curr Biol 17:1275–1285.

Nir Y, Mukamel R, Dinstein I, Privman E, Harel M, Fisch L, Gelbard-Sagiv H, Kipervasser S, Andelman F, Neufeld MY, et al. (2008) Interhemispheric correlations of slow spontaneous neuronal fluctuations revealed in human sensory cortex. Nat Neurosci 11:1100–1108.

Nunez PL, Srinivasan R (2006) Electric fields of the brain: the neurophysics of EEG, 2nd Edition. Oxford, New York: Oxford University Press.

Ogawa S, Lee TM, Kay AR, Tank DW (1990) Brain magnetic resonance imaging with contrast dependent on blood oxygenation. Proc Natl Acad Sci U S A 87:9868–9872.

Palanca BJ, DeAngelis GC (2005) Does neuronal synchrony underlie visual feature grouping? Neuron 46:333–346.

Pesaran B, Pezaris JS, Sahani M, Mitra PP, Andersen RA (2002) Temporal structure in neuronal activity during working memory in macaque parietal cortex. Nat Neurosci 5:805–811.

Pesaran B, Nelson MJ, Andersen RA (2008) Free choice activates a decision circuit between frontal and parietal cortex. Nature 453:406–409.

Pfurtscheller G, Lopes da Silva FH (1999) Event-related EEG/MEG synchronization and desynchronization: basic principles. Clin Neurophysiol 110:1842–1857.

Polonsky A, Blake R, Braun J, Heeger DJ (2000) Neuronal activity in human primary visual cortex correlates with perception during binocular rivalry. Nat Neurosci 3:1153–1159.

Rees G, Friston K, Koch C (2000) A direct quantitative relationship between the functional properties of human and macaque V5. Nat Neurosci 3:716–723.

Ress D, Backus BT, Heeger DJ (2000) Activity in primary visual cortex predicts performance in a visual detection task. Nat Neurosci 3:940–945.

Rickert J, Oliveira SC, Vaadia E, Aertsen A, Rotter S, Mehring C (2005) Encoding of movement direction in different frequency ranges of motor cortical local field potentials. J Neurosci 25:8815–8824.

Riesenhuber M, Poggio T (1999) Are cortical models really bound by the "binding problem"? Neuron 24:87–93 and 111–125.

Rodriguez R, Kallenbach U, Singer W, Munk MH (2004) Short- and long-term effects of cholinergic modulation on gamma oscillations and response synchronization in the visual cortex. J Neurosci 24:10369–10378.

Roelfsema PR, Engel AK, König P, Singer W (1997) Visuomotor integration is associated with zero time-lag synchronization among cortical areas. Nature 385:157–161.

Roelfsema PR, Lamme VA, Spekreijse H (1998) Object-based attention in the primary visual cortex of the macaque monkey. Nature 395:376–381.

Rubino D, Robbins KA, Hatsopoulos NG (2006) Propagating waves mediate information transfer in the motor cortex. Nat Neurosci 9:1549–1557.

Saalmann YB, Pigarev IN, Vidyasagar TR (2007) Neural mechanisms of visual attention: how top-down feedback highlights relevant locations. Science 316:1612–1615.

Salinas E, Sejnowski TJ (2000) Impact of correlated synaptic input on output firing rate and variability in simple neuronal models. J Neurosci 20:6193–6209.

Salinas E, Sejnowski TJ (2001) Correlated neuronal activity and the flow of neural information. Nat Rev Neurosci 2:539–550.

Sapir A, d'Avossa G, McAvoy M, Shulman GL, Corbetta M (2005) Brain signals for spatial attention predict performance in a motion discrimination task. Proc Natl Acad Sci U S A 102:17810–17815.

Sarnthein J, Petsche H, Rappelsberger P, Shaw GL, von Stein A (1998) Synchronization between prefrontal and posterior association cortex during human working memory. Proc Natl Acad Sci U S A 95:7092–7096.

Schall JD (2001) Neural basis of deciding, choosing, and acting. Nat Rev Neurosci 2:33–42.

Schluppeck D, Glimcher P, Heeger DJ (2005) Topographic organization for delayed saccades in human posterior parietal cortex. J Neurophysiol 94:1372–1384.

Sejnowski TJ, Paulsen O (2006) Network oscillations: emerging computational principles. J Neurosci 26:1673–1676.

Serences JT, Yantis S (2006) Selective visual attention and perceptual coherence. Trends Cogn Sci 10:38–45.

Sereno MI, Pitzalis S, Martinez A (2001) Mapping of contralateral space in retinotopic coordinates by a parietal cortical area in humans. Science 294:1350–1354.

Shadlen MN, Movshon JA (1999) Synchrony unbound: a critical evaluation of the temporal binding hypothesis. Neuron 24:67–77 and 111–125.

Shapley R, Hawken M, Ringach DL (2003) Dynamics of orientation selectivity in the primary visual cortex and the importance of cortical inhibition. Neuron 38:689–699.

Shelley M, McLaughlin D, Shapley R, Wielaard J (2002) States of high conductance in a large-scale model of the visual cortex. J Comput Neurosci 13:93–109.

Shulman GL, Ollinger JM, Linenweber M, Petersen SE, Corbetta M (2001) Multiple neural correlates of detection in the human brain. Proc Natl Acad Sci U S A 98:313–318.

Siegel M, König P (2003) A functional gamma-band defined by stimulus-dependent synchronization in area 18 of awake behaving cats. J Neurosci 23:4251–4260.

Siegel M, Donner TH, Oostenveld R, Fries P, Engel AK (2007) High-frequency activity in human visual cortex is modulated by visual motion strength. Cereb Cortex 17:732–741.

Siegel M, Donner TH, Oostenveld R, Fries P, Engel AK (2008) Neuronal synchronization along the dorsal visual pathway reflects the focus of spatial attention. Neuron 60:709–719.

Siegel M, Warden MR, Miller EK (2009) Phase-dependent neuronal coding of objects in short-term memory. Proc Natl Acad Sci USA doi:10.1073/pnas.0908193106.

Silver MA, Ress D, Heeger DJ (2007) Neural correlates of sustained spatial attention in human early visual cortex. J Neurophysiol 97:229–237.

Singer W (1999) Neuronal synchrony: a versatile code for the definition of relations? Neuron 24:49–65 and 111–125.

Sohal VS, Zhang F, Yizhar O, Deisseroth K (2009) Parvalbumin neurons and gamma rhythms enhance cortical circuit performance. Nature 459:698–702.

Somers DC, Dale AM, Seiffert AE, Tootell RB (1999) Functional MRI reveals spatially specific attentional modulation in human primary visual cortex. Proc Natl Acad Sci U S A 96:1663–1668.

Spinks RL, Kraskov A, Brochier T, Umilta MA, Lemon RN (2008) Selectivity for grasp in local field potential and single neuron activity recorded simultaneously from M1 and F5 in the awake macaque monkey. J Neurosci 28:10961–10971.

Steriade M (2000) Corticothalamic resonance, states of vigilance, and mentation. Neuroscience 101:243–276.

Swisher JD, Halko MA, Merabet LB, McMains SA, Somers DC (2007) Visual topography of human intraparietal sulcus. J Neurosci 27:5326–5337.

Tallon-Baudry C, Bertrand O (1999) Oscillatory gamma activity in humans and its role in object representation. Trends Cogn Sci 3:151–162.

Tallon-Baudry C, Bertrand O, Peronnet F, Pernier J (1998) Induced gamma-band activity during the delay of a visual short-term memory task in humans. J Neurosci 18:4244–4254.

Tallon-Baudry C, Bertrand O, Fischer C (2001) Oscillatory synchrony between human extrastriate areas during visual short-term memory maintenance. J Neurosci 21:RC177.

Tallon-Baudry C, Mandon S, Freiwald WA, Kreiter AK (2004) Oscillatory synchrony in the monkey temporal lobe correlates with performance in a visual short-term memory task. Cereb Cortex 14:713–720.

Taylor K, Mandon S, Freiwald WA, Kreiter AK (2005) Coherent oscillatory activity in monkey area v4 predicts successful allocation of attention. Cereb Cortex 15:1424–1437.

Thiele A, Stoner G (2003) Neuronal synchrony does not correlate with motion coherence in cortical area MT. Nature 421:366–370.

Thut G, Nietzel A, Brandt SA, Pascual-Leone A (2006) Alpha-band electroencephalographic activity over occipital cortex indexes visuospatial attention bias and predicts visual target detection. J Neurosci 26:9494–9502.

Tiesinga PH, Fellous JM, Salinas E, Jose JV, Sejnowski TJ (2004) Inhibitory synchrony as a mechanism for attentional gain modulation. J Physiol Paris 98:296–314.

Tong F, Engel SA (2001) Interocular rivalry revealed in the human cortical blind-spot representation. Nature 411:195–199.

Usher M, Cohen JD, Servan-Schreiber D, Rajkowski J, Aston-Jones G (1999) The role of locus coeruleus in the regulation of cognitive performance. Science 283:549–554.

Usrey WM, Reid RC (1999) Synchronous activity in the visual system. Annu Rev Physiol 61:435–456.

Usrey WM, Reppas JB, Reid RC (1998) Paired-spike interactions and synaptic efficacy of retinal inputs to the thalamus. Nature 395:384–387.

Van Der Werf J, Jensen O, Fries P, Medendorp WP (2008) Gamma-band activity in human posterior parietal cortex encodes the motor goal during delayed prosaccades and antisaccades. J Neurosci 28:8397–8405.

Van Veen BD, van Drongelen W, Yuchtman M, Suzuki A (1997) Localization of brain electrical activity via linearly constrained minimum variance spatial filtering. IEEE Trans Biomed Eng 44:867–880.

Wang M, Ramos BP, Paspalas CD, Shu Y, Simen A, Duque A, Vijayraghavan S, Brennan A, Dudley A, Nou E, et al. (2007) Alpha2A-adrenoceptors strengthen working memory networks by inhibiting cAMP-HCN channel signaling in prefrontal cortex. Cell 129:397–410.

Wang XJ (2001) Synaptic reverberation underlying mnemonic persistent activity. Trends Neurosci 24:455–463.

Wang XJ (2003) Neural oscillations. In: Encyclopedia of cognitive science (Nadel L, ed), pp 272–280. London: MacMillan.

Whittington MA, Traub RD, Jefferys JG (1995) Synchronized oscillations in interneuron networks driven by metabotropic glutamate receptor activation. Nature 373:612–615.

Wilke M, Logothetis NK, Leopold DA (2006) Local field potential reflects perceptual suppression in monkey visual cortex. Proc Natl Acad Sci U S A 103:17507–17512.

Womelsdorf T, Fries P, Mitra PP, Desimone R (2006) Gamma-band synchronization in visual cortex predicts speed of change detection. Nature 439:733–736.

Womelsdorf T, Schoffelen JM, Oostenveld R, Singer W, Desimone R, Engel AK, Fries P (2007) Modulation of neuronal interactions through neuronal synchronization. Science 316:1609–1612.

Worden MS, Foxe JJ, Wang N, Simpson GV (2000) Anticipatory biasing of visuospatial attention indexed by retinotopically specific alpha-band electroencephalography increases over occipital cortex. J Neurosci 20:RC63.

Wunderlich K, Schneider KA, Kastner S (2005) Neural correlates of binocular rivalry in the human lateral geniculate nucleus. Nat Neurosci 8:1595–1602.

Wyart V, Tallon-Baudry C (2008) Neural dissociation between visual awareness and spatial attention. J Neurosci 28:2667–2679.

Yu AJ, Dayan P (2005) Uncertainty, neuromodulation, and attention. Neuron 46:681–692.

Yuval-Greenberg S, Tomer O, Keren AS, Nelken I, Deouell LY (2008) Transient induced gamma-band response in EEG as a manifestation of miniature saccades. Neuron 58:429–441.

4.2 Helmut Laufs and Rachel Thornton

Clinical Applications: Epilepsy

Introduction

This book has comprehensively reviewed many of the technical advances and scientific applications of EEG/fMRI. The story of the technique's evolution, however, begins with epileptologists, whose initial aim was to provide a tool for accurate non-invasive seizure localization. It seems logical therefore, to conclude with a discussion of clinical applications of EEG/fMRI, in particular how far the method has come over the 15 years in which it has been used. Unless otherwise mentioned, EEG refers to surface electroencephalography and fMRI to functional MRI based on echo-planar imaging.

The chapter reviews the clinical application of EEG/fMRI to epilepsy at two levels. Initially, the chapter summarizes the body of primary EEG/fMRI patient studies in epilepsy, focusing on the most comprehensive and up-to-date literature available, although in this fast-moving field there have been numerous small studies and case reports that validate the findings of larger work. It then addresses the question of what researchers have learned about the potentials and limitations of this technique, which is still relatively new. Although EEG/fMRI has not lived up to some of its initial expectations, it will be seen that new avenues have appeared. The chapter concludes with a discussion of the immediate next steps and an outlook on the future of the field.

A Brief History of Simultaneous EEG and fMRI

The development of simultaneous EEG/fMRI recording was driven by epileptologists who sought to localize electrical sources of neuronal activity, in particular epileptic discharges (Ives et al., 1993). At first glance, using EEG/fMRI may appear an indirect approach to this clinical question, where EEG electrical source localization should provide a more straightforward solution, especially if constrained by individual anatomy. Yet, while the temporal resolution of EEG is more appropriate for tracking dysfunctional neuronal activity, the precision of fMRI in localizing the spatial topography of neural processes is superior to that of scalp EEG (Ives et al., 1993; Grova et al., 2008).

The great potential of EEG/fMRI as a clinical application led epilepsy researchers to reach methodological milestones including both acquisition hardware and artifact reduction algorithms (Lemieux et al., 1997; Allen et al., 1998). Only later was the methodology extended to physiological human brain function, predominantly the study of event-related potentials (Bonmassar et al., 1999; Kruggel et al., 2000). Prior to the development of artifact reduction methods, EEG/fMRI had to be performed in a way such that readable EEG epochs were obtained inside the MRI scanner. In order to do this, image acquisition was only "triggered" following a trained observer's detection of an EEG change of interest (initially the spike) online, with the EEG recorded continuously in the scanner environment using MRI-compatible equipment exploiting the relative delay in the hemodynamic response to the event. This method resulted in intermittent spike-triggered acquisitions that were then compared to baseline epochs of fMRI, which were assumed not to contain any events of interest. This technique was used for the initial studies in focal epilepsy (Warach et al., 1996; Seeck et al., 1998; Krakow et al., 1999; Patel et al., 1999; Krakow et al., 2000; Lazeyras et al., 2000; Jager et al., 2002). A significant drawback of this technique was that EEG recorded during MR gradient switching could not be evaluated, and absence of interictal epileptic discharges[1] (IED) could not be guaranteed. Researchers considered trying to acquire pharmacologically induced IED-free EEG by means of benzodiazepines (Seeck et al., 1998), but this had the potential of affecting hemodynamic coupling and basic neuronal functioning (Yoshizawa et al., 1997). Thus, researchers developed methods that allowed (1) recovery of

Focal epilepsy – EEG and fMRI

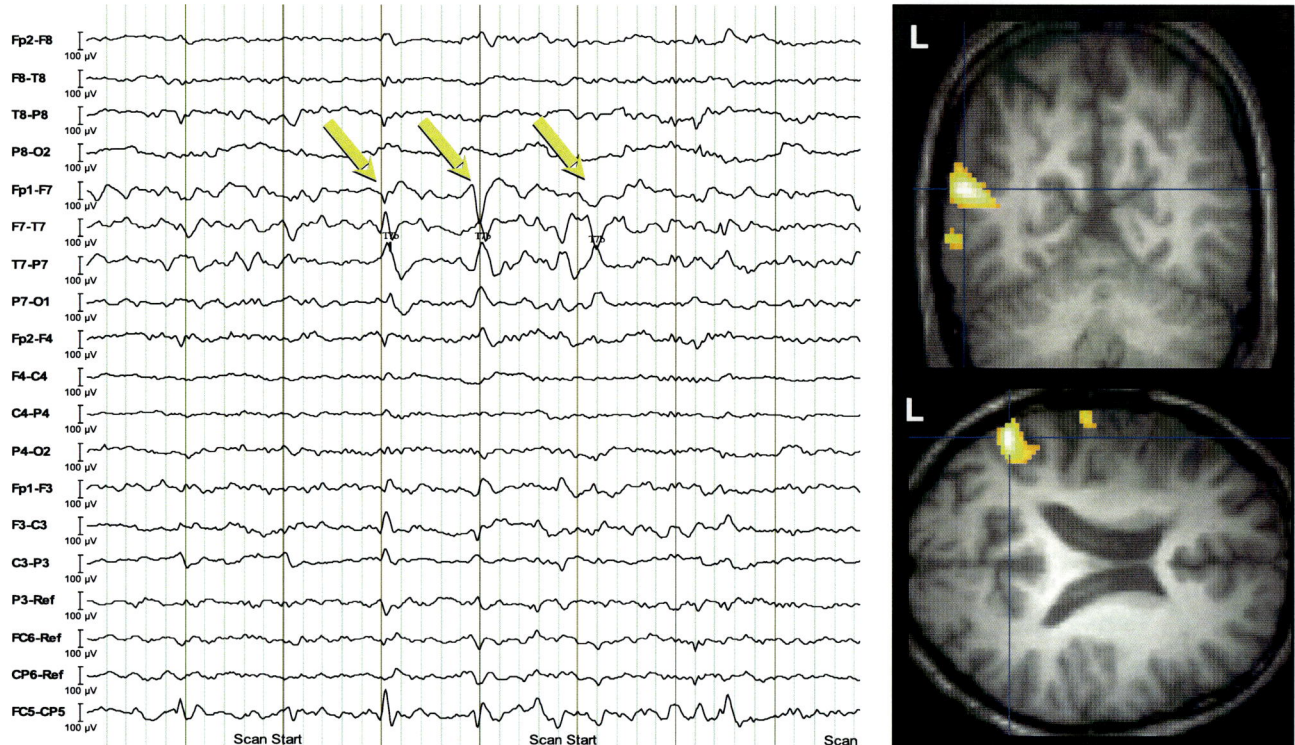

Figure 4.2.1. Mapping of the irritative zone in focal epilepsy. Interictal epileptic discharges (IED, sharp waves, yellow arrows) can be identified in left temporal channels on the EEG obtained during fMRI scanning (Scan Start indicates beginning of volume acquisition) after image and pulse artifact reduction. An IED-based general linear model was created (event-related design) and results were thresholded at $p < 0.05$ (corrected for multiple comparisons, family-wise error) and are displayed overlaid onto a T1-weighted template image. Positive BOLD-signal changes can be seen in the left temporal lobe indicating the irritative zone.

the EEG epochs obscured by pulse and imaging artifact, and, eventually, *(2)* continuous image acquisition during EEG recording, facilitating true event-related IED-based fMRI analysis approaches (Hoffmann et al., 2000; Lemieux et al., 2001). Spike-triggered EEG-fMRI works on the assumption that the hemodynamic response to the interictal event of interest is the same as that to a normal neuronal event, which will be discussed further below.

Following this technical milestone, EEG/fMRI has been applied to series of patients, including children, with different epilepsy syndromes, with the goal of inferring the location of irritative and seizure onset zones (Rosenow and Lüders, 2001), i.e., the brain regions that are thought to be responsible for the patient's epilepsy, and the hope of providing useful clinical information particularly in patients undergoing presurgical evaluation (Figure 4.2.1). Studies have also been undertaken in patient cohorts with syndromes amenable to surgical resection in order to better understand their underlying neurobiology. These clinical studies will be discussed in detail later in the chapter.

Subject safety has been and remains one of the most important technical issues from the inception of EEG/fMRI onward (Lemieux et al., 1997). This is particularly relevant as MR-compatible EEG recording equipment has become readily available and is no longer reserved for the exclusive use of informed experts. It should be understood that as new sequences are developed and the technique is extended to higher field strengths, different coils, and specific patient populations (e.g., children) each change requires rigorous individualized safety testing (Laufs et al., 2008). Efforts are currently underway to establish the safety of clinical and research MRI studies using intracranial electrodes (Georgi et al., 2004; Boucousis et al., 2007; Carmichael et al., 2007; Carmichael et al., 2008b). While this research is highly interesting from a basic science perspective, clinical specialties, particularly epilepsy and movement disorders, motivate and justify research in this area (Zhang et al., 1993; Rezai et al., 2002; Georgi et al., 2004; Mirsattari et al., 2004; van Duinen et al., 2005; Richardson et al., 2006; Carmichael et al., 2008b).

The Motivation: EEG/fMRI in the Presurgical Evaluation of Adult Epilepsy

As has been mentioned, initial studies using EEG-fMRI focused on the non-invasive identification of the seizure onset zone, and the two largest case series performed in focal[2] epilepsy (38 and 63 patients) preselected patients on the basis of having "frequent" IEDs. IEDs were observed in about 50% of patients, and of these approximately half had significant blood oxygen level dependent (BOLD) signal changes concordant with electro-clinical data (Al-Asmi et al., 2003; Salek-Haddadi et al., 2006). In these early studies the ratio of IED-based fMRI results that were classified as concordant (in the same lobe) to those considered discordant with electro-clinical data was referred to as the "yield" of the EEG-fMRI.

The likelihood of a significant fMRI signal change was found to be a function not only of the number of IED but also of morphology and ease of classification (observer bias), and temporal spread: bursts and runs of IED were more likely to generate significant results than separate individual events (Al-Asmi et al., 2003; Liston et al., 2006b; Salek-Haddadi et al., 2006).

The only study to date specifically addressing the role of EEG fMRI in presurgical evaluation looked at a group of 29 patients in whom surgery had been declined in the first instance because of the inability to localize a single source with EEG but who had at least 10 IEDs during 40 minutes of routine EEG (Zijlmans et al., 2007). Results were highly selected before their classification in that only positive BOLD responses in the region "topographically related" to the EEG field of the IED were considered. This did not allow comparison of the results with previous work. Zijlmans and colleagues found that in the complex cases studied, EEG-fMRI either improved source localization or corroborated a negative decision regarding surgical candidacy. The improved source localization led to the reconsidering of two of the 29 patients for exploration with intracranial EEG and potential surgical resection.

Evidence supporting the role of EEG fMRI in presurgical evaluation comes from the limited studies observing the relationship between IED-correlated BOLD signal change and intracranial data. Concordance of IED-related BOLD signal change with intracranially recorded seizure onset has been limited to reports on individual cases (Lazeyras et al., 2000; Bagshaw et al., 2004; Benar et al., 2006; Laufs et al., 2006d; Daunizeau et al., 2007; De Tiege et al., 2007a; Grova et al., 2008; Tyvaert et al., 2008) and a series of 5 patients in whom "active electrodes" on the intracranial EEG were observed to be close to the areas of IED-correlated BOLD activation (Benar et al., 2006). Beyond this, the true value of EEG/fMRI as a tool in presurgical evaluation will only become known where outcome data is available. Currently this is so in the form of case reports within larger series, although longer-term outcomes are becoming available (Al-Asmi et al., 2003; De Tiege et al., 2007a).

EEG/fMRI Studies of Specific Pathologies in Adults

Researchers have sought to identify pathology-specific patterns of IED-correlated BOLD signal changes in focal epilepsies. In six patients with *cerebral cavernous angiomas*, no IED-correlated fMRI response was found in the lesion or its immediate periphery, but diffuse signal changes were detected both near and away from the cavernomas (Kobayashi et al., 2007). The T2*-weighted BOLD signal was compromised by the iron deposits in the lesioned tissue hindering the detection of reliable signals in those areas.

Three EEG/fMRI studies focused on patients with *malformations of cortical development*. One included five individuals with focal cortical dysplasia and one with a ganglioglioma (Federico et al., 2005a). Another included nine patients with polymicrogyria (Kobayashi et al., 2005). Each time, the researchers aimed to test whether EEG/fMRI could help to elucidate the mechanisms of epileptogenicity in malformations of cortical development. Two studies (Kobayashi et al., 2005; Kobayashi et al., 2006b) found either no signal changes or lesional, near-lesional, and subcortical fMRI signal changes, but no particular pathology-specific fMRI pattern (Detre and Crino, 2005). There were similar findings in an EEG/fMRI study of fourteen patients with grey matter heterotopia. In band and nodular heterotopia, BOLD activations and deactivations occurred within, near, or distant from the affected tissue (Kobayashi et al., 2006b). In a third study, the same group tried to distinguish brain regions active during interictal versus ictal EEG discharges in different subtypes of malformations of cortical development (Tyvaert et al., 2008). The dysplastic cortex and the heterotopic cortex of band heterotopia were involved in interictal and seizure processes, whereas nodular heterotopia did not generate seizures, which came from overlying cortex, and were only sometimes involved in interictal activity (Tyvaert et al., 2008). As is often the case with patient studies, efforts were hindered by the limited size of homogeneous patient groups available.

EEG/fMRI in the Pediatric Population

EEG/fMRI is increasingly used in the pediatric population, despite a variety of practical and ethical considerations when applying a research technique to this group. While the data obtained is analyzed from a research perspective, the primary aim—and justification—is to obtain additional information in the context of a presurgical work-up (De Tiege et al., 2007a). EEG/fMRI in children poses challenges, especially when the children have epilepsy (De Tiege et al., 2007a). Subject motion in the scanner is a relevant problem, and in spite of analysis strategies that account for relatively large motion events (Lemieux et al., 2007a), some children cannot be investigated without sedation, which can affect the BOLD signal (Marcar et al., 2006). Quite apart from this, the shape of the hemodynamic response function across the pediatric population has not been extensively studied, but there is evidence of different amplitude and shape to that seen in adults (Richter and Richter, 2003; Schapiro et al., 2004; Jacobs et al., 2008a).

Studies of *benign childhood epilepsy and centro-temporal spikes* have revealed BOLD activations in the (perisylvian) central region (Archer et al., 2003b; S Boor et al., 2003). Multiple-source EEG analysis in children from this patient population localized the centro-temporal spikes close to the fMRI activations, and it was claimed that the spike onset zone could thus be distinguished from propagated epileptic activity (R Boor et al., 2007). Further evidence will be required to confirm this hypothesis. Lengler et al. (2007) studied a similar patient cohort (10 children with a variety of benign focal epilepsies of childhood). They found positive or negative signal changes in perisylvian, central, pre-motor, and prefrontal regions, but these did not reach a level of statistical significance commonly accepted in neuroimaging (Lengler et al., 2007). Studying three children with *occipital lobe epilepsy*, Leal et al. concluded that the location of IED-related BOLD signal changes reflected their semiology well and were similar but not identical to the EEG sources in two patients and entirely different in one (Leal et al., 2006).

A study of 6 children aged 8–15 years, with lesional or non-lesional pharmacoresistant focal epilepsy revealed significant IED-associated BOLD signal changes in 4 of the 6, while both activation and deactivation patterns were found in one child, and widespread deactivation in another. Activations co-localized with the presumed location of the epileptic focus in four children, one of which was confirmed by intracranial EEG. De Tiege et al. concluded that EEG-fMRI can non-invasively localize epileptogenic regions in children with pharmacoresistant focal epilepsy (De Tiege et al., 2007a). Further studies are underway, including children with lesional epilepsy in many centers, and the number of studies of children with generalized epilepsies will also grow (Labate et al., 2005).

Jacobs and colleagues studied a series of five children with *tuberous sclerosis* in order to evaluate the use of EEG/fMRI in the assessment of potential tuber resection (Jacobs et al., 2008b). The findings qualitatively resemble those of the above-mentioned studies of specific pathologies in adults: EEG change-associated BOLD signal changes were revealed around multiple structurally visible lesions both near and distant to the region of the presumed IED source, suggesting complex epileptogenic networks (Jacobs et al., 2008b) and rendering the applied EEG/fMRI method unsuitable as a meaningful presurgical technique.

In addition to the specific hurdles when studying children, EEG/fMRI in the pediatric population faces many of the same difficulties as it does in adults. It may contribute useful data in the presurgical evaluation of selected suitable individuals, but not in every patient; and the appropriate interpretation of relative BOLD signal increases and decreases is still under debate. The hemodynamic response in the maturing brain in general, and the response to IED specifically, requires further investigation

(Jacobs et al., 2007; Jacobs et al., 2008a; Salek-Haddadi et al., 2008). Studies in children, however, may reveal more information regarding specific epilepsy syndromes than may be gathered from adults with long-standing refractory epilepsy.

Lessons from Early Studies: EEG/fMRI Beyond the Irritative Zone

A closer assessment of the directionality of IED-related BOLD signal changes and the location of discordant signal changes suggested a potential extra yield of EEG/fMRI studies beyond the localization of the irritative zone both in focal (Aghakhani et al., 2006; Bagshaw et al., 2006; Gotman et al., 2006; Kobayashi et al., 2006c; Laufs et al., 2006b; Salek-Haddadi et al., 2006) and generalized epilepsy (Archer et al., 2003a; Gotman et al., 2005; Gotman et al., 2006; Hamandi et al., 2006; Laufs et al., 2006a). While group analyses do not benefit individual patients and have not been able to demonstrate BOLD signal change specific to a particular epilepsy syndrome, they provide the potential to image larger-scale cognitive effects coherent with the observed semiology[3] allowing insight into the neurobiology of epilepsy. In particular, the group approach has identified universal epileptic networks[4] in temporal lobe (Kobayashi et al., 2006d; Laufs et al., 2006b) and generalized epilepsies (Archer et al., 2003a; Gotman et al., 2005; Hamandi et al., 2006).

In *generalized epilepsy*, both at the individual subject (Archer et al., 2003a; Salek-Haddadi et al., 2003b; Laufs et al., 2006a; De Tiege et al., 2007b) and the group level (Aghakhani et al., 2004; Gotman et al., 2005; Hamandi et al., 2006; Moeller et al., 2008b; Moeller et al., 2008a), fMRI activations in response to generalized spike and wave activity[5] (GSW) occurred in the thalamus alongside cortical deactivations (Figure 4.2.2)—similar to a pattern already suggested by electrophysiological data from animal studies showing a cortico-thalamic loop of excitatory and inhibitory synaptic activity (Steriade, 2006). The study was also used to attempt to classify epilepsy syndromes; however, group analysis of 30 patients with different *idiopathic* (IGE) and 16 with *secondarily generalized epilepsy*[6] (SGE) did not identify syndrome-specific BOLD patterns (Hamandi et al., 2006). Thalamic activation and deactivation in frontal-parietal cortices and the precuneus were a common pattern for both IGE and SGE in adults (Salek-Haddadi et al., 2003b; Gotman et al., 2005; Hamandi et al., 2006; Laufs et al., 2006a). The particular patterns of cortical deactivation may specifically be related to the features of typical absences[7]: so-called default mode areas of the brain exhibit reduced activity during GSW (Gotman et al., 2005; Laufs et al., 2006a; De Tiege et al., 2007b). The precuneus and bilateral frontal and parietal cortices are normally more active during relaxed wakefulness than during either goal-directed behavior or states of reduced consciousness, such as sleep and anesthesia (Raichle et al., 2001). Impaired

A)   **Generalised epilepsy - EEG**

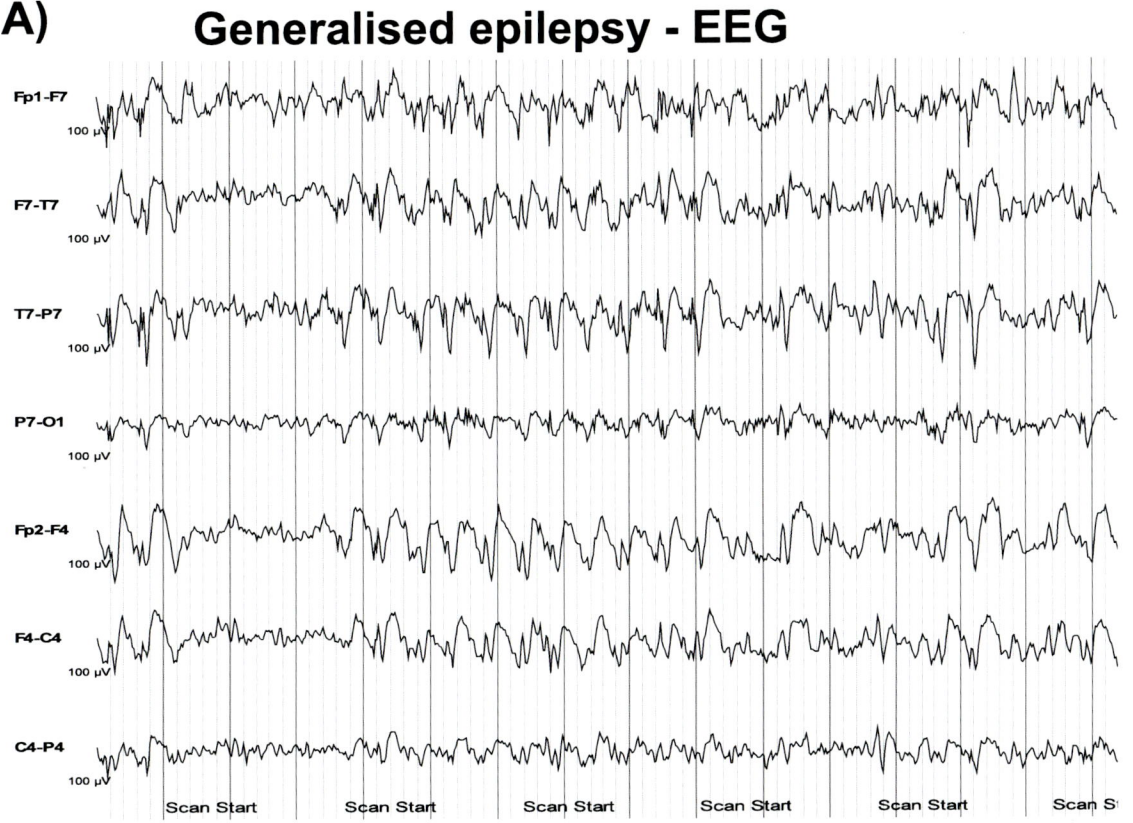

Figure 4.2.2. Mapping of spike and wave activity in generalized epilepsy. A) Generalized spike and wave discharges (GSW) with frontal emphasis recorded during fMRI acquisition (Scan Start indicates beginning of volume) after image and pulse artifact reduction are displayed (Laufs et al., 2006a). B) Statistical maps of GSW-associated fMRI signal decreases are overlaid onto a rendered template T1-weighted brain image (color intensity is a function of depth). A random-effects group analysis of thirty patients with idiopathic generalized epilepsy (Hamandi et al., 2006) revealed BOLD signal decreases in brain regions similar to those known as the "default mode network" (Raichle et al., 2001). Decreased default mode network activity during states of reduced vigilance and the association of GSW with impaired consciousness during absences suggest that the GSW-associated fMRI maps reflect the cognitive state of the patient during GSW or absences. Positive signal changes occurred bilaterally in the thalamus (not shown, compare Figure 4.2.3) as has been demonstrated by animal studies (Steriade, 2006).

B)   **Generalised epilepsy - fMRI**

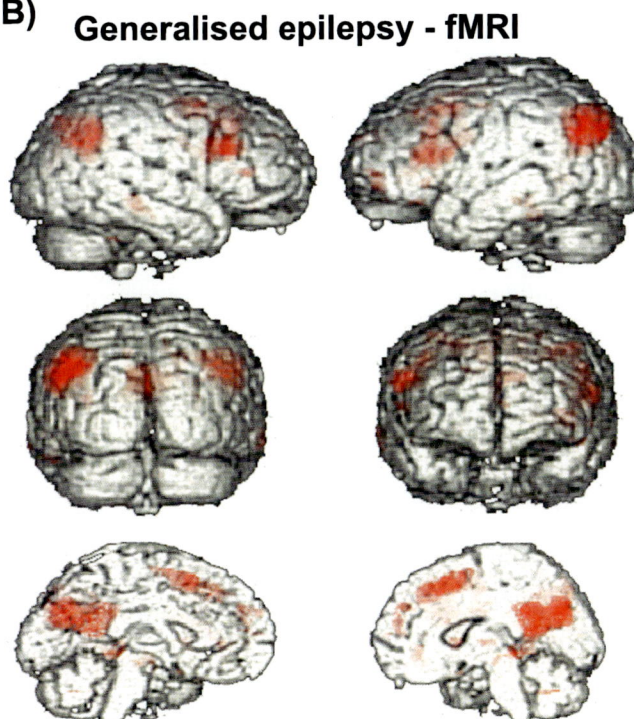

consciousness during absences resembles that during reduced vigilance both phenomenologically and hemodynamically in cortical areas. Owing to the fMRI block design employed in the analysis, only the common relay station, the thalamus, and the lower activity in default mode brain regions may be detected (Laufs et al., 2003), but the BOLD correlates of the sources of the generalized EEG discharges may be missed.

In a group of patients with heterogeneous *temporal lobe epilepsy*[8] syndromes and frequent IED, an analogous pattern of sub-neocortical activation and neocortical deactivation was found: common ipsilateral IED-correlated hippocampal activation and cortical deactivation of default mode brain regions, including areas distant to the temporal lobe (Laufs et al.,

2006b). Remote intra- and extratemporal activations and deactivations, including the contralateral temporal lobe, were also found associated with temporal lobe spikes (Kobayashi et al., 2006d).

It has been suggested that the hippocampus reflects a common relay station in temporal lobe epilepsy with some analogy to the role of the thalamus in generalized epilepsies (Laufs et al., 2006b). The activity decrease of consciousness-subserving default mode areas in response to *inter*ictal epileptic activity might explain the phenomenon of transient cognitive impairment[9] (Binnie, 2003; Laufs et al., 2006b). The widespread deactivations in default mode brain regions both in focal and generalized epilepsy are in keeping with the concept of an "epileptic network" and suggest that the expression "*inter*ictal epileptic activity" might need to be revisited (Figure 4.2.3).

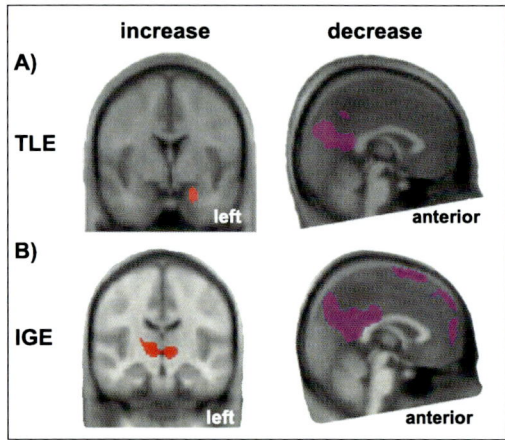

Figure 4.2.3. EEG/fMRI reveals correlates of epileptiform discharges beyond the irritative zone. Electroencephalogram/functional MRI (EEG/fMRI) in epilepsy has been mainly applied to map the area of cortical tissue that generates interictal epileptic discharges (IED), but more and more studies suggest that EEG/fMRI can also map EEG feature-related cognitive "states": (A) A group of patients with left temporal lobe epilepsy (TLE) and heterogeneous EEG features and histopathology was studied using IED-correlated fMRI (Laufs et al., 2006b). Common focal IED-associated blood oxygen level dependent (BOLD) signal increases were detected in the ipsilateral hippocampus, known to play a crucial role in TLE. BOLD signal decreases were commonly observed in the retrosplenium and precuneus, brain areas typically active during conscious rest and less active during states of impaired consciousness, suggesting that focal interictal discharges affect ongoing brain function even when a seizure cannot be observed. (B) In idiopathic generalized epilepsies (IGEs) with absence seizures, similar brain regions exhibit generalized spike- and wave-associated BOLD signal decreases. BOLD signal increases typically occur bilaterally in the thalamus. Hence, there is a parallel between the hippocampus in TLE and the thalamus in IGE each being anti-correlated in activity to "default mode" regions associated with impaired consciousness, a feature of both absence (IGE) and complex partial seizures (TLE).

Methodological Refinement

The notion that IED-correlated BOLD signal changes may have other causes in addition to neuronal activity in the irritative zone led researchers to test more diverse hypotheses, requiring a range of methodological approaches in addition to the classical event-related general linear model (GLM)–based design. Those pertaining to adjusting the hemodynamic response function (HRF) will be discussed in a separate paragraph below. As explained in the preceding paragraph, a possible interpretation of BOLD signal changes remote from the expected electro-clinical focus of pathological activity is that the relatively slow fMRI technique applied may identify cognitive effects, i.e., cerebral activity which are temporally but not necessarily spatially associated with neuronal epileptic activity. The obvious neurophysiological explanation for remote signal changes is IED propagation (Wendling and Bartolomei, 2001; Mirsattari et al., 2007; Bartolomei et al., 2008; Gotz-Trabert et al., 2008; Hamandi et al., 2008b) causing *downstream* effects. However, a *facilitating role* of certain brain states and associated with these the level of activity of the involved brain regions is also possible[10]. Current studies examine the functional and causal connectivity between brain regions at the combined EEG/fMRI level by integrating causal and source modeling of EEG data and fMRI connectivity analyses (Vaudano et al., 2007; Hamandi et al., 2008b; Vulliemoz et al., 2008).

While attention has focused on IED, in analogy to fast activity on intracerebral EEG (Urrestarazu et al., 2006; Urrestarazu et al., 2007), focal slow activity on scalp EEG (Figure 4.2.4) can also be used to model fMRI data, but this is technically challenging (Jirsch et al., 2006; Laufs et al., 2006d; Urrestarazu et al., 2006; Siniatchkin et al., 2007). A relationship exists between physiological brain states and pathological cerebral activity, for example sleep and GSW (Steriade, 2005), suggesting a benefit when integrating this information in an analysis. Brain states (vigilance) as characterized by background EEG are about to be incorporated into the analysis (Gotman et al., 2007) as has been done in healthy subjects (Laufs et al., 2006c).

Human EEG/fMRI studies meanwhile also make use of data-driven methods both from an fMRI (Morgan et al., 2007; Rodionov et al., 2007b) and an EEG standpoint (Jann et al., 2008) in order to increase the sensitivity of the method. This is especially relevant in the absence of visible surface EEG changes. Morgan and colleagues claimed increased sensitivity of an EEG-independent fMRI clustering analysis method for the detection of hemodynamic changes in temporal lobe epilepsy (Morgan et al., 2004). An independent study highlighted relevant shortcomings in comparison with an EEG-based analysis (Hamandi et al., 2005) and was followed by further refinement of the clustering approach (Morgan et al., 2007). Rodionov and colleagues validated spatial independent component analysis (ICA) of fMRI data against a classic EEG-based general linear model analysis. Their findings suggested ICA's capability to reveal areas of epileptic activity in patients with focal epilepsy when abnormalities were not apparent on scalp EEG (Rodionov et al., 2007b). The relevance of these studies will be discussed below.

There has been advancement on both the scanner and the EEG side in terms of higher field strength and number of recordable channels, respectively. High density MRI-compatible EEG is possible and facilitates better source localization (Liston et al., 2006b), but unless the EEG needs to be recorded simultaneously with MRI, conventional unimodal high density EEG or

Multimodal assessment of a patient with focal epilepsy

Reprinted from Magnetic Resonance Imaging, 24/4, Laufs, H., Hamandi, K., Walker, M. C., Scott, C., Smith, S., Duncan, J. S., Lemieux, L., *EEG-fMRI mapping of asymmetrical delta activity in a patient with refractory epilepsy is concordant with the epileptogenic region determined by intracranial EEG*, pp. 367-371, Copyright (2006), with permission from Elsevier.

Figure 4.2.4. Multimodal imaging example of frequency based EEG/fMRI analysis and its validation by intracranial recordings. A patient with refractory focal epilepsy was studied using continuous EEG-correlated fMRI. Seizures were characterized by head turning to the left and clonic jerking of the left arm suggesting a right frontal epileptogenic region. Interictal EEG showed occasional runs of independent, non-lateralized slow activity in the delta band with right fronto-central dominance but without lateralizing value. Ictal scalp EEG suggested right-sided central slow activity preceding some seizures. Structural 3 Tesla MRI was normal. Because there were no clear epileptiform abnormalities during simultaneous EEG-fMRI, asymmetrical 1–3 Hz EEG delta activity near fronto-central electrode positions was modeled in the fMRI analysis (Laufs et al., 2006d). (A) Position of the subdural grid and strips, (B) their approximate relation to fMRI motor mapping and EEG/fMRI activations in response to right fronto-central 1–3 Hz slow activity, and (C) cortical stimulation results. A) Sagittal computed tomography (CT) localizer showing the position of the 48-contact subdural grid over the right anterior frontal lobe and one 8-contact subdural strip overlapping the grid and extending posteriorly. Another 8-contact strip was placed extending medially from contact 34 of the grid (compare C) into the interhemispheric fissure. The insert shows a CT slice reflecting the position of the grid in the axial plane. B) Overlay of fMRI activations onto a surface rendering of a template brain in normalized space, all corrected for multiple comparisons (family-wise error, P < 0.05, extent threshold 30 voxels). Right finger tap fMRI activation is shown in blue (coordinates in Talairach space, maximum at [XYZ] = [-25, -18, 61], left precentral gyrus), left tapping in green ([40,-5, 63], right precentral gyrus and superior frontal gyrus). Indicated in red ([26,7, 65], right superior frontal gyrus) are fMRI signal changes in response to the difference of 1–3 Hz EEG activity recorded at F8-T4 versus F7-T3, masked by signal changes occurring in response to 1–3 Hz EEG slowing at contralateral and posterior electrode positions (T6-O2, T5-O1) and to 4–7 Hz oscillations recorded at F8-T4, F7-T3, T6-O2, and T5-O1. Dashed and dotted lines indicate positions of the subdural grid and strips, respectively. C) Schematic of 48-contact subdural grid with color-coded electrocorticography results. Dark green indicates a motor response from the left hand, lighter green implies the border between motor and somatosensory 75. Stimulation at contact 11 (green circle) provoked stiffening of the left arm. Pink indicates contacts at which seizure onset or early spreading was seen (compare panel D), and red circles mark contacts which by estimation overlie the area of EEG-fMRI activation (compare B, red). (D) Bipolar montage of EEG recorded during seizure onset from the 48-contact subdural grid. An increase in background low amplitude fast activity is seen at contact G20 (pink arrow) evolving into higher amplitude fast activity interspersed with low amplitude (100 µV) spikes, before an underlying semirhythmic slow activity occurs (grey arrow). The discharge is maximal at contact G20, and there is some spread to G12. The bipolar derivations near the suspected area of slowing-associated fMRI activation (G42, G44, red) have a very low amplitude signal, implying synchronous activity at respective electrode pairs. Compare (C) for insert in right lower hand corner.

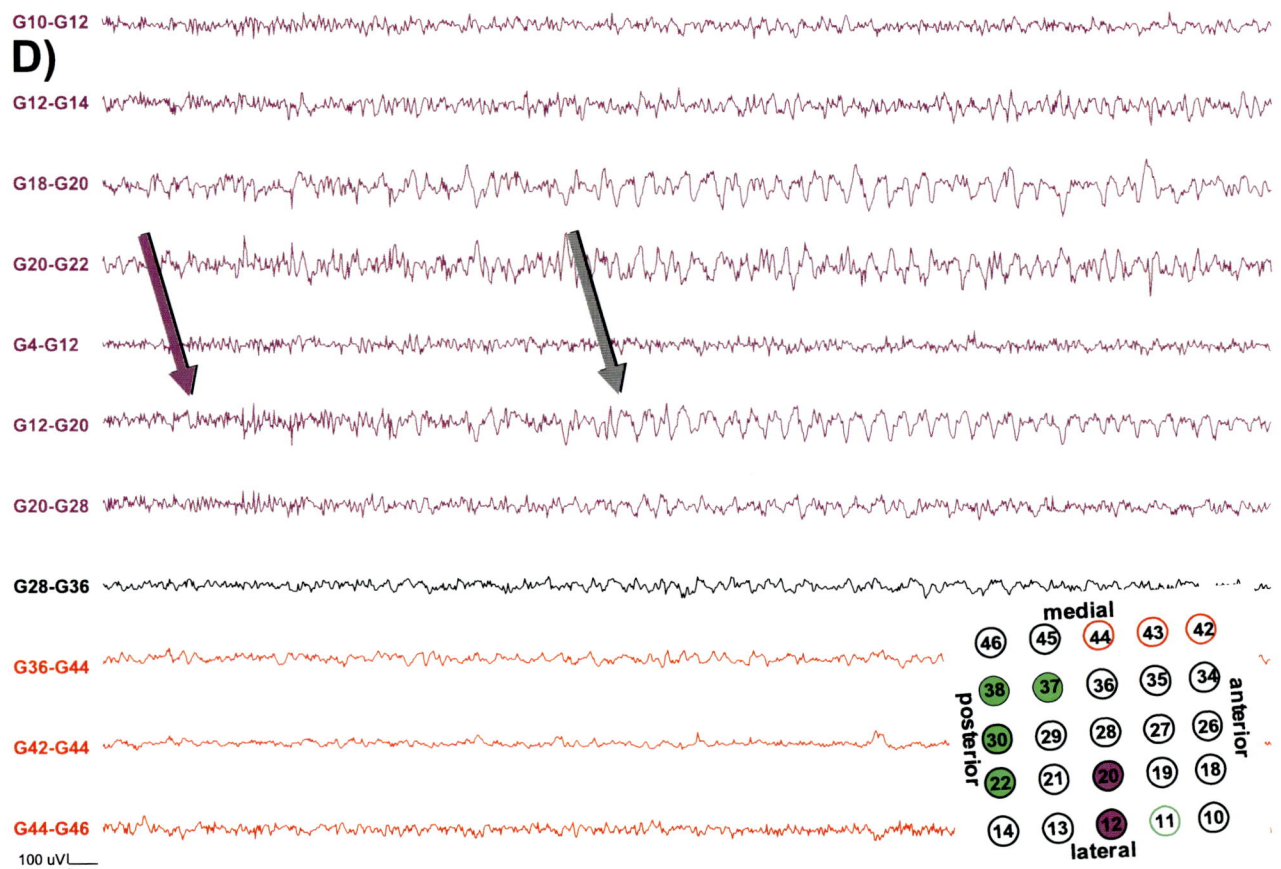

Reprinted from Magnetic Resonance Imaging, 24/4, Laufs, H., Hamandi, K., Walker, M. C., Scott, C., Smith, S., Duncan, J. S., Lemieux, L., *EEG-fMRI mapping of asymmetrical delta activity in a patient with refractory epilepsy is concordant with the epileptogenic region determined by intracranial EEG*, pp. 367-371, Copyright (2006), with permission from Elsevier.

Figure 4.2.4. (Continued)

MEG recordings may still guarantee superior data quality compared to EEG recorded inside an MRI scanner. Large adult patient series conducted at higher field strengths are still scarce (Jann et al., 2008; Liu et al., 2008), and it remains to be shown that fMRI at 3 T will result in a higher yield than studies performed at 1.5 T (Gotman et al., 2006). An anecdotal example of higher sensitivity at 3 T over 1.5 T exists in a single case with generalized epilepsy: EEG/fMRI at 3 T revealed thalamic activation which was not detected at 1.5 T, however, multiple factors in addition to the field strength may have played a role (Laufs et al., 2006a).

The Hemodynamic Response to IED

Up until now, the most common approach to EEG/fMRI data in epilepsy has been based on forward modeling. In most IED-related fMRI studies, beginning with spike-triggered experiments, it was assumed that the hemodynamic response (HR) to IED is analogous to that observed in healthy volunteers (Benar et al., 2002; Salek-Haddadi et al., 2003a; Gotman et al., 2006). As in healthy subjects (Aguirre et al., 1998), some variability of the HR to IED has been observed in patients (Tana et al., 2007), and it was proposed that patient-specific responses need to be taken into account (Kang et al., 2003; Bagshaw et al., 2006; Lu et al., 2006; Lu et al., 2007). However, in scalp EEG–based studies it is difficult to distinguish true altered hemodynamic coupling from timing and propagation effects that lead to an apparent alteration of the HR (Salek-Haddadi et al., 2008): A systematic investigation of the so-called canonical[11] and non-canonical hemodynamic responses to IED (Salek-Haddadi et al., 2006; Lemieux et al., 2007b) revealed that where the shape of the hemodynamic response deviated from the canonical, responses occurred remotely from the suspected focus of epileptic activity, either being a false positive finding or potentially reflecting propagation effects. It was concluded that the BOLD response to IED was primarily canonical in adults (Lemieux et al., 2007b). One animal study suggested a linear relationship between IED and BOLD activity (Mirsattari et al., 2006).

Another perspective on the metabolic changes induced by IED investigates the relationship between blood flow and oxygenation. Initial studies suggest the physiological link between the two measures is preserved in focal and generalized epilepsies both for relative BOLD signal increases and decreases (Stefanovic et al., 2005; Carmichael et al., 2008a; Hamandi et al., 2008a). These findings support the notion that neurovascular coupling in epilepsy per se at least resembles the physiological condition (Krakow, 2008). In the case of symptomatic epilepsy[12] this will vary and depend on the primary lesion type. For example a tumor, angioma, or ischemic lesion (Krainik et al., 2005) will alter the hemodynamic properties of surrounding, potentially epileptogenic tissue.

Ictal Studies in Focal Epilepsy

The basic idea of EEG/fMRI was to study interictal epileptic activity. Several obstacles are in the way of studies of ictal activity. It is currently not readily justified and therefore unethical to induce a seizure during fMRI scanning particularly if it evolves into a seizure with motor symptoms, because the usefulness of the data obtained is then questionable. Very frequently, only (the beginning of) a single seizure is captured during an fMRI session precluding a classical general linear model-based analysis and usually prompting for a visual or data-driven approach lacking the robustness of a formal statistical assessment (Hamandi and Duncan, 2008). Usually, seizure activity will be accompanied by head motion, rendering results during the ictus invalid or at least unreliable (Hajnal et al., 1994; Field et al., 2000; Lund et al., 2005). Nevertheless, in an attempt to maximally exploit the available data a number of studies have been carried out in individual patients with single—or for this purpose ideally—frequent focal seizures. A number of ictal fMRI studies were performed without simultaneous EEG recordings (Jackson et al., 1994; Detre et al., 1995; Detre et al., 1996; Krings et al., 2000; Morocz et al., 2003). Avoiding seizure-induced motion problems, Federico et al. limited their analysis to the BOLD signal time course preceding the clinically judged onsets of seizures in three patients with focal epilepsy. They found BOLD signal changes preceding the clinical seizure and proposed the existence of a pre-ictal state (Federico et al., 2005b).

Salek-Haddadi et al. reported a case of ictal fMRI based on an electrographic seizure recorded on simultaneous continuous EEG (Salek-Haddadi et al., 2002). A left temporal electrographic seizure was modeled in a GLM-based block design alongside realignment parameters as nuisance covariates. An extensive area of left-hemispheric activation was seen. A smaller cluster was also evident within the grey matter of the ipsilateral cingulate gyrus. The mean signal rise was 2.5% followed by a prolonged undershoot interpreted as prolonged oxygen consumption compared to the normal physiological HRF. Kobayashi and colleagues analyzed brief repetitive electrographic seizures during an EEG-

fMRI experiment also by means of a GLM-based block design. The patient showed right hemisphere atrophy and an extensive nodular heterotopia in the right temporo-parietal region reaching subcortically. Ictal EEG-correlated fMRI signal increases were detected in the right angular gyrus, around the heterotopia, and in the contralateral cerebellum, while signal decreases were detected adjacent to the lesional activations and in both occipital regions. The shape of the associated ictal BOLD response showed a maximum signal increase in the range of 6%. A prolonged BOLD undershoot was observed lasting about 20 seconds beyond the one assumed in cognitive activation studies (Kobayashi et al., 2006a). Salek-Haddadi et al. provoked patients with reading epilepsy and found connections between language-induced seizure activity, language processing, and motor control. They speculated that in this type of epilepsy, recruitment of a critical mass of neurons in regions subserving normal (language) function is associated with reflex seizures (Salek-Haddadi et al., 2008). The study by Tyvaert et al. including both ictal and interictal discharges in different types of cortical malformations has been discussed above (Tyvaert et al., 2008). By means of a correlation analysis of EEG/fMRI data obtained during a simple partial seizure, Auer and colleagues underlined the hypothesis of the existence of a preictal state because they found BOLD signal changes to precede the clinical onset of the seizure by around one minute (Auer et al., 2008).

In summary, ictal EEG/fMRI studies have not been able to identify a consistent ictal process, nor a principle common to the variety of syndromes studied. Ictal EEG/fMRI is therefore as of yet of limited benefit in understanding the epileptogenic network. Some explanations for these confines may be found in the following paragraph.

Limitations

Conceptual Limitations of (Inter-)Ictal EEG/fMRI Studies

EEG/fMRI was seen as a promising additional tool for presurgical epilepsy evaluation allowing a precise non-invasive identification of the epileptic foci from the first studies (Seeck et al., 1998). The objective of resective epilepsy surgery is the complete removal or disconnection of the epileptogenic zone, which can be defined as the area of the cortex indispensable for the generation of clinical seizures (Rosenow and Lüders, 2001). Interictal EEG serves to identify the irritative zone (Figure 4.2.1), which may overlap but is not synonymous with the epileptogenic zone. In some cases the two may be spatially distinct. It was thought in the past that EEG/fMRI was a tool which by definition would be capable of imaging the irritative zone (Rosenow and Lüders, 2001), because it was assumed that BOLD signal changes identified the brain regions giving rise to IED (Bagshaw et al., 2006; Grova et al., 2008). As discussed earlier in this chapter (Figure 4.2.3), meanwhile, many studies have suggested that IED-associated BOLD-maps can delineate neuronal activity beyond that of the irritative and probably the epileptogenic zone (Grova et al., 2008; Laufs, 2008). While this may help the epileptologist to enhance their understanding of the epilepsies, it does not tell the surgeon where to cut. Even if EEG/fMRI unequivocally did identify the irritative zone, the relevance of interictal epileptic discharges for epileptogenesis and therefore epilepsy surgery remains unknown (de Curtis and Avanzini, 2001).

The interpretation of BOLD-signal change remains hypothetical in regions distant from the presumed epileptogenic zone.[13] "Cognitive hypotheses" (Figure 4.2.3) derived from EEG/fMRI (de-)activation patterns (Gotman et al., 2005; Laufs et al., 2006b) are difficult to prove, because patients are usually examined at rest without a task (Laufs and Duncan, 2007). The assumption of propagation effects could potentially be tested by means of high-density EEG/ MEG source modeling or invasive recordings (Benar et al., 2006), but with the limitations of insensitivity to deep sources and restricted spatial sampling, respectively.

In principle, information from EEG/fMRI is desirable especially for those patients in whom routine presurgical evaluation does not provide conclusive results. However, in practice, these are cases where interictal surface EEG changes are ambiguous or poorly localized, reducing the chances to obtain a valid EEG/fMRI result. Alternatively, presurgical evaluation may lead to multiple, potentially conflicting spatial hypotheses, but cases where EEG/fMRI could help to select among them remain anecdotal—and most importantly unvalidated (Kobayashi et al., 2005; Kobayashi et al., 2006b; Kobayashi et al., 2007; Jacobs et al., 2008b). Rather, EEG/ fMRI can provide supporting evidence in patients where classical investigations allow the establishment of a good clinical hypothesis with respect to the epileptogenic zone (Salek-Haddadi et al., 2006).

Methodological Limitations of Interictal EEG/ fMRI Studies

While EEG/fMRI can benefit from the combination of these two techniques it is equally vulnerable to the limitations of either one: EEG-based fMRI analyses will be constrained by the sensitivity of the EEG, i.e., its relative blindness to deep sources (e.g., hippocampus, medial frontal cortex) and the related fact that sometimes the only epileptic activity registered on scalp EEG has propagated to the cortical layers from elsewhere (Laufs et al., 2006b). IED-correlated fMRI results will only be as good as the underlying model. In the case of a standard GLM-based forward model this requires accurate IED detection and classification, which is not only hindered technically but is also highly observer-dependent (Liston et al., 2006b; Salek-Haddadi et al., 2006). In essence, finding the ideal

analysis approach of EEG/fMRI data is a work in progress and a gold standard does not exist (Laufs et al., 2008).

MRI is prone to susceptibility artifacts, especially in the mentioned temporal and frontal areas (Fischer and Ladebeck, 1998). Echo planar images are geometrically distorted, requiring sophisticated coregistration algorithms and careful assessment in the clinical context if fMRI maps should serve to be related to structural images and guide surgery (Carmichael et al., 2008a). BOLD-fMRI time-series in particular are sensitive to motion and circulation artifacts, reducing the reliability of EEG/fMRI results if not considered diligently (Lund et al., 2005; Liston et al., 2006a; Lund et al., 2006; Laufs et al., 2007; Lemieux et al., 2007a). Claims that the MRI environment affects neuronal activity and can reduce the frequency of IED currently remain anecdotal.

Despite its non-invasiveness and the wide availability of both MRI scanners and EEG equipment, EEG/fMRI is not only demanding for the patient who has to tolerate lying still and inside the noisy bore for a prolonged time, but also requires laborious preparation and analysis way beyond routine structural MRI or EEG each performed separately. For example, even once potential target zones for epilepsy surgery—or in the first instance for closer investigation with intracranial EEG—have been mapped on BOLD-EPI images, these still need to be coregistered to the structural space of the patient's brain with high accuracy requiring exact coregistration methods.

Finally, it needs to be kept in mind that functional MRI is best at answering a question of the type "where does it happen?" while responses to "how does it happen?" will require input from other modalities.

Potential Solutions

The available MRI-compatible EEG hardware does not currently represent a limitation in EEG/fMRI applied to epilepsy. On the software side, recent efforts were concerned with the refinement of [pulse] artifact reduction methods (see Chapter 2.3 in this book). While visual EEG IED-coding is vastly immune against residual pulse artifact-related false-positive IED detection, automated algorithms may benefit from improved pulse artifact reduction (Laufs et al., 2008).

The practice of studying epilepsy patients at rest without a task in order to localize interictal activity still appears a suitable approach despite the disadvantage of dealing with uncontrolled cognitive and vigilance states. However, in the context of a GLM-based approach, modeling EEG-based information describing these states, e.g., as confounds within the IED-based event-related design, might increase the forward model's sensitivity (Gotman et al., 2007). Of course, it can be equally interesting to model EEG information as an effect of interest beyond discrete events in the presence (Siniatchkin et al., 2007) or absence (Laufs et al.,

2006d) of discrete epileptic discharges. Further attempts aim to improve IED-related forward models by optimizing the assumed HRF as discussed earlier in this chapter. Current research targets the development of symmetrical data fusion models where EEG and fMRI information simultaneously and equally contribute to finding a common solution space for the acquired hemodynamic and electrical data (Laufs et al., 2008), and the first application in epilepsy has been reported (Daunizeau et al., 2007): a strong agreement was found between intracranial EEG and the bioelectrically and hemodynamically active sources of interictal epileptic activity identified using a variational Bayesian data fusion model (Daunizeau et al., 2007).

When probing hypotheses trying to explain IED-associated BOLD signal changes remote to the presumed epileptogenic focus, combining cognitive paradigms with EEG/fMRI experiments might lead to a more realistic characterization of where epileptic EEG activity interferes with the patients' cognitive function (Laufs et al., 2006a). Similarly, impairment of specific cognitive functions induced by IED might be tested by having subjects perform brain region/function-specific tasks during EEG/fMRI (Binnie, 2003; Pressler et al., 2005; Laufs et al., 2006b). Vice versa, as in reflex epilepsies, a stimulus may be used to induce disease-specific changes in the brain (Salek-Haddadi et al., 2008). One could imagine that—provided the existence of normative data—interference of epileptic activity with resting-state brain activity might also hint at pathological brain activity (Rodionov et al., 2007a).

Methods have found their way into routine EEG and neuroimaging analysis techniques that reach beyond the question "where does it happen?" allowing inferences about causality, i.e., "what makes it happen?" for example, by means of effective connectivity analysis (Friston et al., 2003; David et al., 2006; Chen et al., 2008; Hamandi et al., 2008b). Pursuing both functional and effective connectivity analyses allows exploitation of data sets that on first sight appear as if they do not contain useful information in view of epilepsy surgery. Also, group analyses can add extra value. These approaches may help to understand propagation effects among several regions and might reveal those regions playing a causal role in the generation of epileptic discharges. While this is currently only possible using invasive recordings, results obtained by EEG/fMRI with full brain coverage could add valuable complementary information.

Finally, as is common practice in clinical medicine, EEG/fMRI results will be of most value to presurgical evaluation if reviewed in the context of all available information, including clinical assessment, structural imaging, routine EEG, MEG, SPECT, PET, and fMRI, for example. Multimodal data integration both in the clinician's head but also at the technical analysis level has more and more become a requirement in clinical practice (Zijlmans et al., 2007; Hamandi et al., 2008b). As a first step, EEG/fMRI results can be used to generate hypotheses that can then be tested by other methods such as intracranial recordings (Figure 4.2.4).

What Should Be Done Next

Explicit validation studies are lacking that would determine whether a clinical application of EEG/fMRI in epilepsy is reliable, helpful, and hence appropriate. Some reports exist on patients who have been studied with EEG/fMRI and were since operated on (Al-Asmi et al., 2003; De Tiege et al., 2007a). Data with longer periods of postoperative observation will naturally become available over the years (Thornton et al., 2007). Reports exist relating intracranial EEG data to fMRI-BOLD activations (Figure 4.2.4), however these will always be limited by the different spatial coverage achieved by either technique (Lazeyras et al., 2000; Bagshaw et al., 2004; Benar et al., 2006; Laufs et al., 2006d; Daunizeau et al., 2007; De Tiege et al., 2007a; Grova et al., 2008; Tyvaert et al., 2008).

A fundamental challenge posits cases when during fMRI no obvious IED can be detected (Laufs et al., 2006d; Rodionov et al., 2007b). At the same time, these patients are often those for whom the more established investigations also fail to create clear hypotheses, which means that another, full brain, non-invasive analysis technique can be of value. The limitations of data-driven, exclusively fMRI-based analysis techniques have been discussed above. The potential contribution of EEG/fMRI could be that more subtle EEG changes which from a neurophysiologist's perspective would classically be considered nonspecific or of no localizing value might be tested by means of fMRI (Figure 4.2.4) and serve to control primarily data-driven techniques. Of course, the circularity of such an approach would have to be overcome by reviewing the results within the broader picture of the clinical assessment. Closely related to this, further development of the so-called data fusion techniques, weighting EEG and fMRI equally within the model, promise to increase EEG/fMRI's sensitivity (Daunizeau et al., 2007).

Conclusion

As with any clinical test, an optimal balance needs to be struck between its sensitivity and specificity. This has to be kept in mind both at the level of analysis and interpretation. Particularly when EEG/fMRI-based results are presented to clinicians who do not have first-hand experience with the technique, they need to be made aware of its limitations. Conversely, whenever a conservative analysis path is pursued, EEG/fMRI results should be brought to the clinician's attention and incorporated into the presurgical evaluation process—including their use when determining potential implantation sites for invasive EEG. At least for selected cases, this is already current practice in some internationally renowned epilepsy surgery centers around the world (to the knowledge of the authors at least in the United Kingdom, Australia, the United States, The Netherlands, and Germany). Today it appears a reasonable assumption that EEG/fMRI could soon gain equal status among the above-mentioned presurgical investigations. In addition, it has been highlighted that EEG/fMRI cannot only serve its purpose in the presurgical evaluation of epilepsy but is a valuable tool in basic research of epilepsy when studying cognitive effects of (inter-)ictal activity, and its spread and interaction with global brain function. Concurrent recordings of intracranial EEG and fMRI will open even wider avenues (Laufs and Duncan, 2007).

ACKNOWLEDGMENTS

HL was supported by the Bundesministerium für Bildung und Forschung (BMBF grant 01 EV 0703).

NOTES

1. interictal epileptic discharge or ~ activity: waveforms on the EEG which point to or are typically associated with epileptic activity such as spikes, sharp waves, spike and slow wave, poly spikes, focal slow activity or a combination thereof.
2. initial activation of only part of one cerebral hemisphere
3. signs and symptoms associated with an epileptic seizure
4. brain regions which change their activity in association with IED without necessarily being their electrical source
5. generalised, synchronous EEG pattern, consisting of a sharply contoured fast wave followed by a slow wave
6. secondarily generalized: after a focal start, epileptic activity spreads synchronously to both hemispheres
7. a brief (<20 s) generalized seizure characterized by a blank stare and impaired consciousness
8. most common epilepsy of adults, typical clinical features include impairment of consciousness and amnesia
9. term used to describe fleeting cognitive lapses associated with brief epileptic discharges
10. without further modeling, due to the limited temporal resolution of common BOLD applications, the mere activation sequence prohibits any inference on the order of events or directionality of activity spread
11. canonical HR: that generally assumed in the analysis of fMRI studies in healthy volunteers
12. epilepsy secondary to another condition, usually a structural lesion
13. the area of cortex that is indispensable for the generation of epileptic seizures (Rosenow and Lüders, 2001)

REFERENCES

Aghakhani Y, Bagshaw AP, Benar CG, Hawco C, Andermann F, Dubeau F, Gotman J (2004) fMRI activation during spike and wave discharges in idiopathic generalized epilepsy. Brain 127:1127–1144.

Aghakhani Y, Kobayashi E, Bagshaw AP, Hawco C, Benar CG, Dubeau F, Gotman J (2006) Cortical and thalamic fMRI responses in partial epilepsy with focal and bilateral synchronous spikes. Clin Neurophysiol 117:177–191.

Aguirre GK, Zarahn E, D'Esposito M (1998) The variability of human, BOLD hemodynamic responses. Neuroimage 8:360–369.

Al-Asmi A, Benar CG, Gross DW, Khani YA, Andermann F, Pike B, Dubeau F, Gotman J (2003) fMRI activation in continuous and spike-triggered EEG-fMRI studies of epileptic spikes. Epilepsia 44:1328–1339.

Allen PJ, Polizzi G, Krakow K, Fish DR, Lemieux L (1998) Identification of EEG events in the MR scanner: the problem of pulse artifact and a method for its subtraction. Neuroimage 8:229–239.

Archer JS, Abbott DF, Waites AB, Jackson GD (2003a) fMRI "deactivation" of the posterior cingulate during generalized spike and wave. Neuroimage 20:1915–1922.

Archer JS, Briellman RS, Abbott DF, Syngeniotis A, Wellard RM, Jackson GD (2003b) Benign epilepsy with centro-temporal spikes: spike triggered fMRI shows somato-sensory cortex activity. Epilepsia 44:200–204.

Auer T, Veto K, Doczi T, Komoly S, Juhos V, Janszky J, Schwarcz A (2008) Identifying seizure-onset zone and visualizing seizure spread by fMRI: a case report. Epileptic Disord 10:93–100.

Bagshaw AP, Aghakhani Y, Benar CG, Kobayashi E, Hawco C, Dubeau F, Pike GB, Gotman J (2004) EEG-fMRI of focal epileptic spikes: analysis with multiple haemodynamic functions and comparison with gadolinium-enhanced MR angiograms. Hum Brain Mapp 22:179–192.

Bagshaw AP, Kobayashi E, Dubeau F, Pike GB, Gotman J (2006) Correspondence between EEG-fMRI and EEG dipole localisation of interictal discharges in focal epilepsy. Neuroimage 30:417–425.

Bartolomei F, Wendling F, Chauvel P (2008) The concept of an epileptogenic network in human partial epilepsies. Neurochirurgie 54:174–184.

Benar CG, Gross DW, Wang Y, Petre V, Pike B, Dubeau F, Gotman J (2002) The BOLD response to interictal epileptiform discharges. Neuroimage 17:1182–1192.

Benar CG, Grova C, Kobayashi E, Bagshaw AP, Aghakhani Y, Dubeau F, Gotman J (2006) EEG-fMRI of epileptic spikes: concordance with EEG source localization and intracranial EEG. Neuroimage 30:1161–1170.

Binnie CD (2003) Cognitive impairment during epileptiform discharges: is it ever justifiable to treat the EEG? Lancet Neurol 2:725–730.

Bonmassar G, Anami K, Ives J, Belliveau JW (1999) Visual evoked potential (VEP) measured by simultaneous 64-channel EEG and 3T fMRI. Neuroreport 10:1893–1897.

Boor R, Jacobs J, Hinzmann A, Bauermann T, Scherg M, Boor S, Vucurevic G, Pfleiderer C, Kutschke G, Stoeter P (2007) Combined spike-related functional MRI and multiple source analysis in the non-invasive spike localization of benign rolandic epilepsy. Clin Neurophysiol 118:901–909.

Boor S, Vucurevic G, Pfleiderer C, Stoeter P, Kutschke G, Boor R (2003) EEG-related functional MRI in benign childhood epilepsy with centrotemporal spikes. Epilepsia 44:688–692.

Boucousis S, Cunningham CJ, Goodyear B, Federico P (2007) Safety and feasibility of using implanted depth electrodes for intracranial EEG-fMRI at 3 Tesla. In: ISMRM-ESMRMB Joint Annual Meeting, p 1081. Berlin, Germany.

Carmichael DW, Pinto S, Limousin-Dowsey P, Thobois S, Allen PJ, Lemieux L, Yousry T, Thornton JS (2007) Functional MRI with active, fully implanted, deep brain stimulation systems: safety and experimental confounds. Neuroimage 37:508–517.

Carmichael DW, Hamandi K, Laufs H, Duncan JS, Thomas DL, Lemieux L (2008a) An investigation of the relationship between BOLD and perfusion signal changes during epileptic generalised spike wave activity. Magn Reson Imaging 26:870–873.

Carmichael DW, Thornton JS, Rodionov R, Thornton R, McEvoy A, Allen P, Lemieux L (2008b) Safety of localising epilepsy monitoring intracranial EEG electrodes using MRI: RF induced heating. JMRI 28:1233–1244.

Chen CC, Kiebel SJ, Friston KJ (2008) Dynamic causal modelling of induced responses. Neuroimage 41:1293–1312.

Daunizeau J, Grova C, Marrelec G, Mattout J, Jbabdi S, Pelegrini-Issac M, Lina JM, Benali H (2007) Symmetrical event-related EEG/fMRI information fusion in a variational Bayesian framework. Neuroimage 36:69–87.

David O, Kiebel SJ, Harrison LM, Mattout J, Kilner JM, Friston KJ (2006) Dynamic causal modeling of evoked responses in EEG and MEG. Neuroimage 30:1255–1272.

de Curtis M, Avanzini G (2001) Interictal spikes in focal epileptogenesis. Prog Neurobiol 63:541–567.

De Tiege X, Laufs H, Boyd SG, Harkness W, Allen PJ, Clark CA, Connelly A, Cross JH (2007a) EEG-fMRI in children with pharmacoresistant focal epilepsy. Epilepsia 48:385–389.

De Tiege X, Harrison S, Laufs H, Boyd SG, Clark CA, Gadian DG, Neville BG, Vargha-Khadem F, Cross HJ (2007b) Impact of interictal secondary-generalized activity on brain function in epileptic encephalopathy: an EEG-fMRI study. Epilepsy Behav 11:460–465.

Detre JA, Crino PB (2005) A multilayered approach to studying cortical malformations: EEG-fMRI. Neurology 64:1108–1110.

Detre JA, Sirven JI, Alsop DC, O'Connor MJ, French JA (1995) Localization of subclinical ictal activity by functional magnetic resonance imaging: correlation with invasive monitoring. Ann Neurol 38:618–624.

Detre JA, Alsop DC, Aguirre GK, Sperling MR (1996) Coupling of cortical and thalamic ictal activity in human partial epilepsy: demonstration by functional magnetic resonance imaging. Epilepsia 37:657–661.

Federico P, Archer JS, Abbott DF, Jackson GD (2005a) Cortical/subcortical BOLD changes associated with epileptic discharges: an EEG-fMRI study at 3 T. Neurology 64:1125–1130.

Federico P, Abbott DF, Briellmann RS, Harvey AS, Jackson GD (2005b) Functional MRI of the pre-ictal state. Brain 128:1811–1817.

Field AS, Yen YF, Burdette JH, Elster AD (2000) False cerebral activation on BOLD functional MR images: study of low-amplitude motion weakly correlated to stimulus. AJNR Am J Neuroradiol 21:1388–1396.

Fischer H, Ladebeck R (1998) Echo-Planar imaging image artifacts. In: Echo-Planar imaging. Theory, technique, and application (Schmitt F, Stehling MK, Turner R, eds), pp 179–200. Berlin: Springer.

Friston KJ, Harrison L, Penny W (2003) Dynamic causal modelling. Neuroimage 19:1273–1302.

Georgi JC, Stippich C, Tronnier VM, Heiland S (2004) Active deep brain stimulation during MRI: a feasibility study. Magn Reson Med 51:380–388.

Gotman J, Grova C, Bagshaw A, Kobayashi E, Aghakhani Y, Dubeau F (2005) Generalized epileptic discharges show thalamocortical activation and suspension of the default state of the brain. Proc Natl Acad Sci U S A 102:15236–15240.

Gotman J, Kobayashi E, Bagshaw AP, Benar CG, Dubeau F (2006) Combining EEG and fMRI: a multimodal tool for epilepsy research. J Magn Reson Imaging 23:906–920.

Gotman J, Tyvaert L, LeVan P, Grova C, Chassagnon S, Dubeau F (2007) Effects of physiological rhythms on the BOLD signal in epileptic patients. Epilepsia 48:160–161.

Gotz-Trabert K, Hauck C, Wagner K, Fauser S, Schulze-Bonhage A (2008) Spread of ictal activity in focal epilepsy. Epilepsia 49:1594–1601.

Grova C, Daunizeau J, Kobayashi E, Bagshaw AP, Lina JM, Dubeau F, Gotman J (2008) Concordance between distributed EEG source localization and simultaneous EEG-fMRI studies of epileptic spikes. Neuroimage 39:755–774.

Hajnal JV, Myers R, Oatridge A, Schwieso JE, Young IR, Bydder GM (1994) Artifacts due to stimulus correlated motion in functional imaging of the brain. Magn Reson Med 31:283–291.

Hamandi K, Duncan JS (2008) FMRI in the evaluation of the Ictal Onset Zone. In: Textbook of epilepsy surgery (Lüders HO, ed): Chapter 80. London: Informa Healthcare.

Hamandi K, Salek-Haddadi A, Liston A, Laufs H, Fish DR, Lemieux L (2005) fMRI temporal clustering analysis in patients with frequent interictal epileptiform discharges: comparison with EEG-driven analysis. Neuroimage 26:309–316. Hamandi K, Salek-Haddadi A, Laufs H, Liston A, Friston K, Fish DR, Duncan JS, Lemieux L (2006) EEG-fMRI of idiopathic and secondarily generalized epilepsies. Neuroimage 31:1700–1710.

Hamandi K, Laufs H, Noth U, Carmichael DW, Duncan JS, Lemieux L (2008a) BOLD and perfusion changes during epileptic generalised spike wave activity. Neuroimage 39:608–618.

Hamandi K, Powell HW, Laufs H, Symms MR, Barker GJ, Parker GJ, Lemieux L, Duncan JS (2008b) Combined EEG-fMRI and tractography to visualise propagation of epileptic activity. J Neurol Neurosurg Psychiatry 79:594–597.

Hoffmann A, Jager L, Werhahn KJ, Jaschke M, Noachtar S, Reiser M (2000) Electroencephalography during functional echo-planar imaging: detection of epileptic spikes using post-processing methods. Magn Reson Med 44:791–798.

Ives JR, Warach S, Schmitt F, Edelman RR, Schomer DL (1993) Monitoring the patient's EEG during echo planar MRI. Electroencephalogr Clin Neurophysiol 87:417–420.

Jackson GD, Connelly A, Cross JH, Gordon I, Gadian DG (1994) Functional magnetic resonance imaging of focal seizures. Neurology 44:850–856.

Jacobs J, Kobayashi E, Boor R, Muhle H, Stephan W, Hawco C, Dubeau F, Jansen O, Stephani U, Gotman J, Siniatchkin M (2007) Hemodynamic responses to interictal epileptiform discharges in children with symptomatic epilepsy. Epilepsia 48:2068–2078.

Jacobs J, Hawco C, Kobayashi E, Boor R, Levan P, Stephani U, Siniatchkin M, Gotman J (2008a) Variability of the hemodynamic response as a function of age and frequency of epileptic discharge in children with epilepsy. Neuroimage 40:601–614.

Jacobs J, Rohr A, Moeller F, Boor R, Kobayashi E, Levan Meng P, Stephani U, Gotman J, Siniatchkin M (2008b) Evaluation of epileptogenic networks in children with tuberous sclerosis complex using EEG-fMRI. Epilepsia 49:816–825.

Jager L, Werhahn KJ, Hoffmann A, Berthold S, Scholz V, Weber J, Noachtar S, Reiser M (2002) Focal epileptiform activity in the brain: detection with spike-related functional MR imaging: preliminary results. Radiology 223:860–869.

Jann K, Wiest R, Hauf M, Meyer K, Boesch C, Mathis J, Schroth G, Dierks T, Koenig T (2008) BOLD correlates of continuously fluctuating epileptic activity isolated by independent component analysis. Neuroimage 42:635–648.

Jirsch JD, Urrestarazu E, LeVan P, Olivier A, Dubeau F, Gotman J (2006) High-frequency oscillations during human focal seizures. Brain 129:1593–1608.

Kang JK, Benar C, Al-Asmi A, Khani YA, Pike GB, Dubeau F, Gotman J (2003) Using patient-specific hemodynamic response functions in combined EEG-fMRI studies in epilepsy. Neuroimage 20:1162–1170.

Kobayashi E, Bagshaw AP, Jansen A, Andermann F, Andermann E, Gotman J, Dubeau F (2005) Intrinsic epileptogenicity in polymicrogyric cortex suggested by EEG-fMRI BOLD responses. Neurology 64:1263–1266.

Kobayashi E, Hawco CS, Grova C, Dubeau F, Gotman J (2006a) Widespread and intense BOLD changes during brief focal electrographic seizures. Neurology 66:1049–1055.

Kobayashi E, Bagshaw AP, Grova C, Gotman J, Dubeau F (2006b) Grey matter heterotopia: what EEG-fMRI can tell us about epileptogenicity of neuronal migration disorders. Brain 129:366–374.

Kobayashi E, Bagshaw AP, Grova C, Dubeau F, Gotman J (2006c) Negative BOLD responses to epileptic spikes. Hum Brain Mapp 27:488–497.

Kobayashi E, Bagshaw AP, Benar CG, Aghakhani Y, Andermann F, Dubeau F, Gotman J (2006d) Temporal and extratemporal BOLD responses to temporal lobe interictal spikes. Epilepsia 47:343–354.

Kobayashi E, Bagshaw AP, Gotman J, Dubeau F (2007) Metabolic correlates of epileptic spikes in cerebral cavernous angiomas. Epilepsy Res 73:98–103.

Krainik A, Hund-Georgiadis M, Zysset S, von Cramon DY (2005) Regional impairment of cerebrovascular reactivity and BOLD signal in adults after stroke. Stroke 36:1146–1152.

Krakow K (2008) Imaging epileptic activity using functional MRI. Neurodegener Dis 5:286–295.

Krakow K, Woermann FG, Symms MR, Allen PJ, Lemieux L, Barker GJ, Duncan JS, Fish DR (1999) EEG-triggered functional MRI of interictal epileptiform activity in patients with partial seizures. Brain 122 (Pt 9):1679–1688.

Krakow K, Allen PJ, Lemieux L, Symms MR, Fish DR (2000) Methodology: EEG-correlated fMRI. Adv Neurol 83:187–201.

Krings T, Topper R, Reinges MH, Foltys H, Spetzger U, Chiappa KH, Gilsbach JM, Thron A (2000) Hemodynamic changes in simple partial epilepsy: a functional MRI study. Neurology 54:524–527.

Kruggel F, Wiggins CJ, Herrmann CS, von Cramon DY (2000) Recording of the event-related potentials during functional MRI at 3.0 Tesla field strength. Magn Reson Med 44:277–282.

Labate A, Briellmann RS, Abbott DF, Waites AB, Jackson GD (2005) Typical childhood absence seizures are associated with thalamic activation. Epileptic Disord 7:373–377.

Laufs H (2008) Endogenous brain oscillations and related networks detected by surface EEG-combined fMRI. Hum Brain Mapp 29:762–769.

Laufs H, Duncan JS (2007) Electroencephalography/functional MRI in human epilepsy: what it currently can and cannot do. Curr Opin Neurol 20:417–423.

Laufs H, Krakow K, Sterzer P, Eger E, Beyerle A, Salek-Haddadi A, Kleinschmidt A (2003) Electroencephalographic signatures of attentional and cognitive default modes in spontaneous brain activity fluctuations at rest. Proc Natl Acad Sci U S A 100:11053–11058.

Laufs H, Lengler U, Hamandi K, Kleinschmidt A, Krakow K (2006a) Linking generalized spike-and-wave discharges and resting state brain activity by using EEG/fMRI in a patient with absence seizures. Epilepsia 47:444–448.

Laufs H, Hamandi K, Salek-Haddadi A, Kleinschmidt AK, Duncan JS, Lemieux L (2006b) Temporal lobe interictal epileptic discharges affect cerebral activity in "default mode" brain regions. Hum Brain Mapp 28:1923–1932.

Laufs H, Holt JL, Elfont R, Krams M, Paul JS, Krakow K, Kleinschmidt A (2006c) Where the BOLD signal goes when alpha EEG leaves. Neuroimage 31:1408–1418.

Laufs H, Hamandi K, Walker MC, Scott C, Smith S, Duncan JS, Lemieux L (2006d) EEG-fMRI mapping of asymmetrical delta activity in a patient with refractory epilepsy is concordant with the epileptogenic region determined by intracranial EEG. Magn Reson Imaging 24:367–371.

Laufs H, Walker MC, Lund TE (2007) "Brain activation and hypothalamic functional connectivity during human non-rapid eye movement sleep: an EEG/fMRI study"—its limitations and an alternative approach. Brain 130:e75.

Laufs H, Daunizeau J, Carmichael DW, Kleinschmidt A (2008) Recent advances in recording electrophysiological data simultaneously with magnetic resonance imaging. Neuroimage 40:515–528.

Lazeyras F, Blanke O, Perrig S, Zimine I, Golay X, Delavelle J, Michel CM, de Tribolet N, Villemure JG, Seeck M (2000) EEG-triggered functional MRI in patients with pharmacoresistant epilepsy. J Magn Reson Imaging 12:177–185.

Leal A, Dias A, Vieira JP, Secca M, Jordao C (2006) The BOLD effect of interictal spike activity in childhood occipital lobe epilepsy. Epilepsia 47:1536–1542.

Lemieux L, Allen PJ, Franconi F, Symms MR, Fish DR (1997) Recording of EEG during fMRI experiments: patient safety. Magn Reson Med 38:943–952.

Lemieux L, Salek-Haddadi A, Josephs O, Allen P, Toms N, Scott C, Krakow K, Turner R, Fish DR (2001) Event-related fMRI with simultaneous and continuous EEG: description of the method and initial case report. Neuroimage 14:780–787.

Lemieux L, Salek-Haddadi A, Lund TE, Laufs H, Carmichael D (2007a) Modelling large motion events in fMRI studies of patients with epilepsy. Magn Reson Imaging 25:894–901.

Lemieux L, Laufs H, Carmichael D, Paul JS, Walker MC, Duncan JS (2007b) Noncanonical spike-related BOLD responses in focal epilepsy. Hum Brain Mapp 29:329–345.

Lengler U, Kafadar I, Neubauer BA, Krakow K (2007) fMRI correlates of interictal epileptic activity in patients with idiopathic benign focal epilepsy of childhood: a simultaneous EEG-functional MRI study. Epilepsy Res 75:29–38.

Liston AD, Lund TE, Salek-Haddadi A, Hamandi K, Friston KJ, Lemieux L (2006a) Modelling cardiac signal as a confound in EEG-fMRI and its application in focal epilepsy studies. Neuroimage 30:827–834.

Liston AD, De Munck JC, Hamandi K, Laufs H, Ossenblok P, Duncan JS, Lemieux L (2006b) Analysis of EEG-fMRI data in focal epilepsy based on automated spike classification and Signal Space Projection. Neuroimage 31:1015–1024.

Liu Y, Yang T, Yang X, Liu I, Liao W, Lui S, Huang X, Chen H, Gong Q, Zhou D (2008) EEG-fMRI study of the interictal epileptic activity in patients with partial epilepsy. J Neurol Sci 268:117–123.

Lu Y, Bagshaw AP, Grova C, Kobayashi E, Dubeau F, Gotman J (2006) Using voxel-specific hemodynamic response function in EEG-fMRI data analysis. Neuroimage 32:238–247.

Lu Y, Grova C, Kobayashi E, Dubeau F, Gotman J (2007) Using voxel-specific hemodynamic response function in EEG-fMRI data analysis: an estimation and detection model. Neuroimage 34:195–203.

Lund TE, Norgaard MD, Rostrup E, Rowe JB, Paulson OB (2005) Motion or activity: their role in intra- and inter-subject variation in fMRI. Neuroimage 26:960–964.

Lund TE, Madsen KH, Sidaros K, Luo WL, Nichols TE (2006) Non-white noise in fMRI: does modelling have an impact? Neuroimage 29:54–66.

Marcar VL, Schwarz U, Martin E, Loenneker T (2006) How depth of anesthesia influences the blood oxygenation level-dependent signal from the visual cortex of children. AJNR Am J Neuroradiol 27:799–805.

Mirsattari SM, Lee DH, Jones D, Bihari F, Ives JR (2004) MRI compatible EEG electrode system for routine use in the epilepsy monitoring unit and intensive care unit. Clin Neurophysiol 115:2175–2180.

Mirsattari SM, Wang Z, Ives JR, Bihari F, Leung LS, Bartha R, Menon RS (2006) Linear aspects of transformation from interictal epileptic discharges to BOLD fMRI signals in an animal model of occipital epilepsy. Neuroimage 30:1133–1148.

Mirsattari SM, Ives JR, Leung LS, Menon RS (2007) EEG monitoring during functional MRI in animal models. Epilepsia 48 (Suppl 4):37–46.

Moeller F, Siebner HR, Wolff S, Muhle H, Granert O, Jansen O, Stephani U, Siniatchkin M (2008a) Simultaneous EEG-fMRI in drug-naive children with newly diagnosed absence epilepsy. Epilepsia 49:1510–1519.

Moeller F, Siebner HR, Wolff S, Muhle H, Boor R, Granert O, Jansen O, Stephani U, Siniatchkin M (2008b) Changes in activity of striato-thalamo-cortical network precede generalized spike wave discharges. Neuroimage 39:1839–1849.

Morgan VL, Price RR, Arain A, Modur P, Abou-Khalil B (2004) Resting functional MRI with temporal clustering analysis for localization of epileptic activity without EEG. Neuroimage 21:473–481.

Morgan VL, Gore JC, Abou-Khalil B (2007) Cluster analysis detection of functional MRI activity in temporal lobe epilepsy. Epilepsy Res 76:22–33.

Morocz IA, Karni A, Haut S, Lantos G, Liu G (2003) fMRI of triggerable aurae in musicogenic epilepsy. Neurology 60:705–709.

Patel MR, Blum A, Pearlman JD, Yousuf N, Ives JR, Saeteng S, Schomer DL, Edelman RR (1999) Echo-planar functional MR imaging of epilepsy with concurrent EEG monitoring. AJNR Am J Neuroradiol 20:1916–1919.

Pressler RM, Robinson RO, Wilson GA, Binnie CD (2005) Treatment of interictal epileptiform discharges can improve behavior in children with behavioral problems and epilepsy. J Pediatr 146:112–117.

Raichle ME, MacLeod AM, Snyder AZ, Powers WJ, Gusnard DA, Shulman GL (2001) A default mode of brain function. Proc Natl Acad Sci U S A 98:676–682.

Rezai AR, Finelli D, Nyenhuis JA, Hrdlicka G, Tkach J, Sharan A, Rugieri P, Stypulkowski PH, Shellock FG (2002) Neurostimulation systems for deep brain stimulation: in vitro evaluation of magnetic resonance imaging-related heating at 1.5 tesla. J Magn Reson Imaging 15:241–250.

Richardson MP, Grosse P, Allen PJ, Turner R, Brown P (2006) BOLD correlates of EMG spectral density in cortical myoclonus: description of method and case report. Neuroimage 32:558–565.

Richter W, Richter M (2003) The shape of the fMRI BOLD response in children and adults changes systematically with age. Neuroimage 20:1122–1131.

Rodionov R, Laufs H, Thornton R, Chupin M, Duncan JS, Lemieux L (2007a) Analysis of resting state fMRI reveals abnormal hippocampus-precuneus connectivity in patients with temporal lobe epilepsy. Epilepsia 48:253.

Rodionov R, De Martino F, Laufs H, Carmichael DW, Formisano E, Walker M, Duncan JS, Lemieux L (2007b) Independent component analysis of interictal fMRI in focal epilepsy: comparison with general linear model-based EEG-correlated fMRI. Neuroimage 38:488–500.

Rosenow F, Lüders H (2001) Presurgical evaluation of epilepsy. Brain 124:1683–1700.

Salek-Haddadi A, Merschhemke M, Lemieux L, Fish DR (2002) Simultaneous EEG-Correlated Ictal fMRI. Neuroimage 16:32–40.

Salek-Haddadi A, Friston KJ, Lemieux L, Fish DR (2003a) Studying spontaneous EEG activity with fMRI. Brain Res Brain Res Rev 43:110–133.

Salek-Haddadi A, Lemieux L, Merschhemke M, Friston KJ, Duncan JS, Fish DR (2003b) Functional magnetic resonance imaging of human absence seizures. Ann Neurol 53:663–667.

Salek-Haddadi A, Diehl B, Hamandi K, Merschhemke M, Liston A, Friston K, Duncan JS, Fish DR, Lemieux L (2006) Hemodynamic correlates of epileptiform discharges: an EEG-fMRI study of 63 patients with focal epilepsy. Brain Res 1088:148–166.

Salek-Haddadi A, Mayer T, Hamandi K, Symms MR, Josephs O, Fluegel D, Woermann FG, Richardson MP, Noppeney U, Wolff P, Koepp MJ (2008) Imaging seizure activity: a combined EEG/EMG-fMRI study in reading epilepsy. Epilepsia 50:256–264.

Schapiro MB, Schmithorst VJ, Wilke M, Byars AW, Strawsburg RH, Holland SK (2004) BOLD fMRI signal increases with age in selected brain regions in children. Neuroreport 15:2575–2578.

Seeck M, Lazeyras F, Michel CM, Blanke O, Gericke CA, Ives J, Delavelle J, Golay X, Haenggeli CA, de Tribolet N, Landis T (1998) Non-invasive epileptic focus localization using EEG-triggered functional MRI and electromagnetic tomography. Electroencephalogr Clin Neurophysiol 106:508–512.

Siniatchkin M, van Baalen A, Jacobs J, Moeller F, Moehring J, Boor R, Wolff S, Jansen O, Stephani U (2007) Different neuronal networks are associated with spikes and slow activity in hypsarrhythmia. Epilepsia 48:2312–2321.

Stefanovic B, Warnking JM, Kobayashi E, Bagshaw AP, Hawco C, Dubeau F, Gotman J, Pike GB (2005) Hemodynamic and metabolic responses to activation, deactivation and epileptic discharges. Neuroimage 28:205–215.

Steriade M (2005) Sleep, epilepsy, and thalamic reticular inhibitory neurons. Trends Neurosci 28:317–324.

Steriade M (2006) Neuronal substrates of spike-wave seizures and hypsarrhythmia in corticothalamic systems. Adv Neurol 97:149–154.

Tana MG, Bianchi AM, Vitali P, Villani F, Cerutti S (2007) The haemodynamic response to the interictal epileptic spikes. Conf Proc IEEE Eng Med Biol Soc 2007:5223–5226.

Thornton R, Laufs H, Rodionov R, Salek-Haddadi A, Carmichael D, Walker M, Smith S, McEvoy A, Duncan JS, Lemieux L (2007) Correlation of pre-surgical EEG fMRI and postsurgical imaging and outcome in patients with focal epilepsy. Epilepsia 48:397.

Tyvaert L, Hawco C, Kobayashi E, Levan P, Dubeau F, Gotman J (2008) Different structures involved during ictal and interictal epileptic activity in malformations of cortical development: an EEG-fMRI study. Brain 131:2042–2060.

Urrestarazu E, Jirsch JD, LeVan P, Hall J, Avoli M, Dubeau F, Gotman J (2006) High-frequency intracerebral EEG activity (100–500 Hz) following interictal spikes. Epilepsia 47:1465–1476.

Urrestarazu E, Chander R, Dubeau F, Gotman J (2007) Interictal high-frequency oscillations (100–500 Hz) in the intracerebral EEG of epileptic patients. Brain 130:2354–2366.

van Duinen H, Zijdewind I, Hoogduin H, Maurits N (2005) Surface EMG measurements during fMRI at 3T: accurate EMG recordings after artifact correction. Neuroimage 27:240–246.

Vaudano AE, Carmichael DW, Thornton R, Rodionov R, Hamandi K, Kiebel SJ, Duncan JS, Laufs H, Lemieux L (2007) Dynamic causal modelling of fMRI data suggests a balanced cortico-subcortical loop influenced by the precuneal state during generalized spike-wave discharges. Epilepsia 48:157.

Vulliemoz S, Thornton R, Rodionov R, Guye M, Michel CM, Lemieux L (2008) EEG-fMRI activations related to initiation vs propagation of interictal spikes can be discriminated using source localization from EEG inside the MRI scanner. 8th European Congress on Epileptology. Berlin, Germany.

Warach S, Ives JR, Schlaug G, Patel MR, Darby DG, Thangaraj V, Edelman RR, Schomer DL (1996) EEG-triggered echo-planar functional MRI in epilepsy. Neurology 47:89–93.

Wendling F, Bartolomei F (2001) Modeling EEG signals and interpreting measures of relationship during temporal-lobe seizures: an approach to the study of epileptogenic networks. Epileptic Disord 3:SI67–78.

Yoshizawa T, Anno I, Matsumura A, Enomoto T, Yamada H, Muraki S, Itai Y, Nose T (1997) Functional MRI employing diazepam; a proposal of neuropharmacological fMRI. Nippon Rinsho 55:1712–1718.

Zhang J, Wilson CL, Levesque MF, Behnke EJ, Lufkin RB (1993) Temperature changes in nickel-chromium intracranial depth electrodes during MR scanning. AJNR Am J Neuroradiol 14:497–500.

Zijlmans M, Huiskamp G, Hersevoort M, Seppenwoolde JH, van Huffelen AC, Leijten FS (2007) EEG-fMRI in the preoperative work-up for epilepsy surgery. Brain 130:2343–2353.

Index

Note: Page numbers followed by *f* and *t* indicate figures and tables, respectively.